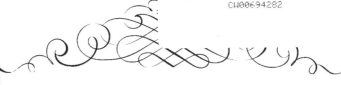

ISBN 978-1-5278-8001-6
PIBN 10896471

For support please visit www.forgottenbooks.com

1 MONTH OF
FREE
READING

at
www.ForgottenBooks.com

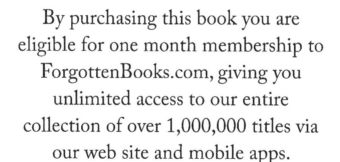

By purchasing this book you are eligible for one month membership to ForgottenBooks.com, giving you unlimited access to our entire collection of over 1,000,000 titles via our web site and mobile apps.

To claim your free month visit: www.forgottenbooks.com/free896471

CYCLOPÆDIA

OF THE

PRACTICE OF MEDICINE.

EDITED BY DR. H. VON ZIEMSSEN,

PROFESSOR OF CLINICAL MEDICINE IN MUNICH, BAVARIA.

VOL. VIII.

DISEASES OF THE CHYLOPOËTIC SYSTEM,

WITH CHAPTERS RELATING TO

DISEASES OF THE BLADDER AND URETHRA,

AND

FUNCTIONAL AFFECTIONS OF THE MALE GENITAL ORGANS.

BY

PROF. F. A. ZENKER, of Erlangen; PROF. H. VON ZIEMSSEN, of Munich;
PROF. F. MOSLER, of Greifswald; PROF. N. FRIEDREICH, of Heidelberg;
DR. G. MERKEL, of Nürnberg; DR. J. BAUER, of Munich; PROF.
H. LEBERT, of Vevey; and DR. H. CURSCHMANN, of Berlin.

Translated by

J. R. GASQUET, M.D., of Burgess Hill, Sussex, England; REUBEN J. HARVEY, M.D., of Dublin;
MR ROBERT W. PARKER, and WARREN TAY, M.D., of London; ROBERT T. EDES. M.D.,
of Boston; and DAVID MAGIE, M.D., and GEORGE G. WHEELOCK, M.D., of New York.

ALBERT H. BUCK, M.D., NEW YORK,

EDITOR OF AMERICAN EDITION.

NEW YORK:
WILLIAM WOOD AND COMPANY,
27 GREAT JONES STREET.
1878.

Trow's Printing and Bookbinding Company,
205 *to* 213 *East Twelfth Street,*
NEW YORK.

CONTENTS.

ZENKER AND VON ZIEMSSEN.

BAUER.

(Translated by Reuben T. Harvey, M.D.)

MOSLER.

(Translated by Robert T. Edes, M.D.)

FRIEDREICH.

                (Translated by Mr. Robert W. Parker.)

MERKEL.

(Translated by Reuben T. Harvey, M.D.)

LEBERT.

CURSCHMANN.

DISEASES OF THE ŒSOPHAGUS.

ZENKER AND VON ZIEMSSEN.

GENERAL STATEMENT.

Literature.

Besides the manuals and text-books of pathological anatomy by *Andral, Rokitansky, Foerster, Klebs, Birch-Hirschfeld*, of special pathology and therapeutics by *Virchow* (chylo-poïetic apparatus, by Bamberger), and of surgery, by *Pitha-Billroth*, (œsophagus, by *Koenig*): *Alexander Monro*, The Morbid Anatomy of the Human Gullet, Stomach, and Intestines. Edinburgh, 1811.—*J. T. Mondière*, Archives gén. de méd. Series I. Vols. XXIV., XXV., XXVII., XXX. Series II. Vol. I. (1833). (Chief work of the earlier literature; contains also very full accounts of the literature preceding it.)—*Blanche*, Du cathétérisme œsoph. chez les aliénés. Thesis. Paris, 1848.—*Oppolzer*, Clinical Reports on Diseases of the Œsophagus. Wiener med. Wochenschr. 1851. Nos. 2, 5, 12. Lectures on Special Pathology and Therapeutics, by the same author, edited by Ritter von Stoffella. Vol. II. Part 1. 1872.—*F. Betz*, Prager Vierteljahrschr. 1854. Vol. XI. 2. p. 106.—*Habershon*, Pathological and Practical Observations on Diseases of the Alimentary Canal. 1857.—*C. Gerhardt*, Deutsche Klinik. 1858. Nos. 16 and 29.— *Waldenburg*, Œsophagoskopie. Berliner klin. Wochenschrift. 1870. No. 48.—*Hamburger*, Klinik der Œsophaguskrankheiten. Erlangen, 1871.—*E. Mouton*, Du calibre de l'œsophage, et du cathéthérisme œsophagéale. Paris, 1874.—*Emminghaus*, Something Concerning Diagnosis and Treatment with the Œsophageal Sound. Deutsch. Archiv f. klin. Med. Vol. XI. p. 304. 1873.—*Idem*, Concerning the Influence of the Respiratory Movements upon the Air in the Œsophageal Sound, in same journal, Vol. XIII. p. 446. 1874.— *Ultzmann*, Folgeerscheinungen nach Sondiren des Œsophagus. Wiener med. Presse. Vol. XV. Nos. 29 and 30. 1874.—*Morell Mackenzie*, Clinical Lecture on Disease of the Œsophagus, with Special Reference to Œsophageal Auscultation. The Lancet. 1874. I. May 30.—*Clifford F. Allbutt*, On Auscultation of the Œsophagus. British Med. Journ. 1875. Oct. 2.—*Gaston Sainte-Marie*, Des différentes modes d'exploration de l'œsophage. Paris, 1875.

The œsophagus is comparatively rarely affected by any serious disturbances. This is explained partly by the nature of the organ, which serves merely the mechanical purpose of a tube for

forwarding the food and drink, and accordingly the tissues composing its walls are of comparatively slight physiological importance, and so exhibit but few varieties of pathological change ;
partly, too, this may be explained by the great protection which
the dense epithelium covering the œsophageal mucous membrane offers against any mechanical or chemical injury to which
it would otherwise be exposed from the food passing over it.
If to the infrequency of the diseases of the œsophagus we add
the trivial character of the symptoms by which many of the
more frequent but slight affections are accompanied, and the
fact that during life the organ is entirely out of sight, we can
understand the very slight interest which has been shown by
physicians in the disturbances of this organ. The result of this
has been that important pathological conditions have failed to
receive the attention they merited, and also many descriptions
have been transmitted from one hand-book to another which bear
but few marks of observation from nature, but present rather the
appearance of having been invented in the study merely to make
up a complete and systematic account. The diseases of the
œsophagus seem to be comparatively independent of the parts
with which it is continuous, and this is particularly noticeable
as regards the stomach. The sharply marked anatomical and
histological differences between the mucous membrane of this
organ and the parts with which it connects at either end, are
usually accompanied by an equally well-defined limitation of
pathological processes, particularly the inflammatory. So, too,
at the boundary line of the pharynx there is not that tendency
to an extension of disease from one part to another which one
might *a priori* expect from the continuity of the same tissues.

Moreover, the anatomical character of the changes in the
mucous membrane of the œsophagus differs in many ways from
that of other mucous membranes, particularly those just mentioned (pharynx and stomach). And Klebs is quite right when
he calls attention to the analogy which many of these affections
bear to those of the skin—an analogy which is sufficiently explained by the similarity in structure of both surfaces (papillæ
and pavement epithelium).

The pathological importance of diseases of the œsophagus

arises from two circumstances: first, from its influence on the process of deglutition, and also from neighboring organs becoming involved in the process originating in this part. In the last point of view the neighboring intrathoracic organs—the trachea, bronchi, pleuræ, lungs, aorta, and pulmonary artery—are especially to be considered.

General Etiology.

As external causes of diseases of the œsophagus we find the mechanical, chemical, or thermal effects of ingesta passing through it ; first, of substances taken as food and drink, then of foreign bodies accidentally swallowed with them, and finally, of corrosive substances, particularly the mineral acids and alkalies, swallowed by mistake, or with suicidal or criminal intent. Then we come to consider as relatively external causes the very frequent diseases of the throat and of the thorax, which secondarily involve the œsophagus. This happens partly by. the pressure exerted by organs enlarged or out of their normal position, and partly by traction or shrinkage going on in the immediate neighborhood ; or it may be pathological new growths, or ulcerative processes, which involve the œsophagus from without, and frequently cause perforation of the tube.

In general diseases it is striking to how trifling an extent the œsophagus is affected. Thus, in constitutional syphilis it is comparatively rare to find it involved. In the most severe and most frequent constitutional affections, as in typhus and general tuberculosis, it usually escapes entirely ; or, if changes are observed, they are of an unimportant character and not specific. Of the acute exanthemata it is only in variola that it is more frequently affected, and then sometimes in a specific manner.

General Symptomatology and Diagnosis.

The symptoms of œsophageal disease are usually of one character, and give little indication of the nature of the pathological processes going on. First among them are *functional disturbances, the anomalies in œsophageal deglutition*, which first attract the attention of the patient and physician. *Difficulty in swallowing* accompanies nearly all severe affections of the œsophagus : inflammatory swelling, and ulceration, as well as cicatricial and cancerous strictures, diverticula, compression of the tube from without, spasm and paralysis of the muscular elements of the œsophagus.

The "sticking fast" and "impossibility of making anything go down," as the patients describe it, which is slowly developed by increasing obstruction, is first noticed as an insignificant symptom easily removed by drinking water after eating. But gradually the opposition is more obstinate, harder to overcome ; most articles of food are regurgitated after a longer or shorter time, accompanied by abundant mucus, and more or less altered in consistency. At last the obstacle is insuperable ; rumination is incessant, and is often aided by efforts by the patient to bring on vomiting. On the other hand, in œsophageal dysphagia arising from the more acute inflammatory or spasmodic affections, the symptoms are much more violent ; every attempt to swallow the food develops anew the impossibility of forcing a passage, and not only excites regurgitation of what has been taken, but also frequently causes reflex spasms of the muscles of the pharynx and larynx.

With the functional disturbances there is now usually found a series of very variable *subjective symptoms.* Above all, *pain* usually localized at a given spot, and, according as the trouble is high up or low down, referred either to the throat, neck, between the shoulder-blades, or behind the lower portion of the sternum. As a rule, it is referred to the anterior portion of the neck, or behind the median line of the sternum, and only exceptionally to the posterior wall of the thorax. According to its character, the pain is sometimes described as a pressure, which is increased on taking food, and sometimes—especially in inflammatory affections, impacted foreign bodies, erosions, or other injuries—as a burning, sticking, or tearing. On taking food (even unirritating fluids, milk not excepted), the pain is increased, often to a considerable extent, and spreads out over other sensitive nerve-fibres, *e. g.*, the intercostal nerves, and is accompanied by reflex spasms of the muscles of the œsophagus and larynx. Otherwise, pain is not a constant symptom, and is frequently wanting throughout the whole course of the disease. Sometimes, however, during slight and transitory disturbances, *e. g.*, in hyperæmia and superficial catarrh of the œsophageal mucous membrane, caused by scalding or chemical irritants, or by mechanical irritation, as *e. g.*, in the first passage of a sound, the pain may be quite severe, and may be recognized by the patient throughout the whole length of the tube.

Besides the pain, other perversions of sensibility are complained of, especially the feeling as if a cord were being tightened about a given part, or as if a foreign body were lodged there; also perversions of the sense of taste, etc.

From the above we can understand how little is the diagnostic value of the subjective symptoms alone.

The objective symptoms, on the other hand, carry much more weight, but even they lack the importance we could wish. In general, it may be said that the diagnosis of œsophageal diseases has made but little progress in the last ten years, and stands not at all on a par with diagnosis of diseases of the upper air-passages and the pharynx.

Œsophagoscopy is still a desideratum, but all attempts hitherto to make the inner surface of the œsophagus accessible to light and to sight have scarcely reached beyond a foretaste of what may be.

Waldenburg seems to have accomplished most in this direction. He experimented with an œsophagoscope made out of a hard rubber cylinder, 1½ ctms. in diameter above, and 1 ctm. below, movably hung in the fork of a metallic handle 14 ctms. in length. (See the plate and description of the instrument in the Berliner klin. Wochenschrift, 1870, p. 580.)

The cylinder was passed into the œsophagus with the handle in the left hand, which at the same time depressed the tongue, while with the right the laryngeal mirror was held in the throat, so that the light passing through the tube should fall on the parts beneath. Generally the instrument was borne by the patient only ten or fifteen seconds, when movements of choking came on and filled the tube with fragments of food from the diverticulum, or with saliva from above. Yet in this short time he succeeded in making out the appearance of the mucous membrane and the stricture. A later instrument by Waldenburg, made of silver, and consisting of two fenestrated tubes sliding the one within the other, like a telescope, each 1 ctm. in diameter and 6 ctms. long, and which by a rivet could be lengthened to 12 ctms.,

seems to have been better adapted to œsophagoscopy; but, so far as we know, later
experiments with this instrument have not been published.

The great obstacle to the introduction of specula into the œsophagus, according
to our experiments (Ziemssen), lies at the narrow spot just below the cricoid cartilage. According to the experiments by Mouton, made by driving fluids through the
tube, and with whose results our own substantially agree, the diameter at this point
does not exceed 14 mm. With forcible distention by fluid (Mouton), or by carbonic acid (Ziemssen), which was driven upward through the œsophagus by firm
pressure on the distended stomach, the lower portion of the tube was enlarged to
from 25 to 35 mm. (40 mm., Ziemssen), and the upper part was enlarged only by a
few mm. (up to 20 mm.). While this narrowing of the upper part of the canal is
a considerable obstacle to the introduction of specula, the difficulty is much
increased by the fact that pressure of the soft parts between the speculum and the
cricoid cartilage in front, and the cervical vertebræ behind, is so irritating to the
patient that he cannot submit to a long examination. Still, the patient may perhaps
become accustomed to it, and we should not abandon the hope that œsophagoscopy
may yet have a future.

For the present, in most cases, inspection with the mirror
must be confined to the parts immediately adjoining the lower
border of the pharynx, the condition of which will give us some
approximate idea, though perhaps only a slight one, of that of
the upper part of the œsophagus.

By reason of the length of the canal, *palpation* can only be employed by the aid of a sound, bougie, or œsophageal tube, and of
all diagnostic procedures, it gives us the most valuable information. First of all, we learn by it the diameter of the tube, the presence of stricture, and the extent of the contraction; and if we employ a good wax bougie, we may even see the shape of the same.

The fenestra in the sound may bring up for us from the lower
part of the œsophagus bits of food, fungus masses, pus, blood,
portions of new growths, or foreign bodies—objects at times of
great assistance in forming our diagnosis. The sound may trans-
mit pulsations when engaged in a stricture caused by the pressure of an aortic aneurism; or, when there are symptoms pointing
to a stenosis, the free passage of the sound may set us right by
giving negative facts on which to base our diagnosis, while, on
the other hand, the fact that sometimes at a given level the
sound strikes an impassable barrier, and at other times freely
passes by the same point, will give us strong ground for suspecting the existence of a diverticulum. Finally, if the sound always

causes pain at a given spot, this, as a rule, indicates the exist-ence of inflammation; and if the fenestra repeatedly brings up pus—or pus and blood mixed—from the spot, it announces the existence of ulceration.

As regards the modus operandi in sounding, we may here say a few words.

The best sounds are the English, which, when moderately warmed, have the proper flexibility, together with sufficient resistance. The bulb at the end, not too spherical, should have one or two fenestræ, the calibre should not be too large, and the tube hollow. The patient should sit erect, with the chest thrown forward, the head bent slightly backward, and the mouth open. In this position, the point of the sound, guided by the index and middle fingers of the left hand, should be pushed over the base of the tongue. If there is any difficulty in passing the cricoid cartilage, twisting the instrument a little is usually sufficient to conduct it readily downward. The introduction of the sound will be greatly aided by carefully oiling it, or smearing it with white of egg (Trousseau). We should push it down very carefully, making many attempts and avoiding any great pressure. If we meet with any opposition, it is best to partly withdraw it and then repeatedly press forward, gently feeling our way. If the contraction is considerable, smaller sounds or bougies should be tried; of the latter, the French, with a soft wire running through them, are the best. The contents of the fenestra, on withdrawing the sound, should be carefully examined macroscopically, microscopically, and chemically.

While the larynx retains its normal sensibility and mobility, we need not fear the entrance of the sound into the air-passages; and this, if it occurred, would quickly be followed by coughing and choking. If, however, you are in doubt whether, in consequence of diminished sensibility, the sound has entered the air-passages, ask the patient to make a sound, which naturally will be impossible if the instrument is between the vocal cords.

If from any cause the patient cannot make a sound, then put a lighted candle before the end of the tube, and this flame, if the instrument is in the larynx, will be drawn in and forced out by the currents of inspired and expired air. It is true this same phenomenon may be observed when the tube is in the œsophagus, but, as we learn from the beautiful experiments of Gerhardt, Emminghaus, and Reincke,[1] only when the open end of the sound is in the intrathoracic portion of the œsophagus. At the time of the inspiratory enlargement of the thorax, all the organs within it are relieved from pressure, or are subjected to negative pressure; yet it is found that air is drawn in, or with expiration is forced out, only from such organs as are con-nected with the outer air by firm and stiff tubes (Gerhardt). While the end of the sound remains in the throat, or after it has passed the cardiac orifice, the flame does not move with the movements of respiration. The forcible escape of air and fluid through the tube, which occurs when the end has entered the stomach and excited

<hr />

[1] Reports of the indoor service of the General Hospital at Hamburg, section of Dr. Engel Reimer. Virchow's Archives, Vol. LI. p. 407.

coughing or movements of strangling, certainly has nothing in common with the respiratory currents of air.

Accordingly, in difficult cases, we can accept the flame movements as an aid in diagnosis when the point of the sound has not passed beyond the first part of the œsophagus, but in doubtful cases we want to know whether the sound has passed into the larynx or œsophagus. If the physician has a long finger, he can, under favorable circumstances, reach with the index down to the entrance of the larynx, and establish by touch the position of the sound. The laryngeal mirror can in doubtful cases, as Emminghaus has proved, help us to decide the question. From what precedes we see how rarely the sound passes unnoticed into the larynx, while the epiglottis and vestibulum retain their normal sensibility and mobility; yet this accident readily occurs when there is paralysis of the superior and inferior laryngeal nerves as a sequel of diphtheria of the fauces, or of diseases of the central nervous system, e. g., tumors in the posterior part of the calvarium, or bulbar paralysis. The immovable epiglottis, bent back upon the base of the tongue, conducts the sound directly into the glottis, and the total loss of sensibility and reflex irritability of the larynx and upper portion of the trachea favors its entrance. (See the complete explanation of this condition under Diseases of Larynx, Vol. VII., p. 921.) In such circumstances the greatest care is necessary in introducing the sound. Also when there is great loss of substance in the epiglottis, when there are ulcers in the entrance of the larynx, or new growths situated there and in the lower part of the pharynx, we must be careful in introducing the instrument and particularly avoid bending the head too far backward.

Certain dangers arise from the contents of the stomach being brought up by the side of the sound, for they may fall into the glottis. Such dangers, however, are only to be feared when the patient is lying down, or is unconscious or deranged. Blanche lost an insane patient by strangulation occurring in this manner; and Emminghaus found, at the post-mortem examination of two persons who had died after vomiting during exploration with the sound, spots of broncho-pneumonia, which he was inclined to believe were occasioned by the inspiration of some of the contents of the stomach. To avoid such accidents it is best to examine all patients, when possible, in the sitting or at least half-upright position, to use a pretty large sound, and to withdraw it immediately if vomiting occurs. This tendency to vomiting during the use of the sound can best be avoided by giving a small hypodermic injection of morphine before the operation.

As regards the largest size of sound which can be employed, we learn from the measurements of the calibre of the œsophagus by Mouton, as well as from our own, that a sound of 14 mm. diameter can be passed through the entrance of the œsophagus without much distending it. The greatest distention of which this portion of the œsophagus is capable—and hence, the maximum diameter of sound—is, according to Mouton, up to 18 mm.; according to my own measurements, up to 20 mm. Special delicacy and care are requisite in exploring the œsophagus under circumstances which cause us to suspect the existence of deep ulcers in the walls, or the presence of an aortic aneurism, since forcible pressure may occasion perforation of the wall.

Sainte-Marie has invented an instrument for *œsophagom-etry, i. e.*, for determining the length and calibre of the normal canal, as well as learning the existence and location of pathological dilatations and contractions of the same; this instrument is cleverly devised, but has not yet given proof of its practical value.

This consists of a hollow œsophageal sound, at the lower end of which an easily compressed rubber bulb is attached, and at the upper end a graduated glass tube. Before introducing the sound it is filled with a colored liquid until the fluid stands without pressure on the bulb at 0° on the scale. On introducing the instrument, any contraction in the œsophagus will cause circular pressure on the bulb and corresponding elevation of the column of fluid, which may be read off on the scale; this will sink to zero as soon as the bulb passes the cardiac orifice. As the sound itself is graduated on its surface in fractions of a metre, we can, after deducting about 15 ctms. for the distance from the incisor teeth to the entrance of the œsophagus, read off in figures the exact depth at which the contraction or dilatation is situated, as well as the extent of the same.

The practical value of this instrument of Sainte-Marie can only be established by experiments on the cadaver, as well as on the living body.

We can gather information by *percussion* of the œsophagus only when it is over-distended with air, or fluid, or solid contents, or when it is the seat of extensive new growths, which is very rarely the case. Such tumors or diverticula filled with food may cause a dull percussion sound on the posterior surface of the thorax beside the vertebral column, which dulness will be permanent in the former case and temporary in the latter. Distended diverticula which are found on the left side of the neck, or sometimes bulge out on both sides of the trachea, in circumstances which favor a development of gas, will give us a clear resonance; and after the gas has escaped, and solid or fluid contents remain behind, a dull sound will be found on percussion.

In stenosis of the œsophagus we (Ziemssen) have sometimes attempted to discern the seat and extent of the stricture and secondary dilatations, by distending the canal above the contraction with carbonic acid gas, developed by introducing a solution of bicarbonate of soda, and following it with a solution of tartaric acid.

We learn from these experiments, which cannot be considered yet as completed, that the œsophagus, forcibly distended by gas, may be accessible to percussion, at least in its lower portion ; and this experiment ought generally to be of assistance in establishing the existence of dilatations, and perhaps also when it is desired to learn the location of contractions without using a sound, or when, for example, after erosions, we suspect multiple strictures, and finally to determine the extent of the contraction by the ease with which gas and fluids pass through it. This procedure may also at times be of value in diagnosticating large diverticula. To *percussion* of the distended œsophagus we should add *auscultation*, for the slow or rapid escape of fluid and gas through the stricture into the stomach can be distinctly appreciated, and will give us an idea of the size of the stricture.

Auscultation of the œsophagus (in the neck on the left side of the trachea, and in the thorax on the left side of the spinal column down to the eighth dorsal vertebra) gives us, when the œsophagus is normal just at the moment of deglutition, sounds of a special character when either solids or fluids are swallowed.

Hamburger, who deserves mention as the founder of the method of œsophageal auscultation, in writing of the auscultatory phenomena developed by swallowing, both in the normal and pathological conditions, has made many statements which are so astounding, that few writers have thought it worth while earnestly to oppose or investigate them.

According to Hamburger, the chief cause of the sound on swallowing is the sudden and forcible pressure of the muscular walls of the œsophagus on the morsel of food. Moreover, as the morsel contains air, the new pressure which it receives at every part of the œsophagus in descent will cause a further admixture of the air and solid portions, which also is a cause of sound.

He claims that on auscultation of the act of swallowing we get the distinct impression that a *small, inverted, egg-shaped body, embraced completely by the œsophagus,* is suddenly driven downward in a vertical direction, accompanied by a sound (râle).

The distinct impression that the morsel, which, by the contraction of the circular muscular fibres of the œsophagus, has become a round and firm body, is of an inverted egg shape, *i. e.,* has its greatest diameter in the middle and tapers at both ends, of which the upper is sharp and the lower more blunt—this picture or image, which the listening ear gains of the shape of the morsel, he asserts is entirely beyond question, and is more distinctly perceived when the morsel is of a partly firm or pap-like consistency.

The sound heard in the normal act of swallowing is that of a something smoothly slipping by, together with the so-called cluck (Glucksen).   The rapidity of the act of swallowing is not always the same; thus, in perfectly healthy persons, by the frequent repetition of the act of swallowing, *e. g.*, during a protracted meal, the irritability of the transverse fibres of the œsophagus is so exhausted that the rapidity of the act is much diminished.   And finally we observe, as he claims, very distinctly how the morsel is forced directly downward, and in a healthy person never laterally or upward.

Still more wonderful are the statements which Hamburger makes concerning the auscultatory phenomena in pathological conditions.

When there is diminished energy in the circular muscular fibres, caused by general marasmus or local disturbances of nutrition in the œsophageal wall, instead of the inverted egg shape, the morsel assumes the inverted funnel shape, because the contraction of the lower fibres becomes weaker.   Hamburger also saw (N. B.— always with his ear) the morsel in regurgitation become sharp-pointed below and blunt above, and, moreover, sometimes observed the long diameter shortened, and sometimes the short diameter bulging forward or laterally (ll), etc., etc.

These eccentricities and physical improbabilities should not, however, nullify the value of Hamburger's services in establishing the basis of a method of examination which promises much in the future.   What of his teachings will remain, what will be set aside, and how much will be superadded to them, can only be learned by a further development of his method at the hands of careful and exact observers.   It will necessarily make but slow progress,—this much we can say already, —and chiefly on account of the lack of proper material for pathological studies.   Accordingly, it will be all the more necessary in any fitting case, even when the diagnosis is established, carefully to prove the auscultatory phenomena.

Among modern writers who have given special attention to œsophageal auscultation we should mention Clifford Albutt, Morell Mackenzie, and Sainte-Marie. For want of space we cannot give the views of each individual writer in detail. Let it suffice briefly to state, after considering their statements and the result of our own experiments, what may be considered as proven up to the present time.

In auscultating the œsophagus we should distinguish the pharyngeal swallowing sound—which, from the admixture of air, is often a very loud gurgling—from the œsophageal, which latter is often obscured by the former in the upper portion of the tube.   For this purpose we auscultate the œsophagus with the stethoscope on the left side of the spinal column, from the upper dorsal vertebra downwards, while the patient, at a given signal, begins to swallow the fluid or solid material which he has taken in his mouth. The best signal, according to Hamburger, is a sudden pressure by the finger on the cornua of the hyoid bone, because, by the raising of that bone, we distinguish the commencement of the act of swallowing and the rapidity with which it is accomplished. In healthy persons, the œsophageal sound is very distinct and of very brief duration ; we appreciate it best when the patient repeatedly swallows food of semi-solid consistency. There is no word to express the impression conveyed to the ear of the auscultator ; we can best state it by saying it seems as if a small body of fluid consistency was rapidly slipping downward.

The cause of the sound is evidently the friction of the morsel against the smooth inner surface of the œsophagus. Sainte-Marie thinks that the separation of the mucous surfaces in front of the descending morsel, which are in contact when at rest, is an additional cause of the sound.

The variations from the normal, which may be observed in disease, and which at times are of importance in diagnosis, are the following: total absence, or great weakness of the sound ; sudden cessation of the same at a given spot; clucking, gurgling, or rubbing sounds ("glouglou," "gargouillement," and "frou-frou" of the French), of shorter or longer duration ; further, diminution in the rapidity of the vanishing of the sound, and, finally, the sound passing upward or laterally instead of downward. To what pathological conditions these variations are due we will explain under the different heads as they arise.

For diagnosis it is very important carefully to examine the regurgitated food. Food retained in diverticula or in dilatations above strictures, will show various changes according to the length of time it has been detained in these localities, which, from their warmth, moisture, and contact with air, favor processes of fermentation and putrefaction ; recently masticated starchy materials are often partly changed into sugar by the saliva swallowed with them, but later show active fermentative processes ; meat, and other albuminous materials after twelve or fourteen hours are simply macerated, and after a longer stay are putrid. The plant-cells are least changed—usually only swollen and macerated. Fissiparous and gemmiparous fungi are found in great quantities in all cases of long-continued obstruction, and we (Ziemssen) often found groups of Leptothrix also in the masses of mucus brought up by the sound from above the stricture, but never Sarcinæ.

General Therapeutics.

The treatment of œsophageal diseases is mostly rational, and more particularly local, since the alimentary tube is accessible to the direct influence of medicaments, physical agents, and mechanical procedures. Still it is far behind the modern treatment of diseases of the pharynx and larynx, in which the eye serves as a guide for therapeutics. The first indication is to make a change in the quantity and character of the food which passes through the canal, adapted to the nature of the disease. In chronic strictures we must limit the patient either partially or entirely to a fluid or half-fluid diet, while in the acute forms we must cut off all food or drink from the œsophagus and nourish the patient by the rectum, according to the well-known method.

Our antiphlogistics are leeches to the neck, etc., and ice-bags applied over the sternum and vertebral column.

The so-called emollients, mucilaginous decoctions, and emulsions with addition of opium, are employed in slight inflammatory troubles. Astringents, particularly nitrate of silver, are useful in chronic catarrh and ulcerations. Antiseptics (boracic and salicylic acids, potassium chlorate, etc.), may be of much service when there is retention of food or mucus in the œsophagus, and also in extension of fungus growths (*muguet*) into the tube.

The mechanical treatment with sounds, bulbs, sponges, and instruments for dilatation, etc., is particularly employed in strictures, but may also have good results at times in cases of hyperæsthesia and spasm. (See farther on, under Treatment of Stenoses and Neuroses.)

The electric current is rarely employed in these diseases, because paralysis and spasms are rarely observed; but when paralysis and spasm occur as a primary affection, the electric current should be used in both forms, by means of single or double-pole electrodes as they are constructed by Duchenne, Tripier, Althaus, and others.

manuals of surgery.

NARROWING OF THE ŒSOPHAGUS.—STENOSIS ŒSOPHAGI.

Literature.

The manuals already cited. The literature of cancerous strictures will be found farther on, under the chapter on "New Formations and Growths."—*Gerardi Blasii*, Observata anatomica. 1674. p. 120.—*Monro*, Morbid Anatomy of the Human Gullet, etc. Edinburgh, 1811. p. 186.—*Mondière*, Archives générales de Méd. Bd. XXV. p. 358 and XXVII. p. 494.—*Cassan*, Archives générales. 1826. p. 79.—*Rokitansky*, Oesterr. Jahrb. 1840.—*Cruveilhier*, Anatomie pathologique. Livr. XXXVIII. Pl. VI.—*Follin*, Des rétrécissements de l'oesophage. Thèse. Paris, 1853.—*Lotzbeck*, Deutsche Klinik. 1859. Nr. 6.—*Virchow*, dessen Archiv. Bd. XV. S. 272. Fall IV. und Krankh. Geschwülste. Bd. II. S. 415.—*J. F. West*, Dublin Quart. Journ. 1860. Febr. Aug. and Lancet. 1872. Aug. p. 291. —*Eras*, Die Canalisationsstörungen der Speiseröhre. Leipsig, 1866.—*Gandais*, Rétréc. cicatr. et cancereux de l'oes. Thèse de Paris, 1869.—*Jon. Hutchinson*, London hospital reports. IV. p. 56. 1867. — *Huber*, Dysphagia strumosa. Deutsch. Arch. f. klin. Med. VI. S. 106. 1869. — *Hamburger*, Klinik der Oesoph.-Krankheiten. Erlangen, 1871. S. 56 ff. — *C. Hilton Fagge*, Guy's Hospital Reports. XVII. p. 413. 1872.—*Bouchard*, De la dilatation graduelle, etc. Gazette des hôpitaux. 1873.—*P. Ferrié*, Études sur les rétréciss. etc. Thèse de Paris 1874. — *Morell Mackenzie*, Clinical lecture, etc. The Lancet, 1874. I. May 30. — *Klob*, Wiener med. Wochenschrift, 1875. 11. S. 210. — *Wernher*, Chron. vollst. Dysphagie veranlasst durch Verdickung des Ringknorpels. Chirurg. Centralblatt II. 30. 1875.—*W. Kebbel*, The Lancet, 1875. I. S. 105. —*Durham*, Dysphagia from Goitre. Med. Times and Gazette, 1876. p. 142.— *J. Dunlop*, Glasgow Med. Journal. N. S. VIII. 2. p. 201. 1876.—*T. Gallard*, Clinique méd. de la Pitié. 1877. p. 187. sqq.—*S. Jaccoud*, Traité de Pathologie int. V. Édit. Tom. II. p. 112. 1877.

Pathology and Etiology.

Narrowings are the most frequent, and clinically the most important, of the affections of the œsophagus. They occur in so many different ways that it seems best to arrange them under some general groups or special heads, according to the manner of their origin. Accordingly we have, 1. *Congenital Stenoses.* 2. *Stenoses by Compression.* 3. *Stenoses by obstruction.* 4. *Strictures.* 5. *Spasmodic Stenoses.*

1. *Congenital Stenosis.*—Congenital atresiæ and partial defects in the œsophagus, since they are incompatible with long life, should not now call for further remark. But, on the other hand, there are stenoses of the œsophagus, although indeed very rare, which from their anatomical structure (a perfectly healthy condition of the tissues and no trace of scars), as well as from their history (the existence of considerable difficulty in swallowing from the earliest childhood and throughout the whole life), must be considered to be congenital, but which, in spite of considerable narrowing of the tube, permit of a prolongation of life even till old age.

a. Simple (congenital) stenosis of the upper portion of the œsophagus. There are only two well-authenticated cases of this kind to be found in the literature of the subject, to which we add a third, which came under our own observation. In all three the stenosis was located at the entrance of the œsophagus ; in two cases it was a simple ring about the tube ; in the third the canal was narrowed for a distance of 8 mm. In all three the patients declared they had suffered from earliest childhood with difficulty in swallowing, which was especially troublesome when solid substances were swallowed. All three died at an advanced age, two by exhaustion from lack of nourishment, in consequence of a great increase in the difficulty of swallowing in the latter part of life, owing to new complications, while death was caused in the third case by disease which had no apparent connection with the stenosis, viz. : carcinoma of the pylorus.

The first case is related by Everard Home [1] The case was that of a lady of fifty-nine years of age, who had from childhood been conscious of a narrowing of the pharynx, which increased gradually and was especially troublesome when solid substances were swallowed, so that at times nothing larger than a pin's head would go down, and hasty swallowing would bring on attacks of suffocation. In the last

---

[1] Article by *Mondière*—Archives Générales, Vol. XXV., p. 369.

eight months before death she complained of a constant pain in the region of the stomach, great nausea and great increase in the secretion of saliva. The patient could no longer swallow anything solid, and died from increasing weakness and symptoms of marasmus. At the autopsy the œsophagus showed " immediately behind the first ring of the trachea a uniform circular contraction formed by the mucous membrane, which presented a perfectly normal and healthy appearance." The stomach was normal.

The second case is related by Cassan (loc. cit.). Patient was a man who from birth had suffered from great difficulty in swallowing, particularly solid food, but was otherwise healthy, and died after a very active life at the age of 77. It was only in the last year of his life, when an inflammation of the buccal mucous membrane caused by an ill-fitting set of false teeth had extended downward, that the difficulty in swallowing was so increased that the patient could only take liquid food.

At the autopsy the lower half of the pharynx was found increased to double its width and filled with a whitish pap. Below this was a sudden narrowing in the form of a circular ring, with a puckered edge and a diameter of one millimetre; this led into an equally narrow canal eight millimetres long, in which the mucous membrane lay in longitudinal folds, and which terminated in a funnel-shaped enlargement below. There was not the least change in the mucous membrane at the seat of the narrowing.

The third case (Zenker) was that of a seamstress, sixty-six years of age. By the courtesy of Prof. Bäumler, who, as assistant at the polyclinic, had carefully observed and treated the patient, she first came for treatment to the Erlanger Polyclinic in August, 1861, suffering from vomiting and diarrhœa. In September she developed thrombosis of both iliac veins, but the evidences of this had entirely disappeared in the November following, in consequence of the establishment of collateral circulation, and the organized thrombi again becoming pervious (as the autopsy showed). In October, 1862, she came again for treatment for frequent vomiting, and died October 30th. During her sickness she complained repeatedly of difficulty in swallowing, and stated that she had suffered all her life from the same trouble, which made it impossible to swallow large pieces of solid food, and the pills that were given her she could not get down. At the autopsy the œsophagus was greatly contracted in its upper portion in a circular form, and would only admit the end of a thick sound; the mucous membrane at the narrow part was pale, delicate, easily movable on the submucosa, and unchanged in anatomical characteristics. From this point down the tube was of normal calibre and the mucous membrane pale and normal. Beyond this, the autopsy revealed an ulcer the size of a dollar at the pylorus, with edges partially infiltrated with cancer, carcinomatous swelling of the epigastric glands, contraction and cavernous degeneration of the iliac veins, etc.

b. *Simple stenosis of the lower portion of the œsophagus.—* Cases of this nature bearing considerable resemblance to each other have been described and pictured by Blasius, Cruveilhier, Hilton Fagge, and Wilks,[1] which must be considered as very probably congenital. Cruveilhier distinctly states that there was no change in the tissues at the seat of the constriction. In all these cases the stricture affected a small region in the lower part of the tube, and immediately above it the canal had suffered saccular dilatation, in which were found in Cruveilhier's case large polypoid vegetations of the mucous membrane, and in Fagge's an epithelial cancer which had perforated the wall.

Unfortunately, in the cases of Blasius and Cruveilhier nothing is known of the symptoms during life.

Fagge's patient, a drinker, forty-eight years of age, had suffered, according to his statement, for more than forty years from difficulty in swallowing, and could only swallow solid food when it was very finely divided. During the last twenty years, in consequence of taking solid food in too large morsels, he had suffered several times from obstruction in the œsophagus, lasting days—indeed, as many as eight days, during which it became impossible to swallow anything even in a liquid form. He stated that he had never suffered from regurgitation. Death ensued from perforation of the wall by cancer situated in the dilated portion. The stenosis would scarcely allow the passage of a lead-pencil.

The case observed before and after death by Wilks (related by Fagge) was that of a man seventy-four years of age, who died of pneumonia. He stated that he had suffered from youth up from difficulty in swallowing and regurgitation, so that every mouthful of solid food had to be washed down with considerable fluid. The stenosed portion at the lower end of the tube would scarcely admit the little finger, while the œsophagus above was enormously distended and hypertrophied.

2. *Stenosis by compression.*—Quite frequently the œsophagus suffers pressure from neighboring tissues or organs which are morbidly changed, enlarged, or displaced, particularly by the glands of the neck and mediastinum (most commonly undergoing caseous degeneration); also by large strumous masses, but only when these extend far back so as, more or less, to surround the tube.

The accompanying cut (Fig. 1, p. 21) taken from a cross-section of the frozen cadaver, prepared by Prof. Ruedinger, gives an admirable representation of the extent to which the œsophagus was displaced and compressed by a goitre which completely surrounded it.

---

[1] *Blasius*, loc. cit., Table XV., Fig. VI. ; and *Cruveilhier*, loc. cit., Part XXXVIII. Pl. VI., Fig. 1 and 1'.

In the same connection we should mention cases described by Lotzbeck, Huber, Durham, and others (loc. cit.).

In a woman, twenty-five years of age, who died of typhus, we (Zenker) observed an enormous parenchymatous struma which completely embraced the trachea and œsophagus for the length of 14 ctms., so that the posterior margins of both lobes of the thyroid gland not only touched, but overlapped one another. The thyroid gland measured 54 ctms. in circumference and 17 ctms. vertically; the mass lying between the œsophagus and vertebral column was 4½ ctms. thick. The pharynx, pressed against the cricoid cartilage, appeared like a narrow transverse fissure through which the sound could scarcely pass, while the tube was also greatly compressed on either side.

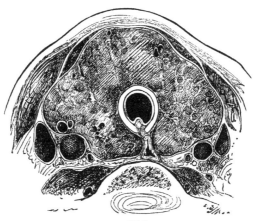

FIG. 1.

Koenig (loc. cit., p. 23) observed in women in similar cases periodical obstructions, caused by increased turgescence of the gland at menstrual epochs.

The thyroid body was found to have caused slight compression of the œsophagus in a very peculiar manner in a case recently observed post-mortem (Zenker); in a woman whose right lobe of the gland was nearly all converted into pus, there were found attached to the posterior and lower margin of the left lobe (which was but slightly enlarged), two adjunct glands, entirely distinct from the cervical glands, and the lower and larger of these, which also showed colloid swelling (5 ctms. long, 3½ ctms. wide, and 1½ ctms. in thickness), was situated entirely between the vertebral column and œsophagus, and had caused distinct pressure on the posterior wall of the tube.

Moreover, there are growths of various kinds which cause pressure, especially sarcoma and carcinoma of the thyroid gland, of the mediastinum, of the lungs, etc. ; also aortic aneurisms, or the rare forms of sacculated diverticula of the pharynx, which, when filled with ingesta, may compress the œsophagus like a tumor ; occasionally also abscesses between the œsophagus and vertebræ. We should mention, however, that the majority of these cases were only discovered post-mortem, and during life occasioned no symptoms, or none worth mentioning, in deglutition. Mondière makes the same statement with regard to aortic aneurisms, viz., that, of twelve cases in which aneurisms had opened into the œsophagus, in at least ten deglutition had not been previously disturbed. This is readily explained by the fact that pressure is usually made only on one side, so that the œsophagus, surrounded only by open connective tissue, easily yields before the pressure, and accordingly its calibre is not interfered with to any extent. It is only when there is general compression on all sides, as, for example, when occasioned in rare cases by enlarged cervical glands pressing in every direction, and in compression by very extensive growths embracing the tube, or when the œsophagus, by previous fixation, is prevented from yielding, that these pathological conditions are of great importance as regards deglutition. And in many such cases in which difficulty in swallowing exists, this is caused less by the narrowing of the tube than by the pain arising from that act in the diseased parts near by.

Dysphagia lusoria.[1]—Among the causes of compression, it has long been customary in hand-books of clinical medicine and pathological anatomy to mention that anomalous course of the right subclavian artery which is sometimes observed, in which it comes off as the last branch from the aorta (to the left of the left subclavian), and from its posterior face, so that, in order to reach its area of distribution, it must cross the œsophagus, in which case

---

[1] *Autenrieth* et *Pfleiderer*, Diss. inaug. De Dysphagia lusor. Tubingen, 1806 ; and Reil's Archiv f. Physiol. 7. Bd. S. 145.—*Fleischmann*, Leichenöffnungen. Erlangen, 1815. S. 213.—*Meckel, J. F.*, Patholog. Anatomie. II. Bd. 1. Abth. S. 98.—*Kirby*, Dublin bospit. reports. T. II. p. 224. Quoted by Mondière. Arch. génér. XXIV. p. 406.—*W. Krause*, in Henle's Handb. d. Anatomie. III. 1. 1868. S. 247.

it usually passes between the œsophagus and vertebral column, and more rarely between the œsophagus and trachea. It is evident that under these circumstances the pulsating artery, with every impulse, must cause slight pressure on the wall of the œsophagus. It is equally clear, however, that this very unimportant pressure could not be considered sufficient to narrow the tube, and hence interfere with deglutition, and accordingly we could not speak of stenosis by compression in such cases unless —which never has been observed—the anomalous artery were enlarged by aneurismal dilatation just at the point of crossing (the case of aneurismal dilatation of the artery shortly to be mentioned implicates that portion immediately before it crosses). Hence we can, without hesitation, strike out this anomalous course of the artery from among the causes of compression.

It is another question, however, whether the reverse is not true, viz., whether the pressure on the artery which must be caused by the œsophagus distended with passing morsels of food, so that the circulation is temporarily interrupted, may not give rise to severe and alarming symptoms, especially when the vessel, as is usually the case, lies behind the tube and is compressed against the vertebræ. It is in this manner that the question was considered by the authors on whose writings the pathological interest in this anomaly depends.

Bayford first reported the case of a woman, sixty-one years of age, who had suffered since childhood from difficulty in swallowing, which gradually increased until with every attempt to swallow she had severe attacks of oppression and palpitation. Finally, in consequence of the very limited nourishment she was able to take on this account, she died in a very emaciated state, and at the autopsy, besides this anomaly (the artery here passed between the trachea and œsophagus), no other anatomical cause could be discerned for the diffiulty in swallowing. As he believed he must attribute the symptom to this freak of nature, he gave it the name of *dysphagia lusoria*. This view of the matter was strengthened by two additional cases by Hulme and Autenrieth, in which the anomalous course of the vessel was found in two individuals who had suffered from a similar difficulty in swallowing. And in another case, on account of the peculiar difficulty of swallowing and other symptoms, Autenrieth felt justified in making a diagnosis of dysphagia lusoria; but as the accuracy of the diagnosis was not established by an autopsy, this case cannot be placed among the others. Finally, we should here quote the case of Kirby, in which a woman having this anomaly swallowed a bone, and afterwards died of "suffocation and a hemorrhage which appeared to come from within the œsophagus." At the autopsy, in addition to fragments of food which compressed the trachea, there was found a splinter of bone which had wounded the œsophagus, and also the right subclavian artery on its way across, between the œsophagus and vertebral column.

Autenrieth accordingly declared that not all cases of this arterial anomaly are accompanied by dysphagia which had been recognized. Since that time the anomalies have been frequently seen, but no case attended by dysphagia has been observed. We (Zenker) have seen a number of such cases, but never could get any history of antecedent dysphagia. Accordingly it seems to be proved that certainly the more severe forms of dysphagia are not the rule in this arterial anomaly, but rather the exception. Supported by this statement, Fleischmann has subjected the theory of dysphagia lusoria to a careful, but certainly not unassailable criticism, which led him to the conclusion that it should be stricken off from the list of diseases. Hamburger more recently expressed the same opinion, and W. Krause described the doctrine as a fable. Though we may admit that the existence of dysphagia lusoria is not established by these three cases, since another cause for the disturbance, though not proven, cannot be wholly excluded, yet it seems rather too sweeping to deny it altogether. For it is not only not improbable, *a priori*, that the circulation should be impeded by this anomalous course of the vessel, but this view is supported by the fact that the first portion of this artery (*i. e.*, before it crosses the œsophagus) is frequently distinctly and often very considerably dilated ("like an aneurism"), as is repeatedly asserted by the older authors, and which we can ourselves confirm. In the four cases of this anomaly in the Erlanger collection of pathological anatomy, this enlargement is distinct in all, and in two very considerable, so that the subclavian seems to come off from the arch with a bulb-shaped dilatation. Now, it does not seem so very improbable that a temporary increase in this disturbance of circulation during the act of swallowing, in individuals otherwise disposed to palpitation, should lead to attacks of oppression, etc. Accordingly it does not seem to us advisable to withdraw attention from this affection.

Finally, I cannot refrain from adding a case observed by myself (Zenker) which perhaps belongs in the same category. A pot-bellied man of seventy-seven years of age, previously in good health apparently, suddenly fell to the ground and within half an hour was dead. The autopsy revealed no sufficient cause for the sudden death. There was found, however, an anomalous course of the aorta, which passed over the right bronchus, backward between the œsophagus and vertebral column towards the left (the first branch from the aorta was a truncus anonymus supplying the left side, then the right carotid and right subclavian as separate trunks). In the pharynx and œsophagus were found an accumulation of fragments of food. Apparently the man was overtaken by the catastrophe in the act of swallowing, and it gave rise to the suspicion that the death had been caused by pressure upon the aorta, and this interference with the circulation, in a man who from advanced age and great obesity probably had a feeble heart, might explain the occurrence.[1]

---

[1] I must here correct a misapprehension regarding this case. *Koenig* ·(loc. cit.

In another similar case recently observed post-mortem, at the Institute of Anatomy and Pathology at Erlangen, in which the descending aorta, after the arch had passed over the right bronchus, ran its whole course between the vertebral column and œsophagus in a patient who had suffered from mental disorder, no difficulty in swallowing had been observed during life.

3. *Obstruction stenoses, i. e.*, narrowings caused by the plugging up of the canal of the œsophagus, arise most frequently from foreign bodies of the most various kinds, which in some cases have remained weeks or even years in situ. In such cases they lie in distended portions like diverticula produced by their own pressure, so that their obstructive nature may be more or less completely removed. The obstruction will naturally be more or less complete, according to the shape and size of the foreign body. In explaining the difficulty in swallowing in such cases, we ought to take into consideration, besides the amount of obstruction, quite as much and perhaps more, the pain caused by the mechanical irritation and actual wounding of the tissues by the foreign body, and the inflammation to which it gives rise. Thus, we are able to explain the apparent incongruity between the symptoms and the size of the foreign body : severe dysphagia in small but sharply irritating bodies, and slight in such as are of larger size, but only moderately irritating. It seems needless to give an enumeration of the objects which have acted as foreign bodies in the œsophagus, since in the literature of the subject we find accounts of substances of all possible kinds which have been swallowed, from insufficiently masticated meat to a live fish, and from a fish-bone to a cellar-door key.

Another special form of obstruction to be mentioned is that

---

p. 59), in treating of foreign bodies in the œsophagus, says : " That is a unique case, in which the aorta is said to have been so compressed by a piece of bone in the œsophagus that sudden death occurred by anæmia. The preparation of this case is to be found, according to Adelmann's written report, in the Bürger Hospital at Dresden." By careful inquiry I find there is no such preparation to be found in the Museum of Anatomy and Pathology at the City Hospital at Dresden, but only the one described above, added by myself to the collection in 1862 ; and doubtless Adelmann's report refers to this specimen, and accordingly the above statement should be corrected. There was no piece of bone found, but only soft pieces of food, and the most important part of the case—the anomalous course of the aorta—is not alluded to by Adelmann.— ZENKER.

caused by the growth of masses of fungus within the œsophagus itself. The thrush fungus (Oidium albicans), which so frequently is found in the œsophagus, in some rare cases grows to such an enormous size that the canal is entirely plugged up and deglutition becomes impossible. (See under *Parasites.*)

Obstructive stenosis may also be caused by pedunculated growths having their attachment to the wall of the œsophagus, or, more frequently, to that of the pharynx. These rarely observed œsophageal polyps, so called, of which very few are found in the literature of the subject, and which, from their texture, as far as any available reports have been made of them, are classed as fibromas with slightly altered covering of mucous membrane, may reach a very considerable size (as much as 20 ctms. in length, and 7 ctms. in thickness).

The end, usually club-shaped, sometimes more or less deeply lobulated, hangs straight downward ; but, on account of the great mobility of the growth with its long pedicle, it may possibly, in efforts at vomiting, be thrown upward into the pharynx or mouth, where, from its overlying the glottis, it may seriously endanger life (Monro). Usually only one polyp has been observed, but sometimes there are several (Schneider, Chas. Bell). As they grow they distend the canal more and more, so that they entirely obstruct it, since the tube contracts firmly around the thickest part of the tumor. But, since the power of distention in the tube remains, sometimes a sound can be passed beside the tumor, and for the same reason, even with growths of large size (as in Rokitansky's case), the dysphagia may be trifling ; from all which it appears that the nature of the obstruction in these cases is similar to that from foreign bodies, and practically there is all the more reason to consider them from the same point of view since the therapeutical indication in both is the same, viz., the mechanical removal of the obstructing body, if possible, by operation. (For further details concerning polyps, see under *Growths.*)

Also in carcinomatous stenoses we have more or less to consider the obstruction occasioned by masses of the new growth, which rise above the mucous membrane and project into the canal. But from their chief characteristic the cancerous stenoses belong in the following category of strictures, and accordingly we shall treat of them under that head.

4. *Strictures.*—Under this head belong all those stenoses which are caused by such a change in the wall of the œsophagus as entirely destroys or greatly limits its power of distention. Here the stiffness of the wall during the act of deglutition has an effect as if an unyielding band surrounded it, and so in this wise is practically a stricture, whether any contraction has occurred or not. Changes of this nature may be either *contracting cicatrices* or *cancerous degeneration*, and the consecutive muscular hypertrophy which may accompany stenosis arising from any cause whatever.

Strictures pure and simple are best represented by the *cicatricial strictures*, *i. e.*, those which remain after the healing of a loss of substance or solution of continuity arising from any cause, when the cicatrix has undergone contraction. Relatively the most frequent and also the most severe are those strictures which sometimes remain after the destructive action of corrosive substances, such as the concentrated mineral acids, particularly sulphuric acid, and caustic alkalies. And yet, since these substances usually cause death, even strictures from this cause are very rare, and these vary in their character according to the depth to which the loss of substance has extended. If the mucous membrane and submucosa have been injured, there is formed a layer of connective tissue which is usually smooth, but here and there projects in little ledges or shelves like valves, sickle-shaped or circular (ledge-shaped strictures). If, on the other hand, the muscular layer is partially or totally destroyed, we then shall have a dense, callous, cicatricial tissue, the contraction of which produces the most extensive and most obstinate strictures (callous strictures [1]). Even when the muscular layer is preserved, the quickly developed hypertrophy serves greatly to increase the stiffness of the wall, to make it unyielding, and so increase the stenosis. With the exception of the pharynx (behind the cricoid cartilage), these strictures, according to Rokitansky, occur most frequently in the vicinity of the cardiac orifice, or even in the muscle which guards

---

Rokitansky, Lehrbuch d. Pathol. Anat., 1861. Vol. III. p. 160.

that opening itself. They may be so tight as only to admit a fine sound, and in their extent they may be several centimetres long or possibly invade nearly the whole length of the tube.

The following case, recently observed (Zenker) may serve as a characteristic example of such a stricture involving the whole length of the œsophagus. It is also of interest as regards the substance which produced the injury, and which has not generally been regarded as highly corrosive in its nature.

A boy, three and three-quarters years old, about seven weeks before his death swallowed a merely nominal quantity of a solution of sulphate of copper (which his father employed in his trade as metal-beater); this was followed by vomiting, which lasted several days. He was brought to the clinic for treatment eleven days before his death (Oct. 23, 1876). At this time the child was greatly emaciated, but free from fever, and complained of pain in his throat and neck, especially on swallowing, and could only take fluid nourishment. Only very small œsophageal sounds (Bougie No. V.) could be passed down to the stomach. Larger-sized instruments met with an obstruction at the level of the lower border of the larynx. In the mouth and pharynx no traces of erosion could be found. On the 30th of October there appeared a swelling at the lower part of the neck anteriorly and somewhat to the left, which was acutely sensitive on pressure, and was accompanied by high fever. At this time the child could not take even fluid nourishment, and since small sounds would no longer pass, we proceeded, on Nov. 1st, to perform œsophagotomy. In the operation we first opened into an abscess lying between the œsophagus and vertebral column, and filled with stinking pus, after emptying which, the sound could be passed somewhat farther downward. No communication between the abscess and the œsophagus could be found. On opening the œsophagus, it was not till after extending the incision to the base of the neck that we succeeded in introducing a fine catheter into the stomach, through which milk was repeatedly injected. Nevertheless, death occurred on the following day.

Autopsy.—Nov. 3, 1876. Twenty hours after death (Zenker). Cicatricial stricture of the whole œsophagus. Œsophagotomy wound. Retro- and para-pharyngo-œsophageal abscess. Purulent inflammation of the anterior and posterior mediastinum.— At the left side of the neck an incised wound, six centimetres long, gaping widely, and opening into the œsophagus; its edges covered with dirty grayish-brown pus. In each pleural sac a few drops only of yellowish serum. Both lungs almost entirely free. On pushing forward the right lung, the pleura, at the level of the lower half of the œsophagus, is seen to bulge forward, pale yellow in color and translucent, covered with a layer of fibrin, which extends some distance on the pleura pulmonalis near the root of the lungs. At this spot the pulmonary tissue over a small region is found empty of air, flabby, containing a viscid material, and apparently compressed; the adjacent tissue of the posterior mediastinum infiltrated with pus. On the left side, at the same level, the pleural tissue is normal. Elsewhere in the lung are found the remains of some earlier pathological changes, in nowise connected with the present trouble. The heart normal. At the highest point of the anterior mediastinum the connective tissue for a distance of one and a half centimetres is infiltrated with pus, partially liquefied. A purulent fistulous canal leads from this spot upward to the left, into the wide bulging cavity of an abscess between the pharynx and vertebral column, which embraces also the side of the pharynx and upper portion of the œsophagus. Its boundary wall, formed partly by callous fibrous tissue and partly by the wall of the pharynx, which is here and there as thin as gauze, and easily torn, is of a dirty yellowish gray color within, and covered with ragged fragments of tissue. This cavity communicates with the upper part of the œsophageal canal by a fissure three centimetres long (wound of operation). No other communication between this cavity and the canal could be found. This cavity also opens downward into a long, very narrow and pretty smooth-walled canal, seven and a half centimetres long, passing behind and to the left of the œsophagus, which farther down, in the region of the posterior mediastinum, grows wider, and here, with a shaggy, sphacelated wall, extends down to the diaphragm. The mucous membrane of the tongue, soft palate, and throat moderately injected, but normal throughout. So likewise is that of the pharynx mostly, which only just before reaching the œsophagus is somewhat livid. The muscular tissue of the pharynx is somewhat thickened and more compact.

The *œsophagus* is contracted throughout its whole length, and its wall is stiff, greatly increased in thickness, up to three millimetres, and this increase is chiefly due to the muscular layer which everywhere is preserved, and which is much hypertrophied, gray in color, translucent, and marked off by bands into little cells or loculi. The wall, when cut open and flattened out, has, at the upper part (in the region of the wound made in œsophagotomy), a breadth of only about thirteen millimetres; the mucous membrane in this portion still remains, but is densely marked with irregular interlacing bands of cicatricial tissue, and here and there with gray and deep red spots of hemorrhagic infiltration; at the edge of the incision the wall is firm, infiltrated, and of a gray color. Next below this follows a portion of mucous membrane two and a half centimetres long, somewhat wider (when laid open, sixteen millimetres in breadth), which shows only a few fine bands of cicatricial tissue and small slate-colored spots. From this point, almost to the cardiac orifice, the tube is most contracted (only eleven to thirteen millimetres wide when laid open). In this section the mucous membrane through nearly all its extent is replaced by a thin, firm, cicatricial tissue, which does not glide over the muscular coat, is partly smooth, partly like net-work, here and there is raised in short, shallow ledges, is spotted with a deep slate color, in two places is livid, and in others has the appearance of being eroded; microscopically this tissue is seen to be made up of fine fibrillæ of connective tissue, and has no epithelial covering. Only just above the cardia a few portions are found where the mucous membrane is intact and the epithelial layer is preserved. The mucous membrane of the stomach is unchanged.

Moreover, cicatricial strictures may remain after the healing

of solutions of continuity caused by foreign bodies, and of ulcerations of the mucous membrane of various kinds.   In many
cases the nature of the ulcers which precede the strictures is
obscure, since the cicatrices show no specific character sufficient
for diagnosis, and the history of the case, as well as the other
post-mortem appearances, throw no light upon it.   The occurrence of cicatricial strictures of syphilitic origin in the œsophagus
was until recently not substantiated, but we can no longer doubt
it after hearing the reported cases, particularly of Virchow, West,
and Klob (loc. cit.), who observed such strictures, both during
and after life, in individuals known to be syphilitic ; and especially after reading Virchow's case, in which, together with a
contracting ulcer, he also found the characteristic gummy tumor
(from which such ulceration proceeds) in a state of fatty degeneration.   Nevertheless, these syphilitic strictures of the œsophagus,
as compared with those frequently seen in the pharynx, are exceedingly rare.   In the cases hitherto reported these strictures
were situated or began in the upper half of the œsophagus (in one
case by West it began four inches below the upper outlet, and
was two and a half inches long).   In only one case did he find
ulceration and narrowing in the lower portion.[1]

Hamburger (loc. cit., p. 146) assumes that cicatricial stenosis may arise from
small-pox, supporting his statements chiefly on a case reported by Lanzoni (Ephe-
merid. natur. curios. Decas II. Anni. 9. p. 80. Obs. XLV. Gulæ et narium coalitus
a variolis) in the year 1688, in which "filiolo cuidam œsophagus a variolis ita
coaluerit, ut denegato cibi potusque per illum transitu, misero puero fame et siti
miserrime pereundum fuerit." As variola undoubtedly does attack the œsophagus,
we cannot entirely deny the possibility of ulceration and subsequent formation of
cicatrices ; yet this case should not be accepted as evidence of the fact, since it was
not proved by autopsy that there was any cicatrix, and since, from the absence of
any statement as to how long after the attack of variola death occurred, we may
fairly infer that the dysphagia was caused by a fresh eruption on the mucous membrane.   Certainly Lanzoni himself thought it was due to cicatricial contraction,
since immediately after it he describes a case, as similar of "coalitus narium"
which was cured by incision.

[1] When Koenig, appealing to Virchow (loc. cit., p. 21), says "the narrowing in rare
cases seems to be caused by the bulging of gummy tumors into the canal," this certainly is a misapprehension of what Virchow intended to say, who refers to the gummy
tumor not as the direct cause of the stenosis, but as the strongest evidence that the
contracting ulcer near by is of syphilitic origin.

Even the simple round ulcer of the stomach, when it is situated, as sometimes happens, immediately at the cardiac orifice, may by its cicatrization cause at that opening tight stricture which extends up on to the lower portion of the œsophagus.

This was the condition in a highly significant case observed by us both, in which death occurred with marked symptoms of perforation of the stomach, after repeated attacks (apparently due to a round ulcer of the stomach) extending over many years, and here the autopsy showed that death was due to softening of the stomach, and not to a fresh ulcer, as was supposed.[1] The evidences of the preceding attacks were found in beautiful contracting ulcers at the pylorus and cardia. Above the narrow stricture of the cardia the canal of the œsophagus showed a funnel-shaped narrowing for a short distance, the mucous membrane was thickened, smooth, firmly fixed and immovable on the hypertrophied muscular tissue underlying it.

Carcinomatous stenoses, from their chief characteristic, come under the head of strictures; for they are essentially caused from the fact that the cancerous degeneration involves the whole periphery of the canal, and that the infiltration, gradually extending from the mucous membrane outward through all the tissues, makes the wall (which is increased to one ctm. and over in thickness) stiff and unyielding, and destroys or seriously impairs the power of distention of the œsophagus. It is true, however, as we have already hinted, that masses of cancer rising above the level of the mucous membrane sometimes cause obstruction and then serve to increase the stenosis. Yet this latter condition is quite secondary to the other in producing stenosis in cancer.

Not only are cancerous strictures the most frequent cause of œsophageal stenosis, but are the cause of more stenoses than all the other forms combined (if we reject the slight compressions which exist without symptoms).[2] Their location is much more frequently in the lower than in the upper part of the œsophagus (most frequently the lower third).[3] They usually involve a con-

[1] See the full report of this case by *W. Mayer*, Gastro-malacia ante-mortem. Deutsch. Archiv. f. klin. med. Vol. IX., p. 105.

[2] Of eighteen cases of œsophageal stenosis found by us at autopsies, nine were carcinomatous strictures, six were compression stenoses (of these several were slight and unattended by symptoms), two were cicatricial strictures, and one was a congenital stenosis.

[3] See the careful collection of cases by *Petri* (Inaugural Dissertation, Berlin, 1868), with whose results our own investigations entirely agree. Of twenty cancerous stric-

siderable portion of the tube (from 5 to 10 ctms. and over), and in rare cases almost the whole length of the canal. As regards the degree of narrowing, they will usually allow the little finger to pass through them, while the worst cases will only admit a fine sound at the narrowest part. It is a fact, however, that in the progress of the disease, from the ulcerative destruction of the cancerous deposit, which is rarely absent, the canal again becomes pervious, and accordingly we can hold out to the patient the deceptive hope that his dysphagia will abate.

Finally, many writers (Albers, Foerster, Niemeyer, Kunze) have reported cases occurring through simple hypertrophy of the muscular tissue, partly extending into the submucosa, which were considered to be a sequel of chronic catarrh. This hypertrophy is described as completely embracing the canal, and involving long portions of it—indeed, the entire length. Nevertheless, the whole matter is involved in considerable doubt. It rests chiefly on the statements of Albers,[1] under whose faulty description we easily detect cases of cancer with subsequent muscular hypertrophy. If there are cases of pure so-called spontaneous hypertrophy, independent of antecedent stenosis, which would give rise to it, they must be very rare. We certainly have never seen a case admitting such an explanation. And in the literature we find no facts to substantiate it. Even in the admirable engraving by Baillie[2] of the preparation in the Hunterian museum, which Albers cites as a characteristic example of this form of narrowing, there was a tight stricture (probably carcinomatous) just at the cardia, which serves to explain this extensive muscular hypertrophy. Accordingly, we can strike out this hypertrophy from the list of *primary* causes of stricture. Nevertheless, the consecutive or secondary hypertrophy (as we have already said), as it serves to injure the power of distention of the tube, will assist in increasing the stenosis already existing, and so cause additional dysphagia.

---

tures (eleven by *Petri*, nine of ours) only two were in the upper third, four in the middle, and fourteen in the lower (lower and middle together).

[1] Explanations of the Atlas of Pathological Anatomy, Part II., p. 237 et seq.

[2] *Baillie*, Series of Engravings, p. 54, copied in Froriep's surgical plates, Plate 179, and in *Albers*, Atlas of Pathological Anatomy, Part II., Plate XXII., Fig. 2.

5. *Spastic Stenosis.*—By this we mean a stenosis caused by painful contraction of the muscular layer, which is transitory, but recurs in a spasmodic form, of greater or less duration, and observed chiefly in hysterical or hypochondriacal patients. Here, in most cases, the anatomical condition of the tube is strictly normal, while in many cases anatomical changes (inflammations or ulcerations) of the mucous membranes are found, producing the abnormal irritability which causes the spasmodic contraction.

As regards the condition of the parts of the canal not involved in the stenosis or the disease which occasions it, the portion below is usually normal, while the parts above generally, though not always, show various changes. Most frequently we find muscular hypertrophy especially involving the circular fibres, often only in a small region, more rarely extending up to the pharynx and constantly diminishing as we ascend. Sometimes it is only trifling, and sometimes very great, and the muscular coat may attain a thickness of five mm., and more, and have the appearance of a firm, jelly-like, translucent layer, marked off into cells by perpendicular bands of white connective tissue, as we have more frequently been accustomed to see it in the stomach and colon.

Moreover, the canal above the stenosis is frequently more or less dilated (though not so frequently as would appear from statements made in manuals upon the subject). Generally this dilatation is insignificant, and only affects the region just above the stenosis. Yet in some cases the process is more advanced, and may extend up to the pharynx.

Finally, we sometimes find with the muscular hypertrophy and dilatation a slight thickening of the mucous membrane and its epithelium.

Symptoms and Diagnosis.

Of the symptoms of œsophageal stenosis, whatever be its cause, the most constant and most important is the functional disturbance of œsophageal deglutition. In stenoses which have a chronic course, in which the narrowing is very gradually developed, as in cicatricial strictures after corrosive processes and ulcerations, after syphilitic affections, in the development of cancers, in compression by aneurisms of the aorta, by strumous glands, or cancer of the thyroid gland, the patient distinctly perceives an increased difficulty in the passage of the morsel, which is usually painless, and it seems merely as if a large and very dry fragment, unmoistened by saliva, were with difficulty finding its way downward. Accordingly the patients moisten their solid food very thoroughly with saliva, and help it along by taking continually a small swallow of water or other fluid after every morsel.

Gradually comes the feeling that the food will not go down, and "sticks fast," and although at first this passes away after waiting and taking a swallow of fluid, yet there comes a time when this is no longer the case, but the bolus, within a shorter or longer time after the patient endeavors to swallow, is regurgitated. At the outset the contents of the œsophagus are not driven up to the pharynx, but only forced up for a certain distance, to sink down again after the fluid portion has passed through the stricture. If nothing, however, will pass through the narrowed portion, the contents of the œsophagus, when it is filled with food, are forced up into the pharynx and mouth.

At the present day we do not need to accept the assumption of an antiperistaltic action in the muscular tissue of the œsophagus, in order to explain the phenomena of regurgitation. The explanation by William Brinton [1] is sufficiently clear and complete, according to whom the peristaltic action, excited by the filling and distention of the canal, exercises a strong circular pressure upon the contents, which slowly proceeds from above downwards. This circular pressure, acting from without and above at the same time upon the periphery of the fluid column, forces the central portion, which is least exposed to pressure, to yield in an upward direction just as a column of fluid in a tube closed at the bottom will behave when pressure is made on its surface by a disc whose centre is perforated (Brinton). In the œsophagus the conditions are much more simple and comprehensible than in the intestine, and there is very little doubt of the accuracy of Brinton's explanation.

---

[1] Intestinal Obstruction. Edited by Thomas Bussard. London. 1867.

The higher up the stricture is situated in the œsophagus, the sooner will regurgitation follow; the nearer it is to the cardia and the more extensive is the dilatation of the canal above the stricture, the later will it be developed. When there is considerable dilatation the food will not be regurgitated for several hours, and will be found mixed with an abundance of mucus.

In rare cases a large morsel of food, inadvertently swallowed, may completely close a very narrow and deeply-seated stenosis for days or weeks without regurgitation, so that for many days not even fluids can be forced through, as occurred in Fagge's case, mentioned above.

In narrowings that have developed acutely, as from corrosion, burns, irritation from foreign bodies, or are caused by primary spasm, etc., the power of deglutition is almost entirely destroyed, and what remains of the canal is generally so completely closed by spasm of the muscles excited by the attempts to swallow, in consequence of the greatly increased reflex irritability of the muscular tissue, that all food which reaches the stricture is immediately regurgitated.

The sound (which, however, in acute cases should never be employed except for urgent reasons in some particular case) will be found to strike at one or more places in the œsophagus against an obstruction through which a moderate-sized pharyngeal bougie may possibly be forced with firm pressure. Gradually we must use smaller and smaller sounds, and in introducing the instrument the fingers perceive that it is firmly grasped by the contraction, and on listening at the back there is heard a friction-sound transmitted through the vertebral column, at the level of the stricture; and finally, nothing will pass through it. The dilatation above the stricture may be recognized by the remarkable mobility of the end of the instrument, and the fenestræ will be found to contain quantities of saliva and mucus, usually of a neutral reaction, and masses of fungus with them. The dilatation will correspond in extent to the rapidity with which the stenosis is developed, and is particularly extensive in medullary cancer of the cardia, because in this disease there is not sufficient time for the development of secondary muscular hypertrophy, and the energy of the parts is exhausted in the process of forming new tissue. In rare cases the neutral reaction of the regurgitated food or of the contents of the fenestræ may aid us in diagnosis when, in consequence of unusual position or condition of the stomach, it is uncertain whether the fragments of food come from the œsophagus or the stomach, *i. e.*, in which of these cavities the end of the sound lies.

On *inspection*, when the narrowing is considerable, we see from the configuration of the abdomen that there is interference with the entrance of food into the alimentary canal ; the whole lower portion of the abdomen is sunken and hollowed like a bowl, and what is particularly diagnostic, the epigastrium and left hypochondrium are deeply sunken, an indication that the access of food to the stomach has reached a minimum.

Auscultation of the œsophagus along the vertebral column in stenoses gives us various phenomena, according to the amount of contraction, the rough or smooth condition of its walls, and the diameter of the part of the canal above the stricture. We may have a clucking, gurgling, or spurting sound, which suddenly ceases at the point of narrowing, or is heard again after a few seconds taking an upward direction, which need not necessarily be accompanied by regurgitation into the mouth. Often we hear the normal œsophageal sound, which suddenly ceases, and always at the same level, sometimes with a pronounced shock. Thus the acoustic phenomena in stenosis may be very varied, as we should naturally expect from the variety in the physical and physiological conditions, yet it is true that the œsophageal râle will suffer changes in quality, intensity, and direction which may be recognized, and will serve as a basis for quite accurate diagnosis in determining the location of the obstruction.

Percussion of the œsophagus, when distended with gas artificially produced (an alkaline solution followed by an acid), not infrequently will give us useful hints concerning the location of the contraction and the amount of dilatation above it.

The *subjective* symptoms are pain (particularly in cancer and strictures caused by a foreign body), sensitiveness on pressure, a feeling of fulness under the sternum, difficulty in breathing in consequence of intra-thoracic accumulation of food above the stricture, a sensation of suffocation, and spasm of the glottis, particularly in the spasmodic stenosis of hysterical patients, hunger and thirst in advanced strictures, or when there is complete immobility of the œsophagus.

The influence of œsophageal stenosis upon the general nutrition of the body varies with the nature, persistency, and tightness of the stricture; it is least, or wholly wanting, in the periodical spasmodic strictures of the hysterical, and greatest in cancerous growths, which gradually lead to a complete occlusion of the canal. In these we observe marasmus most highly developed; the fat is wholly gone, the muscular tissue is atrophied, the expression of the face is that of suffering, and the color of the skin is cachectic.

The *diagnosis* of stenosis as such is not often difficult; the dysphagia, regurgitation of food, auscultation, exploration with the sound, the subjective symptoms, and finally the influence upon nutrition, leave us but little ground for doubt.

On the other hand, the diagnosis of the nature of the stenosis is often much more difficult.

The least difficult cases are those of cicatricial stricture and cancerous stenosis.

In the diagnosis of cicatricial strictures, the following points are important: the history of an antecedent lesion of the œsophagus by a mineral acid, alkali or foreign body, or of injury from without; the gradual development of narrowing (sufficiently remote in time from that of the primary lesion), and the constant increase of the same. The sound recognizes the great resistance of the cicatricial tissue, and treatment by dilatation produces good, and, in many cases, lasting results.

It will be a more difficult matter when we have valve-like or semicircular strictures to deal with, or when several strictures lie one above another. Here we can only decide after repeated examinations.

In the diagnosis of *cancerous* stenosis the age of the patient is of the first importance. Œsophageal stenoses which are developed after forty years of age, without any cause which can be recognized, which constantly increase, accompanied by general marasmus, until the canal is completely closed, are almost always cancerous. By the sound we recognize a more or less extensive narrowing; the resistance is that of a soft or moderately firm body. In many cases by careful dilatation the canal may gradually be so much enlarged that for months solid food can be swallowed.

We should call attention to the frequency of paralysis of the recurrent laryngeal nerves in œsophageal cancer situated high up; since we (Ziemssen) have made it a rule to examine the mobility of the muscles acting on the vocal cords in every case of this nature, the number of paralyses of one or both cords observed by us is greatly increasing. (Consult also the chapter on "Paralyses of the Recurrent Laryngeal," Vol. VII., p. 941.) The occurrence of paralysis is explained by the immediate topographical relations of both recurrents to the œsophagus at the level of the second dorsal vertebra and above, as is illustrated by the accompanying transverse section through the neck, by Braune.

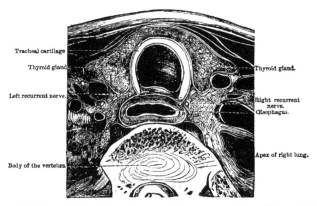

FIG. 2. Cross-section through the neck of a man twenty-five years of age, at the level of the lower border of the first dorsal vertebra. After Braune (Atlas, Plate No. VIII.)

Here, as also in paralysis of the recurrent by aortic aneurism, it is rarely the tumor itself which surrounds and compresses the nerve, but almost always the hyperplasia excited by the new growth and the secondary cicatricial contraction of the peri-œsophageal connective tissue.

In the relatively rapid progress of the stenosis to the most advanced grade of narrowing, cancer of the œsophagus some-times causes considerable dilatation in the canal above the stric-ture, and this arises from the excentric pressure of the accumu-lated food, combined with the diminution of muscular force dependent on cancerous cachexia. Accordingly we shall find the acoustic phenomena and other symptoms of dilatation associated with those of stenosis.

For the diagnosis of *compression stenoses*, which occur next in frequency to the cancerous, we must have first the evidence of a tumor exercising compression. Therefore, we should carefully investigate the condition of the thyroid body, but unfortunately it is only rarely possible to reach by palpation the portions of thyroid tissue which cause pressure from behind.

Accordingly, when strumous enlargement is present, we can admit that it causes the œsophageal compression when the latter is located at the level of the thyroid body and when no other causes for compression can be found. The interesting observa-tion by Koenig (loc. cit.), that in women such stenoses are found to increase during menstruation in consequence of general tur-gescence of the struma, and to diminish again after its cessation, should be of value in the differential diagnosis of difficult cases. The simultaneous compression of the trachea and recurrent nerves, and pushing aside of the œsophagus (recognized by aus-cultation of the direction of the œsophageal murmur) are also of importance in the diagnosis.

The stenosis caused by cancer of the thyroid body is much greater than in simple struma, even when the latter reaches its greatest development.

In two cases of this kind observed by us (Ziemssen), both in females, the steno-sis advanced with considerable rapidity to complete closure, and caused death by inanition.

Compression by aneurism of the aorta is ordinarily accom-panied by compression of neighboring organs, especially of the left recurrent, the trachea or one of the main bronchi, the in-nominate veins or the superior cava, pressing forward of the sternum, etc. ; when the sound is passed down to the aneurism, it will show rhythmical pulsations ; finally, the compression of the œsophagus is rarely very severe. Moreover, the other evidences of aortic aneurism must be present.

Mediastinal tumors, especially cancerous tumors, more easily cause compression, for the tube is ordinarily more or less firmly bound to the vertebral column by hyperplasia of the peri-œsophageal connective tissue. The diagnosis of mediastinal tumors in general is difficult, and only can be accurately made under very favorable circumstances ; and the same is the case with the diagnosis of œsophageal compression caused by such tumors.

The diagnosis of dislocations and narrowings due to the lateral pressure of a diverticulum filled with food requires first that we should establish the existence of a diverticulum. In cicatricial stenoses, above which large diverticula are gradually formed, it becomes doubly difficult to recognize the cause of the narrowing. (See the case of Waldenburg, loc. cit.)

The diagnosis of narrowings due to the presence of foreign bodies which have become firmly fixed in the œsophagus requires either the evidence by anamnesis of the entrance of such a body, or, when this is not possible, as so frequently happens, the discovery of the foreign body by the sound. The acoustic sound of Duplay,[1] although somewhat complicated, is fitted to detect even the smallest foreign body, unless it has escaped into a small diverticulum.

Duplay's sound is armed with a silver olive-shaped bulb at the tip, and at the upper end has a "resonance chamber" (*à la* Koenig), from which a rubber tube leads to the ear, fitted with an ivory ear-piece.

Colin first constructed a sound of this description, and used it successfully in the case of the well-known "fork swallower."

Besides, the severity of the inflammatory symptoms, and of the pain, as well as the acute commencement of the disease, and the lack of other causes, leads us to assume the presence of some foreign body.

Stenosis arising from *syphilis* is, as we have said before, of very rare occurrence, and would be detected by the anamnesis (later forms of the disease in other localities), by the compara-

---

[1] See *Sainte-Marie*, loc. cit. p. 26.

tively slight cachexia, by the results of auscultation (rough friction-sounds when the bougie is passed, or when the patient swallows), and finally, above all, by the favorable results of an antisyphilitic treatment. Yet the diagnosis usually cannot be given as more than "probable."

The diagnosis of *spastic stricture* is chiefly based upon the sudden change from complete impassability of the passage at one time to perfect freedom from obstruction at another, and also upon the recognition of other hysterical or hypochondriacal disturbances, or a general nervous condition, but, above all, upon the evidence by the sound of a normal diameter when free from spasm, while during the attack nothing can be passed through the stricture, or only by using considerable force.

The diagnosis is difficult when we suspect that with the spasm of the œsophagus, and generally as a cause of the same, there is some pathological change in the wall itself, *e. g.*, foreign bodies, ulcerations, or rapidly growing tumors. In such cases we can only clear up the matter by repeated examinations after using remedies to allay spasm, or while employing an anæsthetic.

Termination and Prognosis.

The termination and prognosis of œsophageal stenosis depend upon the gravity of the processes which underlie it.

The prognosis in cicatricial strictures is not very bad when the cicatricial mass is only moderately developed, is high up, and capable of dilatation. Even cases which, at the outset, appear incurable, which scarcely admit the finest sound, and are accompanied by the greatest irritability of the mucous membrane of the throat and œsophagus, sometimes are completely cured. But if we do not succeed in enlarging the opening by methodical dilatation, or if the patient abandons such treatment, then, in consequence of the progressive contraction of the stenosis, associated with dilatation, ulceration, and bulging of the walls in the parts above the stricture, we have inanition, and the danger of perforation of the wall, and escape of the contents of the œsophagus into the peri-œsophageal connective tissue or into neighboring organs which have previously become firmly adherent to it. The subject of perforation will be treated of in a special chapter. Under all circumstances the prognosis of cicatricial strictures should be given with the greatest caution, and with the understanding that the patient shall remain under observation and proper treatment for a considerable length of time.

The cancerous strictures terminate most rapidly and surely in death. The symptoms of inanition appear long before the cancerous cachexia, and, in the general course of the disease, far outweigh the local and general evidences of cancer. It is in young patients we can best assure ourselves of the fact that for a long time the cancer only serves as a mechanical obstacle, and undermines the constitution by the cutting off of nourishment at a time when the symptoms of cancer—above all, pain at the affected spot, swelling of the glands and cachexia—are so little marked that we frequently doubt the accuracy of our diagnosis.

The prognosis is naturally that of a fatal termination, but at the time when the mechanical trouble is the most important, and it seems as if the end would speedily come through inanition, careful and methodical dilatation, and the opportunity thus afforded for the more abundant introduction of food into the stomach will sometimes produce a wonderful improvement in the general condition and prolongation of life for a period of from three to six months.

The termination and prognosis of considerable narrowing from compression by tumors are equally unfavorable, whether this arise from aneurism of the aorta, struma, sarcoma of the mediastinum or pleura, or cancer of the vertebræ. From the recent results of the antiseptic treatment of wounds (Lister's method) we ought to be able to give the best prognosis in strumous growths, since here there is an opportunity for extirpation by operation.

Stenoses from foreign bodies have, in general, a very doubtful prognosis, on account of the danger of perforation, formation of abscess in the peri-œsophageal connective tissue, etc. The literature of foreign bodies is rich in unfavorable terminations in various ways: fatal hemorrhage after perforation of the aorta by a coin in the œsophagus (Bradley); by a bone (Hugues); by a bone penetrating into the vena cava (Coester); into the pleural cavity (Busch) ; into the mediastinum, into the trachea (Adelmann, Predescu) ; and into the left auricle (Bertrand); but, on the other hand, there are found no small number with an unexpectedly favorable termination, in spite of extensive inflammation, and perforation of the œsophagus, and purulent pleuritis (Mayer, Busch, and others), so that the prognosis should not be given as absolutely unfavorable from the outset.

In consequence of the meagreness of our materials thus far, we cannot give any general points for forming a prognosis in *syphilis of the œsophagus.*

Spastic stenosis has almost always a favorable termination in cure, especially when properly treated, yet some fatal terminations have been reported (Pomes). Certainly the proportion of such cases must be very small, compared with the perfect cures.

Yet we should remember the tendency of such stenoses to return, which is often very marked, so that the total duration is sometimes fifteen (Seney), or even thirty years (Lasègue).

The termination and prognosis of the rare form of stenosis by hypertrophy of the cricoid cartilage[1] can be readily imagined. A diminution in the thickening of the cricoid can only be expected through suppurative perichondritis and necrosis of the cartilage. Accordingly, we should esteem ourselves fortunate when no change takes place in the cartilage. In future, our prognosis will be modified by the question whether we can succeed by Wernher's method in rendering the œsophagus, *i. e.*, the lower end of the pharynx, temporarily pervious (see under *Treatment*).

Treatment.

The treatment of œsophageal stenoses requires great prudence and skill on the part of the physician, and faithfulness on the part of the patient. Our first care should be the gradual dilatation of the stenosis, and thereby the improvement in nutrition. The means to this end are naturally varied according to the

---

[1] Properly this form of stenosis affects the lower end of the pharynx, and only concerns the œsophagus in so far as the abnormally developed cartilage, pressing backward, obstructs the entrance of the canal.

cause ; but, since we are powerless against most of them (cancer, compression by tumors), the indicatio causalis will be but little regarded. In stenosis by foreign bodies or polyps, however, we may carry out the causal indication by carefully removing the same—we shall not here enter into the proper methods for removal, since that properly belongs in the hand-books of surgery. In syphilis of the œsophagus we may obtain brilliant results by an antisyphilitic treatment (West, Follin, Morell Mackenzie).

In all other cases the indicatio morbi would lead to a methodical dilatation of the stricture. We can readily understand that we must proceed with the greatest care and precaution at the outset, and, when the instrument passes the stricture, we must employ it for the introduction of liquids into the stomach. In undertaking dilatation, good catgut instruments, elastic bougies with a central wire, then English pharyngeal sounds, and finally the solid conical elastic bougies of Bouchard, are the most serviceable, and in most cases to be preferred to the dilators of Jameson, Fletcher, Trousseau, Bruns, Jaap, Richardson, and others.

When the narrowing is considerable, we must have great patience. Often it is not till after attempts for weeks that we succeed in passing the finest sounds through the canal; after that the progress is usually more rapid.

A statement given by Jonathan Hutchinson is very instructive as regards the method of dilatation and its results. In a case of cicatricial stricture following corrosion by caustic potash, in which, on account of the absolute impermeability of the stricture (not even fluids passing through), he was preparing to perform gastrotomy, another attempt at passing the sound was successful. By repeated dilatation the patient was finally almost completely cured.

Hence, in benign growths or stenoses we should be very cautious in advising gastrotomy, since the result of this operation, according to reports thus far received, is almost surely fatal.

The prognosis of œsophagotomy in stenoses high up is somewhat better (see the statistics of Koenig, loc. cit., p. 69), yet even here we should defer advising the operation while there remains a ray of hope of succeeding with bougies.

We have too little material thus far on which to base an opinion concerning internal œsophagotomy, yet the latest observations by Gillespi, Trélat, and others, lead us to hope for a favorable result when it is employed in cicatricial strictures.

In the stenosis of the lower portion of the pharynx and entrance of the œsophagus by thickening and ossification of the cricoid cartilage, we should follow the method suggested by Wernher, viz. : on introducing the sound, to pull the larynx forward, away from the vertebral column, and direct the point of the instrument towards the left. At present the value of this method rests only on the results in a single case, and requires further confirmation.

DILATATIONS OF THE ŒSOPHAGUS.

Literature.

In addition to the manuals and text-books cited on page 3, and the clinical reports by *Oppolzer*, see *Purton*, Lond. Med. and Phys. Journ. Vol. XLVI. 1821.—*Mondière*, Archives générales de médecine. Sér. II. Tom. I. 1833.—*Hannay*, Edinb. Med. and Surg. Journal. July, 1833.—*Rokitansky*, Oesterr. Jahrb. 1840. S. 219.—*Lindau*, Casper's Wochenschrift, 1840. S. 356.—*Delle Chiage*, Il Progresso. Neapel, 1840.—*Albers*, Atlas d. pathol. Anat. II. T. 24 u. Erläuterungen II.—*Abercrombie*, Die Krankheiten des Magens, deutsch von v. d. Busch. Bremen, 1843. S. 177 ff.—*Spengler*, Wien. med. Wochenschr. 1853. Nr. 25.—*Heschl*, Compendium d. patholog. Anatomie. 1855. S. 396.—*Habershon*, Pathological and Practical Observations on Diseases of the Alimentary Canal. 1857—*Wilks*, Lectures on Patholog. Anatomy. 1859.—*Giesse*, Ueber die einfache gleichmässige Erweiterung des Oesophagus. Diss. Würzburg, 1860.—*Ogle*, Transactions of the Patholog. Society. 1865-66.—*Fridberg*, Ueber Oesophagusdivertikel. Diss. Giessen, 1867.—*Luschka*, Virchow's Archiv. Bd. XI. S. 431 und Bd. XLII. S. 473. 1868.—*Berg*, Die totale spindelförmige Erweiterung der Speiseröhre und das Wiederkäuen bei Menschen. Diss. Tübingen, 1868.—*Waldenburg*, Berl. klin. Wochenschrift. 1870. 48.—*Tiedemann*, Ueber die Ursachen und Wirkungen chronisch-entzündlicher Processe im Mediastin. Diss. Kiel, 1875 und Deutsch. Arch. f. klin. Medicin. XVI. S. 575.—*Davy*, The Med. Press and Circular. 1875. May 5.—*Stern*, Arch. der Heilkunde. Bd. XVII. S. 432. 1876.—*Dave*, Progrès médic. 1877. No. 10. p. 191.—See also the tabular compilation of Pressure-diverticula on p. 53 in this manual.

Pathology and Etiology.

The dilatations of the œsophagus are either diffuse and circular, *simple ektasiæ*, or else protrusions at a single point in the wall, and involving only a small portion of the periphery—*diverticula.*

Simple Ektasiæ.

Simple ektasiæ are most frequently the result of long-continued stenoses of the cardia or of the œsophagus. Yet it was noted above (p. 33) that not nearly all the stenoses are followed by dilatation. On the contrary, frequently enough this is entirely wanting in the most advanced stenoses, and in most other cases is very trifling. It is only in rare cases that we have ektasiæ of any extent. So long as the muscles retain their power of contraction, so long will the food detained in the œsophagus by the stenosis be quickly regurgitated. Accordingly there is little stagnation, and hence little dilatation. When the muscular force gives out from overwork, then the contractile power of the muscular layer, which is usually undergoing hypertrophy, will be more or less affected by degenerative processes, and the ingesta are detained, and we have permanent ektasiæ.

That stenosis of the pylorus should give rise to dilatation of the œsophagus can only be expected in such cases as that described by Klebs, in which, with the stenosis, there was extensive hypertrophy of the whole muscular tissue of the stomach, so that the cavity of the organ was greatly contracted, the power of distention limited, and hence its capacity much diminished. In all other cases, in consequence of the enormous power of distention in the stomach, there could be no considerable stagnation in the œsophagus, and so no permanent dilatation.

These *stagnation ektasiæ* (Stauungs-Ektasieen), as we are accustomed to call them, from the method of their production, are first formed immediately above the stenosis, and here reach their greatest development. From this point they extend generally only over a short portion of the canal above—at the highest only 9 ctms. (Cruveilhier)—and constantly diminish as we ascend. Only in rare cases (in stenosis of the cardia) does the dilatation involve the whole length of the tube, and here it also diminishes usually as we ascend.

It was different, however, in a case reported by Lindau (loc. cit.), in stenosis of the cardia (and also of the pylorus), in which the whole canal was dilated, and the greatest diameter (about four inches) was found at the middle of its course.

The dilatation ordinarily takes place equally all around the periphery. Yet we occasionally see unequal dilatations, in which some portion of the tube, not sharply bounded, protrudes more than the rest, and so bulges towards the neck or the pleura. Indeed, under certain circumstances, a limited diverticulum is sometimes formed (see below).

A case recently reported by Nicoladoni,[1] which, from the method of its production, is a striking instance of stagnation ektasia, but which, from the excessive bulging at one spot, had also the features of a diverticulum, is interesting from many points of view. In a little girl four years of age, who, two years before, after drinking lye, had developed stricture of the œsophagus, for which no treatment had been pursued, it was impossible to pass the sound, for the point continually doubled up. Accordingly, it was believed there was a diverticulum. In consequence of urgent symptoms, Nicoladoni performed œsophagotomy, and came down upon a diverticulum the size of a chestnut, which he cut open. Now the child could be nourished by a tube passed through the opening. Nevertheless, she died of pneumonia six days after the operation. At the autopsy the œsophagus was found to be greatly contracted by cicatrices at its middle portion for a distance of 8 ctms., but above the stricture for 2½ ctms. it bulged unequally, and especially towards the left and anterior portion of the periphery, so that there was here a sack-shaped protrusion applied directly against the stricture, into which one could pass the last phalanx of the index finger. An incision of 2½ ctms. long appeared on the convex surface.

The muscular tissue in stagnation ektasiæ is usually more or less hypertrophied at the seat of the ektasia, and the hypertrophy diminishes as we pass upward. The mucous membrane and submucosa are not unfrequently thickened as well, and the former is sometimes studded with polypoid excrescences (case of Cruveilhier. See above, p. 20).

Besides these stagnation ektasiæ, we find, in rare cases, also considerable, and occasionally enormous ektasiæ, sometimes of the whole canal, and sometimes of only a portion, in which there is no underlying stenosis whatever. In these cases the dilatation is usually greatest near the middle of the tube, and diminishes both upward and downward, so that the œsophagus has the strange appearance of a spindle-shaped sack, with loose walls hanging down between the pleural cavities. In two cases the most dilated portion was the size of a man's arm (in Luschka's case the circumference was 30 ctms.). At the same time the tube

---

[1] Wiener Medicin. Wochenschrift. 1877. No. 25.

is often considerably stretched, so its course is necessarily crooked. The wall is also generally considerably thickened (according to Rokitansky, however, dilatations of less extent are accompanied by thinning of the wall). This thickening is caused chiefly by muscular hypertrophy, especially of the circular layer, yet in one case (Stern) almost entirely by thickening of the mucous membrane. This membrane is sometimes normal, sometimes thickened, sometimes covered with enlarged tufted papillæ, and sometimes with disseminated nodules and plaques. In several cases there were found here and there flat hemorrhagic erosions and ulcers extending down to the muscular tissue, and in one case a star-shaped cicatrix. The tube was filled with a brownish, pulpy mass, or only with small fragments of food.

The greater number of these patients had suffered for many years from severe dysphagia, vomiting, regurgitation of food shortly after eating, and repeatedly from actual rumination.

It seems probable that the causes of these apparently spontaneous ektasiæ must be sought in the diminished contractile power of the muscles—and, in fact, in one such case Klebs found extensive fatty degeneration of the muscular fibres. Yet the remote causes of this affection of the muscles, which must be various in the various cases, are as yet very obscure. In two cases (Purton, Hannay) the trouble came on after a blow upon the breast; in one (Davy), after raising a heavy weight, during which the patient had the feeling "as if something had given way inside;" in one (Spengler), after the patient, eating hastily, had swallowed a hot dumpling which "stuck fast;" in one case (delle Chiage) the dysphagia came on after a "gastric fever;" and in one (Oppolzer), the patient had been treated for gout by causing him to drink great quantities of warm water. The "post hoc ergo propter hoc" may be doubted in all these cases, for in no two was the same cause alleged. Yet there seems to us no real reason why these alleged causes may not be sufficient. That inflammatory processes in the œsophagus, especially catarrhal affections, in so far as they involve the muscular tissue by sympathy, may lead to the formation of ektasiæ, is quite probable, but is not proven, since the evidences of chronic catarrh so repeatedly found at the autopsy may be the result, instead of the cause, of the muscular change. The view of a primary inflammation is best supported by the case of Stern, where there was an early opportunity for post-mortem observation (a man, twenty years old, who died eight months after the commencement of difficulty in swallowing), and where the microscopical examination of the greatly thickened and hypertrophied mucous membrane, in addition to a partial deficiency in the epithelium and raising up of the same by pus-cells, discovered a small-celled infiltration through the whole thickness of the mucous membrane, here and there extending down into the muscular layer. So also as regards the vomiting, which sometimes continues for years before death, it must remain undecided whether it should be considered as a cause or a sequel of the ektasia. Ektasiæ seem to be more frequently developed in youth than at any other time.

Up to the present time seventeen cases of this nature have been described or briefly noted by Purton, Hannay, Rokitansky (two cases), delle Chiage, Abercrombie, Oppolzer, Spengler, Wilks, Giesse (two cases), Ogle, Luschka, Klebs, Davy, Stern, Dave (loc. cit., supra. See particularly those by Rokitansky, Giesse, Luschka, and Stern). We add one also which we ourselves observed (Zenker). The subject of it was a young woman who for a long time had shown symptoms of rumination. The autopsy showed that the œsophagus was considerably dilated from its upper end down to within two ctms. of the cardiac orifice, was spindle-shaped, with loose, flabby walls. The breadth of the tube when split open (in an alcoholic preparation, in which the tissues naturally were considerably shrunken) was 5 ctms. at the greatest width, in the middle of the dilated portion, while it measured only 3 ctms. just below the pharynx and above the cardiac orifice. The muscular tissue throughout the dilated portion was hypertrophied, most so in the middle portion (over 2 mm. thick). The mucous membrane showed nothing abnormal, and particularly no cicatrix underlying the dilatation. With the exception of a slight wart-like hypertrophy of its mucous membrane near the pylorus, the stomach was normal. (Preparation in the museum at the Dresden City Hospital.)

We also should not forget to mention three rare cases, described by Fr. Arnold and Luschka, of partial ektasiæ, with moderate peripheral dilatation, affecting a small region just above the œsophageal opening in the diaphragm, which Luschka terms "vestibule of the stomach" (Vormagen), literally, "coming before the stomach" (to distinguish it from a very similar formation, but situated beneath the diaphragm, which Luschka considers to

appertain to the stomach, and accordingly names "antrum car-
diacum "). The three cases by Arnold were in men who had been
suffering from rumination. Whether these dilatations should in
all cases be considered congenital must remain undecided. They
certainly are sometimes congenital, as the following case under
our own (Zenker) observation will show.

We found the following condition in the body of a seven months child who died
when seven days old, in the Dresden Lying-in Asylum, in consequence of hemorrhage
from the seat of insertion of the cord and from excoriations on the flexures of the
thighs (autopsy, March 31, 1860), viz., at the lower end of the œsophagus a
spherical ektasia, sharply bounded both above and below (next the cardia) with a
very thick, bluish-red wall in consequence of hemorrhagic infiltration. The inner
surface was covered with large-celled pavement epithelium in layers like the normal
epithelium of the tube.

We also (Zenker) observed a very deceptive appearance resembling at first sight
an ektasia, in the body of a patient suffering from mental disease, together with a
slight diffuse ektasia of the lower portion of the œsophagus. The portion of the
diaphragm immediately surrounding the œsophageal opening so bulged into the
thoracic space as to form a sac 7 ctms. long, very wide, reaching to 5½ ctms. in
diameter, into which the œsophagus entered at the upper end, so that, looking from
the cavity of the thorax, it appeared at first as if the œsophagus itself was sacculated
at its lower portion.

Diverticula.

By the name *diverticula*, as already said, we mean those
limited protrusions or bulgings which affect only a small portion
of the periphery of the œsophageal wall. In a strict sense they
are not dilatations, but more properly blind appendages to the
normal canal, and are perceptible externally as limited protrusions. In a careful investigation of the subject we must over-
step the true limit of the œsophagus and consider also the lower
portion of the pharynx at the same time, since one form of these
diverticula, strictly speaking, belongs to the pharynx; but since
it is situated just at the boundary line, and seriously affects the
lower tube by sympathy, in describing œsophageal diseases we
cannot very well omit it. In the literature such pharyngeal
diverticula are repeatedly and erroneously described as œsophageal.

In the laryngeal portion of the pharynx and in the œsophagus are found two different forms of diverticula, and in every point of view—pathogenesis, location, anatomical structure, symptoms, and pathological significance—they are so totally distinct and different that it is impossible by grouping them to give a general description of the disease.

Although this has been done hitherto by nearly all writers (excepting only Rokitansky and Heschl), the only result has been to render the true description of the disease obscure and complex.

Accordingly, it seems best at the outset to distinguish them by different names and descriptions. From the method of their formation we divide them into *pressure diverticula* (Pulsions-Divertikel), which arise from something within the canal pressing outward ; and *traction diverticula*, in which the wall is pulled out by something exercising traction from without.

Pressure Diverticula.

The following table gives a résumé of the cases belonging in this category, upon which our description is based. There are twenty-two cases selected from the literature of the subject which were authenticated by autopsies ; to these are added five which we ourselves observed (one very large, one of medium size, three small), and seven, which, from the symptoms during life, probably belong in this category, but in which the facts were not established by autopsy.

A. *Cases in which an autopsy was made.*

Number of Cases and Date when reported.	Author.	Place where Case is recorded.	Sex.	Age.	Size of Diverticulum.	Died from Diverticulum.	Died from other Causes.	Remarks.
1 (1764)	*Ludlow*	Med. Observ. and Inquir. Vol. III.. 1767, with plate. (See Mondière, Arch. Gén. XXIV. p. 410.)	m	60	Wide sac, reaching down into Thorax.	1	—	Preparation in Hunterian Museum. Plate copied by Baillie. A series of engravings, Part III. Plate 1. Froriep. Surg. Plates. Plate 392. Albers, Atlas of Patholog. Anatomy. Vol. II. Plate XXIII. Fig. 4.
2 (1782)	*Gianella*	Borsieri, Institut. Med. Pract. IV. De Dysphagia. (See Mondière, loc. cit. p. 411.)	m	60	6 or 7 fingers' breadths long.	1	—	—
3 (1783)	*Marz*	Götting. Anz. 1783. p. 2034.	m	73	5 inches long.	1	—	—
4	*De Guise*	Dissert. sur l'anévrysme. Paris. An XII. No. 252. (See Mondière, loc. cit. 1833. Sept. p. 33.)	m	†	—	1	—	—

Number of Cases and Date when reported.	Author.	Place where Case is recorded.	Sex.	Age.	Size of Diverticulum.	Died from Diverticulum.	Died from other Causes.	Remarks.
5 (1806)	*Thilow*	Salzburg. med.-chir. Zeitung. 1806. 2d. Vol. p. 336.	m	52	2¼" long.	?	?	
6	*Monro*	Morbid Anat. of the Gullet, etc. Edinburgh, 1811. p. 12.	?	?	—	?	?	
7	*Chas. Bell*	Surg. Observ. Part. I. 1816. p. 67, with plate.	m	?	Size of a cherry.	—	1	Plate copied in Froriep's Plates. Plate 174.
8 (1821)	*Kühne*	De Dysphagiæ causis. Diss. Berlin, 1831, and Rust's Magazine. Vol. 39. 1833. p. 348, with plate.	m	54	3¼" long.	1	—	Preparation in the Anatom. Museum at Berlin. Plate copied in Froriep, loc. cit. Plate 392, and Albers, loc. cit. Fig. 5.
9 (1837)	*Rokitansky*	Œsterr. med. Jahrbuch. Vol. XXI. 1840. p. 222.	m	66	Over 2" long.	1	—	Preparation in Vienna Museum of Patholog. Anat. Plate in Albers, loc. cit. Fig. 3.
10	*Otto*	Günsburg's Zeitschr. für klin. Med. I. 1850. p. 344, and Albers, Explanations to Atlas of Pathol. Anat. Atlas II. p. 265.	m	78	2½" long.	1	—	Preparation in Anatom. Museum at Breslau. Plate in Albers, loc. cit. Figs. 1 and 2. (The case described in Günsburg Zeitschr. and that pictured by Albers are doubtless identical.
11 (1846)	*Worthington*	Med. Chir. Transact. Vol. 30. 1847. p. 199, with plate.	m	69	3½" long.	1	—	
12 (1848)	*Göppert*	Schleiden and Froriep's Notiz. 3d. Series. No. 177. Jan. 1849. p. 16.	m	80	Very large.	1	—	
13	*Hettich*	Würtemberg Corresp.-Bl. 1851. No. 29.	m	69	Holding at least 2 ounces.	—	1	
14	*Braun*	Würtemberg Corresp.-Bl. 1852. No. 16.	m	75	Size of a child's fist.	1	—	
15	*Cruveilhier*	Traité d'anatomie pathol.génér.Vol. II. 1852. p. 852.	?	?	—	?	?	Cruv. says he has often seen such sacs, but does not give full reports of them.
16 (1859)	*Fridberg* (Gassner)	Diss. concerning Œsoph. Diverticula. Giessen. 1867, with plate.	m	60	3¼" long, holds from 3 to 4 ℥.	1	—	Preparation in the Museum of Patholog. Anatomy at Giessen.
17	*Förster*	Handbook of Spec. Patholog. Anatomy. 2d Edition. 1863. p. 57.	?	?	—	?	?	
18	*Ogle*	Transac. of the Patholog. Soc. 1865–66, with a plate.	m	63	—	—	1	
19 (1867)	*Berg* (Veit)	Die totale spindelförm. Erweiterung d. Speiseröhre u. d. Wiederkäuen beim Menschen. Diss. Tübingen, 1868. p. 26.	m	65	9 ctms. long, holds 5 ℥.	1	—	
20	*Betz*	Memorabilien. XVII. 10. p. 457. 1872.	m	49	6 ctms. long.	—	1	
21 (1875)	*Klob*	Wien. med. Wochenschr. 1875. No. 11. p. 210.	?	?	Size of a goose's egg.	?	?	
22	*Kunze*	Lehrb. d. prakt. Med. 3d Edition. 1877. Vol. I. p. 285.	m	?	Size of a child's hand.	1	—	Died of gangrene of the lung, caused by escape of food from diverticulum into larynx and lungs.
23 (1854)	*Zenker*		m	75	Size of a pea.	—	1	
24 (1862)	*Idem*		m	45	Slight bulging.	—	1	
25 (1864)	*Idem*	Not published hitherto.	m	59	Size of a hazel-nut.	—	1	} Preparations in the Erlanger Museum of Patholog. Anatomy. For plates of No. 26, see Figs. 3 and 4.
26 (1867)	*Idem*		m	77	8 ctms. long.	—	1	
27	*Idem* (Heller)		?	?	Size of a cherry.	?	?	

B. *Cases where no autopsy was made.*

Number of Cases and Date when reported.	Author.	Place where Case is recorded.	Sex.	Age.	Size of Diverticulum.	Died from Diverticulum.	Died from other Causes.	Remarks.
28	*Isenflamm*	Versuch einiger praktischer Anmerkungen über die Muskeln. Erlangen, 1778. § 172.	m	young.	—	—	1	No autopsy could be obtained.
29	*Blücking*	Baldinger's neues Magazin für Aerzte. 1781. Vol. III. p. 242.	m	?	—	—	—	
30	*Collomb*	Œuvres Méd.-Chirurgie. Lyons. 1798. p. 307 (quoted by Mondière).	m	?	—	—	—	
31	*Dendy*	Lancet. June, 1848.	m	?	—	—	—	
32	*Klose* and *Paul*	Günsburg's Zeitschr. für klin. Med. Vol. I. 1850. p. 344.	w	?	—	—	—	
33	?	Edinburgh Med. Journ. 1856 (quoted by Günther. Lehre v. d. blutigen Operationen. 1864. p. 309).	m	55	—	—	—	
34	*Waldenburg*	Berlin. med. Wochenschr. 1870. No. 48. p. 578.	w	40	—	—	—	

The cases of Littré and Roennow, alluded to below (quoted by Mondière), as well as those by Watson and Nicoladoni, are not included in this collection, the first two on account of inadequate description, and the last two for reasons which are given in the notes on pp. 54 and 61.

The *pressure diverticula* (Pulsionsdivertikel) are so rare that few physicians have ever seen a case. Yet, notwithstanding their rare occurrence, they are of great pathological significance, since they occasion the worst form of dysphagia, and through inanition sometimes cause death.

They are located, as it appears, exclusively (certainly only with rare exceptions) at the lowest part of the pharynx, just at the upper boundary of the œsophagus, and on the posterior wall, sometimes exactly in the median line, and sometimes somewhat laterally.[1] There is never more than one such diverticulum present in any given case.

---

[1] *Watson* has briefly described (Journal of Anat. and Physiol. Vol. IX. Part. I. 1875) a pharyngeal diverticulum in an adult male, reaching down to the manubrium sterni, in which the narrow slit-like opening was found on the free border of the posterior pillar of the fauces, immediately behind the tonsil. A diverticulum having a point of origin so entirely different from all other cases should not properly be included with the above without something to identify it.

Concerning the two single cases in which we find it stated that there were several sacs (in one case four, Littré, Roennow), the accounts are not sufficiently full to warrant our including them with certainty in this category.

The smaller ones have the appearance of sharply bounded protrusions of the wall of the pharynx, from the size of a pea to

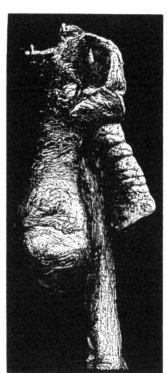

FIG. 3.— *Large pressure diverticulum of the pharynx* (side view), from a man seventy-seven years old (retired clergyman). Preparation in the Museum of Pathological Anatomy at Erlangen. Case No. 26 of the preceding table. Taken from a photograph. The patient, who, two years before his death, was quite a robust and stately man, with strong muscular and bony system, then came under the care of Prof. Wintrich, on account of slight signs of a pharyngeal stenosis. In passing the sound he sometimes succeeded in evading the obstruction and entering the stomach, while at other times the instrument would enter a diverticulum, evidently situated high up in the pharynx. From time to time the patient would eject and eructate food which was undigested, but softened. Towards the end of his life he was not under medical care or observation, and finally died of pneumonia. The autopsy (Oct. 4, 1867, Dr. Heller) showed that the pharynx was prolonged inferiorly into a blind sac of a pear-shape, which was eight centimetres long, and, when distended, five centimetres in breadth, situated a little to the right, and into which the oesophagus entered by a small opening at the upper portion, and somewhat laterally. Besides fragments of food, the sac contained grape-seeds and a piece of slate, rather smaller than a kreuzer. The mucous membrane of the sac was puffed up, and lay in plaits or folds From the preparation of the pharyngeal muscular tissue, it is very beautifully shown that the sac protrudes between the lowest bundles of the inferior constrictor, so that some of the lowest fibres embrace the anterior portion of the neck of the diverticulum. On the posterior face, laterally, at a height of two centimetres, and in the median line (corresponding with the raphé), at a height of one and a half centimetres, are found fibres of the inferior constrictor, greatly arched and drawn downward. Below this there are no muscular fibres whatever on the diverticulum.

that of a hazel-nut, shallow or somewhat deeper (hemispherical), and bulging from the posterior wall. The larger ones have the appearance of a sac directed downward from the pharynx, and hanging between the oesophagus and vertebral column, sometimes spherical, sometimes cylindrical, and sometimes more pear-shaped, with a rounded knob-like end, and a sometimes wide and sometimes comparatively narrow opening. The sac may have a length of thirteen centimetres and more, and a trans-

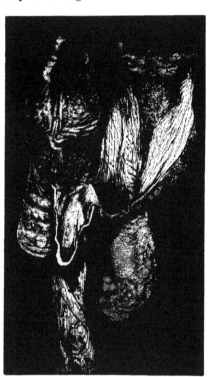

verse diameter of more than five centimetres. The wall of these sacs, at least of the larger ones, is quite thick and firm, as much so as in the rest of the pharynx and œsophagus, a fact which has led the older writers to say that they have the same coverings as the pharynx. A careful dissection a n d preparation, however, will show that they are mostly formed of the greatly thickened mucous membrane, w h i c h within is smooth, or slightly granular from papillary hypertrophy of the *submucosa*, and a layer of connective tissue thickened like

Fig. 4.—Interior view of the same diverticulum as in Fig. 3, in order to show the mouth of the sac.

a fascia, while in the region of the sac the muscular tissue is either wholly wanting, or is present for a short distance at its neck, and elsewhere is not found. From a series of carefully observed cases, it is evident that the sac is formed by the protrusion of the mucous membrane between the separated fibres of muscular tissue, and usually these are the transverse continuous fibres of the inferior constrictor muscle of the pharynx passing over its posterior wall, and accordingly it has been appropriately termed a hernia of the mucous membrane (pharyngocele). In the cases in which muscular fibres are found remaining at the neck of the diverticulum (in one case observed by us, extending one and a half to two centimetres on a sac eight centimetres long), they are usually those of the inferior constrictor, and perhaps also farther down, the upper circular fibres of the œsophagus. The muscular covering of the neck of the diverticulum can readily be explained by the supposition that the sac, gradually enlarging and becoming heavier, has at last involved the muscular fibres adjoining (œsophageal), which were at first not protruded, and secondarily has dragged them down so that now they form the muscular coat of the neck. Whether in addition to these hernia-like diverticula there are any which have a complete muscular layer, is at least highly improbable.

A number of the modern writers distinguish two different kinds of sac-like diverticula, which, resembling each other in their location, shape, etc., are distinguished from one another by the presence or absence of a muscular layer in their wall. They accordingly assert that they arise in different ways, and consider those that have a muscular layer as congenital formations. But, having carefully studied the literature of the subject, and having ourselves investigated four of these very preparations, we consider that this distinction has no adequate basis, but do believe that all diverticula occurring at this place must be considered as identical in anatomy and pathogenesis. Without doubt the reports of many cases by observers do assert the presence of a muscular layer in more or less precise terms. Nevertheless, these statements appear to us highly doubtful, and require careful investigation. These doubts arise not only from the opposite statement of those observers who are the most reliable (Chas. Bell, Rokitansky, Ogle), and the results of our own examination of three preparations in the Museum of Patholog. Anatomy at Erlangen (of which one is the most beautiful specimen of its kind), from which we find that in all three cases (except in a portion of the neck of the largest one) there is no muscular layer whatever, but above all, from the statements, partly indefinite and partly incredible, concerning the arrangement of the muscular fibres in the wall of the sac; and finally, from the result of our own examination of one of these cases, in which the existence of a muscular layer is asserted in the most precise terms. It is that case, so interesting in every respect, reported by Fridberg (observed by Dr. Gassner in Mainz) in his careful dissertation, of which the preparation is to be found in the Museum of Pathological Anatomy at Giessen. In speaking of the large, flask-shaped diverticulum, three and a half inches long, hanging down behind the œsophagus, Fridberg says it is made up " of all the layers of the œsophagus. The muscular layer is moderately developed, and the fibres run in a regular manner entirely around the sac." Although this statement leaves nothing to wish for in precision, yet I could not repress my doubts of its accuracy, and so had recourse to Prof. Perls, with the request that I might prove this point, and he had the kindness to send me the specimen for my own examination. My examination showed in fact that Fridberg's statement concerning the muscular layer was totally incorrect. The mucous membrane, as in the other cases, was found to bulge outward between the lowest separated fibres of the inferior constrictor muscle. Two of the separated fibres reach down to some extent upon the neck of the diverticulum. On all the rest of the sac not a muscular fibre can be found. Accordingly, Fridberg's argument concerning the pathogenesis, which rests upon the presence of the muscular layer, naturally falls to the ground, and the simple and natural explanation, which he opposes, is re-restablished. From what has been said, it is evident that this diverticulum also arises from the pharynx, and not the œsophagus, as Fridberg states.

After this result we shall not be blamed if we believe that the few remaining cases in which a muscular layer was declared to be present are equally incapable of demonstration, as, e. g., the case pictured by Albers (Atlas, Part II., Plate XXIII., Figs. 1 and 2), in which a " thick layer of muscular tissue " was said to exist; but certainly it would not be suspected on examining the plate. In his interesting case, so often quoted, Kuehne only says in general that the outer layer " is made up of muscular fibres of considerable thickness coming from the œsophagus, which spread out like a web over the surface of the sac," which certainly cannot be interpreted as meaning a continuous muscular layer. And in Worthington's case, in which "nearly two-thirds of the sac is covered with muscular fibres from the constrictor of the pharynx," at least a considerable portion of the sac, according to this statement, must have been free from such fibres. Other cases are less capable of proof on account of even less complete statements.[1]

But the assumption that the muscular layer, when wanting, may have formerly been there, but has become atrophied by the enlargement of the sac (Klebs, Koenig), is not only entirely gratuitous — for the statement by Klebs, in opposition to our

---

[1] In the case of *Marx*, in which the sac is described as " made up of coats like those of the pharynx," *Wrisberg*, who reported the case before the society at Göttingen, laments in so many words " that more pains were not taken, in preparing the specimen, carefully to investigate the condition of the constrictor muscles, which would have materially assisted in clearing up the nature of the affection." And as regards the case of *Watson*, quoted above (foot-note on page 54), in which the wall of the diverticulum was described as made up of tough mucous membrane and "a layer of red, striped, longitudinal muscular fibres " (while the circular fibres were entirely wanting), we have already remarked that, in consequence of its unusual and totally different point of origin, it could not properly be included in this series.

experience, that most of the smaller sacs present all the coats, finds no proof in the literature of the subject—but also, for the cases which we have investigated, would be entirely untenable, when we consider the arrangement and origin of the fibres of the inferior constrictor through which the mucous coat protrudes.

Concerning the *etiology* and *pathogenesis* of these diverticula, we can only make hypothetical statements, since in most cases the patients are unable to give any cause for this malady so gradually and slowly developed over a period of years. Still, in some of the cases most accurately described, very credible assertions are made concerning the cause and development. And these point to a mode of origin so entirely probable, and theoretically so comprehensible, that we without hesitation may base our views upon them.

Here we may lay down the following principle of the method of origin of these diverticula, under which the various empirical causes are easily comprised : a limited region or spot on the wall of the pharynx loses its power of resistance against the pressure exercised upon it in each act of swallowing, because it has lost the support of the muscular fibres which usually sustain it, in consequence of some local influence upon the same. Now, with each act of swallowing, the morsel of food (or the fluid swallowed), compressed by the rest of the pharyngeal muscles, will press most forcibly against that spot which most readily yields ; the mucous membrane begins to bulge slightly, and, with this constant and frequently repeated act, gradually protrudes more and more, until finally a sac is formed, in which food may remain at other times than during deglutition. Then, from the weight of the masses detained in it, the sac will be distended and dragged downward ; and so, in the course of years, it is developed into one of those sacs which hang down behind the œsophagus, between it and the vertebral column, and which, when distended, must press the œsophagus forward, so that now the cavity of the diverticulum is a direct continuation of the pharynx, and thus all ingesta fall into the diverticulum, while the compressed œsophagus, whose opening into the pharynx is thrown out of the axis, receives no more food, unless, with great difficulty, by means of artificial manipulation (manual compression of the diverticulum, or the introduction of a sound).

Now, as regards the most frequent causes of the interference with the play of the muscles at this limited spot, they are, as far as we can gather them from reported cases: *imprisonment of a foreign body* or a firm morsel in the pharynx, which presses hard against the mucous membrane, and separates some of the muscular fibres, between which the mucous membrane protrudes. In one case it was a cherry-pit, which remained *in situ* for three days and then was ejected (Ludlow); in another it was a peppercorn, which remained eight days (Dendy); in a third, a piece of crust of bread or a small chicken-bone (Kuehne); all which, with certainty, were claimed to be the cause, since the symptoms were gradually developed from the time of their ingestion. Ludlow's admirably reported case seems to leave no room for doubt of the immediate connection between the two. Perhaps this is the most frequent method of their origin. Or an injury may lead to a rupture of some of the muscular fibres of the œsophagus. This surely must have been what occurred in the interesting case of Gassner (Fridberg). The patient was an officer, who was thrown from his horse during some military manœuvres, and remained unconscious for twenty-four hours. Immediately after the fall a swelling was observed between the sterno-kleido-mastoid muscle and the trachea, and as soon as he could take nourishment again he was troubled with dysphagia. While the swelling gradually disappeared the dysphagia increased, and in the course of years the diverticulum, with all its sequelæ, followed, which finally caused death by inanition. In this case we cannot doubt that the swelling which occurred immediately after the fall was not caused by the diverticulum, but was a hemorrhage and inflammation directly caused by the injury. Accordingly this case, with the probable rupture of the pharyngeal muscles—which would explain the immediate dysphagia as well as the subsequent formation of a diverticulum—naturally has a bearing upon the method of causation we are considering. We have already corrected Fridberg's anatomical mistake, in consequence of which he considered this very probable explanation as entirely inadmissible, and replaced it by an artificial hypothesis.[1]

---

[1] In *Waldenburg's* case, seen only during life (No. 34 in the preceding table), in

Finally, the muscular fibres may be destroyed by other influences of various kinds. Thus we must interpret the case in which the patient ascribed his trouble to his once having burned the pharynx by eating a piece of hot beef.

Naturally, various other possible causes might be suggested, but we wish here to introduce only such as are capable of proof.

If there is already a stenosis of the upper end of the œsophagus before the occurrence of any of these causes, it may be readily understood that this would favor the formation of a diverticulum, for not only would a foreign body in this case be more easily detained in the canal, but also, in consequence of the stasis of food caused by the stenosis, the pressure on the weak spot must be increased. The stenosis, however, can only be considered as a favoring cause, since by itself it would only give rise to a diffuse ectasia. As a fact, two cases are reported (Gianella, reported by Borsieri, and Worthington), in which there existed at the same time a stenosis at the upper part of the œsophagus. However, in these cases it may be doubted whether it was not a secondary stenosis, caused by the diverticulum, which was believed to be primary. Yet, in Gianella's case, dysphagia had existed from early youth, so that here we have reason to suspect the presence of one of those congenital stenoses alluded to above.[1]

In two cases (Marx, Rokitansky) there was at the same time a considerable enlargement and induration of the right lobe of the thyroid body, which reached round to the pharynx and œsophagus, and, as Marx says, must have compressed the pharynx. So also in Rokitansky's case, according to the patient's statement, the dysphagia came on during the period of the degeneration of the thyroid gland ; accordingly, we are warranted here in assum

which, from the accurately described symptoms, it is very probable that a pressure diverticulum existed, the patient ascribed the origin of the trouble, which had lasted eight months, to severe pressure upon the left side of her neck, which she suffered in a quarrel which led to violence. This also would seem to be of traumatic origin. In *Klose* and *Paul's* case (No. 32 of the table) a fish-bone is stated to have originated the trouble, so that an internal wound was probably the cause.

[1] *Nicoladoni's* case (see p. 48), in which the stricture certainly was primary, might also be included here, but since it is represented as not being a pure pressure diverticulum, but rather chiefly a stagnation ectasia, it were better not to include it in this category.

ing a causal connection, though perhaps not immediate. Again, in two cases (Kuehne, Buecking) the patients attributed their trouble to wearing too tight clothing about the neck, and, in fact, such a habit would seem to be well adapted to occasion delay of the morsel from the backward pressure brought upon the larynx.

It remains still to mention the assumption only hinted at by some of the older writers, but distinctly laid down by many of the more modern (Klebs, Koenig), that the greater part of these diverticula are congenital, and have only increased in size in later life. In so far as this assumption rests upon the pretended presence of a complete muscular layer, we have shown above that no such case is sufficiently authenticated. And so long as not a single case is observed in a new-born child, or even in childhood, so long must this assumption remain unverified.

A case recently related by Monti, in the person of a child a year old, under the title of "Laryngeal Stenosis caused by a Foreign Body Engaged in a Diverticulum of the Œsophagus" (Jahrbuch für Kinderheilkunde. New series. Vol. IX., p. 168. 1875), is clearly a misconception. It is a case where a foreign body (seal ring) detained in the pharynx was the source of considerable ulceration. But whether besides this there was actually a diverticulum present could not be gathered from the description, which is obscure in many respects. If there was any such, it pertained not to the œsophagus but to the pharynx, and not to the lower portion even of that. The case of Mayr, quoted by Koenig (Jahrb. d. Kinderheilk. Vol. IV. Part 3. p. 209. 1861; Schmidt's Jahrb. 113. p. 75), of a girl six years of age with a congenital fistula of the neck, in whom symptoms were observed during life very similar to those produced by large diverticula, proves nothing, since it was not established by dissection that any diverticulum existed, and the symptoms may very easily be capable of another interpretation. The improvement which took place in her condition makes it very improbable that a diverticulum was present. If it was a diverticulum, it may possibly have been a traction diverticulum (see farther on) and hardly a congenital one.[1] The small tent-like diverticulum observed by Klebs, of which the congenital nature is also not proven, certainly from its form does not belong in this category.

Accordingly we believe that all the diverticula here described

---

[1] The interesting case by *Kurz*, published while these sheets are in press (Deutsche Zeitschr. f. prakt. Med. 1877. No. 48),of a girl three years old, gives symptoms which most evidently point to a true congenital ectasia. Concerning the form of this— whether it is a diverticulum in our meaning of the word, or what seems more probable to us at first sight, a "Vormagen" or vestibule of the stomach as explained above—we cannot speak decidedly, since the child is still living.

which anatomically and clinically are alike, are acquired and developed (not congenital) formations, and in accordance with the principles laid down above, from their nature are properly described by the name pressure diverticula. If, however, in most cases no such cause has come to our knowledge, we need not wonder. Since the first disturbances, when they do not immediately leave behind them permanent disorders, quickly subside, such circumstances easily escape the mind. If the troubles only begin years after the occurrence to be seriously felt, so that the patient has to seek medical aid, the circumstance has long since been forgotten, or else the patient does not associate it with this sickness apparently just developed, and hence says nothing about it to the physician. Negative statements by less intelligent patients are of no value whatever. Moreover, in a portion of the cases the report is merely fragmentary.

The development of the pressure diverticula exclusively (or nearly so) on the posterior wall of the lowest part of the pharynx, at the boundary between the latter and the œsophagus, is easily explained on anatomical grounds. For nowhere is the muscular tissue of the pharynx so thin as in the region of the lower transverse fibres of the inferior constrictor, and nowhere does the arrangement of its fibres so favor a separation between the bundles as at this spot, where they run in parallel lines in a very thin layer transversely from one side to the other, while above they are oblique and freely interlaced, and below on the œsophagus the circular and longitudinal fibres overlie one another, and hence in both places are better adapted to resist pressure from within. On the œsophagus it is only the triangular space on the posterior wall, just below the boundary of the pharynx unprovided with longitudinal fibres, which offers less resistance. While this spot seems anatomically disposed to the formation of diverticula, it is also the spot which is most exposed to the causes likely to produce them, because just here the canal is the narrowest, and on account of its immobility from the pressure of its anterior wall against the cricoid cartilage morsels of food and foreign bodies are very easily lodged here.

A very striking fact, which appears from a comparison of the cases which certainly belong in this category (established by autopsy) is this, that of the twenty-two cases in which the sex is given, not one was a female—all were men. And of the seven cases which, from symptoms during life, probably belonged in this list, though it was not proven by autopsy, we find that five are men and two women. Such a proportion can hardly appear to be a matter of chance. It is not easy to state with accuracy the causes for this immunity of the female sex. The larynx is smaller than in man; is later in undergoing ossification, and hence is more yielding; perhaps the freedom of the neck in opposition to the stiff and tight dressing of the neck in men, so imperative particularly in earlier days, ought also to be considered. In the two single cases of women the cause was alleged to be, in one, an actual injury (violent pressure upon the throat), and in the other, a fish-bone which stuck in the gullet (probably also a wound within the tube), from both which the above mentioned peculiarities of the sex would give them no immunity. Accordingly, these apparent exceptions would only prove the rule.

We learn further, that of nineteen cases in which the age of the patient is given, seventeen died after fifty years of age, and of these fourteen after sixty. There died:

Between the 40th and 50th years............ 2
   " 50th " 60th " 3
   " 60th " 70th " 8
   " 70th " 80th " 5
     In the 80th year............ 1

From this we cannot draw the conclusion that the trouble only comes on in old age, for it is usually a slow, tedious affair, and in a number of cases is reported to have lasted from twenty to thirty years, and in one case even forty-nine years. Accordingly we see that the duration of life is not seriously affected by this severe disorder—a fact which deserves consideration when in a new case the question arises whether the operative procedure, which certainly is practicable but not free from danger, should be undertaken for the relief of the patient.

A further analysis, however, of ten cases in which the date of commencement of the trouble was accurately known or could be very nearly approximated, shows that in eight out of the ten it originated after forty years of age. The first symptoms appeared:

In the 17th year............ 1
" 35th " 1
Between the 40th and 50th years............ 3
" " 50th " 60th " 4
In the 66th year............ 1

It is therefore distinctly a disease of later life. The case in which the dysphagia began in the seventeenth year (Rokitansky's case, with a duration of forty-nine years) is, as we have suggested, capable of another explanation, since the earlier disturbances may with great probability be referred to the struma which was then forming, so that the diverticulum was only afterward superadded. We have already suggested that in Gianella's case the dysphagia, from earliest childhood, should be referred not to the diverticulum, but to the probably congenital stenosis. But the patient who acquired the trouble in the thirty-fifth year was the Gassner-Fridberg case, and this arose from an injury. If, therefore, a disposition to this trouble increases after the fortieth year, the question naturally arises whether it is not the ossification of the larynx which is the weightiest factor in its production, since this change begins between the fortieth and fiftieth year in men, and much later, and in general much more rarely in women.[1]

It is evident also from these facts that there is no foundation left for the theory of a congenital origin for diverticula.

As regards the subsequent increase of the trouble and the symptoms occasioned thereby, we have given an outline of the former above. So soon as the bulging mucous membrane, at first only a shallow depression within, has enlarged to the shape of a sac, the ingesta entering with every act of swallowing will necessarily be longer and longer detained, since the sac, unprovided with any muscular layer, cannot eject them, and hence by their continuous presence and pressure they will gradually enlarge it. If this wall were provided with a muscular layer no such danger would exist, as is proven by the true intestinal diverticula (remains of the unobliterated *vitelline duct*) so frequently seen,

---

[1] See *Henle's* Handbook of Systematic Anatomy. Vol. II., p. 230. 1862.

which doubtless are congenital and possess a complete muscular coat ; in them the subsequent formation of a sac-shaped diverticulum is never seen. The distention requisite to form the large sacs always takes place slowly, and after many years of gradual increase.

While at the commencement of the formation of the diverticulum, often no difficulties in swallowing, or very slight ones, and then but little characteristic, are observed, which may lead us to suspect a slight stenosis ; the more severe symptoms commence with increasing violence and in a more characteristic form, when the sac has assumed such a size and position that, when full, must cause it to compress the œsophagus. Now the diverticulum is quickly filled up at the beginning of each meal, and by the compression exercised, entirely prevents the entrance of food into the œsophagus. The food subsequenly introduced, which can find no escape downward, and is detained in the pharynx, will soon be thrown out again. The ingesta which have fallen into the diverticulum may remain there one or many hours (perhaps even for days, case of Collomb), when, apparently involuntarily in part (probably by compression of the sac laterally by the contraction of the muscles of the neck), and partly by pressure with the hand upon the neck, they are again brought up into the mouth, sometimes entirely unchanged and sometimes only softened and mixed with mucus. Then they are either ejected from the mouth, or the patient attempts to swallow them again, so that in many cases there is actual rumination. This symptom is most characteristic, although, as we saw, it occurs also in diffuse dilatations. Often there is actual vomiting also. Only by painful efforts do they sometimes succeed in introducing small portions of food into the stomach. Finally, nothing will go down, and life is only sustained by the use of a sound, which sometimes fails, or by nutritive enemata. The patients die with most profound marasmus and constantly increasing emaciation, unless some intercurrent disease comes to put an end to their sufferings.

Of the twenty-seven cases proven by autopsy, in thirteen the patients died in consequence of the diverticulum, in eight of other diseases. In six cases nothing is said of the mode of their death.

The objective signs in these later stages of the disease are a diffuse or circumscribed tumor of the neck in the œsophageal region, which is perceptible by inspection and palpation, and is sometimes unilateral, sometimes bilateral. By pressure upon this swelling we can force the food which has been taken, up into the mouth again, and the swelling collapses. When the sound is introduced it enters at once into the diverticulum, and meets an impassable barrier, which may cause us to suspect the existence of a stenosis unless we are able to move the end of the sound freely in the sac (Gassner-Fridberg). It is only by very skilful manipulation that we sometimes succeed in passing by the opening and carrying the instrument down to the stomach. And it is just this varying success or failure in introducing the sound, when successful meeting no obstacle whatever (Ch. Bell and Prof. Wintrich, statement in our case), which will guide us to the true diagnosis. In the Gassner-Fridberg case the patient himself had learned to introduce the sound, and through it to carry nourishment to the stomach, until finally he could no longer pass the obstacle, when, tired of life, he made no further attempt to introduce nourishment, and died of inanition.

The irritation set up by the ingesta detained in the sac brings on a chronic catarrhal condition of the mucous membrane, with abundant secretion of mucus ; as a result of which the mucous membrane in the larger diverticula is almost always greatly thickened, sometimes with a smooth inner surface and sometimes granular, in consequence of considerable papillary growth and development, as we found it in two cases. No other changes are found in the mucous membrane ; and particularly no ulcerations or perforations of the wall, with their sequelæ, have been observed in any of these cases. (The softened spots in the case of Veit-Berg certainly must be considered *post-mortem* changes.)

Hard foreign bodies which fall into the diverticulum may easily remain there a long time. Thus in Foerster's case several pieces of buckshot were found in the sac, which had become smooth by attrition ; in the case of Veit-Berg a piece of coarse corn was found, and in our case a little piece of slate, somewhat larger than a kreuzer. In Ludlow's case the sac contained a great quantity of quicksilver, which the patient had been caused to swallow fourteen days before his death.

Traction Diverticula.

The traction diverticula are, as we have already said, in every respect quite different formations from the pressure diverticula, and only resemble them in being also protrusions of mucous membrane.

Compared with the great rarity of pressure diverticula, the traction diverticula, as we can state from our own extensive experience, are of very frequent occurrence. It is only in consequence of the little attention paid to the œsophagus at autopsies that we are able to explain the fact that they have been so rarely observed; and although, in most of the cases, they have been entirely latent, without occasioning any disturbances whatever, so that they are only discovered by chance, *post-mortem*, yet their existence is a source of great danger to the individual. For the cases are not very rare in which, by their perforation, they formed the nucleus for a variety of severe and ultimately fatal symptoms, which first found a satisfactory and generally unsuspected explanation, at the autopsy, by the discovery of a diverticulum. Hence, considering their frequency, they have a much more practical significance than the pressure diverticula, which certainly offer a richer field for speculation, and from their strange nature form a very striking disorder, but yet must be classed in the cabinet of rarities, and are also less dangerous to life.

Traction diverticula of the œsophagus were first described and properly recognized, from their nature and mode of formation, by Rokitansky, based originally on one case only (Oesterreich. Jahrbuch. 1840. p. 230. Case 4. Handbuch der Patholog. Anat. Vol. III. p. 160. 1842). But already, in an Erlangen dissertation, written under Dittrich's instructions, but which had lain unnoticed (Greiner, Diseases of the Bronchial Glands. 1851) it is stated that, in Dittrich's experience, these diverticula are very frequently found. Heschl also (loc. cit. 1855) describes them as not very rare. Later, Rokitansky, in the new edition of his work (Lehrbuch, Vol. III. 1861. p. 127), while mentioning the frequency of their occurrence, clearly sketches the whole pathology in a few brief, sharp, and striking lines (referring particularly to a recent very marked and fatal case. Ibid. p. 38). Based on these statements, ever since that time the manuals of clinical medicine and pathological anatomy refer to the traction exercised by bronchial glands, while contracting, as a special cause of the formation of diverticula of the œsophagus. But this statement always appears in one single form, which shows that the authors are not acquainted with these diverticula from their own observation, and consider them as a rare occurrence. More recently Klebs (Manual of Pathological Anat. 1st Part. 1868. p. 163) has laid down his teaching in a form which resembles a theory carefully excogitated at his desk, but to which only a conditional authenticity should be allowed. Openly resting for a basis on this representation, one of the most recent clinical handbooks speaks in these words: such "protrusions might arise by traction from without." Such a doubtful endorsement of the correctness of the observation certainly is not warranted in the presence of these reported cases. Conscientious reports of well-marked cases are very scarce. We would refer to two cases briefly related by W. Mueller (Jen. Zeitschrift für Med. u. Naturw. Vol. IV. 1868. p. 164), and one described and pictured by Fridberg, in his dissertation (Giessen, 1867), of which the preparation is in the museum at Giessen. Two cases from the Institute of Pathological Anatomy at Erlangen, which we ourselves observed, were very opportunely published at the same time (Deutsch. Archiv f. klin. Med. Vol. V. pp. 18 and 255). Thus it is seen that the doctrine has not made any progress since the first reports, and generally has not received the recognition it merited. This recognition we hope to enforce by the following presentation of the subject. As it is now many years since we first turned our attention to the subject, we are able to support our views by more than sixty cases, which we ourselves (Zenker) have seen and investigated, and of them we have the records of fifty-four lying before us. Rokitansky's statements are verified on all sides by these reports, and enlarged in several directions. Fifteen more cases were reported briefly in Tiedemann's Dissertation at Kiel, alluded to above. This dissertation was written under the observation of Prof. Heller, who, as former assistant at the Erlangen Institute of Pathological Anatomy, had learned to recognize and appreciate the condition. These observations are, therefore, incorporated directly with our own.

The location of traction diverticula is exclusively on the œsophagus, and up to this time no such case has been observed affecting the pharynx. They are always found on the anterior wall, and in the greatest number of cases at a point corresponding to the bifurcation of the trachea, or else close by, above or below it; sometimes in the median line and sometimes laterally, directed towards one or the other of the bronchi. Yet they do occur also, though much less frequently, higher up and lower down.

Usually only one sac is found. Yet there are cases in which

two and even three were found, either close together or remote, and this not very rarely.

Of fifty-four cases, in forty there was one only; in eleven, there were two; and in three, there were found three diverticula.

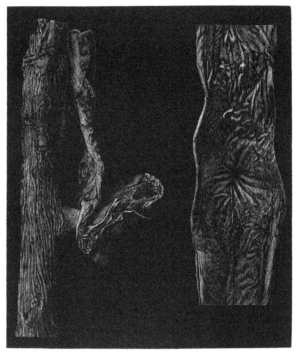

Fig. 5.—Traction diverticulum of the œso-phagus. Side view: the apex held fast to the bifurcation of the trachea by contracted glands. Taken from a photograph.

Fig. 6.—Inner view of another traction diver-ticulum of the œsophagus, in order to show the opening.

Their shape, with rare exceptions, is that of a narrow or some-what wider funnel of only moderate depth. Most frequently we found them from two to eight millimetres deep; yet in a few cases they attain a depth of nine to twelve millimetres. Larger diverticula than this certainly are very rare exceptions.[1] Their opening is sometimes narrow, sometimes wider, with a diameter of from six to eight millimetres. The apex of the funnel looks sometimes directly forward or laterally, and sometimes up or down, and is held fast by indurated tissue, usually to the bifurcation of the trachea, or to one bronchus, and more rarely to the root of the lung, and is imbedded in this cicatricial tissue without any sharp boundary-line between them. In exceptional cases they have the shape of a more or less shallow fossa, whose flat base is held over a considerable extent fastened to the limiting induration ; or else they are like a pouch, shaped like a half-moon, with a slit-like opening, or entrance. We saw one of this latter form situated in the upper part of the œsophagus, and here the cul-de-sac was tied to a remote bronchial gland, which was contracted, by only a single, thin, but tense and firm cord of connective tissue, so that pulling the gland brought traction on the diverticulum as well.

The wall of the diverticulum is made up either entirely of mucous membrane alone, or with the muscular layer superadded, which also has been dragged forward. The mucous membrane is sometimes laid in plaits or folds in the diverticulum, but is otherwise generally normal. But in many cases it has, particularly at the bottom of the funnel, a distinctly cicatricial appearance, and frequently is blackish in color at that spot. Not infrequently we find in the diverticulum, or at its mouth, a little bridge of mucous membrane, which would seem to be the remains of a cicatrized ulcer which had undermined the membrane. The relation of the muscular layer to the diverticulum is various. In many cases it is as Rokitansky described it ; the mucous membrane, protruding between muscular fibres, has no muscular covering whatever. In one case we found the mucous membrane, which protruded between the separated longitudinal fibres, crossed by a few fine fibres from the circular muscle. In other cases, and, it would appear, in a majority indeed, the muscular layer, as Tiedemann rightly describes it, is drawn out together with the mucous membrane. In such cases

---

[1] The traction diverticulum in the Giessen collection, described by *Fridberg*, is stated to be one and a half inches (?) long.

we can distinctly see the longitudinal fibres, which are stretched and drawn out of their course, continuing at an angle down on to the diverticulum, and either losing themselves in the cicatricial tissue at the apex, with which they are fused, or else bending at an acute angle over the apex, and returning to their course down the œsophagus. And yet, with this arrangement, it sometimes happens that at the apex of the diverticulum the mucous membrane protrudes uncovered at some gap in the muscular wall. These differences may be easily explained by unimportant variations in the course of the disease, and by the various ways in which the adhesion takes place between the œsophagus and the contracting cicatricial tissue. Accordingly, it would be quite incorrect on pure anatomical grounds to make a distinction between such as are and such as are not provided with a muscular layer, since in their mode of formation they are identical. The most important matter, in order to comprehend these diverticula, is the *condition of the neighboring parts which bound it.* In this respect, we see in the most unequivocal manner that a firm and distinctly contracted tissue lies directly against the apex of the diverticulum, and is more or less firmly adherent to it, indeed entirely surrounds it, or reaches out to it only with its radiating prolongations or bands. In by far the greatest number of cases we find circumscribed, firm, black nodules, which, lying against the bronchi or trachea, more frequently at the bifurcation, from their position, form and coloring, are recognized as shrunken bronchial glands, and they not unfrequently enclose calcareous deposits, or sometimes a decaying black mass. The surrounding connective tissue is generally distinctly drawn towards it in lines, radiating from it as a centre. Frequently these nodules are so contracted that it is only by their black pigmentation that they can be recognized as the remains of bronchial glands. Sometimes the contracted gland, and the surrounding connective tissue, also contracted, and occasionally other swollen glands, are involved in one diffused cicatricial mass of considerable extent.

In some cases, but rarely, we fail to find any evidence of antecedent contraction of bronchial glands, but instead we find radiating cicatricial fibres of connective tissue, whose extensive connection with the diverticulum is equally clear, and which must be considered as the remains of a chronic mediastinitis originating in some way unknown, and resulting in induration.

Finally, we certainly have observed single cases in which no contracted tissue could be found on the periphery of the diverticulum, while the condition and appearance of the latter, as regards its location, form, etc., caused us to consider it a traction diverticulum. We will not deny that possibly another explanation might be offered for one or the other of these cases, and that possibly it is wrong to include them here. But since it is well known that very distinct cicatrices may vanish entirely after a number of years, and since many of these diverticula have surely been in existence for several decades before being observed postmortem, it is certainly not unfair to assume in these cases that a less distinct cicatrix has in time totally disappeared.[1]

The pathogenesis of traction-diverticula is easily gathered from the above anatomical description. The starting-point is an inflammatory swelling of the parts immediately adjoining the œsophagus, which leads to a firm adhesion between this inflamed region and a limited portion of the wall of the œsophagus. If cicatricial induration and contraction follow in these inflamed regions, since they are also adherent to less yielding structures (particularly the wall of a bronchus), they must draw that portion of the œsophageal wall outward. This method of origin in the great proportion of cases is so evident from the anatomical appearances, that in the presence of such preparations there can be no dispute about it. Experience tells us that it is disease of the tracheal and bronchial glands, especially those at the bifurcation, which is the most frequent cause of such inflammation; and it is the dense accumulation of these glands at the bifurcation, which makes the corresponding portion of the œsophagus the seat of election for the formation of these diverticula.

It may be a simple inflammatory swelling of these glands, or suppuration, or cheesy degeneration and subsequent softening,

---

[1] This explanation seems the most probable also for the case observed by *Klebs*, which he considered a small tent-like diverticulum, of congenital origin, and which was connected with the trachea at the bifurcation by a firm band, but near which no contracted gland could be found.

which, through the periadenitis they excite, cause adhesion to the wall of the œsophagus, and then, when they contract, produce the diverticulum. The original nature of the process cannot always be accurately determined from an observation of the completely formed cicatrix.

The method of union of the gland with the œsophageal wall is various, and accordingly will be accompanied by varying appearances in the diverticulum. Either the gland is adherent only to the outer surface of the muscular layer, or the periadenitic thickening penetrates into the muscular layer; in both cases the contraction will first pull the muscular layer outward and the mucous membrane will follow; or else the condensation may have extended through the muscle down to the mucous membrane, when both coats will be drawn out together. In all these cases the diverticulum is made up of the mucous and muscular layers. Or it may be that the gland is glued fast immediately to the mucous membrane through a gap in the muscular fibres, and this we can explain by supposing that a periadenitic suppuration has destroyed a portion of the muscular fibres and pressed forward down to the mucous membrane.

Certainly in many such cases, during the early period of the disease, we have the abscess breaking into the œsophagus. If contraction of the remaining glandular tissue follows quickly upon the escape of pus, the opening of perforation will soon be closed, and the mucous membrane will be drawn out through the opening in the muscular fibres; we shall then have a funnel of mucous membrane without any muscular covering, which, from the continuous contraction, will be drawn out more and more, and may also press aside the neighboring muscular fibres.[1] Thus we can best explain the diverticula in which the mucous membrane, particularly at the deepest part, is cicatrized, and which appear black from the black substance of the gland glued fast to them at that point.

In an analogous way the cause of a diverticulum is more rarely found to lie in contracting bands of connective tissue,

---

[1] Preparation No. IV. in *Tiedemann's* dissertation shows a case in process of formation.

which are attached to a limited spot on the œsophageal wall. Although this chronic mediastinitis in most cases is associated with disease of the glands, yet it may occur independently, *e. g.*, as an accompaniment of pleuritis or of caries of the vertebræ,[1] and as such deserves special mention.

The remote causes of the disease which produces the trouble are not, in most cases, to be found. A priori, it is probable in many cases that it is scrofulous in its nature from the simultaneous affection of the lymphatic glands, and in some cases it has been proven.

See Preparation No. IV. in Tiedemann, and one case which we observed in a child one and a half years old, who died of caseous pneumonia.

This fact also supports the same view, viz., that in adults the largest contingent of cases of diverticula has been furnished by those who died of phthisis and those affected with caries. Another cause, which not unfrequently seems to give rise to the formation of traction diverticula is the inhalation of gritty particles in the air (Chalicosis). We, as well as Heller, found diverticula repeatedly in cases which showed the characteristic changes of chalicosis in the lungs. The most beautiful as well as the clearest case of the kind was that published by Immermann,[2] observed in the polyclinic at Erlangen, in which, among other pathological conditions resulting from contraction at the root of the lung and in the mediastinum (stricture of branches of the pulmonary artery, traction diverticulum of the right bronchus), we found also a most beautiful traction diverticulum of the œsophagus, and a subsequent chemical examination of the lungs verified our suspicion at the autopsy that the trouble originated from chalicosis.

As regards the period of life when traction diverticula are formed, the well-known frequency of affections of the bronchial glands in childhood made us suspect that they were often developed at this time. Experience confirms our view, for both we and Heller (Tiedemann) found diverticula existing already in childhood.

---

[1] In one case a traction diverticulum was found associated with caries of the dorsal vertebræ, and in two cases with caries of the lumbar vertebræ and psoas abscess.

[2] Deutsch Archiv für klin. Med. Vol. V. 1869. p. 235.

We have seen them in children of one and a half, six, and eleven years of age; Heller in children of three and eight years.

We met with six cases occurring between puberty and the thirtieth year. All other cases (forty-three in number) were found between the thirtieth and eighty-sixth years of age, which tells us nothing, however, concerning the period at which they were formed, but only shows that in most cases they do not interfere with life or health. From the method of their formation we should suppose that sex would have little influence as a predisposing cause. In fact, we found that of 54 cases, 29 occurred in men, and 25 in women.

Now, as regards the subsequent history of these diverticula and their pathological significance, it would appear that, after the cicatricial contraction of the connective tissue is over, and the diverticulum is formed, it ordinarily remains stationary. Its depth is entirely dependent upon the amount of contraction. It has no tendency whatever to enlargement, which is so marked in the subsequent history of pressure diverticula. The small quantities of food and drink which enter it in the act of swallowing are not calculated by their weight to cause any enlargement in the sac, the less so because the sac is directed more frequently upward or horizontally, and directly forward, than downward. The fact also that it is frequently imbedded in indurated tissue, and has a firm wall when the muscular layer is involved, would be unfavorable to any further enlargement. So they never form those extensive sacs which could cause pressure by their size, and give rise to further disturbances.[1] And since they do not seem calculated to produce any dysphagia, and in our experience do not produce any, we might suppose that no pathological significance worth speaking of could be attached to formations of so little importance as harmless cicatrices. But there is a danger underlying them, which, pregnant with many further dangers, makes them worthy of the most earnest attention of pathologists,

---

[1] The statement by *Rokitansky*, that "these diverticula may by extensive enlargement become imbedded in the lung," we can only explain as follows, viz., that by an unusual and relatively considerable development induced by great shrinkage of surrounding parts, they may extend to the lung, and perhaps also between the bronchial glands at the root of the lung.

and that is, as we have said at the outset, the not unfrequent occurrence of perforation of the apex. Usually we cannot, by direct observation, tell what leads to this perforation; *a priori* we might suppose it could take place from within outward, or the reverse, from without inward. And both forms may occur, but the former must be the more frequent manner. At least one cannot clearly see what should give rise to ulceration or necrosis in these masses of indurated tissue which bound them, which are so indolent in character, and so little prone to inflammatory processes, unless it be some source of irritation from the cavity acting upon the mucous membrane. That this latter may lead to ulcerative destruction, and so to perforation, is not only clear *a priori*, but is proved from experience by the important case of Rokitansky, who first exposed to us the deleterious results of these diverticula.[1] In this case it was a small, flat piece of bone with sharp angles, which was found caught in the opening of the diverticulum, and had led to perforation and extensive suppuration.[2] In analogous cases observed by us we did not succeed in finding any foreign body. Besides pieces of bone, it may be fruit-pits or other hard substances, which, imprisoned in the diverticulum, set up the same trouble, but after they have been discharged through the perforation may easily escape observation. But soft portions of food also may remain in the diverticulum, undergo putrefaction, and become a source of inflammation and ulceration.

When the inflammation, thus established, has led to ulcerative destruction of the apex of the diverticulum, it spreads first into the adjacent induration, glued fast to it, *i. e.*, generally into the shrunken bronchial glands. Then, as we have often observed, a fine sound will pass through the apex of the sac, into a cavity just in the region of the bronchial glands, encapsulated, and

---

[1] Lehrbuch d. patholog. Anatom. Vol. III. 1861. p. 38.

[2] A case reported by *Coester* (Berlin. klin. Wochenschr. 1870. No. 43), of perforation of the œsophagus and of the vena cava by a piece of bone, perhaps also belongs here, since he states that "the piece of bone was caught in a protrusion of the mucous membrane of the œsophagus, like a diverticulum;" but, as the diverticulum is not particularly described, we cannot be sure about it. Perhaps he refers only to a bulging or protrusion caused simply by the bone itself. Its unusually deep situation (one and a half inches above the diaphragm) would be in favor of the latter view.

filled with a black, crumbling and pap-like mass, which, by pressure, can be made to flow back into the diverticulum. This state of things we found by chance in a patient who had died of another disease, and had given no evidence during life of any such condition. Accordingly, it would appear that in this stage also it may be entirely latent. But sooner or later the cavity, which freely receives air and soft food undergoing fermentation, will become ichorous, and now the process extends beyond the region of the bronchial glands into the mediastinal connective tissue, and an irregular, sinuous and ichorous cavity is formed, which, creeping along through the whole breadth of the mediastinal space, attains considerable dimensions, and contains, besides ichorous pus, black fragments (remains of bronchial glands) either lying free or attached to the wall, and also calcareous particles from the same source. For some time, even such ichorous cavities as these may exist without producing severe symptoms, but now the process extends on all sides in the direction of organs most important to life, viz., bronchi, pleura, lungs, pericardium, pulmonary artery, and aorta—all of these may be involved, and into any of them it may break; and thus the most various and severe diseases are set up, apparently spontaneously, which lead to death—sometimes slowly, sometimes more rapidly, and sometimes instantaneously—and are only explained at the autopsy, and perhaps not even then, if the œsophagus, as frequently happens, is not thought worthy of investigation.

From our experience, these subsequent diseases with a fatal issue are usually as follows in frequency : the most frequent occurrence is *perforation into one of the bronchi*, and as the ichorous cavity is just at the bifurcation, *often into both* of the main bronchial tubes. On opening these near the bifurcation, we find the wall perforated by one or more apertures usually the size of a pin's head, but sometimes larger, through which, by pressure on the surrounding tissues, blackish ichorous pus will be seen to exude into the lumen of the bronchus, and now by means of the ichorous cavity a fistulous communication is established between the œsophagus and bronchus, which, on account of its irregular course, cannot always be easily found with the sound.

Around the orifice of the perforation, and extending beyond it, we find the bronchial mucous membrane most intensely reddened and quite spongy; nowhere have we seen it so beautifully granulated as at such spots (granular bronchitis). It may be that the force of the inflammation will now be spent on the bronchitis, without involving the lung, and we cannot deny that possibly restoration may yet occur. Perforations of the bronchial wall which have been closed by cicatrization are frequently found; but usually these are direct perforations by softening of bronchial glands, without any communication with the œsophagus, which latter materially enhances the danger.

But, further, the ichorous matter in the bronchial tube may be drawn into the lung, and the portion of lung supplied by that bronchus will become the seat of gangrene, from contact with the foul products, and the end will be fatal.

A woman, sixty-six years of age (Erlangen, October, 1864), died of a very obscure disease, which did not admit of accurate diagnosis. The autopsy showed the cause of death to be a very extensive double gangrenous pneumonia, and a slight (right) ichorous pleuritis. In the right bronchus were found numerous perforations extending from an ichorous region in the mediastinum, into which, on the opposite side, opened a funnel-shaped diverticulum of the œsophagus, situated at the level of the bifurcation of the trachea.

When caverns already exist in the lung, fistulous communication may be formed between them and the perforated diverticulum, and particles of food entering from the œsophagus, and undergoing putrefaction, may set up gangrenous destruction.

Heller observed a very wonderful case of this kind (Case XIII. in Tiedemann's dissertation): a man, seventy years old, had bronchiectatic caverns in the apices of both lungs, of which one communicated directly by a fistulous tract, and the other indirectly through a periœsophageal ichorous tract, with a perforated traction diverticulum in the œsophagus. In one of the caverns and in the suppurating area, besides fat-crystals, bacteria, etc., there were found striped muscular fibres, as an evidence that portions of food had penetrated there, and the wall of the caverns showed advanced gangrenous destruction.

Or else death follows from an *ichorous pleuritis*, set up either by the suppurating area which immediately bounds the pleura, or possibly breaks through into its cavity, or perhaps by the foul material drawn into the lung (before the lung itself becomes gangrenous).

By the first of these methods we must explain the case of Rokitansky already quoted, in which the conical diverticulum, perforated by a sharp-edged piece of bone, dipped into an ichorous accumulation, which had laid bare some of the ribs, and at the same time the pleural covering of the left lower lobe of the lung was gangrenous.

The latter method seems the most probable explanation of the following case: a laborer on the railroad, fifty-four years old, after undergoing surgical treatment for a chronic inflammation of the shoulder-joint, was transferred to the medical division, on account of symptoms of scurvy, and there was attacked with pleuritis of the right side and bronchial catarrh, from which he died (Dresden, March, 1860). The autopsy showed an extensive pleuritic exudation on the right side, which was purulent and ichorous, and greatly compressed the lung. The compressed lung was of a bad color, and had a gangrenous odor. The bronchi of the right side contained a dirty gray material. In the right main bronchus was found a beautiful granular bronchitis, spreading from a perforation the size of a pea, which led into a bulging ichorous cavity the size of a cherry, situated in the mediastinum, at the level of the bifurcation of the trachea. In the œsophagus there were found at the same level two small funnel-shaped diverticula, which communicated by perforation with the ichorous cavity. Beside this there was found a total adhesion of both layers of the pericardium, apparently quite recent.

Pericarditis also may be caused, just as is the pleuritis, by the neighboring ichorous region, sometimes with and sometimes without perforation of the pericardium—in the former case accompanied by entrance of air into the sac (*pneumopericardium*). Apparently pericarditis occurs more frequently than pleuritis, which may be explained by the nearer relations of the pericardium to the region of the bifurcation. While this pericarditis in many cases tends to death, in others restoration seems to take place. At all events, we found adhesion of the pericardial layers associated with traction diverticula, a remarkably frequent occurrence (in eighty-four cases it occurred nine times; in eight was total, and in only one partial), without in most cases finding at the autopsy any other explanation for this pericarditis.

In the case just reported, the clearly recent character of the adhesion ("apparently fresh, delicate connective tissue, with a jelly-like infiltration") would seem to indicate a causal connection of the pericarditis with the fatal sickness. In the other cases, in which the appearance of the adhesions gives no clue to their age, there is only the frequency of its occurrence simultaneously with diverticula, and the lack of any other explanation of the pericarditis, which would indicate the causal relation of the two. Yet we should not, for this reason, suppose that the pericarditis can only be caused by perforation of the diverticulum, for it might be occasioned, at the time of the formation of the diverticulum, by fresh disease of the bronchial glands, which, by their subsequent cicatrization, exercised the traction on the œsophagus. But that perforation of the diverticulum may lead to pericarditis, and to death by this means, was proved by a case which G. Merkel observed at Nuremberg, and afterwards examined post-mortem in our presence. Here, together with a diverticulum of the œsophagus perforating into the mediastinum, the cause of death was found to be an enormous fibrinous and hemorrhagic (and at the same time tuberculous) pericarditis. No perforation of the pericardial sac could be found.

As an example of pneumopericardium resulting from perforation of the œsophagus, I would cite a recently reported case by Forsyth Meigs (American Journ. of Med. Sci. 1875. See Centralbl. f. d. med. Wiss. 1875. No. 34). A man, eighteen years old, was attacked with a double pleurisy as a result of getting his feet wet (?). Four weeks later tympanitic percussion-sound and loud, gurgling râles were heard over the pericardial space. Two days later he died. At the autopsy the pericardium was found distended with gas, containing also a reddish brown fluid and clots; was thickened, rough, and shaggy. In the œsophagus, one quarter of an inch below the bifurcation of the trachea, was found a hole half an inch in diameter, with irregular, ulcerated margins, which led directly into the pericardium. Dr. Meigs thinks that the rupture took place from the pericardium into the œsophagus. The reverse, however, is far more probable. Certainly, from the report, we cannot say that the case surely was one of perforated diverticulum, but it is quite possible that the protrusion was overlooked, for when the surrounding disturbance is extensive, it may become indistinct.

Finally, the immediate vicinity of the large blood-vessels is a further source of danger to life. Death may instantly carry off individuals who were apparently in perfect health, by perforation of the arterial trunks (the pulmonary artery as well as the aorta) which have been undermined and corroded by the ichorous condition of the adjoining parts.

We can quote authentic cases of perforation of the aorta and also of the pulmonary artery arising from a diverticulum. Perforation of the aorta, and of the bronchus as well, was observed by G. Merkel, as I learn from his own lips. I saw a sudden death from perforation of the pulmonary artery in a case which was very interesting from many points of view (Erlangen, March, 1871). A servant, seventy years of age, who, in his latter days, busied himself about the railway station, but who for several days had raised a little blood, suddenly fell fainting, with a severe hemorrhage, recovered himself again, but died at one o'clock at night. We found a perforated traction diverticulum of the œsophagus, which led into an ichorous cavity in the mediastinum; this had undermined and corroded the left pulmonary artery for a considerable distance, which was perforated by a rent one and a half centimetres long into the mediastinal cavity. Both pulmonary branches were narrowed at the root of the lung. The stomach was distended by an enormous blood-clot. In this case also there was total obliteration of the pericardial sac.

Thus we see how health and life are surrounded by most serious dangers in individuals who are the subjects of these insignificant formations, and from the outset the occurrences which call forth this danger are not less insignificant. Accordingly, one will be well repaid by an attempt to bring to light and make accessible these insidious enemies of diagnosis hidden away in a corner. But, alas ! thus far there is but little prospect of it. The depth at which they are usually situated makes them inaccessible by œsophagoscopy. An investigation with a sound, preferably a fine one (and the greatest precaution is urged in their use, especially in these diverticula), will best give us information, and perhaps render a pretty accurate diagnosis possible, but certainly only in those cases in which the cavity of the diverticulum is directed downward. When it is directed horizontally or upward, the sound will pass by unimpeded.

Thus far we cannot expect to get much help for our diagnosis from indirect symptoms. No dysphagia has been observed to arise from the existence of the diverticulum *per se*. In none of our cases was anything known of such difficulty, and dysphagia is not even a probable symptom, since the passage of food and drink cannot be impeded by the presence of the diverticulum—indeed, can scarcely be made painful. At most it is possible that large, firm morsels, pieces of meat, or the like, may by chance become caught in the diverticulum. These, however, will usually soon pass down. And it is only in swallowing firm bodies that there is danger lest they be caught in or puncture the diverticulum. Yet it is possible that the awakened attention, when once the interest of the practitioner in this condition has been aroused, may discover many apparently insignificant symptoms which will be of value in diagnosis. A frequent detention of

food at a fixed spot, pretty .ow down, particularly the slight
delay of granular food, like barley or rice (to which Tiedemann
calls attention), when we can exclude the existence of stenosis,
should be held to be suspicious, although such symptoms may
have several explanations.

When the sequelæ already described (upon the symptomatology and diagnosis of which this is not the place to speak) have
come on apparently without any external cause, the observing
and cautious physician, familiar with the facts here laid down,
will consider this possibility, even though a sure diagnosis can
scarcely ever be made, and when the autopsy clears up the
nature of the disorder, which remained so obscure during life,
he will perhaps not fail to investigate the condition of the all-
important region. As regards the perforation of the ichorous
region into the bronchus, which, as we saw, sometimes accompanies and sometimes actually produces the more severe symptoms, a somewhat sudden expectoration of sputa of an intense
black color will be a very suspicious sign, since the ichorous
fluid is always intensely black from the coloring matter of the
necrosed and crumbling bronchial glands.

As regards *treatment*, there naturally can be none directed
towards the removal of the diverticulum, or closure of its cavity,
even if we succeeded in diagnosticating its presence. The hopeless attempt to close the diverticulum by the employment of irritants, as was actually proposed for pressure diverticula (Dendy),
might here be followed by the most disastrous results, by assisting the perforation. Accordingly, our only resource would be
by prophylaxis to avoid the approach of danger, to make it a
matter of duty with the patient to use the greatest caution in
eating and drinking, carefully to avoid swallowing hard substances, and mostly to subsist on soft food or fluid nourishment.
It might be well also to recommend to the patient to drink
immediately after his meal, in order to wash out any remains of
food from the diverticulum.

When the secondary affections have appeared, it would
scarcely be possible to vary the treatment appropriate to each
disease, in consequence of a knowledge of the underlying cause,
and hence we ought to succeed, early in the disease, before the

ichorous region is greatly extended, in introducing antiseptic substances through the œsophagus, which of itself would not be impossible. These are only suggestions and hints, but yet they do not seem superfluous. By following them, we may in time perhaps succeed in making the demon of disease fight for another inch of his domain.

Symptoms, Diagnosis, and Termination.

a. Simple diffuse ectasiæ, without stenosis of the œsophagus, whether they arise from chronic inflammation, from an injury, or from nerve-paralysis, cause so great an obstruction to the regular ingestion of food that, as we learn from the above reported observations of these rare cases, they must give rise to the most severe dysphagia, vomiting, regurgitation of the greater part of the ingesta, pain, a sense of constriction in the chest, and labored respiration. The intensity and constancy of these symptoms will depend upon the size and distention of the ectasia, and not less on the condition of the muscular coat of the œsophagus.

Slight partial dilatations of the œsophagus when the muscular coat is in good condition, frequently enough will not be recognized during life, or will only cause a slight trouble while eating, easily removed by drinking, and of this neither the patient nor those about him will be conscious, nor will it be brought to the attention of his physician. In ectasiæ of medium size, from the mild character of the symptoms, the diagnosis cannot go beyond the region of the possible, or, at most, the probable. But even the more serious disturbances in ectasiæ of large size will hardly authorize a precise diagnosis ; it will only be a probable diagnosis, arrived at by exclusion. If we can recognize the absence of stenosis, or any other obstruction in the œsophagus, that would be in support of the existence of a simple diffuse ectasia, yet the absence of any obstruction to the passage of the sound should be established as a constant condition by repeated examinations, in order to avoid mistaking it for a diverticulum, in which it sometimes happens that the sound will several times in succession pass freely by the opening of the sac without hinderance. Moreover, in using the sound, the abnormal readiness with which the tip will be found to enter the ectasia, and to be freely moved about when there, is not unimportant.

As regards the auscultatory phenomena and their aid in diagnosis, we must wait for further observations. *A priori* it is not improbable that a change in the acoustic phenomena may accompany a change in the calibre of the tube during the act of swallowing, but the statements of Hamburger are not calculated to awaken in us confidence in the accuracy of his observations.

"Relaxations of lesser grade," says Hamburger (loc. cit. p. 182), "are recognized from the fact that the bolus is perceived to be not contracted, but enlarged at its lower end, so that, instead of the inverted egg shape, it assumes a shape like a funnel. If the loss of muscular activity increases, then the bolus no longer has this form, but gives one the impresson as if a long, thin cord were passing through the œsophagus. The diameter of this cord depends upon the condition of the upper third of the œsophagus. If this is in a healthy condition, then it seems to be a moderately thick cord, which is driven pretty rapidly through the lower diseased portion. But if the muscular energy in the upper third is also diminished, then we seem to hear a threadlike cord slowly running through. In limited dilatations, particularly when circular, we hear distinctly how the bolus is driven into the cavity of the ectasia by removal of all muscular opposition, as rain is driven by the wind, so that we are in a position, by our ear, to recognize the depth and breadth of the ectasiæ in all their dimensions."

How, in single cases of diffuse ectasia, the symptoms of dilatation may entirely disappear, to return again with their original or even increased intensity, can only be explained by supposing that the force of the muscular tissue of the œsophagus, which has suffered from one or several of the above-mentioned injurious influences, *e. g.*, acute or chronic inflammation, can, for a long time, be completely restored. Return of the old or new noxious influences will sooner or later cause renewal of the trouble, which finally destroys the power of the muscular tissue of the œsophagus. These occurrences are analogous to the fluctuations so frequently observed in functional disturbances of the heart, intestine, and bladder.

The enormous œsophageal ectasia which Davy observed in a farmer thirty-eight years of age, and which, as it appeared, arose from lifting a heavy weight, did not cause death until ten years later. At first he had pain in the course of the œsophagus, vomiting of food, mucus, etc., then an improvement took place, and *for five years the patient was entirely free from all disturbances.* But then they returned with violence, and death followed from inanition in consequence of obstruction to the introduction of food. Besides the enormous ectasia (circumference at the cardia 9″, farther up, 6″), there were found numerous white spots upon the mucous membrane, which were believed to be cicatrized ulcers. The cardia would admit two fingers, and the stomach was also dilated.

b. Partial ectasiæ or diverticula, when of moderate size, may also entirely escape observation ; the reasons for this we have given in full on page 82. It is quite different, however, when the diverticula have attained such a size that portions of food and foreign bodies may be caught and concealed in them. The disturbances, though very slight at first, will soon become intense, and very often the interference with nutrition, owing to the diverticulum, will terminate ultimately in death. The disturbances are various, according to the location and size of the ectasia, as well as the condition of the mucous membrane. The leading symptom is the detention of food at a fixed spot, with regurgitation of the same sooner or later, while at other times no dysphagia, or none worth mentioning, exists. At one time the sound will strike against an impassable barrier at a given spot, through which even the finest instruments will not pass, while at another time (particularly when the sac is entirely empty) the largest sounds will pass through the affected spot without the least difficulty. The smaller the diverticulum, the narrower its mouth, and the emptier of food is the sac, the more frequently will the latter condition be found, while the former condition —*i. e.*, imprisonment of the sound in the sac—will be more constant when the sac is of large dimensions, has an opening of considerable size, and is filled with food. The large and distended diverticulum places itself in the vertical axis of the œsophagus, and pushes aside the normal walls of the œsophagus from their true direction. Under these circumstances, nine times out of ten, the sound will pass directly into the sac, and only when the same is completely emptied (a rare occurrence in large diverticula), and now hangs as a flabby appendix outside of the vertical axis, will the sound pass into the portion of the œsophagus below the entrance of the sac. The accompanying diagrammatic figures show the passage of the sound in cases of large diverticula when filled and when empty. But it is just this variation in the results of passing an instrument in the same individual, and the continuous absence of evidences of stenosis, which form the strong points in the diagnosis of a diverticulum.

Next in order come a series of important symptoms : first of all, the recognition of a *swelling in the neck*, coming on after eating, and diminishing or disappearing after vomiting or eructation ; the same may be unilateral or bilateral, beside the trachea, pushing it forward and looking like a tumor.

Pressure on the tumor, particularly by patients who have acquired skill in doing it, will partially or completely evacuate it, and a splashing or gurgling sound will be heard at the time. In such cases the patient sometimes has the power of preventing the filling of the sac at the time of eating, by making pressure upon the neck at the level of its entrance into the œsophagus.

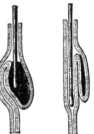

Fig. 7.—Passage of the sound when the diverticulum is full. Fig. 8.—Passage of the sound when the diverticulum is empty.

In the case observed by Betz[1] (stenosis of the œsophagus, and a diverticulum between the œsophagus and vertebral column, 6 ctms. deep, and almost the same wide), by making pressure at the base of the neck, a gurgling sound was produced which was audible all over the room. The same was produced in a less degree by swallowing also.

If the sac is large and tense, by the pressure it exercises on surrounding parts, *e. g.*, the nerves passing down the neck (the pneumogastrics, the recurrent laryngeals, the phrenics, etc.), next upon the vessels, particularly the veins, and finally upon the trachea itself, it may cause serious disturbances in innervation, in the circulation and respiration. These troubles are not wanting in diverticula which hang down into the thorax, but they are more rare in consequence of the more yielding nature of the surrounding organs. Accordingly observations are on record where pressure was exerted upon the innominate veins, the venæ cavæ, the pulmonary arteries and the auricles, the trachea, and bronchi.

---

[1] A contribution to Œsophageal Rāles. Memorabilien. 1872. No. 10.

The regurgitation of food from the sac is common to all the larger sacculated dilatations. The food is more or less changed, according to the length of time it has remained in the sac, and to the patient has either a sweetish, insipid, or foul taste. The change of starchy food into grape sugar by the action of the saliva takes place very rapidly in the sac, while the putrefaction of albuminous elements requires a longer time, and only occurs when the sac is large, or of such a shape and so situated as not to discharge its contents till some time after eating. In these cases there is a formation of sulphuretted hydrogen gas and other foul gases, which render the patient's breath fœtid.

The termination of œsophageal dilatations of large size is almost always unfavorable, though death may not occur till after years of suffering.

The dangers which these troubles induce in their subsequent course are: first, diminished introduction of food, which, since the diverticula from the constantly repeated entrance of food, and the degenerative processes in the tissues of the walls steadily increase in size, finally leads to total inanition, especially when we cannot succeed any longer in passing the sound into the stomach and thus introducing nourishment. Under such circumstances the sufferings become unendurable, and are calculated to drive the patient to suicide.

There may be also, in rare cases, a sudden termination of life by the compression of vital organs within the thorax.

Prognosis and Treatment.

From what precedes, it will be seen that the prognosis will always be very grave when the existence of an extensive diffuse or partial ektasia has been established.

In treatment, our first endeavor will naturally be to properly nourish the patient, and for this purpose the exclusive use of fluids, and the introduction of fluid nourishment through the sound when we succeed in introducing it, is indicated. It is sometimes necessary in desperate cases to leave a soft sound for many days in the stomach, when we have fortunately been successful in passing it, although the irritation caused by long retention of the sound may result in ulceration. Artificial nourishment by the rectum must also be employed at an early stage.

Electric irritation of the œsophageal muscles by the aid of an œsophageal electrode, with the object of producing a cure, is to be recommended, and promises favorable results in paralyzed conditions of the muscular tissue (see under the head of Neuroses of the Œsophagus). From the favorable results in Waldenburg's case (loc. cit.), the percutaneous introduction of the electric current directly upon the sac should be tried even in diverticula.

The radical cure of diverticula by operative procedure from without is at the present time one of our vain wishes ; yet we should hope that even this operation, conducted on Lister's plan, might at some future day be performed without danger. Nothing is to be hoped from attempts to destroy the diverticula by the introduction of astringent or irritating materials through the pharynx—at least from our experience thus far, and from consideration of the fact that we cannot, by compression or any other procedure, prevent the entrance of food, or of mucus and saliva, into the diverticulum, even for a short time.

SOLUTIONS OF CONTINUITY IN THE ŒSOPHAGUS.

RUPTURES AND PERFORATIONS.

Pathology and Etiology.

Among the solutions of continuity in the œsophageal wall through its whole thickness (and it is only such that we consider here), we are accustomed to distinguish between rents by violence and occurring suddenly, in a wall previously healthy, but arising from causes within the tube—*i. e., ruptures* (traumatic lacerations by bullet-wounds or perforating wounds are not here included)—and the more gradual piercing of the wall by morbid processes—*perforations*.

Solutions of continuity caused by swallowing foreign bodies, in so far as these foreign bodies serve to wound the wall, and not merely to destroy it by inflammation or by pressure, are best distinguished from perforations by the term *internal wounds*. These also we shall not consider here, for they belong properly in the domain of surgery, and are fully considered in surgical text-books. See particularly Koenig, loc. cit. p. 51.

1. Ruptures (including Softening).

Ruptures of the œsophagus, which take place in a healthy or relatively healthy condition in the form of a sudden catastrophe, with the most alarming symptoms, and forming the only cause of death, are certainly of rare occurrence, but yet are authenticated by a number of trustworthy observations.

The number of well-established cases—*i. e.*, those in which the symptoms during life, together with the post-mortem discoveries, distinctly prove that the rupture of the œsophagus found at the autopsy took place during life, and must be considered as the only cause of death, amount to nine. They are as follows: *Boerhaave*, Atrocis nec descripti prius morbi historia. Lugd. Batav., 1724 (Opuscula omnia. 1738. No. X. p. 98).—*Dryden*, Med. Commentaries. Edinburgh, 1788. Vol. III. p. 308.—*Oppolzer*, Wiener med. Wochenschr. 1851. p. 65.—*Habershon*, Patholog. and Practical Observ. on Diseases of the Alimentary Canal. London, 1857 (Schmidt's Jahrb. Vol. 100. p. 259). The same was previously reported by *King* and *Comley*, Guy's Hospital Reports. Apr., 1843. Schmidt's Jahrb. Supplementary Vol. No. IV. p. 275).—*Jos. Meyer* (case from Schoenlein's clinic), Pr. Ver. Zeitung. N. F. I. 39-41. 1858 (Schmidt's Jahrb. Vol. 101. p. 182).—*Gramatzki* (case from Leyden's clinic), Koenigsberger Inaugur.-Dissert. 1867.—*Griffin*, Lancet. 1869. Vol. II. p. 337. Sept. 4.—*Charles*, Dublin Quart. Journ. of Med. Sci. 1870. Vol. I. p. 311.—*Fitz*, Americ. Journ. of the Med. Sci. Jan., 1877. p. 17. (Archives Gén. April, May, 1877.)

The work last named, besides the very full report of his own case, contains an almost complete collection of all reported cases, with an excellent criticism upon them, which is only here and there a little wide of the mark. As a result of his studies, he only admits two or three of the above as belonging properly in the list. Our own view, which does not accord fully with that, we shall elaborate in what follows. Oppolzer, unfortunately, has described his case so aphoristically, that only his high authority and well known accuracy would cause us to place it here without hesitation. Other cases cited as examples of rupture of the œsophagus surely may be excluded, since in them death clearly was caused by other diseases, no symptoms during life led to a suspicion of rupture, and the rent found at the autopsy must be considered as an accidental discovery, and dependent upon antecedent softening of the œsophagus. In this class belong the cases of *Thilow*, Baldinger's neues Magazin für Aerzte. Vol. 12. 1790. p. 114. *Kade*, De morbis ventriculi. Halæ, 1798. p. 17. *Guersent*, Bulletin de la Faculté de Médecine de Paris. 1812. Vol. I. p. 73. *Bouillaud*, Archives générales. Vol. I. 1823. p. 531.

The case of Boerhaave is so wonderful in itself, and was so carefully observed and described, that it demands a complete report here as a typical example of this rare form of disease; and this all the more, since it is often quoted, but appears to be but little understood, and since Fitz, who has learned it from a very incomplete epitome, casts doubt on the accuracy of Boerhaave's explanation. One will be repaid, while laboriously studying out in dull Latin the account of the case, in which none of the least important particulars are omitted, by the clear insight he will gain into the thought and action of this great physician in this case—so astonishing, from its strange nature, to the man of large experience. We see him, with all the acuteness of his intellect, vainly endeavoring during life to discover the nature of this sickness, which burst forth with such violence; we follow him step by step at the autopsy, conducted by himself with exemplary care and the greatest attention, up to the final discovery of the underlying cause of this obscure disease, never hitherto observed.

The case was that of the great Admiral Baron Wassenaer, a man fifty years of age, and distinguished for his personal and mental characteristics in the best society of Holland, who in general enjoyed very good health, had suffered somewhat from attacks of gout in the winter, and after some of his heavy dinners (from which this otherwise very temperate man, in consequence of his social relations, could not absent himself) he had frequently been attacked with a ·disagreeable feeling in the region of the cardia. From these he got relief most readily by the use of emetics. He became accustomed to their use, and, contrary to his physician's advice, resorted to them at unseasonable times. On the day of his severe attack, in the best of health, he had eaten a good, but not a very large dinner (his bill of fare is spread out before us). In the afternoon he ate nothing further, and, apparently in perfect health, took a ride on horseback with his son. After returning, according to his custom, he ate nothing more, but, as he had this annoying feeling at the cardia, at half-past nine he took three cups of warm tea to induce vomiting, but he threw up little, and only with great difficulty. Then he drank four cups more, but did not vomit. While sitting there, trying to vomit, he suddenly uttered a terrible cry. To the attendants, who quickly hastened to him, he said that something had burst in the region of his stomach, high up, and that his pain was so unutterable that death must be near; said that the physician's aid would not avail, for he should die before the doctor could reach him. Cold sweat broke out, and he turned pale. When carried to bed, he allowed himself to be rubbed with warm cloths, etc. After half an hour he drank four ounces of sweet-oil, of which he brought up a part, after exciting vomiting with his finger. After taking two more ounces of sweet-oil, he threw up nothing, and had no tendency to vomiting, but the pain constantly increased. Again, half an hour later, he took about six ounces of warm "Joopenbier," which, as well as everything he afterwards took, he retained. The nearest doctor, who now came, gave him mucilaginous drinks and put on poultices. Soon Boerhaave himself arrived. Examination of the mouth and throat and palpation of the abdomen revealed nothing abnormal. No nausea; scarce any eructation. Drinks were swallowed easily, and without causing pain. No hiccough throughout the sickness. The vomited material showed only the ingesta. The body had its usual warmth; the pulse was rather weak, but regular; the breathing easy and natural; consciousness undisturbed. The sole complaint was of the very violent pain, which was constant and unceasing, and referred with accuracy by the patient to the region of the cardia just above the diaphragm, and the very distinct sensation as if some change had taken place in the position of the organs within the chest. Later the pain extended to the back, on both sides. The patient said that nothing so increased the pain as eructation, and afterwards movements of the spinal column. On the most careful consideration of these symptoms, it was impossible to refer them to any known form of disease, and particularly as no poisoning could be admitted. Accordingly, with so obscure a diagnosis, from general indications for the alleviation of suffering, the patient was bled, warm fomentations were applied, mild drinks given, etc.—all without the least relief. About 9 o'clock A.M., after a clyster had been given, followed by a natural passage, a second bleeding was resorted to, equally without result. In spite of the great quantity of fluid swallowed, the patient only passed a few drops of urine. After three o'clock in the afternoon dyspnœa came on, the extremities grew cold. With the belief that the great quantities of fluid drunk had accumulated in the stomach, and must be retained by constriction of both orifices, the only hope lay in inducing vomiting. Accordingly they gave him two ounces of almond-oil, followed by seven ounces of warm water, and tickled the fauces with a feather, and he threw up a small quantity of fluid, but none of the oil. The skin became cold and pale, and a cold sweat broke out, and at about five o'clock P.M. (nineteen hours after the sudden attack of pain) he died. Boerhaave made the autopsy twenty-four hours after death. He found first a very extensive emphysema of the skin; the abdomen inflated, tense. On carefully opening the greatly distended belly, a quantity of air escaped. Abdominal cavity normal throughout, and with the exception of a stomach and intestine greatly distended with gas, the same was true of all the abdominal viscera. Bladder empty. Diaphragm and mesentery uninjured.

The stomach contained, besides gas, only a little reddish yellow fluid, no blood, no bile, and scarcely any food. On carefully opening the thorax a quantity of air escaped. Both lungs greatly collapsed, but otherwise entirely normal. The heart also normal. On opening the thorax a peculiar odor was perceived, which Boerhaave's acute sense of smell, with a culinary education, diagnosticated as the roast duck eaten at the last meal, and in both pleural cavities was found a quantity of a reddish yellow fluid (in all 104 ounces), the color of which was due to the beer mixed with water which the patient had taken, and upon its surface the oil was swimming. Not a drop of blood was seen. On pulling forward the left lung, there was found on the pleura covering the œsophagus, two inches above the diaphragm, a round, flabby, blackish spot, about three inches in diameter, distended with air, and at its centre a gaping rent one and a half inches long by about three lines wide, from which, by pressure on the surrounding parts, there flowed a fluid similar to that in the pleural cavities, with which also the subserous cellular tissue in the neighborhood was infiltrated. The finger carefully introduced into this rent, passed through a soft tissue into the right pleural cavity without touching the œsophagus. After withdrawing the finger part way it could be passed into the œsophagus, whose continuity had been sundered, and the two portions had been dragged respectively upward and downward. Boerhaave, in consequence of this discovery, decided that the condition had not been caused by any of the food eaten at the last meal; that no poisoning had occurred; also that the rupture had not been caused by any long-standing ulcerative process; and accordingly nothing remained but to assume that a fresh rent had taken place in an œsophageal wall previously healthy. The lower part of the œsophagus had been dragged downward by the distended stomach, and yet more by the vain attempts at vomiting, and the upper part had been dragged upward in consequence of contractions caused by introducing the finger into the pharynx. Hence, a non-penetrating rent had taken place, which,

from the continuous strain (by weight) and repeated traction (by attempts at vomiting), had finally torn through entirely.

As in this case, so in all the others, the catastrophe occurred
suddenly and with such terrible violence that there was no room
for doubt that some very serious internal lesion had instantly
occurred. Many of the patients, like Boerhaave's, declared that
something had burst at a point corresponding to the rupture,
and they complained especially of violent pain just at this spot.
In two patients this was increased particularly by movements of
the vertebral column. In others the violent pain was less precisely located, or changed its position. Fitz's case is the only
one in which, from the outset, pain was not a prominent symptom;
but here it was not wanting subsequently. The catastrophe was
brought about in two cases by violent retching in order to remove a morsel of food caught in the œsophagus or pharynx (once
successfully, and once without success), and a little blood was
raised at the time. In the other cases the attack was preceded
by nausea and vomiting, but not at all violent, or only attempts
at vomiting, or more or less violent retching, by which some
blood (but never much) was raised. Usually no vomiting occurred
afterwards, in spite of attempts and therapeutical measures to
that end.

In many cases this was followed by profound collapse (pallor
of the face, cold sweat, and cold extremities).

In a diagnostic point of view a very important symptom is
the almost constant [1] appearance of a rapidly developed emphysema of the skin, which, appearing first on the neck above the
clavicles, soon extended over a large area, and sometimes involved
the whole surface of the body.

Later, more or less severe dyspnœa appeared, sometimes violent orthopnœa and distress ; the pulse, hitherto quiet, was much
accelerated, and, with a continuous increase of all the symptoms,
death followed generally in less than twenty-four hours (7–19) ;
in one case (Meyer) after fifty hours, and in one (Fitz) on the
eighth day.

---

[1] Of eight cases there is but one in which it is not alluded to. The ninth (*Oppolzer's*)
case cannot be considered in this analysis of symptoms, on account of its lack of all
particulars.

At the autopsy in all the cases a rent was found in the œsophagus, sometimes five centimetres in length and involving all the layers, always in the lower part of the canal, and beginning a short distance above the cardia, or even extending into the mucous membrane of the stomach. In Boerhaave's case the œsophagus was torn completely across, so that the two parts were drawn respectively upward and downward. In all the other cases it was a longitudinal rent; in one case (Gramatzki) a second longitudinal rent was found on the opposite side, only extending down to the submucosa.

Through the rent the fingers usually passed into a cavity in the mediastinum, filled with a discolored fluid, fragments of food and also some blood, and the cellular tissue surrounding it was saturated with the same fluid. In many cases this cavity communicated by a rent in the pleura with one (the left) or both of the pleural sacs. The latter contained a quantity of cloudy fluid (104 ounces, Boerhaave; three quarts, Griffin) which from its character, odor, and appearance, and particularly from the fat or undigested food it contained, was evidently an overflow from the stomach, increased by the great quantities of drink sometimes taken, which gave it a characteristic appearance, while on opening the thorax an escape of gas was observed. In none of these cases was any tissue-change found which could be considered as a remote cause of the laceration (ulceration, cancer), so that we must consider it a rupture of an organ hitherto normal.[1] Although this anatomical condition is considerably obscured by the group of symptoms sketched above, yet while these latter are totally unexplained by the supposition that the rent in the

---

[1] In *Gramatzki's* case it certainly was assumed in the clinical explanation that the two rents of the œsophagus found at the autopsy were due to a sharp body (piece of bone) which he may have swallowed six weeks before his death, at which period he suffered for a short time from pain in the stomach; and that the rapidly fatal rupture which occurred at the seat of the larger laceration was induced by the old injury. If this supposition were true, the case would necessarily be excluded from this list, which contains only ruptures of the healthy œsophagus. Nevertheless, no foreign body was found at the autopsy, nor did the history reveal any account of such a body being swallowed. And since it seems very improbable that a patient with so severe an internal injury unhealed, could "in the best of health" have undertaken a sea-voyage as engineer on a steamship, as he did, we do not consider the assumption warranted, and believe rather that the case should come in the same category as the rest.

œsophagus took place merely in consequence of post-mortem softening, it seems wrong, while fully recognizing the propriety of a profound scepticism in the presence of such unusual occurrences, totally to deny the existence of rupture of the œsophagus during life so long as there is any possibility of explaining it. Now, in fact, it is scarcely credible that an œsophagus with tissues intact could be lacerated merely by its own contraction or by traction exercised by neighboring parts (diaphragm, stomach), nor could we accept this explanation even for the cases (Meyer, Fitz) in which a not very large morsel of food engaged in the canal brought on violent contractions. For though, under such circumstances, the tense muscular tissue might give way, yet the same would scarcely occur with the firm mucous membrane which, by the contraction of the muscular layer, is more than ever relaxed. Nor would this explain the laceration of the pleura so loosely joined to the œsophagus. Moreover, in most of the cases there was no such violent contraction preceding the trouble, for in vomiting the œsophagus is relaxed.

In order to ascertain how much force was requisite to tear a healthy œsophagus, we made the following experiment: the healthy œsophagus of a powerful man, fifty-five years of age, who was suddenly killed by a railroad accident, was hung up uninjured nine hours after death, by means of a band firmly attached to its upper end, while a weight was fastened to a band similarly attached to its lower end. It bore the weight without tearing up to five kilogrammes, while the tube between the bands was stretched from seventeen centimetres up to twenty-four centimetres in length. When five kilogrammes were used, after about a minute, the muscular layer, together with the thin cellular coat, tore in a circular form just above the lower band, and retracted from the totally uninjured mucous membrane. Now, the lower band was fastened on to the lower portion of the mucous membrane which alone remained at that part. The muscular layer again tore just below the upper band when twelve and a half kilogrammes were used (also in a circular form). Then the upper band was fastened to the upper portion of the mucous membrane, which was all that now remained at this part, but was totally uninjured. For some time it bore a weight of five kilogrammes without injury. Not until ten kilogrammes were used, and after stretching considerably for several seconds, did the mucous membrane give way at about its middle, with a ragged circular rent.

Is it comprehensible that by contraction of the œsophagus itself, or by the distention or traction exercised by neighboring parts, any force at all approaching this could be brought to bear on the organ?

Accordingly, we are forced to assume, as the true underlying cause of the catastrophe, the existence of some change which seriously affects the firmness of these tissues; and, in fact, such a condition was proven in two of the cases, and very probably existed in the others. Fitz has with great propriety emphasized the fact that in two of the cases (Habershon, Charles), according to the statements of the authors, signs were present which pointed to œsophago-malacia (in Habershon's case the greater curvature of the stomach was very much softened), and that in most of the other cases in which the authors do not allude to it—in Boerhaave's time this condition was not recognized—the description of the anatomical changes in the neighborhood of the rupture is quite in accord with the assumption of softening; indeed, when we consider the tearing of the pleura, we are forced to accept it. We fully agree with him, but must add that the two cases (Meyer, Fitz), in which Fitz does not allude to this possibility, should not be excluded, since we can point to the fact that the condition described in both cases, viz., the lack of epithelium below the rupture, corresponds with that appearance which King has accurately described as the commencement of œsophago-malacia.

Although this point is sufficient to cause Fitz to reject all these cases as untrustworthy, yet we hold quite a different opinion. Such radical skepticism might be justified if we had not strong proofs of the possibility of rupture of the stomach during life as a sequel of gastro-malacia. But since the proof of this, in our judgment, has been brought forward with the greatest clearness and accuracy by the case reported by W. Mayer, which we ourselves observed,[1] there can be no doubt that the same might occur in the œsophagus. Accordingly, instead of rejecting them, we feel justified in believing *that all these cases of so-called spontaneous rupture of the œsophagus may be referred to an antecedent vital œsophago-malacia — arising while the patient is in a healthy condition*—very rapidly developed *by special circumstances or surroundings.*

---

[1] Deutsches. Archiv. f. klin. Med. Vol. IX. p. 105. 1871, and this Hand-book. Vol. VII. p. 261.

Since we accept the œsophago-malacia as an explanation of the ruptures, in justification of this assumption it is only right to insert here what we have to say concerning this tissue-change in general, which seems all the more proper from the fact that it is only in consequence of its relation to ruptures, which we are now considering, that it assumes a real pathological interest.

Softening of the Œsophagus—Œsophago-Malacia

occurs not unfrequently—though less frequently than softening of the stomach—under the same form and practically the same conditions as the latter, and in general is more frequently combined with it, but sometimes is found alone. It always invades the lower half of the œsophagus to a greater or less extent, beginning just above the cardiac orifice. In the lowest grades the epithelium is thrown off either over large regions, or here and there in the form of little islands, or in parallel longitudinal bands corresponding to the furrows between the folds of the contracted œsophagus. The mucous membrane, stripped of epithelium, is smooth, shining, and watery, discolored gray or yellowish, and crossed here and there by a few blackish lines marking the course of vessels, but not much altered in consistency; the muscular layer is as yet intact.

In the higher grades the mucous membrane, and usually the muscular layer as well, are very soft, generally translucent, with a jelly-like appearance (exactly like a piece of tissue when thrown into vinegar), more rarely blackish in color, and pulpy. The whole wall tears on the slightest traction, or, more commonly, in spite of the greatest precaution in handling, is separated into longitudinal strips by fissures. In the latter stage the neighboring connective tissue of the posterior mediastinum is discolored over a large space, soft, and pulpy, and frequently the pleura in this region is torn on one or both sides. Then we find in the corresponding pleural sac a more or less copious accumulation of fluid, evidently the contents of the stomach, of a dirty brown or grayish red color, and apparently mixed with blood (by which at the autopsy our attention is first called to the pathological change which has taken place), the softening influence of which upon the adjacent parts is very evident. The pleura pulmonalis of the lower lobe of the lung is often much macerated, or here and there entirely thrown off, while on the portions still remaining not unfrequently livid spots are found, which are easily distinguished from those portions which are merely discolored and œdematous. We have observed similar livid spots also in other portions affected by the softening, e. g., in the mediastinum and on the adventitia of the aorta. A more or less extensive subpleural emphysema is also ordinarily observed in such cases. The rest of the œsophageal wall above is ordinarily normal. Yet in one case we found the mucous membrane bordering on the softened and ruptured spot deeply injected, and in another case freshly ecchymosed for a distance of three centimetres. But still we have never seen the great hemorrhagic infiltration of the œsophageal mucous membrane which C. E. E. Hoffmann observed in two cases.[1] Now, as regards the nature and pathological significance of œsophago-malacia, there can be no doubt that the process is identical with that change which takes place in the stomach under the same name, and what is true of the latter is equally true of the former. And since these very interesting questions now in dispute are fully considered by Leube in this Hand-book, under Diseases of the Stomach,[2] we will refrain from entering into the matter here, as the views there laid down fully coincide with our own. With Leube, we hold firmly to the opinion expressed particularly by Hunter and Elsaesser, and defended chiefly by King (loc. cit.), as regards the œsophagus, that the softening in the great majority of cases is a post-mortem process which then takes place, because the contents of the stomach, which contain pepsin and at the same time sufficient acid, are in contact for a long time, while the body is sufficiently warm, with tissues in which the circulation has stopped, and which therefore can no longer offer resistance to their softening influence. In order that such a state of affairs should exist in the œsophagus, it would be necessary that a regurgitation of the contents of the stomach should have taken place before death, and that in con-

---

[1] Virchow's Archiv. Vol. 44. p. 352 ; Vol. 46. p. 124.

[2] This Hand-book. Vol. VII. p. 264. See also there the appropriate literature of the subject.

sequence of diminished contractile power in the œsophagus they should have remained there some time. We believe, however, with Leube, that the softening does not always occur after death, so to speak, is completed, *i. e.*, is not entirely cadaveric, but that in other cases, and we think frequently, it begins during life, *i. e.*, during the long agony, and may advance to the highest grades, even to perforation, and that it should therefore be described not as post-mortem, but as an *intra-mortem* process. This belief is not at all inconsistent with our holding to the above-mentioned method of its development, for the great slackening and weakening of the circulation which is doubtless present in many cases during the agony of approaching death (especially with the prostrating forms of sickness with which malacia is apt to be associated) may be considered sufficient to remove the opposition to "self-digestion," which is in force while the circulation is unimpaired. But we cannot, from our experience, accept the view that a hemorrhagic infiltration of the œsophageal mucous membrane always or even ordinarily forms the underlying cause of the softening. The hemorrhages observed by Hoffmann, in two of his cases, may be considered the result of the softening quite as well as the cause.

The proofs that the softening and perforation in a part of the cases occurred before life was fully extinct may be found in what is said above concerning the anatomical appearances. The ecchymoses there described, located in the various tissues exposed to the destructive effects of the contents of the stomach (which we have often seen both in œsophago- and gastro-malacia), are totally incomprehensible on the basis of a purely cadaveric origin, but are readily explained if we suppose that the softening of the tissues, and also of the walls of the vessels, occurred at a time when the circulation, however feeble, was still going on. Accordingly, we fully agree with Hoffmann, who considers this a very important indication that the softening occurred during life.

But hemorrhages also occur during life, and Elsaesser rightly considers this one of the strongest proofs of intra-vital softening.[1]

---

[1] "Softening of the Stomach in Nursing Children." Stuttgart and Tübingen, 1846. p. 8. "If the colloid softening takes place during life, it is very strange that a child

The following case may serve as an example of it. A boy, nine years old, who died from bilateral parenchymatous nephritis, had, according to the statement of his physician, vomited a considerable quantity of bloody fluid several hours before death. The autopsy (July 1, 1875, twenty-eight hours after death) showed, besides the affection of the kidneys, *colloid softening and perforation of the œsophagus, with an escape of the contents of the stomach into the left pleural cavity, and subpleural emphysema*. The appearance was as follows: in the left pleural cavity a great quantity of a dirty, dark brown, cloudy fluid. The pleura ruptured on the left side above the diaphragm for a distance of four centimetres, in the region of the posterior mediastinum, and an opening in the œsophagus of great extent, with pulpy, softened margins. The diaphragm also pulpy, and soft at the œsophageal opening. The pleura pulmonalis of the left lower lobe, and partly also the corresponding portion of the pleura costalis covered with large subpleural emphysematous sacs. In the right pleural cavity a few teaspoonfuls of bloody fluid (no emphysematous sacs found on the right pleura). The œsophagus (for a distance of seven centimetres from its upper portion) entirely normal (with the exception of two superficial erosions, lying opposite one another at the highest part); from here downward the mucous membranes very much discolored, and crossed by brownish and blackish blood-vessels, and farther down to just above the cardia the whole wall deeply affected with colloid softening, with partial longitudinal separations, and torn into the left pleura. The stomach, moderately distended, only showed slight traces of commencing softening on its greater curvature.

In another case, which is significant in many respects, no hemorrhages were observed during life, but it is distinctly stated that blood was found in the stomach and upper intestinal tract. The case was that of a boy, six years old, who had long been confined to his bed, suffering severely from caries of the right hip-joint and ilium, and who died of general tuberculosis. Two days before his death he was troubled with vomiting, and the epigastric region was very sensitive on pressure. The next day he was soporose, took no more nourishment, and vomited frequently. In the evening there was loud tympanitic resonance on percussion over all the left half of the thorax. He died at three o'clock the next morning.

Autopsy, November 29, 1876, eight hours after death.—*Diagnosis from examination of the cadaver. Caries of the right hip-joint and ilium; cheesy abscess on the inner surface of the right ilium; tubercular basilar meningitis, with acute hydrocephalus; partly softened tuberculous nodules in the substance of the brain; tubercular meningitis spinalis; miliary tuberculosis of the lungs, liver, spleen, kidneys, and abdomen; traction diverticulum of the œsophagus;* SOFTENING OF THE ŒSOPHAGUS WITH PERFORATION OF THE PLEURA; CONTENTS OF STOMACH AND UPPER INTESTINE BLOODY; *ascaris lumbricoides; tricocephalus dispar; oxyuris vermicularis:* the portion of the report pertaining to the subject under consideration is as follows. In the left pleural cavity some bloody fluid; left lung entirely free. On raising this

suffering from gastro-malacia has never vomited blood, and that nothing of the kind is found in the contents of the stomach."

lung the pleura over the aorta and lower portion of the œsophagus is found to be imperfect for a distance of 5 ctms. The uncovered œsophagus is here of a brownish color, and torn by fissures in various places. On the adventitia of the exposed aorta are seen two ecchymotic spots the size of a bean, and of a bluish red color. On laying open the œsophagus, there are seen at the upper part, at corresponding points on the anterior and posterior surfaces, oval spots 7 mm. in diameter, where the epithelium is wanting (commencing decubitus); with this exception the mucous membrane, for a distance of 5 ctms. from the top, is normal. Throughout the rest of the tube, for a distance of 10 ctms., the epithelium is wanting and the mucous membrane is in part of a yellowish color. In this region are three longitudinal fissures, the upper 2 ctms., and the lower 5½ ctms. in length. On their edges the tissues are deeply affected with colloid softening, and of a yellow color; the muscular layer looks as if its meshes were opened in consequence of the colloid condition of the tissues between them, and several of the circular fibres are separated. Above the upper fissure the mucous membrane of the upper part of the tube, otherwise healthy, is deeply injected. The mediastinal connective tissue which bounds one of the lower fissures is greatly ecchymosed. One of the lower fissures ends 1 ctm. above the cardiac orifice, where also the discoloration of the mucous membrane abruptly terminates. At the level of the bifurcation of the trachea, between the upper and lower fissures, a traction-diverticulum 3 mm. deep is found. The pleura pulmonalis of both lungs, particularly posteriorly and inferiorly, is covered with numerous ecchymoses; on the posterior surface of the left lower lobe a subpleural interstitial emphysema with very small air-sacs (which is not present on the right side). The stomach, but little distended, with pretty thick walls, contains at the fundus a moderate quantity of black, turbid, and very acid material, with the appearance of coffee-grounds. The mucous membrane covered with a thin layer of mucus, moderately injected, and nowhere softened. In the upper coils of the jejunum a dark, blackish brown, viscid material like tar; the mucous membrane here but slightly injected. Farther down, partly greenish chyme, and pale yellow masses of mucus. The contents of the stomach, subjected to microscopical examination, showed very numerous red blood-corpuscles, partly well preserved, partly shrunken, and partly decolorized, while in the tarry mass in the jejunum none such could be discovered. But the presence of blood was proven, by the test for hæmin, both here and in the stomach. In both these cases, if we consider the softening of the œsophagus as a purely post-mortem change, and accordingly reject it (as the cause of intra-vital rupture), no cause could be discovered for the blood discharged during life, and observed after death in the alimentary canal, which escape must have occurred shortly before death, but certainly before death took place. The dark, grayish red or brown coloring of the contents of the stomach which had escaped into the pleural cavity, is in favor of an ante-mortem hemorrhage, but yet it requires further proof in future cases.

Why such hemorrhages are not constantly found and are not more considerable in quantity, is explained, on the one hand, by the fact (which we have assigned as a cause of the softening) that in patients thus affected there is already a great falling off in the force of the circulation, and on the other, as we freely admit, by the fact that in a portion of the cases it is simply a post-mortem occurrence.

The subpleural emphysema also, in the cases of perforation, would seem to be a strong evidence, since it occurs so soon after death, and, considering the antiseptic character of the contents of the stomach, as well as the lack of other evidences of putrefaction, it could scarcely be considered as induced by that process.

The lack of inflammatory reaction in the neighborhood of the softening, on which Elsaesser lays great stress, would not avail against the view here supported, since such reaction could scarcely be expected within the few hours of life at a low ebb which we consider a prerequisite for the development of the whole pathological process.

The final and unassailable proof, however, must come from clinical observations, for by these we shall, at some future time, succeed in proving, by physical exploration during the last agony, that fluid or air has suddenly entered the pleural sac. Therefore, in this connection, we would recommend the most careful investigation of patients suffering from tubercular basilar meningitis during the agony (since, in our experience, softening occurs very frequently in such patients), and at the same time we would urge the greatest delicacy in handling the patient, since, when softening is already present, any movement, and particularly putting the patient in an upright position, may cause a rupture of the œsophagus. All other symptoms—such as pain, sensitiveness on pressure in the epigastrium, even the hemorrhages already discussed — are of secondary importance on account of their doubtful testimony.

The symptoms observed before death in the second of the above cases are of importance in this connection, but are yet too incomplete and of too doubtful interpretation to be considered absolute proofs. And in particular the tympanitic resonance over the left half of the thorax, observed the night before death, which suggested pneumothorax, cannot, unfortunately, be accepted as a proof, since, at the autopsy, the presence of air in the pleural cavity was not recognized—perhaps only because no such change was anticipated, and accordingly was not carefully sought for.

Why destruction of the œsophageal wall is not accompanied by a much more striking group of symptoms, which could not possibly be overlooked (as in the cases above described of true rupture in the narrower sense), is very readily explained by the general condition of the patient at the time of the final agony.

There can be no doubt, according to our experience, of the causal connection between softening of the stomach and œsophagus, on the one hand, and diseases of the brain—particularly tubercular basilar meningitis—on the other, a connection which has been emphasized by Jaeger, and later by Rokitansky, based upon the most extensive experience, but is denied by Elsaesser; our own experiences, particularly as regards the œsophagus, are very striking.

In 2,587 autopsies made at the Institute of Pathological Anatomy at Erlangen, from 1362 to 1876, advanced œsophago-malacia was observed nine times (six times accompanied by perforation of the pleural sac). In these nine cases the stomach was very much softened only in two (once ruptured), in three slightly softened, and not at all in four. Of these nine, in one the head was not opened (death by diffuse nephritis—boy nine years old—see above); in all of the other eight cases, together with the other pathological changes, there were diseases of the brain, viz.: four times basilar meningitis with acute hydrocephalus (at the ages of six, ten, forty-one, and fifty-eight); in one an enormous congenital hydrocephalus (boy fifteen years old); in one, a cicatrix in the corpus striatum with slight chronic hydrocephalus (in a tubercular patient twenty-three years old); in one, excessive hyperæmia of the brain with slight internal hydrocephalus (boy three months old); in one, moderate hyperæmia and œdema of the brain (death from croupous pneumonia—girl nine years old). These figures, few as they are, are yet sufficient to exclude the belief that the simultaneous appearance of the two affections was merely a fortuitous occurrence.

From this statement it certainly is not possible to consider the softening as purely an accidental discovery at the autopsy, which has no causal relation to the fatal disease. We are forced, rather, to assume that diseases of the brain, and, above all, hydrocephalus, favor the development of conditions likely to produce softening of the stomach and œsophagus. Whether the affection of the brain produces this effect by its influence on the secretions of the stomach (as Rokitansky suggests), or—which to us seems more probable — on the circulation in the affected parts, or in some other way, must remain undetermined.

It is clear that the view we are here defending has nothing in common with the purely vitalistic theory, entirely overthrown by Elsaesser, according to which the softening is considered as an independent disease of long duration, accompanied by a special group of symptoms, and forming the only cause of death. On the other hand, it accords fully in principle with the theory of Hunter and Elsaesser, and is a modification of the same only in so far as the latter represents the softening in all cases as the digestive destruction of dead tissues in the cadaver, which we fully accept as true for a portion of the cases, but not for another portion, in which we consider it equally a digestive process, not of tissues completely dead, but rather taking place in a body while in the agony of death arising from other diseases.

The practical significance of this affection will be somewhat, but not essentially, modified by this manner of looking at it, for in the cases here reported the fatal termination was inevitable through other diseases before the softening began. Yet in many cases death may be hastened by minutes, or even hours, in consequence of perforation (as was, perhaps, true in Hoffmann's case, in which death occurred during an attack of coughing). Hence, therapeutically, it should be our special care, in endeavoring to make death easy in cases where softening is suspected, to avoid everything which might lead to perforation (avoidance of all movement of the patient, or any operative or mechanical interference).

These considerations acquire the greatest pathological significance since they form the connecting link with that opinion above laid down, that œsophago-malacia may be developed in rare cases, *intra vitam*, in a patient in a perfectly healthy condition, without any connection with any preceding serious disease, and form the basis of the so-called spontaneous rupture of the œsophagus described above. We must return therefore to these cases and see how far the circumstances, under which those ruptures occurred, serve to support this view.

If we hold fast to the principles of the theory laid down concerning œsophago-malacia, is it possible to understand the sudden occurrence of this affection during life and health? This question we must answer affirmatively. For if we carefully consider the various things which, in our judgment, are prerequisite: 1. The presence of stomach-contents, rich in pepsin and acid; 2. Regurgitation; and 3. Protracted retention of regurgitated food in the œsophagus; 4. Sufficient warmth of the body; 5. Cessation or great weakness of the circulation of blood in the œsophagus—we shall see that 1 and 4 are present in the healthy condition during every normal process of digestion, 2 occurs frequently enough when the stomach is over-distended, but can only be effective when 3 is associated with it, since protracted contact of the œsophageal wall with the gastric juice seems to be absolutely necessary to produce softening. But in a perfectly healthy condition this is not apt to occur, since by subsequent contractions the regurgitated material is apt to be forced upward or downward. For the realization, therefore, of Number 3, a diminished muscular energy in the œsophagus, arising from any cause whatever, is necessary. There is no doubt that such diminution may exist under morbid conditions, and may also be rapidly developed in the healthy state as a sequel of continuous and violent vomiting. There remains, therefore, only Number 5, the diminished force of the circulation; and it certainly requires no proof that this also may be rapidly developed over a limited region by various influences. Accordingly, there is no inconsistency in the assumption that this process, which ordinarily belongs to the period just preceding or following death, may under special circumstances be developed in practically the same manner during healthy life, and it only remains for us to see if these requisites were actually present in the cases of rupture of the œsophagus.

Now, the etiological relations of these cases do afford the most striking support to our theory.

All the eight cases in which the particulars were known were *men* at the most vigorous time of life, from twenty-four to fifty years of age.[1] With the exception of Boerhaave's patient, who

---

[1] Only in *Oppolzer's* case does it seem to have been a woman, since the rupture is said to have occurred " while ironing."

is described as a man of striking characteristics both of mind
and body, and of temperate habits, all seem to have been habitual
drinkers (five are distinctly described as such and as intemperate, and what is said of the others would lead us to the same
conclusion). Moreover, all of them were essentially healthy. It
is worthy of mention only that two (Meyer, Charles) had suffered
since childhood from occasional dysphagia, as a cause of which
there was found at the autopsy of one, in whom it was referred
to having swallowed lye, a narrow spot just above the cardia,
"without distinct cicatricial formation."

The occurrence of the catastrophe in all the cases either followed immediately upon a more or less abundant meal, or a few
hours after a drinking-bout. In four cases it occurred while
eating, and twice (as we have said) at the time of detention of a
morsel in the œsophagus (Meyer, Fitz), and twice (Habershon,
Griffin) accompanied by nausea, apparently on account of a
meal which disagreed with them (Griffin's patient distinctly laid
it to the plum-pudding he had eaten, which he said always made
him sick). In two other cases (Boerhaave, Charles) it occurred
either immediately after or during a horseback ride taken just
after the meal; and finally, in the last two (Dryden, Gramatzki)
it occurred early in the morning, after a bout of drinking the
evening before, which probably extended into the night.

We have already stated that the first symptoms in all the
cases were nausea, retching and vomiting, and the sudden pain,
and the other terrifying symptoms followed more or less quickly
thereafter.

Thus it is seen that, as with the symptoms during life, and
the post-mortem appearances, so the etiological conditions are
strikingly similar in all; and hence, notwithstanding the small
number of cases, accurate conclusions can yet be formed.

Now, as regards a predisposition to rupture, it is a very important circumstance that in nearly all cases the victims have
been habitual drinkers, and the fact that they were with scarcely an exception men, may be referred to the same circumstance.
Now, to make out from the complicated physical condition of a
drinker, just that particular pathological peculiarity which
would serve as a disposing cause, it is best to compare their cor-

poreal condition with that of Boerhaave's patient (who is the only exception), and see if both agree in any one particular. From this we learn that the man, naturally of such temperate habits, from his social relations, was obliged frequently to partake of heavy dinners, and particularly after such he was wont to feel a very disagreeable and annoying sensation in the region of the cardia, and from this he usually relieved himself by taking an emetic, and was accustomed to use them at improper times, contrary to the advice of his physician. Since no old anatomical changes in the cardia were found at the autopsy, this troublesome feeling was most probably due to atony of the muscular layer of the œsophagus, particularly at the cardia, induced or increased by the abuse of emetics, in consequence of which regurgitation would easily take place when the stomach was overloaded, and the material would remain for a long time in the œsophagus, causing that annoying sensation which was so easily removed by an emetic.

Now, eructation and vomiting, partly as direct results of a debauch, and partly as sequels of chronic gastritis, are among the most frequent symptoms, and the use of emetics one of the most common procedures amongst professional drinkers. And since in many of our cases repeated tedious antecedent attacks of gastritis were distinctly remembered (the short sickness with pain in the stomach in Gramatzki's case needs no other explanation), and mention was made of the frequent use of emetics, there is in fact, in this respect, the most complete harmony between Boerhaave's case and the others. Therefore, we shall not go wrong in considering that *atony of the muscular tissues of the œsophagus and cardia, caused by the habitual use of emetics, and a tendency to regurgitation, form the disposing causes of rupture.*

As *accidental* causes of rupture, we find in all the cases, occurrences of various kinds, either during or shortly after a more or less full meal or drinking-bout, which caused eructations, retching, or vomiting, and hence regurgitation of the contents of the stomach, which at the time contained pepsin and an acid. It seems worthy of note that on two occasions the trouble began during or just after a horseback ride on a full stomach, since no movement would seem so well adapted to cause regurgitation as the jolting while riding. As a result of continued retching and futile attempts at vomiting, we should expect a delay of the regurgitated food in the œsophagus. In both the cases in which a morsel of food was stuck fast in the œsophagus, the way out was closed, and the detention must occur (unless the morsel was just at the cardiac orifice) more surely yet, as in Meyer's case, where also escape was cut off below by the existing contraction above the cardia.[1]

So the prerequisites for the development of intra-vital œsophago-malacia have been most completely realized, except the weakening of the circulation. We cannot conclude that this existed from anything in the history of the sickness, or from any discovery post-mortem—a fact which need not astonish us, even if we suppose it to have existed, for many such disturbances give no sign either during life or at the autopsy. Accordingly, it only remains for us to see if such weakening of the circulation could be likely to exist in these cases. First we are to consider that, if the protection against "self-digestion" lies in the rapid neutralization of the acids by the alkaline blood coursing through the part, the œsophagus, on account of its much less abundant blood-supply, and the necessarily less copious secretion, has much less protection against the gastric juices than the stomach. But it requires much less protection, since ordinarily it does not come in contact with them. In the stomach, it must be supposed, such protection is in excess, so that the circulation may be greatly diminished without exposing the wall to self-digestion; otherwise it would be constantly in danger. In the œsophagus there is no such superfluous supply, and hence a much more moderate diminution in the circulation would be sufficient to destroy the equilibrium and allow self-digestion to begin.

As regards the nature of the disturbance in the circulation, we must reject the hemorrhagic infarction of the œsophageal wall, which Hoffmann assigns as a cause in his intra-mortal cases,

---

[1] This case of *Meyer's* shows the most complete analogy to our case of rupture of the stomach, quoted above (reported by *Mayer*), in which the escape of the destructive contents of the stomach was prevented on either side by the existence of strictures both at the cardiac and pyloric orifices.

since in all the reports of autopsies no allusion is made to such a discovery; and since we cannot refer it to embolism, we naturally turn to *spastic ischæmia*. The occurrence of such spasmodic ischæmia we cannot consider as fortuitous and independent of the rest, but shall rather suppose that it has causal relations with all the other conditions necessary to softening and rupture, and which have been shown to exist. And hence, accepting Andral's witty remark, that, in consequence of the varied emotions, the stomach, quite as well as the skin, may now turn pale, and now be suffused, we certainly shall ask whether the striking pallor of the face and lips during vomiting does not extend to the stomach and œsophagus. This ischæmia may not ordinarily extend to a degree where the tissues would be exposed to the action of the gastric juice, but an unwonted increase in the same would open the door for a catastrophe.

After all that we have said, we hold that the view is well founded, that all cases of spontaneous rupture of the œsophagus may be referred to an intra-vital œsophago-malacia.[1]

Perforations of the Œsophagus.

Bibliography.

Oppolzer, Hamburger, ll. cc.—*Mondière*, Archiv. génér. de Méd. II. Sér. T. III. 1833. p. 50.—*Vigla*, Communications accidentelles de l'œsophage avec les poumons et les bronches. Arch. génér. de Méd. 4. Sér. T. XII. 1846. pp. 129 and 314.— *Habershon*, Guy's Hosp. Reports. 3. Series. Vol. II.—*Eras*, Die anatom. Canalisationsstörungen d. Speiseröhre. Dissert. Leipzig. 1866.—*Schneider*, Berl. klin. Wochenschr. 1868. Nos. 31 and 32 (Communicationen des Œs. mit den Luftwegen). — *Murchison*, Oesophageal Cancer. Tracheal Fistula. Transact. Path. Soc. Vol. XIX. p. 224. 1869.—*M. Mackenzie*, Oesophageal Cancer. Tracheal Fistula. Ibid. Vol. XIX. p. 213. 1869.—*Greenhow*, Ibidem. Vol. XXII. p. 120. 1871.—*J. S. Bristowe*, Tracheal Fistula. Death from Erosion of the Left Common Carotid Artery. Paralysis of Left Vocal Cords. Ibid. XXII. p. 134. 1871. *Saussier* and *Carteron*, Obs. de fistule œsophago-trachéale. Bull. de l'Acad. de Méd. XXXV. p. 841. 1871.—*G. Freudenhammer*, Oesoph.-Carcinom. commu. nicirt mit Bronchus sinister. Diss. Berlin, 1873.— *W. Kebbel*, Perfor. in Bronchus. Lancet, 1875. I. Jan. 16.—*Chalybaeus*, Krebs-Perfor. in Lungencavernen.

---

[1] *Andral*, Précis d'anatomie pathologique. Vol. I. p. 76. 1829.

Deutsch. Klinik. 1868. No. 23.—*Reincke*, Oes.-Krebs, mit Lungencavernen comm. Virchow's Archiv. L. I. 1870.—*Adelmann*, Prager Vierteljahrschrift. 1867. IV.—*Gaudais*, Rétréciss. de l'œsoph. (Pleura-Perforation). Thèse de Paris, 1869.—*F. Busch*, Ueber Perforation d. Oesoph. durch fremde Körper. Arch. f. klin. Chirurgie. 1874. XVI. p. 68.—*Léger*, Pleura-Perfor. Bull. de la Société Anat. 1876. 4 S. I. 2. 1876. p. 411.—*Ti eulich*, Pyopneumothorax nach Perfor. eines Oes.-Geschwüres. Prager Vierteljahrschrift. 129. p. 132. 1876.— *Luermann*, Oes.-Fistel u. sec. Mediastinalabscess. Berl. klin. Wochenschrift. 1876. No. 19.—*J. C. S. Coghill*, Oesophageal Fistula leading to Lateral Wall of the Thorax. Brit. Med. Journ. Jan. 20, 1877.—*Leudet*, Gaz. Méd. de Paris. 1864. Nos. 25, 26, and Schmidt's Jahrb. Bd. 125. p. 247 (Perforationen von Aortenaneurysmen in den Oes.).—*Amodru*, Carc. d l'œsoph. Perfor. der Aorta. Bull. de la Soc. Anat. 3 S. X. 2. p. 219.—*Bradley*, Foreign Bodies (coins). Perforation into the Aorta. Med. Times and Gazette. 1868. Oct. 17.—*Beckers*, De Pneumopericardio. Dissert. Greifswald, 1860 (Perfor. in den Herzbeutel).— *Tuetel*, Ein Fall von Pneumopericardium. Deutsche Klinik. 1860. p. 359.— Ueber Perforation von Tractionsdivertikeln, vide *Rokitansky* and *Tiedemann*, ll. supra cc.

As has been already stated, we designate as perforations the solutions of continuity in the œsophagus produced by destructive morbid processes. These *morbid processes* may belong primarily *to the œsophagus itself*, and then, as the destruction generally begins in the mucous membrane and invades successively the external layers, lead to perforation *from within outward ;* cases of this kind we denominate *primary perforations*. Opposed to them are the *secondary perforations*, produced by *diseases of the neighboring parts*, which secondarily involve the œsophagus in one of two ways: either the degeneration, beginning in them, extends to the œsophageal wall, and so gradually makes its way through the latter *from without inward*, or the wall of the œsophagus, although not actually destroyed, becomes so much softened (from atrophy due to pressure, or from sloughing) that it finally *tears* from some slight cause. It is customary to include these latter cases in the perforations, because the morbid processes preparing the way for the opening perform the chief part, while, from the manner in which the rent finally takes place, they belong more properly to ruptures, and form, as it were, the connecting link between the two.[1] A sharp boun-

---

[1] If our theory, developed above, of the spontaneous ruptures proves to be correct, then the whole difference between them and the perforations of this kind would be

dary line cannot, therefore, be drawn between the two forms of solution of continuity (rupture and perforation).

Primary and *secondary* perforations may occur with about the same frequency (perhaps, with a slight majority, in favor of the primary). Of the *sexes*, the male furnishes by far the larger quota. As regards *age*, they occur occasionally at all periods of life, but are much more frequent in older persons.

Of twenty-four cases of perforation of the œsophagus seen by us (Zenker), twelve certainly belonged to the primary form, nine to the secondary, while in three the form was doubtful. Nineteen cases occurred in men, five in women. In regard to age, all decades, from one to seventy years, were represented; however, only eight cases (one-third) fell within the first four, and sixteen cases (two-thirds) within the last three decades. The greatest number (eight) occurred between the ages of forty and fifty years.

The statistics furnished by Vigla do not compare in every respect with our own, for the reason that they were not made out from material limited strictly to observation, but from a series of cases collected from publications—hence, only the singularly remarkable cases; and for the reason, moreover, that they refer only to perforations of the œsophagus *into the air-passages*. In regard to these, Vigla is perfectly correct when he declares (contrary to our statement) the primary perforation of the œsophagus to be the rule, and the secondary to be the very rare exception. In all other respects the harmony between his statements and our own is worthy of notice. Thus, he found the proportion in the male sex very great (fourteen men, four women). According to him, almost all ages were represented, and (although not so great as with us) the majority occurred in persons more advanced in years. An analysis, undertaken by us, of 114 cases of perforation of the œsophagus of the most varied kind (our own cases and those collected by Vigla included) gives a similar result. Of these 114 cases, seventy-seven occurred in the male and twenty-five in the female (in twelve the sex was unknown). Thirty-five cases occurred under forty, and fifty-nine over forty years of age (in twenty the age was not known). And here also the largest number (nineteen) occurred between the ages of forty and fifty.

In this collection the number of *primary* perforations considerably exceeds that of the *secondary* (seventy-six primary, twenty-eight secondary, ten doubtful), and this depends again upon the fact that, in publishing these cases, special preference is given to communications between the œsophagus and air-passages (to which this proportion applies), because they so often lead to a fatal termination under the gravest symptoms, while other perforations, frequent enough in themselves, and often secondary (*e. g.*, from the mediastinal glands), are only very inadequately given, on account partly of their very latent, and partly of their insignificant

reduced principally to the different kind and degree of the softening in the œsophageal wall.

course. Hence, in order to obtain a correct idea of the relative frequency of these two forms of perforation, we can only retain cases, strictly limited to observation, in examination of which these proportions were kept in view. On this account we believe that greater importance must be attached to our own figures, given above, even though they are somewhat small.

According to our experience, traction diverticula constitute the most frequent basis of *primary perforations*, inasmuch as their wall, becoming inflamed by the impaction of small foreign bodies, etc., is occasionally ruptured by ulceration. These perforations, generally very small at first, are on that account often enough closed again by cicatrization, but may, on the other hand (*vide supra*), lead to very extensive and dangerous losses of substance. Next to these in frequency would stand the perforations caused by *carcinomatous ulcers*, which likewise lead to very extensive losses of substance. Then come larger *foreign bodies* that have been swallowed, which, if they do not immediately, as sharp-pointed or angular bodies, produce a perforating wound, may, by remaining for a longer time, lead to ulceration and sloughing of the mucous membrane, and thereby, at a longer or shorter period after their introduction, to perforation. In rare cases the action of *corrosive substances* may be the cause of complete solution of continuity in the wall. Finally, *ulcerations not of any particular kind* are the cause of perforation. Many of these ulcers may have been produced by foreign bodies, which were already removed at the time of the autopsy. Others are certainly to be referred to traction diverticula, which were not recognized, or, on account of the total destruction of their wall, were actually no longer recognizable. Carcinomatous ulcers, with slight cancerous infiltration of their edges, have certainly now and then been described as simple ulcers. On this account there is no reason to suppose that any other specific form of ulcer is inclined to perforation. The theory of a "perforating ulcer of the œsophagus," analogous to the round ulcer of the stomach, expressed by several authors, depends apparently on the observation merely of such perforations of no definite character. For an ulcer with anatomical appearances so characteristic as this form of ulcer possesses, has never, up to the present time, been seen by anybody (see Ulcers).

· ·The cancerous perforations are generally believed to be by far the most fre·· quent; in fact, this seems to stand out in a striking manner from the statistics of published cases; for of sixty-four published cases ascribed to primary· perforation, there are found no less than thirty-eight cases of cancerous perforation, while eleven are to be traced to the action of foreign bodies, nine to ulcers of indefinite kind, and only six to diverticula. This calculation, however, is fallacious, for there is no doubt that the cases of carcinomatous perforation, by reason of the magnitude of the lesion, and the gravity which this gives to the form of the disease, have been much more frequently published than the so much less apparent diverticula, to which until recently attention has not been at all directed, and which have undoubtedly often been overlooked entirely, or wrongly interpreted. According to · our own observations, the matter stands thus, that of twelve cases of primary perforation, eight were from diverticula and only two from carcinoma, while two were from ulcers of doubtful character. These figures might be somewhat modified by a larger number of cases, but they certainly would not be reversed.

The processes which lie at the foundation of *secondary perforations* are of various kinds. Most frequently they are *diseases of the bronchial and tracheal lymphatic glands,* as glandular abscesses, softening of caseous or highly carbuncular glands; furthermore, by suppuration in the mediastinum or in the retro-œsophageal connective tissue in the neck, due to *caries of the vertebræ.* Rarely they are primary *ulcerations of the trachea,* and *gangrenous masses in the lung,* which become firmly adherent to the œsophagus, and subsequently lead to perforation. We saw it perforated by a suppurating cyst of the thyroid gland.[1] Finally, by continuous, strong *pressure from without,* the wall of the œsophagus may be eroded even to the extent of complete perforation. Thus, in a large substernal bronchocele, which compressed the trachea very much and crowded it against the œsophagus, we saw the wall of the latter completely pierced by the posterior extremity of the fifth cartilaginous ring of the trachea, so that the denuded cartilage projected freely into the canal. Hamburger (l. c., p. 185) quotes an entirely analogous case, in which the ossified larynx was pressed backward by a considerable tumor of the neck, and the anterior and posterior walls of the œsophagus (pharynx) were perforated by the cricoid cartilage pressing against the spine. But this

---

[1] *Mondière* (Arch. génér. XXX. p. 507), on the other hand, publishes a case of primary (carcinomatous) perforation of the œsophagus in a cyst of the thyroid gland. ·

effect of pressure especially applies to *aneurisms of the aorta descendens thoracica*, rupture of which into the œsophagus (sometimes with simultaneous erosion of the vertebræ) has been occasionally observed (9 times in 114 cases of perforation of the œsophagus). In some of these cases the process is complicated, as the aneurism, pressing against the œsophagus, causes by such pressure a circumscribed sloughing of the mucous membrane. By separation of the slough an ulcer now forms *(gangrenous ulcer, from pressure)*, perforation of which establishes the communication with the aorta. Two destructive processes meet here, and we have to deal, in a certain measure, with a combination of secondary and primary perforation.

This complicated kind of origin in a communication between aneurisms of the aorta and the œsophagus has been placed in a proper light by Leudet (l. c.), based upon several authentic cases. We are able to add one of our own, also very authentic.[1]

Allabach, sixty-nine years, male. Sudden death from severe hemorrhage. Autopsy (March 8, 1864) revealed aneurism of the arch of the aorta, with erosion of the vertebræ, circumscribed sloughing of the mucous membrane of the œsophagus (not yet perforated), and perforation of the left bronchus. Atrophy of the recurrent nerves (notably the left) from pressure. The result of the examination of the œsophagus was as follows: "in the *œsophagus*, immediately below the bifurcation of the trachea, a circumscribed prominent space, 12 mms. in diameter, with several pale gray, sharply defined, sloughy spots, and slight zone of redness, but without solution of continuity. This space corresponded with a bulging and extremely thin portion of the aneurismal sac. In the *left bronchus*, immediately at the bifurcation, a sharply defined opening, size of a lentil, which leads directly into the aneurismal sac, but is covered there by thin layers of fibrinous membrane."

Hanot (Arch. génér., July, 1876, p. 22) believes that the pressure of the aneurism on the filaments of the pneumogastric nerve supplying the œsophagus (as was true in our case) is to be regarded as the cause of the ulceration in the mucous membrane. The more simple explanation, however, of direct pressure upon the wall of the œsophagus, seems quite sufficient. But if Leudet considers this complicated kind of perforation by aortic aneurisms to be the only one that exists, his theory does not appear to be well supported.

In the great majority of cases there is only *one* perforation, sometimes two, and rarely still more. In the event of more than

---

[1] The case is given in detail by Prof. Ziemssen, in "Laryngoskopisches und Laryngotherapeutisches." Deutsch. Arch. f. klin. Med. Bd. IV. p. 878.

one perforation, they are generally situated close together, since one and the same diseased mass merely breaks through in several places. This occurs most frequently in carcinoma of the œsophagus.

The location and size of the perforation are naturally very different according to the fundamental disease. Perforations occur in all parts of the œsophagus, but are much more frequent in the intrathoracic than in the cervical portion. A point of predilection—in consequence of the frequent direct or indirect implication of the bronchial glands—is the anterior wall in the region of the bifurcation of the trachea.

The size varies from a small opening, pervious only to a fine bougie, up to deficiencies in the wall of 2, 3, or more ctms. in diameter. They are mostly round, but in isolated cases (rupture from without) they are in the form of a slit.

In primary perforations, the surrounding mucous membrane shows the changes peculiar to the fundamental trouble, while in the secondary form it is generally quite normal, or gangrenous only in small spaces. In rare cases, simple inflammatory or some other kind of morbid process extends secondarily, from the point of perforation, over larger portions of the œsophageal wall.

We saw not long ago, in rapid succession, two cases of extensive secondary perforation of the œsophagus, produced by softening of caseous bronchial glands. In one case there was found in addition a severe phlegmonous inflammation of the œsophagus, extending over the entire length of the tube, which was certainly excited by the perforation. In the other case, the mucous membrane around the perforation, for a distance of 3 ctms., was thickly strewed with small, round ulcers, extending only as far as the submucous cellular tissue.

In regard now to the changes in the neighboring parts, produced by primary perforations, they are limited in many cases to the destruction by ulceration, sometimes of small, at other times of more or less extensive portions, of the mediastinal connective tissue. As a rule, however, in the event of a chronic or comparatively long-continued morbid process (as by the impaction of foreign bodies), before the stage of perforation is reached, an inflammatory thickening, not unfrequently callous induration or cancerous infiltration of the contiguous cellular tissue, will take place, so that the ulcerated cavity in the mediastinum will, to a certain extent, be enclosed in a capsule. This explains the fact that the final rupture is not, as a rule, immediately followed by symptoms so grave and lesions extending so rapidly as we saw them occur in spontaneous rupture of the healthy œsophagus. In particular, the emphysema of the skin, which is apparently of constant occurrence in those cases, extending rapidly over large portions of the surface, is never seen here. Hence, such perforations at first—indeed, as long as they continue—may exist in a latent form, and that too in patients who are under the most careful medical observation. And if the fundamental process has no progressive tendency, as it has in cancer, these perforations may heal by cicatrization, as has been certainly verified by the cicatrices occasionally found in post-mortem examinations.

On the other hand, however, the ulceration, once begun, extends frequently in a slow manner, but sometimes rapidly, farther and farther around itself, and thus leads to the formation of very large, sinuous cavities which penetrate the mediastinum in various directions, even in its entire length.

What an enormous circumference these cavities may attain, and at the same time what little authority there is for describing perforation of the œsophagus as in and for itself a necessarily fatal affection, the case from Bartels' clinique in Kiel, published by Luermann (l. c.) teaches, which—as recovery at the time of publication was expected—is not made out by post-mortem examination, but by model clinical observation. In a patient, twenty-four years old, a mediastinal abscess had formed in consequence of a perforation of the upper third of the œsophagus, arising from some unknown cause (impaction of a foreign body was suspected); this abscess extended from the neck, where it was opened by incision, down as far as the diaphragm, and in front bordered immediately on the heart. The cavity, which at first contained two quarts of fluid, projected when full far into the left side of the thorax. After treatment, continued three-quarters of a year, the mediastinal cavity was considerably reduced in size, but the communication with the œsophagus still existed. Closure of the œsophageal fistula by operation was contemplated. Nothing is thus far known by us of the subsequent history of the case.

These cavities now enter into relation with all the vital parts situated in and contiguous to the mediastinum, and all the hollow viscera found here are exposed to perforation from them. If, as frequently happens, the cavity extends directly to the pericardium or one of the pleuræ, pericarditis[1] or pleuritis very generally supervenes, and that when the serous membrane is not perforated. Most frequently the perforation involves one of the *bronchi* (right or left about equally), or both at the same time, or the *trachea*. The *lungs* especially (much more frequently the right), upper as well as lower lobes, are liable to perforation, mostly by the establishment of fistulæ, which either open directly into a pre-existent cavern, or make their way into the substance of the lung and form cavities there by the process of ulceration. The perforations into the *pleural cavity* (also the right in a large proportion) and *pericardium* are more unfrequent, and may (but apparently only rarely) lead to pneumothorax and pneumo-pericarditis. Finally, perforations of large *arteries* are not unfrequent, notably that of the aorta desc. thorac. Moreover, the pulmonary artery (*vide supra*), intercostal, carotid, right subclavian (once in the latter when it pursued an anomalous course between the œsophagus and vertebral column —dysphagia lusoria,—from the point of a bone, Kirby, another time from carcinoma), and inferior thyroid arteries have been found perforated. Perforations into the larger veins, on the contrary, appear to happen only occasionally. In one instance the left azygos vein was apparently the source of a fatal hemorrhage from perforation by a bone swallowed; in another case it was, with all probability, the vena cava.[2] In one case there was found an opening in the *left auricle.*[3]

While now the occurrence of a communication with a large blood-vessel (whether from primary or secondary perforation) always, with symptoms of severe hemorrhage or internal loss of

---

[1] *Von Dumreicher* (Wien. med. Presse. VII. 15. 16. 18. 1866) describes the pericarditis following perforation of the œsophagus from a foreign body as " almost constant."

[2] *Vide* these cases, described by *Mondière*, Arch. génér. T. XXIV. p. 404, 406, 407.

[3] *Bertrand* et *Bussard*, Gaz. hebdomad. 1874. p. 459. In this case, very carefully observed and described before and after death, the sinuous cavity, situated at the bifurcation, had perforated first into the right bronchus, and then into the left auricle. On the anterior wall of the œsophagus there was found a cul-de-sac, separated from the gangrenous cavity by a thin layer of cellular tissue (probably a traction diverticulum). At the same time there existed a recent pericarditis. The patient, twenty-four years old, died after a three weeks' illness, from repeated attacks of severe hæmatemesis.

blood, tends to a fatal result, suddenly or after a speedy recurrence of the first attack, communication with the other organs mentioned proves rapidly fatal only in exceptional cases, and is much more likely to continue for a longer time. But the entrance of pieces of food, in a state of putrefaction, and of gases from the œsophagus into the perforated part, acts as an intense cause of inflammation and produces at the same time putrid decomposition of the inflammatory products. It gives rise to purulent pleuritis or pericarditis, putrid bronchitis with velvet-like softening, or even granular thickening of the mucous membrane about the point of perforation. By inspiration of the putrid contents of the bronchus there are developed gangrenous patches in the lungs, which may of themselves lead to purulent pleuritis. Moreover, the ulcerations caused by perforation of the lung itself, or the cavities which have opened into the œsophagus, always assume a gangrenous character.

· As might be expected, these processes, in a majority of cases, end fatally, although sometimes after considerable time has elapsed. Nevertheless, even these fistulous communications with neighboring organs, especially the bronchi, may in rare instances close by cicatrization, as is proved by the cicatrices occasionally found after death at corresponding points in the œsophagus and bronchus, together with cicatrized conditions in the mediastinum. Indeed, recovery (by incision) was reported (Busch, loc. cit.) in a case of perforation of the œsophagus from the sharp end of a bone, in which an opening into the pleura had led to pneumothorax and pleuritic exudation. Small secondary perforations, caused by abscesses of lymphatic glands and the like, of course heal more easily. And that recovery not so seldom occurs in cases of pericarditis dependent on œsophageal perforation, is proved by the remarkably frequent coincidence, already emphasized above (*vide* Traction Diverticula), of pericardial adhesions with traction diverticula in the œsophagus. Hence the œsophageal perforations proper (in so far as they do not result from carcinoma) should not be considered as an objective form of disease, which, from the very beginning, is unamenable to every mode of treatment.

An analysis of 120 cases of perforation of the œsophagus (primary and secondary included), arranged with reference to the frequency of communication with the different neighboring viscera—in which it is to be noted that in some cases communication with several viscera took place—shows the following figures. The œsophagus communicated with:

R. bronchus.	L. bronchus.	Trachea.	R. lung.	L. lung.	R. pleura.	L. pleura.
14	12	21	17	6	10	1
26			23		11	

Pericard.	L. auricle.	Aorta.	Pulm. artery.	Carotid.	Subclav. art.	Inf. thyroid art.
7	1	18	1	1	2	1

Intercost. art.	Vena cava.	Left vena azygos.	Cyst of thyroid gland.
1	1 ?	1	2

In seventeen cases the communication occurred merely with the mediastinum or peri-œsophageal cellular tissue in the neck.

Symptomatology and Diagnosis.

The *symptoms* of *rupture* of the œsophagus, so far as such can be gathered from a meagre supply of cases, are specified above (p. 94). The *diagnosis* of this rare occurrence is established with some degree of probability when, on the one hand, the preliminary conditions, viz., the stomach filled with food, and energetic efforts in vomiting or choking, are present ; when, on the other hand, in attempting to vomit, and in connection with the sensation of an internal laceration, a sudden, violent and fixed pain occurs in the course of the œsophagus, which is sometimes increased by movements of the spine ; when, furthermore, *subcutaneous emphysema*, beginning above the clavicles and extending farther and farther, occurs with rapidly increasing collapse, acceleration of the pulse, and dyspnœa to the extent of orthopnœa, extreme precordial oppression, constant attempts to vomit and choking with bloody mucus, without actual vomiting of the contents of the stomach. Special value must be attached to this phenomenon of subcutaneous emphysema, since it appears to be a constant occurrence. As auscultatory phenomena, Hamburger would have us observe extinction of the sound produced by swallowing at the point of rupture, and a whistling noise. Then if perforation of the stomach, pneumothorax from any other cause, and internal hemorrhage, can be excluded in this complicated symptomatology, a rupture of the œsophagus may, with probability, be assumed to exist.

The *symptoms and diagnosis of primary perforation of the œsophagus* are composed of the phenomena of the primary affection in the œsophagus (carcinoma, ulcerations from corrosive substances, foreign bodies, etc.), and added to these, the symptoms of inflammation due to perforation in the neighboring organs and its results. With the comparative frequency of primary perforation, especially by foreign bodies and cancers in the œsophagus, the physician must always be prepared for its occurrence in the course of any destructive affection of the œsophagus, and under such circumstances he will in the majority of cases be able to establish the diagnosis of perforation with greater probability, although not with certainty, if he finds signs of a purulent pleuritis, pneumothorax, purulent mediastinitis, or tracheo-bronchitis, with expectoration of food, etc.

The beginning of the perforation is characterized either by the sudden appearance of severe inflammatory symptoms, with the sensation of internal rupture, then of an acute pneumothorax, pneumo-pericardium, mediastinitis, etc.—especially in perforations from foreign bodies—or the process goes on slowly, firm adhesions connect the wall of the œsophagus with some neighboring organ, and the perforation takes place quite imperceptibly, or without violent symptoms, so that the lesion is made out only by very careful observation.

Sudden diminution or cessation of the dysphagia and apparent freedom from stricture, after complete impermeability had previously existed, have not unfrequently been observed in the œsophagus, as the fluid swallowed, in the same manner as the sound, henceforth enters by the "false passage" into the adjacent organ. In regard to the phenomena of auscultation and percussion, von Reincke, in his case of communication between the œsophagus and a cavity in the lung caused by cancer (which acted more like a diverticulum), has made the following observation:

When we listened posteriorly to the right of the vertebral column, while the patient was drinking slowly, there was heard, with every swallow, a short tinkling noise down to the stricture; *but after every sixth or eighth swallow, the fluid passed through the contraction with a lengthened, shuffling roar, as when a flood-gate is suddenly*

opened.   In following up this phenomenon, attention was directed to a slight dulness, previously made out, which extended over a space about as large as a silver
dollar, and was situated on the right side of the spinal column, at the level of the
seventh cervical vertebra.   _When percussion was made over this spot, while the patient
was drinking, the dulness gradually increased to a remarkable degree in intensity, and
somewhat in extent, to diminish again rapidly from the moment when, by simultaneous
somewhat deeper auscultation, the beginning of the roaring sound was announced._   The
phenomenon did not occur when the patient took solid food.

So soon as the conditions for a perforation of the œsophagus
are fulfilled, the occurrence of violent coughing after swallowing,
and the quality of the expectoration, deserve particular attention.
When in such cases a fluid of peculiar properties, as milk,
whortleberry soup, and the like, is expectorated, there is without doubt a communication between the œsophagus and lung-
tissue or bronchi.   It was so in the following case seen by us
(Ziemssen).

G. B., mechanic, thirty-seven years old, presented himself, October 23, 1867, at
the Medical Clinique in Erlangen, with symptoms of advanced carcinoma of the
lower third of the œsophagus, as well as of the stomach and liver.   The patient has
been suffering for one year; for the past six months has vomited solid food,
and for the past ten days fluid food as well.   At a point forty-five centimetres
from the incisor teeth the sound encounters an insuperable obstruction, and causes
pain behind the ensiform cartilage.   From Oct. 24th, a sound, five millimetres
in diameter, was passed through the stricture daily, and since the 25th the patient
was able to swallow fluid food without difficulty; introduction of sound caused no
pain, and from Nov. 10th a sound one centimetre in diameter passed easily through
the stricture, when made to take a somewhat spiral direction, so that the point was
pushed more to the left side in its downward course.   By Nov. 16th, patient could
swallow meat and potatoes cut up in small pieces, and Nov. 18th he left the hospital, having increased twelve pounds in weight.

The patient returned Nov. 23d, stating that for the last twenty-four hours he had
not been able to swallow fluids.   The weight of the body is diminished by eleven
pounds.   The sound, even the smallest size, would not pass at first, but on the following day its introduction was again successfully accomplished, and from the 27th
the sound one centimetre in diameter was passed through the stricture.   An intercurrent carbuncle in the neck was opened, and healed slowly.   From Dec. 1st the
sound no longer passed through the stricture, but, after being introduced for the
distance of forty-two centimetres, encountered a resistance of softer material than
that which existed previously at a point three centimetres lower down.   The patient,
however, was able to swallow fluids, and even finely minced meat and bread.

Dec. 7th he was discharged from the hospital at his own request, and treated as an out-patient. The introduction of the sound was regularly continued.

At the beginning of February the closure of the œsophagus was complete, the emaciation extreme, and the tumor, as large as an apple, previously recognized in the liver, could now be distinctly felt. Epigastrium and left hypochondrium much sunken, and the whole abdomen was in the form of a tray.

He entered the hospital again Feb. 5th. The smallest sound sometimes reached the stomach, at other times it was caught as in a funnel. At the lower lobe of the right lung, near the vertebral column, there was slight dulness on percussion, without essential change in the respiratory murmur. The noise in swallowing ceased suddenly at the upper part of the stricture. The patient was kept alive on milk and gruel. From Feb. 9th there was violent cough, with abundant yellowish white expectoration, without pain in the thorax, and without dyspnœa or increased frequency of respiration. *Spasmodic cough invariably followed the drinking of milk, and by the cough a small portion of the milk was expectorated.* This phenomenon continued unchanged until death, which occurred Feb. 12th.

The autopsy (Zenker) revealed, in the upper third of the œsophagus, two isolated cancerous nodes, larger than a hazel-nut. The canal was contracted in the lower third for a distance of four centimetres, so that the little finger did not pass through; the mucous membrane adherent, at first whitish gray, farther down slate-colored, uneven, apparently cicatrized, and studded with single, whitish gray nodules, and one lobulated tumor one and a half centimetres long and attached by a pedicle. Immediately above the cardiac extremity the lumen was only large enough to admit a pea, with resistant wall and muscular tissue very much hypertrophied. *From the beginning of the stricture, going off to the right by an opening about the size of a pea, was a fistula which led through the callous mediastinal tissue into the lower lobe of the right lung, where it opened posteriorly into several cavities, varying in size from a cherry-stone to a hazel-nut, with smooth internal surface, and grayish red fluid contents.* The substance of the lung around these cavities collapsed, solid, and bright gray. There were found, besides, disseminated nodes of cancer, size of a pea, in the mucous membrane of the stomach about the cardiac orifice, some of which were ulcerated, and communicated by a fistula with a cavity, produced by ulceration, in the hypertrophied left lobe of the liver. A cancerous gland was found in the upper third of the œsophagus, small metastatic nodes of cancer in liver and kidneys, and an almost completely stiff spinal column from superficial exostoses of the vertebræ.

In this case a fistula, pervious to fluids, had formed between the œsophagus and the secondary cavity, produced by ulceration, in the lower lobe of the right lung. The communication between the cavity and the bronchi leading to it appeared to have been established at a late date, as the milk conveyed during inspiration from the œsophagus into the cavity produced cough only a short time before death, and was partially expectorated. Whether the introduction of the sound was the cause of the unrecognized perforation could not be made out; life was certainly prolonged for several months by the persistent use of the sound.

In other cases the perforation into the pulmonary tissue is the immediate cause of gangrene of the lung, while if the opening be into the trachea, or one of the principal bronchi, symptoms of purulent tracheitis, or bronchitis, with secondary gangrene of the lung, or lobular pneumonia from inspiration of foreign substances, may appear. Communication with the pleura is generally followed by very acute empyema or pyopneumothorax. The severity and quantity of the exudation and the purulent or ichorous nature of the fluid, as proved by the introduction of a trocar, taken in connection with the previous œsophageal trouble, confirm the diagnosis.

Rapidly fatal hemorrhage naturally follows perforation into the aorta or one of the large vessels. The question whether the perforation is due to the action of a foreign body, which has made its way unobserved into the œsophagus, is commonly not cleared up until the autopsy, since, as frequently happens, not one of the necessary grounds of presumption existed during life.

Perforation into the *pericardium* presents such characteristic symptoms that its recognition is seldom difficult. The acute purulent effusion, with mixture of air from the œsophagus, *pyopneumo-pericardium*, has thus far been observed only a few times ; and in the cases of Chambers[1] and Tuetel[2] (Niemeyer), a perforated ulcer of the œsophagus was the fundamental cause, while in the case of Thompson and Walshe,[3] the point of a knife, which was swallowed, had pierced the pericardium.[4]

In all three cases air had entered the pericardial sac, which (in case there are no valves nor valve-like deposits at the point of perforation, which prevent the entrance of air) may be described as a constant occurrence, and may be looked for in all future cases. As mentioned before, the air is drawn into the œsophagus by the normal inspiratory act, and thence into the pericardial sac by the elastic traction of the lungs upon the latter, as well as by the diminution of the heart during systole.

---

[1] London Med. Journ. July, 1852.

[2] Deutsche Klinik. 1860. No. 37. This case has also been appropriated by *Beckers*, for his inaugural dissertation, "De Pneumopericardio. Gryphiæ. 1860."

[3] Treatise on the Diseases of the Lungs, Heart, and the Aorta. II. ed. London, 1854. pp. 201 and 627.

[4] See " Pneumopericardium." Vol. VI. p. 657.

The extraneous substances (blood, pus, mucus, remnants of food, particles of cancer) making their way with the air into the pericardial sac, set up at once a purulent pericarditis, which speedily causes a moderate exudation.

The subjective symptoms are often unimportant: slight dyspnœa, oppression and pain in the region of the pericardium; the objective symptoms, on the contrary, possess great weight, and are very apparent. In addition to the signs of general collapse and cardiac debility, there exists a bulging in the region of the heart, which in the supine position gives a clear, tympanitic percussion-sound with a metallic tinkling, the pitch of which may vary with the systole and diastole of the heart. In sitting, or by bending forward, there is absolute dulness in place of the tympanitic sound, from the gravitation of the fluid which has been exuded.

Metallic phenomena of very great intensity are presented to the ear, and that at great distances from the patient. The cardiac sounds have a metallic ring like a chime, or there is heard a rhythmical succussion sound produced by the shaking of the fluid from the action of the heart, a metallic splashing, the bruit de moulin, bruit de roue hydraulique of the French. This murmur is so loud that it can be heard throughout the room, and, indeed, in the case from Niemeyer's clinique in Greifswald (October, 1859), seen by me, and described by Tuetel, the attendant in an adjoining room was awakened at night by the noise. This case, as being a good example, deserves reproduction here in abstract form.

T. W., forty-six years old, laborer, was admitted October 16, 1859, to the Medical Clinique in Greifswald, stating that he had suffered for three years from vomiting directly after swallowing, and that more recently he had lost strength and flesh to a considerable extent. After a few days, although the pharyngeal sound had not been used, there was suddenly heard, in the evening, a rhythmical splashing sound with every cardiac systole. The apex beat feeble, but in the normal situation. The region of cardiac dulness not essentially changed.

The splashing sound continued without intermission during the night, and was so loud that the attendant heard it in the next room, although the door was closed. On the following morning the patient was comatose, the cardiac dulness had entirely disappeared, and in its place was a full, though not tympanitic percussion-sound. The apex-beat could not be felt. The metallic tinkling continued with every contraction of the heart, and was audible through the whole room. The breath extremely fetid. Death occurred about noon.

Autopsy (Professor Grohe) revealed: pericardium tightly stretched by air, much distended, and contained about six hundred cubic centimetres of fetid fluid. Behind the base of the left ventricle, in the pericardium, which is much thickened at this point, was a cleft-shaped opening, which communicated with the interior of the œsophagus by a canal three-quarters of an inch in length. In the œsophagus, beginning half an inch above the cardiac extremity and extending upwards for five inches, was a cancerous ulcer, in the middle of which, and on the anterior wall of the œsophagus, was the perforation. The pleuræ on both sides adherent to the œsophagus, and partially eroded; slight infiltration in both lungs.

Perforation into the *mediastinum*, or into the peri-œsophageal tissue in the neck, may be recognized by pain in the chest, limited motion in the vertebral column, fever, and especially by *subcutaneous emphysema* in the neck. The last symptom, though so constantly observed in ruptures of the œsophagus, is an extremely rare phenomenon in perforations, and seems to occur only in lesion of the œsophagus produced by foreign bodies (compare Busch, loc. cit., and Adelmann, loc. cit.). When it does occur in these cases, it is naturally of the greatest value in diagnosis. It may subsequently proceed to formation of abscess, and to fistulous communications between the œsophagus and surface of the neck, through which the fluids swallowed make their appearance.

The *prognosis* of a perforation, when the diagnosis has been made out, is always unfavorable, and in the majority of cases fatal, partly on account of the fundamental affection, partly on account of the secondary lesions which the perforations produce in a neighboring organ. The small perforations, which certainly heal frequently, run their course with such slight or indistinct symptoms, that in them the question of diagnosis, and consequently of prognosis, is excluded. As for the rest, the perforations produced by foreign bodies, especially into the pleural cavity, present the most favorable outlook, since in such individual cases recovery follows the early operation for the empyema, etc. (Adelmann, Busch). The perforation by needles offers decidedly the most favorable outlook, as these can make their way into neighboring cervical or thoracic organs, and finally appear on the surface. But these perforations, as Busch correctly observes, can scarcely be described as such, since sharp-pointed needles only push asunder the tissue of the œsophagus, but do not destroy it.

Treatment.

The treatment of ruptures, as well as of perforations, can only be symptomatic, and must be limited chiefly to combating the secondary lesions in neighboring organs.

As a matter of course, the introduction of food and drink is to be suspended entirely, in order to prevent their entrance into the opening, and thereby, as much as in our power lies, to help along the closure of the perforation. The supply of water and food must take place exclusively through the rectum.

HEMORRHAGES.

Pathology and Etiology.

Hemorrhages rarely occur in the tissue of the œsophageal wall. They are confined to the mucous membrane in almost every instance, and appear sometimes as more or less numerous ecchymoses. Such ecchymoses are found in certain severe hyperæmiæ, as, for example, that resulting from stasis in diseases of the heart, in the eruptions of small-pox, in softening of the œsophagus, when the ecchymoses are found at the point where the softening and rupture occur (*vide supra*), and in rapidly fatal cases of poisoning.

Thus, in a case of poisoning by ammonia (man, æt. sixty-six), proving fatal in four hours from œdema of the glottis, the mucous membrane of the œsophagus, nearly throughout, was found studded with ecchymoses, and its epithelial covering clouded and partially detached. Again, in a case of poisoning by cyanide of potassium (man, æt. fifty-four), the mucous membrane of the œsophagus, as well as that of the stomach and duodenum, was ecchymosed.

At other times these hemorrhages appear as large or small livid spots, which most frequently result from the impaction of foreign bodies, but have likewise been observed (C. E. E. Hoffmann) in softening of the œsophagus. More extensive hemorrhagic infarctions of the mucous membrane belong to an extremely rare hemorrhagic form of inflammation of the œsophagus. These hemorrhages, however, inasmuch as they give rise to no symptoms whatever, are far less momentous than those copious effusions of blood in the œsophageal canal, which immediately after they occur make their appearance in the form of hæmatemesis, or, at a later date, as bloody evacuations. Such hemorrhages may result in sudden death, when the autopsy reveals the hemorrhagic contents of the stomach and intestines, and when—as not unfrequently happens—in the absence during life of all signs of disease of the œsophagus, any conjecture as to the probable source of the hemorrhage was out of the question.

The most important of these hemorrhages are those already mentioned in the preceding chapter, where sudden communication is established between the œsophagus and one of the large blood-vessels of the thorax, neck, or with the heart itself, and death occurs, with symptoms of fatal hemorrhage, immediately, or after a speedy recurrence of the effusion, which had been arrested for a time by the intervention of a clot. The blood-vessel by far the most frequently involved, viz., the aorta (thoracic descend.), is quite as liable to perforation from the œsophagus, as conversely the latter is liable from the aorta. In cases where the perforation occurs from the aorta, the cause will be found, almost without exception, in the rupture of an aneurism of that vessel, and such an aneurism may be true, false, or sacculated (without necessarily being of large size).

A very characteristic case has been described by Pick (Transact. of the Patholog. Soc. London, 1867, p. 477), in which an aneurism of the thoracic aorta, situated at the root of the great vessels, by ulceration of its coats, led to an effusion of blood in the walls of the œsophagus, which passed downward in its muscular coat as far as the cardiac extremity of the stomach, and, by a rent in the serous membrane, escaped finally into the peritoneal cavity.

Bristowe (ibid. X. p. 88) gives the particulars of a case of aneurism of the abdominal aorta, near the cœliac axis, in which the effused blood pursued an upward course, displacing the œsophagus, and producing obstruction of the lower three inches of this tube.

Perforations have likewise been found in other blood-vessels (pulmonary, intercostal, carotid, right subclavian arteries, vena cava (?), left azygos vein and left auricle), all resulting from lesion of the œsophagus. So also all the varieties of primary perforation (*vide supra*), whether produced by foreign bodies, diverticula produced by traction, carcinomatous and other ulcerations, may occasionally terminate in fatal hemorrhage.

Moreover, severe and even fatal hemorrhage may take place from the vessels of the œsophagus itself, by internal wounds and ruptures, but above all by ulceration, especially when the latter is due to the presence of cancer.

Neureutter and Salmon saw a fatal hemorrhage follow the separation of diph-theritic membrane from the œsophagus of a girl æt. six, suffering from scarlet fever (Oesterr. Jahrb. f. Pädiatrik. N. F. VII. I. 1876). In another case described by the same authors (p. 114), blood was found mixed with the fæces eight days before death, which the autopsy showed to depend on no other cause than a per-forating ulcer of the œsophagus. No complaint of pain on the part of the patient, or any other symptom, had existed during life to arouse suspicion of disease of the œsophagus. E. Wagner observed a profuse effusion of blood in a case of œsopha-gitis complicating variola (Arch. d. Heilk. XIII. Bd. p. 113).

Finally, there remains to be mentioned another very impor-tant source of these severe and even fatal hemorrhages, to which the attention of the profession has only very recently been called; we refer to *varices of the œsophagus*. These varices, situated in the submucous cellular tissue, are quite a common occurrence in elderly persons. Single, or distributed in greater or less number over the entire length of the canal, but, as a rule, more frequently in its upper portion, they appear as sharply-defined, bluish red spots, varying in size from the head of a pin to a lentil, shining through the mucous membrane, or producing mammillation of the same. The blood which they contain can easily be pressed into the plexus of veins, which are normal in size or slightly dilated, by which fact the diagnosis between varix and extravasation is easily established. The mucous membrane itself preserves its normal condition. In certain in-stances, however, these venous dilatations attain an unusual size, particularly in the lowest portion of the tube, where the tortuous and varicose veins may attain the size of a goose-quill, raising the mucous membrane in folds. As a result of rupture of one of these varices, or in consequence of erosion taking place by means of very small ulcers situated at the summit of the varix (*varicose ulcers*, which do not differ essentially from catarrhal ulcers), important hemorrhages (mostly by the mouth) are appa-rently not very unfrequent, and although their arrest is possible, they generally prove rapidly fatal.

Hemorrhage from this cause has been observed very largely—though not exclusively—in cases of *cirrhosis of the liver*. Other forms of atrophy of the liver, as syphilitic hepatitis (Klebs), advanced senile atrophy, and atrophy of the liver produced by tight lacing (Schnuerleber, our own observation) seem also to lead to a still greater development of these varices. There is no reason to doubt that in these cases of cirrhosis of the liver we have to deal with a collateral dilatation of the lower œsophageal veins, which anastomose with the gastric vein, and that through this new channel the obstructed portal blood escapes into the azygos vein.

These hemorrhages have been observed in males and females between the ages of thirty-nine and seventy-one.

The earliest information concerning fatal hemorrhage from varix of the œsophagus is derived from Rokitansky (Medicin. Jahrb. d. oesterr. Staates. Neueste Folge. XXI. Bd. p. 230. 1840). A second case described by Rokitansky (Lehrb. d. path. Anat. 3 Bd. p. 126, 1861), in which frequent attacks of hæmatemesis occurred for two years, probably belongs here, although, in addition to the varices in the dilated œsophagus, there were found hemorrhagic erosions in the stomach. In a previous year (1838) Fauvel saw a similar case, which also occurred with cirrhosis of the liver, and which was afterwards published with another case by Le Diberder (Recueil des trav. de la Soc. méd. d'observat. Fasc. III. 1858. Schmidt's Jahrb. CI. 207). In this last case the patient had already survived one severe attack of hæmatemesis, which first recurred after an interval of fifteen years, and from which the patient seemed to be recovering, when pneumonia set in and caused death. Cirrhosis here, as in a case of Bristowe's (Transact. of the Path. Soc. of London. Vol. VIII. p. 175. 1859. Schmidt's Jahrb. CII. 289). did not exist. Similar cases are communicated by Ebstein (Schmidt's Jahrb. CLXIV. 160. 1874); Fioupe (Bull. de la Soc. anatomique. 1874. p. 100); Hanot (Ibid. 1875. February. Case from Herard's division); Dusaussay (Thèse, Paris, 1877. No. 60. Case from Millard's division); in all of which cirrhosis of the liver existed; vide also Klebs, Handb. d. path. Anat. I. Bd. p. 162. 1868. The whole subject of varices, with their relation to cirrhosis, which Gubler (De la cirrhose, Thèse pour l'aggrégation. Paris, 1853), beginning with Fauvel's case, discussed, has been more minutely treated in the thesis of Dusaussay, already mentioned, as well as in the theses of Audibert (Paris, 1874. No. 146) and Chautemps (1875). Charcot alludes to the subject in his lectures on diseases of the liver (Progrès. médic. 1876. No. 42. p. 703). Finally, Duret (Progrès médic. 1877. No. 16. p. 306), after a very thorough examination of the subject, discusses the anatomical relations of the œsophageal veins, and explains the mechanism of these varices, laying particular emphasis on the close analogy which exists between them and varices of the rectum and anus.

The causal relation of these hemorrhages to cirrhosis of the liver seems, then, from these concordant observations, to be well established. At all events, one occurs very rarely without the other. In Bristowe's very complete case the liver was normal; considerable ascites and marked enlargement of the spleen did exist, however; unfortunately, the portal vein was not examined. In Rokitansky's and Le Diberder's cases the condition of the liver is not mentioned. With respect to the relation existing between other forms of atrophy of the liver and œsophageal varices, the concurrence of the two conditions is, according to our (Zenker) experience, certainly very frequent. In 178 cases in which the autopsy revealed advanced stages of chronic atrophy of the liver in its different forms (especially senile atrophy, and that produced by tight lacing and cicatricial contractions, etc., not including cirrhosis). œsophageal varices were found conjointly forty-three times = twenty-four per cent. (in eighteen cases of cirrhosis only once = five and one-half per cent.). However, these figures do not prove conclusively the dependence of these varices on atrophy of the liver, because the senile atrophies furnish the chief quota of the cases, and a very large proportion of the varices occur in advanced life. Both may well be regarded as effects of one and the same cause, viz., old age, and this is especially true as we found the varices more frequently in the upper portions of the œsophagus.

Diagnosis and Prognosis.

The *diagnosis* of œsophageal hemorrhages is seldom more than a conjecture, and this is based usually on the knowledge of some destructive process taking place in the œsophagus itself, or in its vicinity (cancerous ulcer, ulceration by foreign body). In hemorrhages resulting from varices in the submucous cellular tissue, especially those cases which depend on disturbances in the portal circulation (cirrhosis, syphilis, advanced atrophy of the liver), the diagnosis is exceedingly difficult and almost impossible. The much greater frequency of hemorrhages from the stomach in these diseases will, inasmuch as the source cannot be made out by differential diagnosis, lead us to suppose that they always originate in that organ.

The concurrence of varices in the pharynx with those in the œsophagus is not constant, and does not aid in the diagnosis of the latter, nor of the hemorrhages resulting from them. Equally inconstant are dysphagia and cardialgia, which, according to Frank, taken in connection with pharyngeal varices and hemorrhage, establish the diagnosis of varices of the œsophagus.

The diagnosis of these varicose hemorrhages is rendered still more difficult by the fact, strongly insisted upon by the latest French writers (Audibert, Dusaussay, Charcot), that the clinical phase of hepatic disease is very materially changed, and even obliterated at first, by the collateral dilatation of the veins in the lower third of the œsophagus. Consequently the diagnosis of cirrhosis of the liver, hard enough without this, is made extremely difficult, and often impossible.

The collateral circulation between the gastric vein (which empties into the portal) and the vena azygos, established through the dilated œsophageal veins, may for a long time relieve the portal system to such an extent that ascites does not appear until late in the disease, and remains inconsiderable, as also does œdema of the lower extremities, and that also without any collateral enlargement of the superficial veins of the abdomen. The enlargement of the spleen, however, generally exists in spite of the collateral circulation.

The *prognosis* is always unfavorable if the hemorrhage is at all considerable. In the majority of cases the first or second attack causes death, or at least hastens the already threatening fatal issue.

Treatment.

The treatment of these hemorrhages coincides precisely with that of hemorrhages from the stomach : cold in the form of bladders containing ice to the sternum and epigastrium, or, if the source of the hemorrhage is higher up, to the upper portion of the spine and neck ; also small pieces of ice and ice-water internally. In obstinate cases styptics, especially tincture of the chloride of iron, in doses of five to ten drops, with syrup, may be administered.

The introduction of food through the œsophagus must at first be entirely suspended, and, when the hemorrhage has ceased, milk, especially iced milk, may be allowed, and its use continued for a long time, every other form of nourishment being excluded. According to the observations of Dusaussay, some cases progress favorably on a pure milk diet, and this is especially true of cases in which the hemorrhage recurs. The milk fulfils two important indications : it serves as an excellent means of subsistence, and causes the least possible irritation of the mucous membrane. In the majority of cases it will be necessary to resort to nourishing enemata, since, as might be expected, the copious hemorrhages rapidly reduce the strength of the patient.

INFLAMMATIONS OF THE ŒSOPHAGUS (ŒSOPHAGITIS). ULCERS. GANGRENE.

Bibliography.

Mondière, Arch. génér. T. XXIV. p. 543. 1830; and II. Série. T. III. p. 34. 1833.
—*Oppolzer, Bamberger, Hamburger*, ll. cc.—Hand- und Lehrbücher der path.
Anatomie von *Andral, Rokitansky, Foerster, Klebs, Birch-Hirschfeld.—E. Wagner*, Beitr. z. pathol. Anat. d. Oesophagus. Archiv der Heilk. VIII. Bd. p. 449.
—*Steffen*, Krankheiten des Oesophagus. Jahrb. f. Kinderheilkunde. N. F. 2.
Bd. p. 142. 1869.

Pathology and Etiology.

The mucous membrane of the œsophagus, being well protected by its thick epithelial covering, is very little disposed to inflammatory affections. Such affections do occur, however, in very different forms, but in all these forms they are rare, and in some, extremely rare events. Of the few cases of inflammation observed after death, a considerable number manifested no symptoms whatever during life. The same is true of the remaining coats of the œsophagus, if we except the chronic inflammation of the external cellular covering which results from perforation.

Of the *causes of œsophagitis*, considered as a whole, we may mention, first, the *mechanical, thermal,* and *chemical irritants* of every kind which pass through the canal ; next, the more severe irritations produced by the lodgment of *foreign bodies*, and the destructive action of *corrosive substances* swallowed by accident or design. Besides these may be mentioned *inflammations of neighboring parts*, which extend to the œsophagus either from adjacent mucous surfaces by continuity, or entirely from without (as from the vertebræ, mediastinal connective tissue, lymphatic glands). Finally, inflammation of the œsophagus occasionally occurs as a local manifestation of certain *general diseases*, as cholera, typhus, pyæmia, the acute exanthemata (variola, scarlatina). We have already seen, when speaking of strictures, that the œsophagus is not entirely exempt from syphilis.

In proceeding to discuss the individual forms of inflammation of the œsophageal mucous membrane, anatomically considered, we find the three forms peculiar to inflammation of mucous membranes in general—the catarrhal, the fibrinous (croupons), and the diphtheritic. In addition to these are several other forms, well characterized by their distinct location or their special cause.

Catarrhal Inflammation of the Œsophagus. Desquamative Catarrh of the Œsophagus.

Catarrhal inflammation of the œsophagus, as Klebs very correctly remarks, must be regarded as a type of catarrh very different from that of other mucous membranes, especially that of the stomach. The marked hyperæmia, with the swollen and velvet-like softened mucous membrane and adherent layer of mucus, will not be found. The general proposition, emphasized by Klebs, that lesions of the œsophagus differ in a striking manner from those of other mucous membranes, and bear a certain resemblance to diseases of the skin, possesses peculiar force when applied to this so-called catarrh. Even the name itself, in the absence of any secretion, is not strictly correct, and has been adopted merely because this condition results from the same causes which produce true catarrhs in other mucous membranes. In point of fact, however, when slight inflammatory changes in two mucous membranes are produced by one and the same exciting cause, it seems proper enough to describe both by the same name, even though the appearances underneath the surface are not precisely similar.

Desquamative catarrh of the œsophagus occurs as an acute or chronic affection. The causes of inflammation, specified above in general terms, apply equally to this form. Prominent among these causes are the swallowing of acrid or hot food and drink —whether the direct action of cold by water (Béhier) or ice (Hamburger [1]) produces this form of inflammation, must remain an open question ; the swallowing of foreign bodies, and corrosive substances, which may be comparatively mild in their action—as ammonia, or violent in themselves, but which come in contact with portions of the œsophagus better able to resist their effects. The catarrh may likewise extend from the pharynx and stomach to the œsophagus. It may occur as a non-specific local affection in certain general diseases, by the side of specific lesions, or without such. Finally may be added the catarrhs depending on venous congestion in chronic diseases of the heart. The result of these causes, acting for a short time and not repeated, is the acute form, while the long-continued and recurring causes (as in the intemperate) produce the chronic form. The changes in the calibre of the œsophagus, mentioned in former chapters, act as very strong predisposing causes of the chronic form, inasmuch as they favor the constant accumulation of ingesta ; the same applies to strictures, dilatations, and diverticula of the œsophagus. These conditions may exist for many years, and chronic catarrh then assumes its highest degree of development.

Acute catarrh, which is certainly much more frequent than its insignificant symptoms during life and few well-marked lesions after death would lead us to suppose, consists of a hyperæmia, more or less intense, of the mucous membrane, with thickening, softening, and abundant exfoliation of its epithelial covering, essentially desquamative in its nature. The epithelium presents a dull white, opaque appearance, which has the effect after death to still further conceal the hyperæmic injection of the membrane. A thick layer of mucus, lying on the mucous membrane, is wanting in most cases, but in a certain proportion —and then never in large quantity—it will be found as a compli-

---

[1] Vide *Hamburger*, l. c., pages 63 and 71. The statement that " catching cold," in the ordinary sense, can produce such catarrh, is not proved.

cation when the few mucous glands of the œsophagus, contrary to the general rule, become implicated and swollen (*vide infra*). In many cases the softening of the epithelial covering advances to complete separation of the same in small spots. It is true that the extensive solutions of continuity in the epithelial layer, occasionally found in post-mortem examinations, and principally in the lower third (where the denuded membrane appears smooth, shining, discolored, and tinged with bile), may have originated after death by regurgitation of the contents of the stomach ; the same applies to the longitudinal fissures in the mucous membrane of the contracted œsophagus. But the early appearance of these phenomena after death forces us to conclude that in many cases the separation existed during life ; and certainly those small, sharply defined defects, of the size of a pin-head or lentil, round or longitudinal in form, which are observed in the softened, but otherwise healthy epithelial layer, are true pathological phenomena. These denuded spots then become superficial ulcers (*catarrhal erosion*), and the loss of substance thus commenced may extend to the deeper layers, or may increase in circumference, especially in a longitudinal direction. When the attendant catarrh has pursued a favorable course, these *catarrhal ulcers* are marked by negative signs, especially by the entire absence of all thickening of their edges, and by their smooth, yellowish, cloudy base, confined to the mucous membrane entirely. Under ordinary circumstances they do not involve the deeper layers, and do not lead to perforation. Closely resembling these catarrhal ulcers, and, like them, marked by negative signs only, but, on the other hand, often leading to perforation, are the *ulcerations resulting from* the *impaction* of *foreign bodies* (*Fremdkörpergeschwüre*) and the ulcerations which destroy the wall of a traction diverticulum. These ulcerations will always be accompanied by a local catarrhal inflammation, depending in the one case upon the constant and increasing irritation of the foreign body, and in the other upon the local trouble due to the bulging and partial separation of the mucous membrane from the muscular coat. In the case of a foreign body, it has been observed that the irritation produced by one that is small often causes deeper ulceration and perforation.

These catarrhal erosions and ulcers are especially frequent in pulmonary tuberculosis and phthisis (mostly associated with laryngeal ulcers), and in a large proportion of cases are found in the upper portion, on the anterior wall. There is no doubt, as has occasionally been shown by post-mortem examination, that the simple ulcers, when nothing more than erosions, heal without any visible scar, and that the deeper ulcers leave behind them, on healing, small radiating cicatrices. In certain cases, especially in a traction diverticulum, we find short bands of mucous membrane stretched across the cicatrix, showing that the membrane has been undermined by the ulceration (hence the preference shown by these cicatrices for the point corresponding to the bifurcation of the trachea). When these occur independently of such a diverticulum, they may be traced to a cicatrized ulcer produced by a foreign body.

Chronic catarrh presents essentially the same appearance. It is marked in the beginning by a more intense (livid) hyperæmia, which in time gradually subsides, leaving the epithelial layer much thicker than in the acute form. The secretion from the mucous follicles is more abundant in the chronic form. The brown or slate-colored pigmentation of the membrane, however, which nearly all text-books on pathology and clinical medicine declare to be characteristic of chronic catarrh of the œsophagus (as in the case of the stomach), we are compelled positively to deny. The mucous membrane of the œsophagus is in no way disposed to such pigmentations. We have never in a single case (excluding the small, black spots and livid discoloration caused by carbuncular glands) seen this slate-colored pigmentation ; and when in these instances, as in Luschka's case of enormous diffuse dilatation, "slate-colored stripes and spots" are mentioned (which are not described in the majority of analogous cases), the phenomena presented by such an unusual case ought not to enter into the general description of the disease. This view has been derived from the current and accurate description of chronic catarrh of the stomach, which in this, as in other respects, differs very widely from chronic catarrh of the œsophagus.

In a catarrh which has continued for several years, there is developed, then, a chronic hypertrophied thickening of the mucous membrane, and in rare cases (Cruveilhier, Luschka) it progresses to the formation of polypous, villous, and papillary growths (in this respect the analogy with chronic catarrh of the stomach is complete). With this thickening of the mucous membrane is associated, in most cases, an hypertrophy of the muscular coat which is generally inconsiderable, but sometimes, and especially when complicated with dilatation of the tube, is well marked.

Finally, ulcers sometimes form in chronic catarrh, and resemble in every essential particular those already described ; but in some instances, where the irritation is continuous and intense—as in diffuse dilatation from the presence of the decomposed ingesta —they attain a more considerable development, as regards number, size, and depth, and by the invasion of one of the larger blood-vessels give rise to hemorrhages. These chronic catarrhal ulcers have never in any noticeable manner led to perforation of the wall of the œsophagus, as also in the case of pressure diverticula, when the mucous membrane is intensely affected by the catarrh, perforation has never been observed. The great thickening and consolidation of the coats from hypertrophy, especially of the external cellular coat, may account for the remarkable resistance which they show against such constant and powerful exciting causes.

As a more remote result of severe chronic catarrh, we see now and then a relaxation of the entire tube, in consequence of which it loses its perpendicular course and inclines with a slight curvature to the right side of the thorax. This condition depends upon impaired power of contraction in the hypertrophied muscular coat, and hence the supposition that chronic catarrh may lie at the bottom of diffuse dilatation is quite probable, although not clearly demonstrable, since the catarrh in such cases may also be regarded as the result of the dilatation.

The opposite theory, which the text-books have somewhat reluctantly advanced, that simple catarrh, by the consecutive hypertrophy, especially of the muscular coat, may lead to a special form of stricture of the œsophagus—a theory which rests upon certain statements of Albers, which Foerster has accepted without objection—we have already (vide Stenoses) estimated at its true value.

Intimately connected with catarrhal, and, as we have seen, desquamative œsophagitis, is another form of inflammation, represented thus far by *one* case which has been published by Birch-Hirschfeld,[1] in which the most rapid and complete exfoliation of the epithelial layer, very different from the gradual, imperceptible exfoliation of catarrh, took place.

A hysterical, but otherwise healthy woman, without any suspicion of poisoning, was taken sick with pain in the neck, dysphagia, malaise, and febrile symptoms; on the third day, after considerable choking, there came up a membranous tube, about 20 ctms. in length (corresponding to two-thirds of the length of the œsophagus), which Birch-Hirschfeld showed by microscopical examination to be the epithelial covering in toto, normal in its upper layers, but thickly studded with round cells in the lower layers. Complete recovery gradually followed. This was a case of very acute subepithelial suppuration, which led to removal of the epithelial covering.

It is very probable that many cases hitherto regarded as true croup of the œsophagus are to be ascribed to this pseudo-croupous form of inflammation[2] which, as a matter of course, can be distinguished from the former only by microscopical examination.

Follicular Inflammation of the Œsophagus. (Inflammation folliculeuse, *Mondière.*) Follicular Catarrh.

Mondière, Arch. génér. II. Série. T. III. p. 34. 1833.

The mucous follicles of the œsophagus, few in number, as is well known, irregularly distributed over the mucous membrane, and arranged in short, longitudinal rows, are occasionally found perceptibly swollen, either singly or in groups, and more frequently in the upper portion of the tube. They form, then, according to the shape of the follicle, somewhat hard, conical, or oblong nodules, which cause the mucous membrane to project above its level. By pressure, a drop of viscid mucus can be made to exude from them upon the mucous surface, and when the

---

[1] Lehrb. d. pathol. Anatomie. p. 818. 1877.

[2] This term, used by *Birch-Hirschfeld*, may suffice in this one case, but the use of these pseudo names, which only signify what the thing appears, but is not, and not what it is, is somewhat uncertain and slightly confusing.

number of follicles thus affected is small, there will be found a slight quantity only of mucus adhering to the mucous membrane. Microscopical examination shows very distinctly the excretory duct of the follicle occluded by mucus and cells, and sometimes the connective tissue about the same infiltrated with round cells. The mucous membrane over the nodules is either normal, pallid, or it shows (in rare cases) a ring of congestion about the nodule ; or, finally, ulcers about the size of a pin-head or somewhat larger may form, so that the gland is exposed and more or less destroyed by ulcerative process (*follicular ulcers*). Whether these ulcers increase in size, or involve the deeper tissues, it is scarcely possible to ascertain, because they differ in no respect, after destruction of the follicle, from the catarrhal ulcers above described, and moreover, the two forms may exist side by side.

In doubtful cases the arrangement of the little ulcers, as sometimes occurs, in short longitudinal rows (corresponding to the similar arrangement of the follicles), proves them to be follicular.

Follicular catarrh may occur, as before remarked, in connection with acute or chronic desquamative catarrh. But it occurs quite independently, as Mondière very correctly emphasizes, without any change whatever in the rest of the mucous membrane, and hence must be regarded as a special form of disease. Concerning its etiology, nothing more can be said now than was said in the time of Mondière. Roederer and Wagler saw several cases in the well-known epidemic of typhus fever at Göttingen, and Mondière suspected, probably with good reason, that the œsophageal ulcers, seen by Louis in typhus fever patients, were referable to this cause. However, it cannot occur frequently in typhus, since it is not once mentioned by the latest authorities on this affection, notably C. E. E. Hoffmann [1] in his careful analysis of two hundred and fifty autopsies of typhoid fever. We saw it in a case of tubercular basilar meningitis, in an adult, but we have seen it more frequently in other cases, where no special relation could be proved between this and any distinct forms of

---

[1] Untersuch. üb. d. path.-anat. Veränderungen der Organe beim Abdominaltyphus. Leipzig, 18C9.

disease. Mondière mentions the frequent occurrence of this affection in croup. Billard saw it very well marked in a new-born
infant, which survived only one day. The occurrence of follicular
catarrh in mania, which many of the earlier authors assert, and
upon which they lay great stress, does not appear to be confirmed
in recent times, since we find no mention of it whatever in the
latest reports on this subject, or in modern systematic treatises
on this disease (Virchow, Reder, Bollinger). Further careful
attention to the subject must throw much light on the etiology
of this affection.

Fibrinous (Croupous) and Diphtheritic Inflammations of the Œsophagus.

These two forms of inflammation—the names being taken in
the ordinary anatomical sense: the former being characterized by
the fibrinous false membrane on the mucous surface, the latter
by thick, firm infiltration of the tissue of the mucous membrane,
with consecutive ulceration — occur in the œsophagus, seldom
involving its whole extent, generally a very limited portion. Inasmuch as these two forms are frequently combined, or in a
certain sense alternate with one another, so that by the side of
a fibrinous deposit on one mucous membrane, diphtheritic infiltration will be found simultaneously on another, showing that
both forms are due to the same cause, we shall include both in
one common description.

Fibrinous membranes, as well as diphtheritic infiltrations, are
found scattered over the mucous membrane, more frequently in
its upper portion, and appear almost invariably either as irregularly defined islands, or as longitudinal stripes, which correspond
to the height of the mucous folds. Very rarely they are diffused
over a larger extent of surface, and include even the entire periphery of the tube.

In many published cases of extensive croupous membrane, involving the entire
length of the œsophagus, it has undoubtedly been mistaken for thrush, which can
be distinguished from the soft croupous membrane, not always with certainty by
the naked eye, but very easily by the microscope. A further source of fallacy

has been disclosed by establishing the existence of the "pseudo-croupous inflammation" above described.

The diphtheritic deposits are occasionally liable to erosion, or, by complete separation of the dried exudation, may be converted into deep, irregular ulcers (*diphtheritic ulcers*), the nature of which is made out from the fibrinous deposits or exudation adhering to the edge of the ulcer, or existing in other parts of the œsophagus or pharynx ; these ulcers can give rise to dangerous hemorrhages (*vide* Hemorrhages). Underneath these more or less adherent, gray or brownish gray deposits, the mucous membrane is sometimes reddened, at other times apparently quite normal, and rarely infiltrated by the diphtheritic process.

The two cases described by E. Wagner as phlegmonous œsophagitis (Arch. d. Heilk. VIII. Bd. p. 464), may well be regarded as a modified hemorrhagic form of diphtheritic inflammation.

In regard to the *occurrence* and *etiology* of fibrino-diphtheritic œsophagitis, it may be stated that it is never a primary form of disease, produced by causes acting directly on the mucous membrane, but invariably a secondary affection—sometimes being directly continued from the pharynx, the more frequent location of this form of inflammation, and the upper portion only of the œsophagus will then be involved—sometimes independently of any pharyngeal trouble, which may or may not exist, but widely separated from such, it appears as the expression of an acute or chronic general disease. Of the acute general diseases to which it is incident may be mentioned *typhus* [abdominalis] *fever*, *cholera* (in the stage of reaction, although it does sometimes occur early in the disease : we saw it in a man seventy-three years of age, who died twenty-four hours after the invasion), *measles*, *scarlatina* (in which it may be the continued, and hence, in a more restricted sense, the diphtheritic form), *small-pox* (Andral, Bamberger, who saw the most extensive croupous deposits in this disease, E. Wagner), and *pyæmia* (E. Wagner). Among chronic general diseases, or local diseases which become general, we ourselves and others (especially E. Wagner and Steffen) have seen it in *pulmonary tuberculosis ;* in an insane person with *cardiac disease*, who died of croupous pneumonia ; in *Bright's disease*, car-

cinoma, suppurative arthritis, suppurative pyelitis ; in *infil-tration of urine* following stricture of the urethra with croupous diphtheritic pyelitis ; and finally, to a greater extent in an *atro-phied* girl, six weeks old, who died from obstruction of the air-passages, caused by inspiration of the contents of the stomach. Steffen,[1] who observed this form of inflammation very frequently in children, saw it repeatedly in *circumscribed pneumonia* and *intestinal catarrh.*

From true *diphtheria* (in its clinical sense), however, the œso-phagus shows a remarkable degree of exemption. As a rule, in the very worst cases, the line of demarcation is sharply drawn at the inferior boundary of the pharynx, and the œsophagus escapes. This exemption is very strikingly exhibited in cases where the inflammation, after spreading extensively over the air-passages, fauces, and pharynx, jumps over the œsophagus entirely, and attacks the mucous membrane of the stomach, which is so little liable to this affection.

We saw this in one of the worst cases of diphtheria that ever occurred to us : a strong woman (thirty-nine years of age, who had taken care of her two children, both of whom died from diphtheria), was herself taken down by the disease four-teen days after, and on the fifth day tracheotomy was performed on account of the severe dyspnœa, but she died on the second day after the operation. In this case the larynx, trachea, soft palate, fauces and pharynx were found entirely covered with thick false membrane, with a distinct line of demarcation at the beginning of the œsophagus, which was perfectly normal throughout, while at the cardiac ex-tremity of the stomach were found several well-marked croupous deposits, about the size of a pea, on the intensely red mucous membrane. A very similar case is quoted by E. Wagner, from West.

This exemption, however, is by no means complete. On the contrary, the disease occasionally extends from the pharynx to the upper portion of the œsophagus, or stretches as far as the cardiac extremity of the same (West[2]), or, passing this boundary, even to the stomach itself (Andral,[3] girl twelve years old).

---

[1] *Steffen* (l. c.) reports 44 autopsies in children, in 15 of which disease of the œso-phagus in some form was observed. The statistics on this point, however, are not sufficient as yet to decide the question whether the œsophagus of the child is, in so large a proportion, predisposed to disease.

[2] Pathol. u. Therapie d. Kinderkrankh. Deutsch von Wegner. Berlin, 1853. p. 217.

[3] Anatomie pathologique. T. II. Paris, 1829. p. 161.

E. Wagner (l. c.) found this extension of the deposit to the upper portion of the œsophagus in two out of about eighty autopsies, where death occurred from diphtheria. We found it (in a much smaller number of examinations) only twice; in one case, a woman forty-two years old, there were gray membranous deposits in abundance in the upper portion, single clusters below, with similar deposits in the pharynx, while the larynx and trachea escaped entirely; in the other case, a boy eleven years old, were found superficial ulcers, some small and round, others in the form of longitudinal stripes, together with similar ulcers, covered with bacteria, in the pharynx, and ulcers with membranous deposits in the larynx (besides ichorous infiltration of the sub-maxillary glands and cellular tissue of the neck, nephritis, pneumonia, etc.).

Whether the cicatrization of these diphtheritic ulcers is fol lowed by narrowing of the œsophagus, as Leube and Penzoldt[1] suppose, on the ground of a case observed by them, and cured by the introduction of the sound, and, as seems in point of fact very probable, must from lack of evidence remain an open question. But certainly, after what has been stated above, it must be acknowledged as possible.

The case occurred in a young woman twenty-one years old, who had complained of slight difficulty in swallowing for four years. After an illness diagnosed "Quinsy sore throat," which followed a severe pneumonia, she noticed, as convalescence began, an increasing dysphagia, so that finally she was able to swallow fluids only, and became perceptibly emaciated. On the surface of the palate were found white cicatricial marks, and on the fauces the same were found thicker and convergent. The introduction of a sound proved conclusively the existence of numerous contractions in the lower portion of the œsophagus. After treatment by the use of the sound, continued for five weeks, and commenced with the finest bougie, she recovered entirely.

Variolous (or Pustulous) Inflammation of the Œsophagus. Œsophageal Pock.

In addition to the non-specific form of catarrh, or croupousdiphtheritic inflammation of the œsophagus, already mentioned, as seen in variola, there occurs not unfrequently a specific variolous eruption in this same tube.

---

[1] Klinische Berichte von der medicin. Abtheil. des Landkrankenhauses zu Jena. Erlangen, Besold. 1875. p. 125.

E. Wagner (Arch. d. Heilk. XIII. Bd. p. 112) found pock in the œsophagus twenty times in about 170 examinations of small-pox patients, and that in considerable number. We saw them twice in a small number of such examinations, both times in old people (sixty and sixty-eight years).

The eruption appears in the œsophagus as elevations (papules), about the size of a hemp-seed, scattered over the entire mucous membrane, and sometimes, especially in the upper portion of the tube, standing close together; the mucous membrane between them retains its normal condition. These papules consist of circumscribed red spots in the mucous membrane, due to congestion or hemorrhage, infiltrated on their surface or slightly granular, while the epithelial covering is thickened, softened, and clouded (but not raised in the form of vesicles). The slightly adherent epithelial layer is easily removed, and then, in place of the papules, will be found small, round imperfections in the otherwise intact membrane; the red spots are laid bare, and by erosion are converted into small, flat, *variolous ulcers*. At no stage in this affection is there any vesicular elevation of the epithelial layer — because the exudation forces itself between the loose layers of epithelium—and therefore the designation of these eruptions as pustules is very erroneous, as Virchow[1] demonstrated long ago. In their nature, however, they are unquestionably identical with the eruptions as they appear on the skin, and consequently their description as œsophageal pock is entirely correct.

When such cases recover, scarcely any traces whatever of the disease remain, inasmuch as losses of substance so superficial as these can heal without visible cicatrices. The statement made by Hamburger (l. c., p. 146), that this cicatrization can produce fatal contraction, is founded, as we remarked above (*vide* Stenoses), solely upon a wrong interpretation of an old and very imperfect publication by Lanzoni.

A "pustular" eruption, similar in all essential respects to that of variola, but confluent as well, occurs, according to Rokitansky, in the lower third of the œsophagus, as a consequence of the internal administration of tartar emetic in large doses.

---

[1] Deutsche Klinik. 1858. No. 31. p. 306.

Phlegmonous (Purulent) Inflammation of the Œsophagus.

Purulent inflammation of the submucous cellular tissue, as described in current phraseology, assumes the same form in the œsophagus as it does in the stomach (Vol. VII. p. 392), and, like the latter, is an extremely rare occurrence, at least in its more severe forms. In the œsophagus, however, the disease is limited at times to smaller, more circumscribed spaces ; at other times it extends over large tracts — in fact, over the entire length and periphery of the tube, and may continue, through the cardiac orifice, far into the stomach itself (Belfrage and Hedenius[1]), as conversely phlegmonous gastritis may secondarily attack the œsophagus (Ackermann[2]). The circumscribed and diffuse forms of the disease differ only in extent.

The process begins with a purulent infiltration, by which the submucous layer becomes very much thickened (even to the extent of 9 mm., Belfrage and Hedenius), and its tissue so disguised that it appears as a pure layer of pus, while microscopical examination shows the bundles of cellular tissue between the purulent masses to be still intact. As the disease advances the tissue breaks down completely, and in place of the submucous layer there exists a cavity, in the form of a crevice, filled with pus. In consequence of the forcible distention of the submucous cellular tissue, the mucous membrane will, when the purulent collections are small, be thrown into little prominences, or, in case the infiltration involves the entire periphery, it will project inward on all sides. While in the former case there is no actual stricture, inasmuch as the greatest part of the tube is still capable of dilatation at the level of the purulent collection, and allows the food to pass; in the latter, contraction may exist to such an extent that the end of the little finger can only with difficulty be introduced into the canal.

The mucous membrane is not essentially involved in the process. It is either normal or divested of its epithelium, or con-

---

[1] Upsala läkarefören. förhandl. VIII. 3 p. 245. 1873. Schmidt's Jahrb. Bd. 160. p. 33.

[2] Virchow's Archiv. Bd. 45. p. 39.

gested on account of a fresh infiltration and covered with more
or less mucus.

In a single case only (in a tuberculous patient) we found the mucous membrane,
in the lowest portion of the œsophagus, over a group of small abscesses, extensively
diphtheritic, which is either to be regarded as an accidental combination, or else the
abscesses are to be considered as secondary to the diphtheria (never the reverse).

The muscular coat, likewise, appears intact to the naked eye,
but microscopical examination shows that the smaller purulent
deposits have encroached upon it from the submucous layer.

After a time this purulent infiltration results either in degeneration and complete destruction of the pus-corpuscles, or in
bacterian vegetations (for which, in this affection, scarcely any
cause can be ascribed), or in inspissation of the pus. On the
other hand, the suppurative process may result in the pus bursting through the mucous membrane, which in the more extensive
infiltrations takes place at several points unequally distributed
over the collection, so that when these perforations lie close
together the membrane presents a sieve-like appearance (phlegmonous ulcer).

The pus having made its escape in this way, recovery generally follows. In the case of the smaller abscesses this takes place
in such a manner, that by cicatrization of the perforation the
undermined mucous membrane assumes its normal relation to
the muscular coat, and scarcely anything remains but the small
cicatrices (at the most a slight thickening of the submucous
layer). In cases, however, where the undermining has been
more extensive, recovery takes place in a different way, and
leaves behind certain singular and characteristic effects, which
again resemble, in a high degree, those remaining after recovery
from phlegmonous gastritis. The crevice-like cavity, produced
by the purulent degeneration of the submucous cellular tissue,
which undermines the mucous membrane, remains, as also do the
openings in this membrane. The internal surface of the cavity,
sometimes spanned by single bridge-like cords, is quite smooth,
and lined throughout with an epithelial layer precisely similar to
that of the œsophagus, which extends also to the openings; even
the papillæ seem not to be wanting. Thus, then, the cavity

remains with its completely organized wall, communicating with the lumen of the œsophagus by several round, sharply defined apertures, varying in size from the head of a pin to a cherry-stone—to a certain extent like an intraparietal diverticulum with several mouths. No secondary dilatation of these cavities (as in diverticula produced by pressure) seems to occur. Moreover, other disastrous results of this condition (either from foreign bodies becoming lodged, or decomposition of the ingesta) appear at least not to be frequent. At all events, in the four cases observed by us, there was nothing of the kind to be seen.

Extensive sloughs, burrowings in the mediastina, perforation of the pleura, etc. (Klebs), such as frequently occur after complete rupture of the œsophageal wall from different causes (*vide supra*), have not been seen by us as results of phleg-monous œsophagitis, and we can find no proofs of their occurrence in the literature of the subject. Such a theory is devoid of probability, since it is scarcely possible, in this form of disease, for the pus to make its way outward into the mediastinum (excluding only such cases as result from sulphuric acid poisoning, in which it is a question of more complicated events). Where, then, a perforation of the external layers exists, it appears, as we shall presently see, that this itself is the primary cause, which introduces the phlegmonous œsophagitis.

With regard now to the *causes* of the phlegmonous œsopha-gitis, first of all to be mentioned is the irritation produced by the impaction of foreign bodies, and that, whether they have actually penetrated the submucous layer, or have caused no wound what-ever capable of demonstration (case of Belfrage and Hedenius : fish-bone sticking fast, with no wound of the mucous membrane visible after death).

More frequently, however, the cause appears to lie in the bursting of the peri-œsophageal collections of pus (glandular abscesses, perichondritis cricoidea, abscess of the vertebræ, Klebs), and especially of softened masses of caseous lymphatic glands, into the external coverings of the œsophagus. In these perforations, which extend by layers from without inward, the submucous appears to be the only covering in the œsophageal wall which is adapted to the diffusion of pus. Moreover, this diffusion takes place before the perforation has made its way through the mucous membrane. Then, when the phlegmonous inflammation is fully established, but not dependent on this in any way, the mucous membrane is finally perforated, as the result solely of the extension inward of the original morbid process. We find, then, on making the autopsy, phlegmonous inflammation and perforation of the mucous membrane side by side, not dependent the one on the other, but both as effects of the same cause (Compare Case I., given below). It is now generally conceded that these peri-œsophageal collections of pus and softened glands, while they burst in the direction of the œsophagus, may at the same time force their way in another direction and perforate a second hollow organ, as the larynx (by perichondritis laryngea), or the trachea (from softened glands). In this way direct communication is established between the œsophagus on one side, and the larynx or trachea on the other, which, after the cure of the coexistent inflammation, may continue as narrow fistulous openings between the two (compare Case II., given below); and yet the fistula is not to be regarded as the result of the œsophagitis. Here, too, it is a question only of co-effects of the same cause.

Furthermore, phlegmonous œsophagitis occurs as a partial phenomenon of corrosive inflammation (*vide infra*), and peculiarly so in severe cases of sulphuric acid poisoning, when it will be found under the gangrenous mucous membrane. Whether other inflammations of the mucous membrane can superinduce this, as an advanced form, must remain in doubt. The case already mentioned, of diphtheritic infiltration combined with small abscesses, admits of such construction, but can, as remarked, be regarded also as an accidental coincidence.

Moreover, as was already mentioned, this form of inflammation occurs as an extension of phlegmonous *gastritis* to the œsophagus (Ackermann).

In conclusion, we found the changes in question, especially the circumscribed abscesses, in some cases where the autopsy failed to demonstrate any local cause, and nearly all these occurred in phthisical patients.

The single exception to this rule occurred in a syphilitic woman, forty-one years old, in whom the above described residua of a cicatrized abscess were found in the lowest portion of the œsophagus, along with specific lesions in numerous parts (cicatrices in the pharynx, larynx, etc.); a chronic mediastinitis postica, the results of which were found in the form of a hard cord, uniting the vena azygos and right lung firmly together, might possibly have had some connection with the disease of the œsophagus.

The preceding description of phlegmonous œsophagitis is founded upon the typical case of Belfrage and Hedenius, already quoted several times,—closely observed and described by them clinically and anatomically,—upon ten of our own cases (Zenker), which presented the different forms and degrees of the disease, and upon a few brief notices elsewhere published. These eleven cases occurred in individuals between the ages of 24 and 71, about equally distributed within these limits, and of these nine were men and two women, so that (as Leube maintains concerning phlegmonous gastritis, Vol. VII. p. 157) its remarkable predominance in the male sex is fully established. Two of our cases exhibited diffuse purulent infiltration, more or less recent (in one involving the entire œsophagus) ; four cases showed circumscribed abscesses (from the size of a pea to the length of 2 ctms., and breadth of 1 ctm.) ; four cases showed the characteristic results of purulent undermining. In regard to causes, one case resulted from corrosion by sulphuric acid, one case certainly (probably three cases) from perforation by a softened caseous gland, and the rest without any special cause that could be made out (phthisical persons, and one in a case of syphilis of long standing).

Inasmuch as so little has been published concerning *phlegmonous œsophagitis* in general, we may be allowed to give in detail the reports of the two most important of our cases, and to add a short epitome of the case seen by Belfrage and Hedenius.

Case I.—Anna K., thirty years old, unmarried, an inmate of the asylum at Erlangen, on account of epileptic insanity of long standing, was taken ill the last of April, 1877, coughed considerably, and physical examination, very incomplete, owing to the struggles of the patient, revealed extensive bronchial respiration posteriorly. From June, since which time no further epileptic attacks have occurred, she kept her bed most of the time, and took scarcely anything but liquid food (wine, meatbroths, and a large quantity of water) ; at times sweet things and a little meat. No difficulty in swallowing was ever noticed. Whether her refusal to take food depended on pain in swallowing could not be made out, because she very often threw the food aside untouched, when she did not wish to eat. Profuse diarrhœa supervened ; during the last eight days she vomited twice. Marked fœtor from the mouth. Fluids could still be taken on the day before her death. Died July 19th.

Autopsy (July 20, 1877, thirty hours after death, Zenker) revealed the following surprising condition of the œsophagus and its surroundings ; and to show the bearing of this on the more complex results of the autopsy, we premise all the lesions found :

Slight recent pachymeningitis hæmorrhagica. Marked anæmia of the brain and its membranes. Small cicatrix in the cortical substance of the brain. Double cheesy pneumonia. Slight pleuritis on left side. Diminished size of heart and large vessels. Anomaly of the right subclavian artery (dysphagia lusoria). Purulent, cheesy, phlegmonous inflammation of the œsophagus. Perforation of the œsophagus, as also of the trachea and both bronchi, from cheesy tracheal and bronchial glands. Cheesy enlargement of the mesenteric glands. Slight tubercular ulceration of the small intestine. Simple atrophy of the liver and kidneys. Extensive obstructive thrombosis, of long standing, of the vena cava inferior, iliac, and femoral veins. Œdema of both lower extremities. Trichocephalus dispar.

Mucous membrane of *pharynx* slightly congested, normal. From the pharynx the little finger enters with some difficulty the opening of the *œsophagus*. The latter is much contracted in its entire length, decreasing towards the lower portion. Externally its wall, posteriorly, is discolored, somewhat black. On section, the œsophageal wall appears thickened in its upper portion to the extent of 7-8 mm., somewhat less below, by a dirty yellowish gray infiltration of the submucous tissue, soft and caseous above, softer farther down, and finally, purulent entirely. The mucous membrane, in its upper portion, is of a light slate color, with some slightly enlarged veins, otherwise normal; the lower half is much injected, and covered with thin gray mucus. 5.5 ctms. below the inferior border of the cricoid cartilage (exactly at the spot where the right subclavian artery, arising abnormally as the last branch to the left of the arch of the aorta, crosses the œsophagus on the left side of the anterior wall), is a perforation 1.5 ctms. long and about 5 mm. broad, with a smooth border of mucous membrane, not thickened. This leads into a cavity, about the size of a cherry-stone, which contains some yellowish, cheesy fragments, partly loose and partly adherent to the wall. Outside this cavity is a border of callous, slate-colored cellular tissue, and a couple of caseous tracheal glands, about the size of a cherry-stone. From this cavity the mucous membrane is partially undermined for about 8 mm., but without communication with any neighboring part, especially the trachea. Immediately below the perforation is a superficial ulcer, 6 mm. long and 3 mm. broad, with a border somewhat ecchymosed. Microscopical examination of the fluid purulent infiltration of the submucous tissue shows numerous (although not crowded together), delicate spherical cells, with a single nucleus (pus globules), besides a very large number of the finest molecules with well-marked dancing motion (detritus mixed with numerous micrococci), with larger globules consisting of short stelliform needle-crystals; and finally, numerous triple phosphate crystals in the cellular tissue. In the dry, cheesy portion of the infiltration scarcely any distinct pus-corpuscles were found, but simply the finely granular masses (detritus with micrococci); and everywhere, obscuring the preparation entirely, were found numerous thick needles of fatty acid, some very long, and not affected by the addition of soda.

The mucous membrane of the *larynx* is pale, but normal; that of the *trachea* mostly normal, except on the posterior wall, opposite the perforation of the œsophagus, where it is of a grayish color. In the lowest portion of the trachea, exactly over the beginning of the right bronchus, on the right wall, are two sharply-defined perforations, one large enough to admit a probe, the other the size of a lentil, around which the mucous membrane is much congested and somewhat ecchymosed. These openings lead into a narrow, crevice-like cavity, immediately adjacent to the tracheal and bronchial walls, which is bounded on other sides by a nodular, cheesy

mass, larger than a cherry. This mass proves to be a caseous tracheal gland, surrounded by a tough capsule, the cheesy parenchyma of which is closely adherent
to the capsule, but in the direction of the trachea is entirely detached from it by a
cleft in the mass, whereby the crevice-like cavity is produced. The mucous membrane of the *right bronchus*, in its middle portion, is ulcerated, with ill-defined
limits, to the extent of 1.5 ctms. in length, and 4–7 mm. in breadth; the base of
the ulcer consists of detached portions of caseous glands; one cartilaginous ring is
exposed and necrosed. Beneath the point where the bronchus of the right upper
lobe is given off is a well-defined perforation, size of a pea, which leads into a cavity, lying on the bronchus, and enclosed by lung-tissue (softened bronchial gland);
in this cavity lie two rough, chalky concretions. In the *left bronchus*, near its bifurcation, is a perforation, size of the head of a pin, from which cheesy fragments of
a gland exude. In the bronchi is abundant tough mucus; mucous membrane of
same, for the most part, intensely congested. The bifurcation distended by large
conglomerations of glands, which press very strongly upon the pericardium, and on
the other side upon the œsophagus. Other bronchial and tracheal glands, especially
on the right side, combined in large parcels, enlarged, caseous to a great extent, and
softened in places; the pleura covering them extremely vascular in parts, ruptured in one place, and intensely livid about the point of rupture. In the anterior
mediastinum, under the manubrium sterni, is a large mass of caseous glands.

There can be no doubt that in this case there existed primarily a perforation of
the trachea and bronchi on one side, and of the œsophagus on the other, produced
by caseous degeneration of the bronchial glands; and secondarily, a phlegmonous
œsophagitis was set up at the point of rupture, which extended over the whole tube.
Examination of the purulent infiltration, with or without the microscope, showed
that this condition had existed for a long time, certainly for weeks.

Case II.—John F., fifty-four years old, teacher, was treated at the Medical Clinique in Erlangen, for disease of the vertebræ and myelitis, and died June 20, 1874.
Autopsy sixteen hours after death (Zenker).

Lesions : *Caseous ostitis, periostitis and caries of the seventh to ninth cervical vertebræ. Caseous pachymeningitis externa spinalis. Softening of the spinal cord, with
displacement. Moderate chronic hydrocephalus. Hemorrhagic cicatrix in left corpus
striatum. Small amount of recent encephalitis in left hemisphere. Miliary tubercles
in pleuræ (corresponding to the periosteal cheesy collections). Pulmonary tuberculosis.
Emphysema and œdema of lungs. Ulceration of surface of lungs (from the cheesy collections). Perforation of trachea from peri-tracheal collection of pus. Miliary tubercles on the mucous membrane of the trachea, at the point of bifurcation. Cured phlegmonous œsophagitis. Liver moderately fatty. Enlargement of spleen. Tubercles in
the kidneys. Catarrh of the bladder. Cheesy nodules in the mucous membrane of the
small intestine. Enlargement and partial caseous degeneration of the mesenteric
glands. United fracture of the tibia.*

The phenomena relating to the œsophagus were as follows: mucous membrane
of *pharynx* pale, normal. *Œsophagus* slightly dilated, especially in its upper half;
mucous membrane slightly congested, studded with numerous papillæ, about the

size of the head of a pin. Over its upper half are distributed irregularly seven well-defined round openings in the mucous membrane, varying in size from the head of a pin to a cherry-stone; around some of these openings the mucous membrane is undermined in all directions, while in other places the undermining extends only in one direction. The largest of these submucous cavities, produced by the undermining, is 2 ctms. long, 1 ctm. wide, and communicates by three openings with the œsophagus. The edges of these openings have a superficial covering, and the inner surface of the cavities is smooth throughout, white, covered with a thick layer of epithelium, which resembles exactly that of the œsophagus (also shows characteristic ribbed cells), and is directly continuous with it. The papillæ are very distinct. At the bottom of some of these cavities are found one or more fine openings, entering which a very fine probe passes through narrow fistulous passages into peri-œsophageal cavities, bounded by thickened tendinous cellular tissue, the largest of which cavities (2 ctms. long, 5 mm. wide) lies between the œsophagus and thyroid gland, while the rest are lodged more deeply between the œsophagus and the trachea. One of the latter, in which an ossified cartilaginous ring of the trachea is exposed, opens on the other side into the *trachea* by a fistula large enough to admit a fine probe, about in the middle of its left wall, so that communication exists between the œsophagus and trachea. The mucous membrane of the trachea is about 5 mm. thick in the vicinity of this fistulous opening, studded with miliary tubercles, while the remaining portion shows bright red injection, increasing lower down. The *glands* at the bifurcation are detached, spotted black and gray. The soft parts covering the *vertebral column* from the fourth dorsal vertebra to the diaphragm project forward and towards both sides in the form of a tumor. The pleuræ studded with miliary tubercles. The subpleural cellular tissue much thickened. On section, we come to a very extensive, conglomerate, caseous collection, anterior to as well as by the side of the vertebræ, in which are found numerous cheesy fragments of bone, some detached, others loosely adherent, and through which the finger introduced passes into the carious and fissured vertebræ.

From the result of the autopsy it was very evident that a purulent mediastinitis had developed as a consequence of the caries of the spine, and this had led to rupture into the trachea on one side, and into the œsophagus on the other. From these various perforations a phlegmonous inflammation had spread over large spaces, which, after rupture of the mucous membrane and evacuation of the pus, had subsided, leaving behind the sinuous cavities.

Case described by Belfrage and Hedenius (loc cit.): A woman, forty-two years old, of good constitution, in her fifth month of pregnancy, stated that in consequence of lodgment of a fish-bone, which caused a sensation of scraping, she had a severe chill, and simultaneously sharp pain in the chest, with considerable fever. They were described as sharp pains, starting from the stomach and lower part of the œsophagus, and extending around the left side as far as the back. There were occasional attempts, but no actual vomiting. Epigastrium very tender. The patient said nothing more about the fish-bone; she did not complain specially of difficulty in swallowing, and no foreign body could be detected. The remedies employed caused no improvement in her condition. The pains, which became more spasmodic, were very severe, so that she was obliged to sit up from fear of suffocation. On the third day she was much worse; increased pains, cyanosis, dyspnœa, pulse small and frequent, skin hot, urine moderately albuminous. In the evening premature delivery occurred, with pretty considerable loss of blood. Death took place on the morning of the fourth day of the disease. The *autopsy* revealed (besides aortic stenosis and large fluid effusion tinged with blood in both pleural cavities) the following condition of the *œsophagus* (nothing unusual outside): its wall, commencing at a point about 6 ctms. below the cricoid cartilage and extending to the cardiac extremity of the stomach, was much thickened (8–12 mm., and that exclusively by thickening of the submucous tissue [5–9 mm.]), which on section was homogeneous, grayish yellow, smooth, shining and pulpy, and on pressure gave exit to considerable grayish yellow, dark pus. The internal surface presented slight knoll-like prominences. Mucous membrane of normal thickness, smooth and even, anæmic, but without other change, notably without any sign of irritation by a foreign body. The purulent infiltration extended 8 ctms. beyond the cardiac extremity upon the small curvature of the stomach. Microscopical examination showed only slight traces of epithelium in the œsophagus; in the submucous tissue the cellular-tissue bundles were very perceptible, but widely separated by pus; the pus-corpuscles were in part well preserved, in part fatty. The purulent infiltration had likewise extended between the bundles of muscular tissue.

Corrosive Inflammation of the Œsophagus.

Rokitansky, Lehrb. d. pathol. Anat. 3 Bd. p. 158. 1861.

The intensely corrosive fluids, which chiefly come to our notice in this connection in the form of the concentrated mineral acids (especially sulphuric and nitric), and the salts of potash and soda, produce direct action upon the mucous membranes with which they come in close contact, and in cases where these reagents have been swallowed this action is plainly seen in the œsophagus, not altogether as inflammation, but as direct sloughing. Notwithstanding the fact that the portions of mucous membrane which do not always slough are less intimately affected than the parts lying underneath the gangrenous layer, they still exhibit evident signs of inflammatory changes so soon after the occurrence, and if life continues can be so much further developed, that we are justified in regarding it as a complicated and modified process of inflammation, caused by sloughing of a part of the tissue. This we shall describe as corrosive inflammation.

The effects of *sulphuric acid*, which come most frequently under observation, are (next to the stomach, which shows the most marked changes owing to longer contact with the acid) most intensely developed in the œsophagus. The explanation of this is that the fluid, in spite of its rapid passage, comes into the closest contact with the mucous membrane, owing to the narrowness of the tube ; while in the mouth, throat and pharynx, where the cavity is wider and the contact less intimate, a lower degree of change is generally found. In exceptional cases, when only a small quantity of acid reaches the stomach, the œsopha-gus may be the part most severely affected. As a matter of course there will be different degrees of intensity and extent of the lesion, according to the quantity and concentration of the acid. The inflammation, however, generally extends about equally over the entire length of the œsophagus, beginning with a well-defined line of demarcation at the lower border of the cricoid cartilage and extending to the cardiac extremity of the stomach ; on the other hand, it does not always involve the entire periphery, and sometimes assumes the form of more or less wide stripes, which run from above downward.

In the *mildest degree* of corrosion the effect is limited to destruction of the epithelium only, which is converted into a thick, grayish white, rugous membrane, peeling off here and there (not unlike croupous membrane), under which the mucous membrane appears pale.

In the *more advanced degrees* the mucous membrane itself, in its entire thickness, is converted into a dirty gray or grayish yellow soft slough, traversed by black blood-vessels with smooth surface (being divested of its epithelium), and the submucous cellular tissue is infiltrated first with serum, afterwards with pus, and ecchymosed. The muscular coat is shrivelled, pale, or fawn-colored, and the loss of tone which results causes the whole tube to hang like an unstrung bow towards the right pleural cavity. The external cellular covering is of a red, livid color, and traversed by black vessels.

In the *highest degrees* the mucous membrane and submucous cellular tissue are converted into a black, rotten mass, distended by a sanguinolent fluid, and the muscular coat is either changed in the same manner, or is simply converted into a pale, gelatinous mass.

While the highest degrees always prove very rapidly fatal, life may, in less severe cases, be prolonged for days, weeks, and even permanently, and then we find a further development of the inflammatory lesions. At first the line of demarcation forms between the blackened mucous membrane and the parts of the same which are less involved, and the gangrenous portion is soon detached from its subjacent layer by the undermining, purulent (phlegmonous) infiltration of the submucous cellular tissue ; thus detached, it is generally expelled in single shreds, but sometimes it remains complete, and the whole or nearly the whole length of the tube, to the extent of a foot, is thrown off, together with a portion of the mucous membrane of the stomach.

Such cases of tubular expulsion of the whole mucous membrane of the œsophagus following sulphuric acid poisoning are published by Trier in Copenhagen (Hospitals-Meddelelser, Bd. V. H. 1. Schmidt's Jahrb. Bd. 76. p. 310. 1852); Mansière (Des rétrecissements intrinsèques de l'œsophage. Thèse de Paris. 1866. Canstatt's Jahresber. 1866. II. p. 128); Laboulbène (Progrès médic. 1876. No. 52. p. 901).

When these large losses of substance with suppurating base (corrosive ulcers) have formed in the manner described, the suppuration may continue, and, in the form of hollow passages and collections of pus, may extend down even into the mediastinum, and cause perforation of the trachea or bronchus, and subsequently produce death. Recovery can take place, even in such cases, with the establishment of a broncho-œsophageal fistula. More commonly, however, the suppuration ceases after separation of the mucous membrane, and recovery takes place by cicatrization, leaving behind those extensive strictures which involve more or less equally the entire length of the canal, and which have been already described (vide Stenoses). The most considerable strictures, and at the same time most easily overcome, are found in cases where the muscular coat has been totally or in great part destroyed. The narrowest are those which occur at the entrance to the œsophagus (behind the cricoid cartilage) and at the cardiac extremity of the stomach ; .also at points where the œsophagus, in its normal condition, is very narrow, and on that account very intensely affected by the corrosive action.

Other mineral acids (*nitric* and *hydrochloric*) produce the same, only less intense effects. *Salts of potassa and soda* may lead to complete sloughing and separation of the œsophageal mucous membrane and to inflammation of the submucous cellular tissue, with subsequent stricture produced by cicatrization. Concentrated *solutions* of *sulphate of copper* act in the same way (compare case described above, under Stenoses). On the other hand, *ammonia* produces merely a fibrinous exudation, or congestion with ecchymosis and slight cloudiness and separation of the epithelial layer (*vide* case mentioned above, under Hemorrhages).

We give the following case as a characteristic instance of corrosive inflammation of the œsophagus produced by sulphuric acid: A hotel-keeper, fifty years old, was admitted to the Dresden Hospital, June 19, 1862, with delirium tremens and symptoms of sulphuric acid poisoning, and died on the following day. The autopsy, made June 21st (Zenker), gave the following results relating to the action of the acid:

Mucous membrane of *tongue* normal in its anterior portion, without marked congestion; farther back in the middle, divested of epithelium, whitish, the papillæ red at some points; still farther back, much congested and somewhat ecchymosed. *Uvula* much swollen, infiltrated with yellow pus, and relaxed. Mucous membrane of *hard palate* and *pharynx* intensely congested in some places, and covered in others by a thick, yellow, moderately adherent, but easily separable membrane, in the form of large islands, with yellow infiltration underneath these; in other places, again, covered with thin pus, with purulent infiltration of the tissues beneath, and very much softened. The edge of the *epiglottis* covered with thick membrane; mucous membrane underneath and over the whole remaining surface much congested, of a rose-red color, and ecchymosed in some places. The rest of the mucous membrane of the *larynx* covered with thin pus, and intensely congested throughout. Mucous membrane of *trachea* covered with a somewhat frothy mucus, and moderately congested. *Œsophagus* very much relaxed, forming a bow which inclines towards the right pleural cavity; somewhat discolored on the external surface, of a livid red color, its larger veins filled with black, slightly coagulated blood. The mucous membrane shows on its anterior surface a well-defined stripe, small above, but 1¼ ctms. wide below, beginning exactly at the lower border of the cricoid cartilage, and extending to the stomach. This stripe is formed by the mucous membrane being converted, in its entire thickness, into a soft, grayish yellow slough, with smooth surface. This slough is partially separated from the adjoining mucous membrane by a rather deep furrow. Underneath is found a layer, about 1 mm. thick, infiltrated in part with yellow pus. The remaining posterior portion of the mucous membrane in some places little, in others very much congested, but otherwise normal. The adjacent aorta unchanged. In the *abdominal cavity* no sign of peritonitis. *Stomach* contracted in the form of a sausage; external surface of a somewhat gray color, with rather rigid wall; hemorrhagic stripes along the small curvature. On being opened, there is found about one ounce of thin, dirty brownish red fluid in the fundus. The entire posterior surface (increasing from the fundus towards the pylorus) is converted into an irregularly rugous surface, which consists partly of brownish gray and partly of dark red rugæ, 1 ctm. high, close together, and projecting like the teeth of a comb. On section, the tissue throughout is thick, very red or livid, and the vessels filled with blackish blood. Muscular coat mostly normal. The border of this rugous surface is indicated partly by the membranous deposits on the rest of the normal mucous membrane, and partly by the shallowness of the furrows. Near the pylorus the mucous membrane is studded with emphysematous sacs, for the most part relaxed, of a brownish color, with some ecchymoses, and traversed thickly by black vessels. On the anterior surface, mucous membrane only slightly softened and moderately congested in spots. The line of demarcation is sharply drawn at the pylorus. Mucous membrane of the *duodenum* slightly congested, with isolated, somewhat more numerous ecchymoses farther on, and some thin, reticulated membranous deposits. In the *upper loop of the small intestine* are numerous ecchymosed tufts.

Remaining small and large intestine normal. Further examination showed nothing worthy of mention, except marked congestion of the kidneys. Microscopical examination of the kidney revealed peculiar yellowish brown clots in the vessels, which could only be explained as fragments of the carbonized blood coming from the vessels of the œsophagus or stomach, and conveyed there as emboli.

Ulcers.

The forms of ulcer occurring in the œsophagus are very numerous, and can generally be distinguished according to their etiology and pathogenesis, whereas anatomical distinction is not easy in some of them, when fully developed.

If we adhere to the nomenclature which is based upon their causes and modes of development (these names agreeing in the main with those which have already been more or less in use), the following varieties of ulcers may be enumerated:

1. Ulcers produced by foreign bodies (*vide* p. 137).

2. Catarrhal ulcers (*vide* pp. 137 and 139).

3. Varicose ulcers (which differ from 2 only in being situated over varices (*vide* p. 130).

4. Follicular ulcers (*vide* p. 141).

5. Diphtheritic ulcers (*vide* p. 143).
6. Variolous ulcers (*vide* p. 146).
7. Phlegmonous ulcers (*vide* p. 148).
8. Corrosive ulcers (*vide* p. 157).
9. Gangrenous ulcers, from pressure (*vide* p. 115).
10. Ulcers of the pharynx, from decubitus—decubitus pharyngis.
11. Gangrenous ulcers, by extension from neighboring parts.
12. Syphilitic ulcers.
13. Carcinomatous ulcers. } Neoplastic forms of ulcer.
14. Tubercular ulcers. }

Inasmuch as the first eight forms have all been described in previous sections (in the places designated), and Nos. 13 and 14 will be discussed in the chapter that follows, on Morbid Growths, it only remains for us to say something of Nos. 9–12, inclusive.

Gangrenous ulcers may be produced by continuous pressure exerted upon the œsophagus, from within or without, which first causes necrosis of the mucous membrane, then of the other layers, and finally losses of substance by separation of the slough. In this way hard foreign bodies, forcibly introduced, sometimes act from the inside, so that a portion of the ulcers produced by foreign bodies may be included under this title, From the outside it is chiefly aneurisms of the aorta which cause this form of ulcer, and directly lead to perforation (p. 115).

As *ulcers from decubitus* we designate a not uncommon form of ulcer, which is very distinctly characterized by its peculiar situation and other phenomena, which point very clearly to its pathogenesis. It does not belong to the œsophagus exclusively, but may be found in the pharynx, and, strictly speaking, it lies on the other side of the boundary line (generally adhered to in these pages) between the two. We insert it here for the reason that no mention of it is found in "Diseases of the Pharynx."

The situation of this ulcer is at the lowest portion of the pharynx, directly behind the cricoid cartilage. In point of fact, however, there are always two ulcers on the anterior and posterior walls, directly opposite, and about the size of a five-cent piece, which appear at the same time and in the same form, so that one seems to be an impression of the other. The mucous membrane in these places is converted into a sharply defined, dirty gray, soft slough, with a line of demarcation partially formed. In place of this there may be found, after more or less complete removal of the slough, round ulcers with but slightly elevated edges and discolored, pulpy base, which in isolated cases can extend to such a depth as to expose in places the cricoid cartilage in front or the vertebral column behind. The remaining portions of the pharynx are usually free from ulcers.

These ulcers are found only in persons very much reduced by disease, who are exceedingly feeble, and have been kept in bed for a long time. Their pathogenesis is, without doubt, to be found in the fact that, in consequence of the general muscular atony, the larynx in the recumbent position falls back, and, in connection with the cartilaginous rings of the trachea, presses the two mucous surfaces together and against the vertebral column. This pressure is sufficient to interrupt completely the circulation, already enfeebled in the highest degree, at certain points in the mucous membrane, and thereby to induce necrosis. In point of fact we have to deal with a gangrene from pressure, caused *by the recumbent position*, and accordingly we are justified in giving it a name, which, by the peculiarity of its cause, as well as its situation, distinguishes it from other gangrenous ulcers produced by pressure (No. 9).

Owing to the fact that these ulcers do not appear until the last days or weeks before death, nothing can be said of further development or retrograde action.

The case above quoted by Hamburger (p. 114) is evidently of this type, in which, however, the larynx must have been "pressed backward by a considerable tumor in the neck." Unfortunately, Hamburger does not state the source from which the case is derived. Liouville has recently published a case in the Société anatomique de Paris (Feb. 12, 1875), which apparently belongs to this class; but, inasmuch as it occurred in a tuberculous patient, he regarded it as tubercular.

Gangrenous ulcers (by extension from neighboring parts) may spread from the pharynx to the œsophagus. Klebs observed deep ulcers, of a gangrenous character, following gangrenous pharyngitis and tonsillitis of scarlatina, probably from the diphtheritic process being transmitted from these regions. Steffen likewise (l. c.) saw, in a case of noma of the left cheek (girl seven years old), the mucous membrane of the mouth, larynx, upper half of the trachea, pharynx and œsophagus as far down as a point below the cricoid cartilage, swollen, discolored, friable, in a condition of gangrene, although not as yet ulcerated.

That *syphilitic ulcers*, although rarely, do likewise occur in the œsophagus, has been proved to a certainty by the cicatricial contractions, undoubtedly syphilitic (*vide* Stenoses), observed by Virchow, West, and Klob. As regards the earlier stages of these ulcers, however, only *one* authentic case has thus far been recorded by Virchow, who saw, "in addition to an ulcer in the process of contracting, yellow gummata undergoing fatty degeneration, from which the ulceration resulted."

A "superficial ulcer with fatty base," found in another case, is mentioned by Virchow as probably belonging to this class, but the history of the case is too uncertain to warrant us in introducing it here. In like manner, a case published by Bryant (*Lancet*, July 7, 1877, p. 9, from Habershon's wards in Guy's Hospital, 1866) of a "stricture of the œsophagus from syphilitic ulceration, in a tuberculous patient," gives occasion for the gravest doubts as to the correctness of the diagnosis. In a man, forty-eight years old, who died from phthisis, and who had syphilis at the age of twenty, but apparently without secondary symptoms, there was found "in the posterior portion of the pharynx, extending downward, an oval, indolent ulcer, two inches long, almost surrounding the canal, without elevated edges, and with base formed by the degenerated muscular layer." In the larynx were found "ulcers peculiar to the syphilitic larynx."

Finally, we must return to the mooted question, whether the existence of a *perforating ulcer of the œsophagus*, analogous to "perforating ulcer of the stomach," is admissible. As authors who pronounce in favor of the occurrence of this specific form of ulcer, and who thus explain their reported cases of perforation of the œsophagus, may be mentioned Albers,[1] Reeves,[2] Flower,[3] Vigla,[4] Eras.[5] Rokitansky also, in the latest edition of his

[1] Graefe's u. Walther's Jour. f. Chir. u. Augenheilk. 19. Bd. u. Erläuterungen z. Atlas d. path. Anat. II. p. 204.
[2] Associat. Med. Journ. 7 Oct., 1853.
[3] Med.-chir. Transact. 36. Bd. 1854. Schmidt's Jahrb. 85. Bd. p. 294.
[4] L'Union. 1855. Schmidt's Jahrb. 88. Bd. p. 46.
[5] Die anat. Canalisationsstörungen der Speiseröhre. Leipziger Dissert. 1866. p. 21.

Pathological Anatomy, admits the occurrence of this form of ulcer, on the ground of such statements (apparently not from his own observations), as an exceedingly rare phenomenon. All these statements, however, do not bear rigid criticism. In no one of them are the phenomena described sufficient to prove the existence of this form of ulcer. In many of such cases the anatomical appearance bears no resemblance whatever to the typical form of perforating ulcer of the stomach. Moreover, all of them can easily be traced back to one or other of the forms of perforation of the œsophagus mentioned above (*vide* Perforation) —ulcers produced by foreign bodies, perforated diverticula due to traction, cancerous ulceration, or rupture from without. Agreeing, then, with the majority of the later writers on this subject, we are compelled to pronounce decidedly against the occurrence of this form of ulcer in the œsophagus.

Allusion has already been made to the *gangrenous* processes (sloughs, gangrene) which occur in the œsophagus. As an independent process, gangrene is not found in the œsophagus. Many cases described as such in earlier times are probably to be traced to softening (œsophago-malacia).

Symptomatology and Diagnosis.

Catarrhal inflammation of the mucous membrane of the œsophagus, in mild cases, gives rise to no symptoms at all, or they are so slight and ambiguous that the disease is overlooked entirely or merely suspected.

Acute catarrh of a mild grade, whether the irritation be chemical, thermal, or mechanical, produces *pain* in the œsophagus, which is felt only when the patient swallows, and is distinctly localized in one spot, or extends over the entire length of the canal, according to the situation and extent of the exciting cause. Deglutition is seldom interfered with, and the pain rarely continues more than a few days.

In the higher degrees of the inflammation, the pain is more permanent, oppressive, and spasmodic; during the act of swallowing, especially of hard or dry morsels of food, and of very hot or very cold fluids, the pain is considerably augmented.

Mechanical irritation applied to the œsophagus by pressure on the neck, blows on the vertebral column, forcible bending of the body, extension or twisting of the spine, and notably the introduction of a sound, increase this pain. The reflex spasm of the muscular coat, produced by swallowing, ceases with the downward movement of the morsel of food, leaving behind an exceedingly painful sensation of something sticking, or renders the passage of food quite impossible, so that it is immediately regurgitated. On close examination the masses thrown off show a thick mucous or muco-purulent covering. The admixture of blood, when constant, points generally to the existence of ulcers.

The introduction of the sound (which should be used with the greatest care, and never without urgent need) encounters no obstruction at any point, unless such as is produced by reflex spasm, but calls forth very painful sensations in the inflamed region, which may be complained of frequently and for a long time after the removal of the instrument. The material found in the fenestra of the sound (mucus, pus, blood) is naturally of great value in diagnosis.

The inflammation can only be recognized as *croupous* in form, when shreds of false membrane are brought to light either by the sound or by spontaneous vomiting (Abercrombie, Bleuland). Moreover, this form of inflammation may be inferred with some probability when symptoms of œsophagitis are associated with a pharyngeal croup.

It is scarcely possible to recognize *phlegmonous inflammation of the œsophagus*. The presumption in favor of the existence of such an inflammation is very great in cases of vomiting of large masses of pus or ichorous material, but the diagnosis is not established, because the pus may come from the peri-œsophageal cellular tissue or from neighboring organs, and by perforation make its way into the œsophagus.

Corrosive inflammation of the œsophagus can generally be made out from the history of the case, and inspection of the mouth and throat. The pains are sometimes very severe along the course of the œsophagus; at other times and in the worst cases, the pains are slight or entirely wanting; the mucous membrane in severe cases is generally in a sloughy condition.

Course. Results. Prognosis.

The course of catarrhal inflammation is almost invariably rapid and favorable. The pain and difficulty of swallowing disappear in a few hours or days.

In the more severe forms of inflammation which arise from corrosion, scalding, foreign bodies, etc., the course of the disease is much more protracted and the prognosis always doubtful, or account of the danger of its resulting in ulceration, perforation, formation of abscess, and gangrene. Again, in such cases, where the inflammation, with or without ulceration, extends to the deeper layers, there is the special danger of stricture from cicatricial contraction of the ulcers, and, on the other hand, in protracted chronic catarrhs, the possibility of consecutive dilatation must be kept in mind.

The diagnosis and prognosis of these sequelæ have been given in the chapters devoted to their special consideration.

Treatment.

The treatment can be directed to the cause only, when the inflammation is due to the impaction or piercing of foreign bodies, syphilitic ulceration, or the action of corrosive substances. In the last-mentioned form, however, something more than removal of the cause will be required, for the reason that antidotes, if they are successful, must be administered immediately, and this is almost never possible. The removal of foreign bodies must be undertaken as soon as possible, and prosecuted with the greatest care and patience. In all other cases the treatment is symptomatic and antiphlogistic : application of ice-bags to the chest, neck, or back, according to the location of the pain ; local bloodletting at points on the surface corresponding to the situation of the inflammation; small pieces of ice, small quantities of ice-water or ice-cream internally. The introduction of solid food into the œsophagus must be stopped entirely ; the nutrition of the patient must be kept up by way of the rectum in long-continued dysphagia resulting from inflammation. Feeding through the œsophageal tube is excluded, as a matter of course, for the reason that it augments the inflammation, and increases the danger of perforation where corrosion and ulceration extend to any depth.

When the inflammation becomes protracted, and the dysphagia exists in greater or less degree, the use of powerful revulsives (iodine, croton oil, setons), and the internal administration of iodide of potassium and astringents, especially nitrate of silver, will be indicated. The treatment of cases resulting in cicatricial contraction, perforation, etc., will be found in the chapters where they are described.

MORBID GROWTHS—VEGETATIONS.

Pathology and Etiology.

The morbid growths and vegetations occurring in the œsophagus are not very numerous, and, with exception of carcinomata, possess very little pathological interest; certain forms, although somewhat frequent, are associated with no functional disturbance of any kind, while others, although they do occasionally lead to severe disturbances, are so exceedingly rare that the great majority of practitioners, even those most engaged in clinical work, never see such a case. Metastatic tumors seem never to have been observed in the œsophagus. The following forms do occur here:

Warts of the œsophagus, Verrucœ œsophagi.—These are formations which in their structure so much resemble the ordinary cutaneous warts, that they may properly be described by the same name, and illustrate very forcibly the analogy, emphasized by Klebs, between diseases of the mucous membrane of the œsophagus and those of the skin. They present themselves to the naked eye as slight conical projections of the mucous membrane, varying in size from the head of a pin to that of a lentil, which are outlined still more against their surroundings by the cloudiness of the thickened epithelial covering. Microscopical examination shows that each of these projections is caused by a simple elongation of a group of normal mucous membrane papillæ, with simultaneous thickening of their epithelial covering, and complete preservation of their typical arrangement, so that, exactly like simple cutaneous warts, they are to be regarded as circumscribed papillary and epithelial hypertrophies.

Such warts are found very frequently, especially in elderly persons—sometimes single, at other times in large numbers—scattered over the entire length of the tube (the circumscribed thickening of the epithelial covering, mentioned by Birch-Hirschfeld as occurring in chronic catarrh, probably belongs here). They do not seem to undergo any further changes. When the epithelial covering is removed by reason of post-mortem changes, it is sometimes found still adherent to these warts, making them very perceptible. We have never been able to learn that their existence in large numbers has given rise to any symptoms whatever during life—(œsophagismus thus far unexplained anatomically might be thought of in this connection). No relation has ever been made out between these papillary growths and the production of carcinoma,—a relation analogous to that between papillary tumors of the lip and epithelioma. They appear insignificant, at least in the beginning.

Lúschka observed larger *tuft-like papillæ*, visible to the naked eye, in a case of general dilatation of the œsophagus resulting from chronic catarrh. The caruncular excrescences which Hamburger, according to Lieutaud and Palletta, mentions, may have been similar, but larger formations.

In animals such papillary growths are found in much greater development and extent. The pathological museum in Erlangen contains the œsophagus of an ox, which is covered in its entire length with flaccid papillomata, several centimetres long, with thin pedicles and numerous branches.

Once in a great while there are found small *retention cysts* of the mucous follicles, situated in the submucous cellular tissue, usually not larger than a pea (perhaps as large as a hazel-nut, Klebs), which cause conical projections of the mucous membrane. They contain a very clear, colorless viscid fluid. As a rule, there will be found only one or two, and usually in the uppermost portion of the tube, but occasionally the number will be larger. Even the largest of these cysts, however, cause no trouble.

Closely connected with these cysts is a tumor designated *adenoma polyposum* by Weigert,[1] and recently described by him as found on the anterior wall of the lower third of the œsophagus.

---

[1] Virchow's Archiv. Bd. 67. p. 516.

It was an oblong tumor, 3½ ctms. long, 2 ctms. oroad, and 1 ctm. high, which hung down as a pedunculated, pyriform appendix, as large as a hazel-nut, and consisted of numerous hollow spaces, clothed with cylinder-epithelium and surrounded by a stroma of connective tissue. It might well have arisen from the mucous follicles.

Fibromata, lipomata and *myomata* are occasionally found as well-defined tumors, which cause conical projection of the mucous membrane into the lumen; the first two arise from the submucous cellular tissue, the latter from the muscular coat. They commonly attain the size of a pea or hazel-nut, but in exceptional cases are considerably larger. However, even the largest (with the rarest exceptions) cause no difficulty in swallowing. The same remark applies to these as to other affections of the œsophagus (*e. g.*, compression by aneurisms, etc.), in which, from the anatomical construction, it would appear that dysphagia could scarcely fail to exist—viz., that so long as the greater part of the periphery of the tube is dilatable, the food easily makes its way through the obstruction.

Eberth found (Virchow's Archiv. Bd. 43. p. 137) in a melancholic woman, fifty years old, a pure myoma, 9.1 ctms. long, 11.9 ctms. broad, 3.5 ctms. thick, immediately over the cardiac extremity; it arose from the circular muscular fibres, and involved one-half the circumference of the œsophagus, leaving the anterior wall free; no symptoms pointing to the tumor existed during life.

Fagge (Med. Times and Gazette, 28 November, 1874) exhibited at the Pathological Society of London a myoma œsophagi, two inches long, one inch thick, and situated below the bifurcation of the trachea, which never gave rise to dysphagia. On the other hand, Coats (Glasgow Med. Journ. Febr. 1872. Virchow-Hirsch's Jahresber. für 1872. Bd. II. p. 154) has described a myoma, four and three-quarter inches long, two inches broad, its upper border six and three-quarter inches below the cavity of the glottis, which was attached to the posterior wall of the œsophagus by a thin, fibrous pedicle one and three-quarter inches long (in its external appearance resembling the polypi presently to be described), and which caused the death of the patient, a man sixty-one years old, by inanition.

A case of *sarcoma* (alveolar) at the entrance of the œsophagus has been published by Chapman.[1] Several tumors partially connected, varying from one-half of an inch to two inches in diameter, apparently arising from the submucous cellular tissue

---

[1] American Jour. of the Med. Sciences. 1877. Oct. p. 433.

of the œsophagus, and growing upward and outward, occupied the lowermost part of the pharynx and uppermost part of the œsophagus, and had completely closed the entrance to the latter, so that the woman, forty-five years old, died from inanition.

Fibrous Polypi of the Œsophagus (and Pharynx).

Bibliography.

Voigtel, Handb. d. pathol. Anat. 2. Bd. 1804. p. 427 (contains cases from *Schmiæder*, *Hofer*, *Vater* (?), *Dallas*).—*Monro*, Morbid Anatomy of the Human Gullet, etc. Edinburgh, 1811. p. 186.—*Mondière*, Arch. génér. 2. Sér. T. III. 53. 1833 (with cases from *de Graef*, *Baillie*, *Schneider*, *Pringle*, *Monro*).—*Ch. Bell*, Surgical Observ. I. p. 76 (drawings copied in Froriep's surgical prints, 174. Fig. 4. —*Rokitansky*, Oesterreich. medicin. Jahrb. N. F. 21. Bd. p. 225. 1840.—*Middeldorpff*, De polypis œsophagi. Vratislav. 1857 (Schmidt's Jahrb. Bd. 99. p. 130). —Two cases from *Roeser*, Würtemb. Corr. Bl. 1859. 21. Schmidt's Jahrb. Bd. 103. p. 341.— *Warren* and *Holt*, Schmidt's Jahrb. Bd. 139. p. 131.—*Coats*, loc. cit. (myoma).—For surgical reference, vide *Koenig* in particular, loc. cit. p. 37.

Presenting much greater pathological interest, especially from a surgical point of view, are the so-called *fibrous polypi of the œsophagus*, which are indeed very rare, and the majority of which certainly do not belong to the œsophagus, so far as their origin is concerned, but are simply lodged there. They may be described as soft tumors, knobby or more cylindrical in form, with their pedicles generally originating[1] in the submucous cellular tissue, on the anterior wall of the lower portion of the pharynx; from this pedicle, which is only a few lines in thickness, they swell out to considerable size; their surface is smooth, flat, or deeply lobulated, and from their point of attachment they

---

[1] The statement, repeatedly copied, that these polypi take root "as a rule in the perichondrium of the cricoid cartilage," is found only in the first edition of *Rokitansky's* text-book, when he refers to the description of his own case. In this description it is mentioned explicitly that the polypus arose from the submucous cellular tissue. In the later editions of his book, he says the polypi "come principally from above, *e. g.*, from the cricoid cartilage," by which is certainly meant the neighborhood of this cartilage. Hence, we are obliged to adhere to the original statement as really the most probable.

hang down more or less in the œsophagus, and at times stretch it to a considerable extent, so that the œsophagus compresses it at its greatest circumference. One of the largest of these polypi (Rokitansky's case) measured seven and a half inches in length; and at the blunt end, which was situated two and a half inches above the cardiac orifice of the stomach, it was two and a half inches thick. In their structure they resemble fibromata, sometimes with more or less abundant cell-formation. Myomata may appear in the same form (*vide* Coats' case). The mucous membrane covering these polypi is partly smooth, partly studded with papillary growths; it has also been found much congested, and even ulcerated in places.

As a rule, there is found only *one* polypus. Charles Bell found a group of comparatively small polypi, some of which apparently originated in the œsophagus itself.

It seems very probable, as Middeldorpff has shown, that the cause of these polypi is to be looked for in the passage of the food through the narrow portion of the pharynx, where the transverse folds of the mucous membrane are but feebly developed. When such a fold is pushed out of place, it can be more and more stretched and irritated by the constantly recurring distention, and thus become the starting-point of the growth. These polypi are developed in advanced life, and occur more frequently in men than in women.

Of eleven cases in which the sex and in part the age are given, ten occurred in men from thirty-six to seventy years old, and only one in a woman, fifty-four years old.

These enormous growths, however, sometimes exist for a long time without giving rise to any difficulty in swallowing. Bell's patient, as well as Rokitansky's, experienced no dysphagia until a few months before death, and in the latter it soon ceased. Yet the growths must certainly have attained a considerable size long before this symptom appeared. In other cases, as in those of de Graef, Monro, and again in Middeldorpff's patient, where the tumor was successfully removed by an operation, the dysphagia had certainly existed for years, and was accompanied by urgent dyspnœa. When the polypus is not removed, these patients finally die from exhaustion brought on by arrest of deglutition, resulting from the extreme stenosis.

We add the first case seen and published by Monro (l. c.), as a very typical example of this form of tumor. It was first published in the Edinburgh Physical and Literary Essays, Vol. III., p. 525, where a drawing of the tumor, as preserved in the Anatomical Museum of Edinburgh, is to be found.

A man, sixty-eight years old, entered the Edinburgh Hospital, April, 1763, to undergo an operation for polypus of the pharynx. This polypus was not generally visible on simple inspection of the pharynx, but by movements of vomiting, artificially induced, and sometimes by coughing, it was thrown forward as far as the front teeth, and appeared then as a hard, fleshy tumor, consisting of four lobes, attached by a common root. As the tumor covered the entrance to the larynx, the patient could suffer it to remain in the mouth scarcely half a minute, and was obliged to swallow it again as soon as possible. He had suffered for several years from dysphagia and cough, and could neither breathe nor speak as formerly. After tracheotomy, which was first performed in order to keep up respiration during the operation, a large portion of the tumor was removed by a loop of thread placed around it, and it was allowed to come away *per anum*. Two years later (1765) the patient returned to the hospital much emaciated and excessively weak, owing to the fact that for several months he had been able to swallow nothing but fluids, and these only with difficulty. The polypus was not to be seen as before. After his death, which occurred shortly after admission to the hospital, the œsophagus was found much dilated by an enormous fleshy polypus, arising by a single root from the anterior wall of the œsophagus (described, however, as arising from the pharynx, p. 183), three inches below the glottis, divided in its lower portion into several lobes, the longest of which reached the cardiac extremity of the stomach. At the lower extremity of this last-mentioned lobe was found the cicatrix resulting from the operation.

Carcinoma of the Œsophagus.

Bibliography.

Lebert, Traité prat. des malad. cancér. 1851.—*Koehler*, Krebs- und Scheinkrebs-Krankheiten. 1853.—*Oppolzer*, *Bamberger*, *Hamburger*, *Koenig*, ll. cc.—*Rokitansky*, *Foerster*, *Klebs*, *Birch-Hirschfeld*, ll. cc.—*Deininger*, Fall von Epithelkrebs im Oesophagus. Erlanger Diss. 1860.—*Petri*, Krebs der Speiseröhre. Berlin. Diss. 1868.—*Fritsche*, Ueb. d. Krebs d. Speiseröhre. Berlin. Diss. 1872.

Of all tumors occurring in the œsophagus, as regards relative frequency as well as gravity of symptoms, carcinoma is by far the most important. It is not, however, an absolutely frequent disease. It occurs as a *primary* disease, taking its origin in the œsophagus itself, and as a *secondary* form, extending from neighboring parts to the œsophagus. Its pathological interest is connected entirely with the primary, which is really the more frequent form. We will speak first only of primary cancer, and at the close add the little that is to be said of the secondary form.

From our own observations in 5,079 autopsies, we found *primary cancer of the œsophagus* 13 times = 0.25 per cent. ; besides 6 cases of the *secondary* form = 0.11 per cent.

The form in which *primary carcinoma* appears *in the œsophagus*—and apparently the only form in which it appears—is the *flat-celled epithelioma* (cancroid). It presents here the typical microscopical structure of this form of cancer, as we have learned to recognize it in the lip, which is by far its most frequent location. Here, as there, are the same well-defined, large, differently shaped, flat epithelial cells ; here, too, do we find the same grouping together of these cells in well-defined plugs or more spherical bodies, which fill up the alveolar spaces in the connective-tissue frame, and which can be squeezed out of the cut surface as little corks, in the form of a worm or comedo ; the same groups of cells, arranged in concentric layers (described as epithelial pearls or nests of cells) in the interior of each plug. According to the more or less powerful development, and the firmer or more delicate organization of the stroma, the tumor may exhibit all transitions, from the hardest, dry (scirrhous), to the softest, juicy (medullary) forms, and yet this difference in consistence does not afford any basis for the establishment of essentially different forms of cancer, in the sense of the older writers on pathology.

In regard to the early development of carcinoma of the œsophagus, Carmalt[1] has made investigations in three cases, which convinced him that the cancerous growth originated partly in the deeper epithelial layers of the mucous membrane itself, and partly in the epithelium of the excretory ducts of the mucous follicles.

Virchow's Archiv. Bd. 55. p. 481. 1872.

Until the beginning of 1860, very few cases of epithelial cancer of the œsophagus had been described or mentioned, viz., those by Bruch, Lebert, Hannover, Schuh, Foerster, Robin, Habershon, Deininger, Neumann. As compared with other forms of cancer in the œsophageal canal, it was regarded as rare. Later and more numerous investigations have entirely overthrown this view. Foerster, in the second edition of his text-book (1863), emphasizes the frequency of epithelial cancer in comparison with every other form (among sixteen cases he found only three of his "carcinoma vulgare"), and even these—since the latest phase in the development of the cancer doctrine had not at that time been divulged—would be looked upon by him to-day, perhaps, as very doubtful. Petri, who worked under Virchow's direction, states that the forty-four cases in the Berlin Pathological Institute, collected by himself, all belong to the cancroid form. Numerous single cases give the same result. In like manner the latest manuals and text-books of pathological anatomy (Klebs, Birch-Hirschfeld) teach that the epithelial is the only form of cancer which occurs in the œsophagus. We have always seen it in this form. Accordingly, when more recent clinical text-books (including the new editions of Foerster's Text-book of Pathological Anatomy, which here, as elsewhere, retain unchanged the original text of Foerster) represent scirrhus and medullary sarcoma as occurring in the œsophagus, in addition to epithelial cancer, the statement depends upon a mixture of modern and ancient nomenclature that is necessarily quite confusing. If we still make use of the old expressions, scirrhus and medullary cancer (Markschwamm), which originally indicated only coarse anatomical differences, but the same histological structure, then it must be in the old established sense (as Koenig very properly uses them), in which the solid form, with abundant, thick stroma, is regarded as scirrhus, and the soft variety, with delicate, loose frame, as medullary cancer; besides, the histological (and pathogenetic?) character of the tumor must be indicated by the special name given to it in modern nomenclature. The proper name, then, for cancer of the œsophagus —as it now appears, for every case without exception—is *flat-celled epithelioma* (Plattenepithelkrebs).

As regards the location of carcinoma, it may occur in any part of the œsophagus. In extremely rare cases it involves the whole or nearly the whole length of the tube (cases by Baillie, Ribbentrop, Petri, Zenker).

In the case observed by us there was only one place, 4 ctms. long, in the middle of the canal, which was entirely free from cancer, while the remainder, above and below, was completely occupied by it, so that two distinct cancerous masses existed. We shall return to this very rare case in another connection (p. 180).

Sometimes, although quite rarely, one-half of the tube will be involved, but most frequently only a small space, from 3 to 10 ctms. in length. If we divide the œsophagus into three parts of equal length, in order to fix more closely the location of these spaces occupied by cancer, the great majority is found in the lower third, a considerably smaller number in the middle third, and by far the smallest number in the upper third.

The statements hitherto published concerning this ratio are partly true, and partly (in consequence of the different mode of expression), but only seemingly, as contradictory as they well could be. While Rokitansky makes the upper half of the thoracic portion the most frequent location, and "less frequent the terminal portion next to the cardiac extremity," Koehler, and subsequently Foerster, designate the lower end of the canal as the most frequently (according to Foerster, in one-half of the cases), and the middle portion as less frequently involved (according to F., in one-quarter of the cases, exactly as in the upper portion). According to Klebs and Rindfleisch, the middle portion, especially the part corresponding to the bifurcation of the trachea, is the most common location. This last statement agrees pretty well with that of Rokitansky concerning the upper half, since the "middle portion" of the œsophagus coincides partially with the "upper half of his thoracic portion." Both these statements, however, are quite contradictory to that made by Foerster, and supported by figures, and still more so to the accurate statement of Petri, who has prepared the subjoined table from his own and from our data, which essentially agree with his. Birch-Hirschfeld gives the same table (but erroneously ascribes it to Foerster). The clinical authors naturally follow the statements made by the pathologists. Oppolzer and Bamberger follow Rokitansky word for word. Niemeyer apparently follows him (8th Edition), but not exactly, as he concludes that "the location of the cancer is most frequently the upper and lower thirds, more rarely the middle third," which no pathologist has stated in this way. In the ninth edition of the same work Seitz makes the cancer to appear "by preference in the portion opposite the bifurcation of the trachea," but "rarely in the middle region" (!). Kunze, however, following Rindfleisch on this point, designates the middle third as the chief seat of the cancer. So then the confusion is at its height in the two clinical text-books most in use at the present time! The practitioner can choose between the upper, middle, or lower third, as he feels inclined.

This confusion can, of course, only be gotten rid of by statistics, denoted by figures, since a simple estimate from memory, in a form of disease so very rare, is hazardous even for the most experienced observers. Petri has (under Virchow's direction) made an excellent beginning. We annex our own more meagre material (fifteen cases, including two preparations sent to us), which, in all the most essential points, has led to the same results. Moreover, since Foerster has arrived at a like conclusion in regard to the most important point, viz., the very frequent invasion of the lower third, our foregoing statement is sufficiently well founded. In order to test this, we give Petri's figures and our own.

Carcinoma is situated:

	According to Petri.		Zenker.		Petri and Zenker together.	
In the upper third................	In 2 cases = 4.5 %	In 2 cases = 13.3 %.		In 4 cases = 6.9 %		
" middle third..................	" 13 " = 29.5 "	" 1 " = 6.6 "		" 14 " = 34.1 "		
" lower third....................	" 18 " = 40.9 "	" 6 " = 40.0 "		" 24 " = 41.3 "		
" upper and middle thirds......	" 1 " = 2.2 "	" 2 " = 13.3 "		" 3 " = 5.1 "		
" middle and lower thirds......	" 8 " = 18.1 "	" 3 " = 20.0 "		" 11 " = 18.9 "		
In all three thirds	" 1 " = 2.2 "	" 1 " = 6.6 "		" 2 " = 3.4 "		
	43 " 1	15 "		58 "		

If we calculate, besides, how often in these fifty-eight cases each one of the three portions was involved, it results as follows:

The upper third was involved 9 times = 15.5 per cent.
" middle " " 30 " = 51.7 "
" lower " " 37 " = 63.8 "

These figures find their expression in the statement contained above in the text. Further statistics in addition to these, which are meagre, arranged in the same manner, and obtained from other sources, especially the large pathological schools, are much to be desired. But certainly statistics, although meagre, made up from individual, so to speak, pure material, possess greater value than the more ample statistics which are gathered from published cases, in which the various motives for publication on the part of the authors lead them to misrepresent the facts. However, even such statistics might be of some service.

The cancerous mass is sometimes in the *form of an island,*[2] inasmuch as it is entirely surrounded by healthy mucous membrane, or in the *form of a belt*—i. e., surrounding the whole tube, so that the mucous membrane above is separated from that below by this interposed cancerous mass (insular and belt-shaped form). *Post-mortem* examination of cases of œsophageal cancer almost always shows the belt-shaped form in larger or smaller spaces, and sometimes the cancerous belt is found to project, like a peninsula, more or less into the healthy mucous membrane. The purely insular form is observed after death from other diseases. At first the cancer invariably assumes the

[1] The percentage is estimated by *Petri* on 44 cases, in one of which the situation was unknown.

[2] We avoid the term annular [wandständig], applied to this form by others. This expression, quite familiar in the description of thrombus, is not opposed to anything belt-shaped, but to something causing obstruction (obturirende). The belt-shaped cancer is also annular.

insular form, but even then shows a tendency towards the belt-shaped extension, precisely as in other portions of the digestive tract (pylorus, rectum). It is scarcely possible to determine how soon this transition to the belt-form ensues, for the reason that the smaller insular cancers, as a rule, give rise to no troublesome symptoms. Moreover, forms of transition naturally occur in which a belt-shaped cancer surrounds the canal almost completely, leaving simply a narrow longitudinal stripe, a few millimetres wide, free from the disease. In regard to results, such cases rank with the complete belt-shaped forms. Most frequently by far only *one* such cancerous mass is found. Occasionally, however, in addition to the principal mass, there will be found one or two smaller islands, quite distinct from the first, which most probably are to be regarded as secondary masses derived from the original cancer. When two distinct masses about equally developed exist (as in the case already mentioned by us, in which almost the entire œsophagus was involved), it is impossible to decide whether we have to deal with an unusually early and more highly developed dissemination, or with two masses independent from the very beginning.

At first the cancer projects above the level of the mucous membrane in the form of a wall or hillock, with more or less perpendicular border, and with a surface sometimes smooth, at other times papillary and even villous in some places. The whitish gray, infiltrated mucous membrane, inseparably blended with the submucous cellular tissue, has lost by this fusion its power of shifting and arranging itself in folds. At an early date the muscular coat becomes hypertrophied at and above the place where the cancer occurs. Later in the disease the cancerous infiltration attacks the hypertrophied muscular coat in the form of irregular, whitish gray stripes, by which the characteristic fan-shaped appearance of this layer is more and more effaced. Finally, the external cellular coat is invaded by the cancerous infiltration, and becomes thick and dense. The entire wall, the different layers of which can no longer be made out, or at least very imperfectly, attains a thickness of one centimetre or more, and becomes very rigid. Arising in this way, and chiefly from the rigidity and loss of expansive power in the œsophageal wall (less frequently from the moderate projections into the canal), *stricture* is formed, and when the cancer has nearly or quite assumed the belt-like form, this becomes the most important feature in the whole picture of the disease. In accordance with the tables given above, which show the relative frequency of cancer in the different portions of the canal, such a stricture will be found most frequently in the lower third, more rarely in the middle third, and most rarely in the upper third. (For further description concerning these strictures, *vide* Stenoses.) In the less extensive insular cancers, where the greater portion of the wall is still exempt and capable of expansion, the question of stricture does not arise.

Ulceration is apt to begin at an early date, as in cancers of other mucous membranes exposed to various mechanical injuries, and will be found in the insular as well as in the belt form, but especially in the latter. The cancerous tumor becomes converted, in whole or in part, into a deep, sinuous ulcer, with an edge projecting like a rampart. This edge often undergoes degeneration, leaving the canal open again (and causing a deceptive improvement in the condition of the patient). As a rule, the base of the ulcer is covered distinctly with small portions of the cancerous mass, in the form of granules, or floating tufts, and the edge shows a distinct layer of cancerous infiltration. In rare cases the cancerous mass can be so completely destroyed and removed that the ulcer resembles more the simple gangrenous form, and the discovery of the smallest portion of cancer on the edge, or the identification of secondary cancer in neighboring parts, reveals the cancerous nature of the ulcer.

See cases of this kind given by Petri, Nos. 28 and 34, and one seen by us (dissected by Dr. Bostroem), Deutsches Arch. f. klin. Med. Bd. XVIII. p. 500, where it serves another purpose. Rokitansky (Lehrb. d. path. Anat. I. Bd. 1855. p. 278) states that radical cure, with resulting cicatricial contraction, may follow these cases of complete destruction by ulceration. Unfortunately, no individual observations establish this certainly not impossible result.

The deeper ulcerations lead finally to complete *perforation of the œsophageal wall*, in greater or less extent, sometimes into the contiguous connective tissue, indurated by inflammation and infiltrated with cancer, at other times into the hollow viscera, with which the œsophagus had first become firmly united. The cancerous infiltration can either extend to the wall of such viscus and dispose it to perforation, or the ulceration, after breaking through the cancerous layer, proceeds to a neighboring organ and makes its way into it. The parts liable to these perforations are, first of all, the larger air-passages, trachea and bronchi, then the lungs, pleuræ, and pericardium, and, in cancer over the cardiac extremity of the œsophagus, the peritoneum itself (Petri, Case 4); finally, the large blood-vessels, aorta and pulmonary, carotid and subclavian arteries, etc. (for particulars, *vide* Perforations).

Petri found single or multiple perforation twenty-seven times in his forty-four cases.

Secondary extension of œsophageal cancer, as in other cancers, although of less frequent occurrence, takes place in three ways: by direct extension, by dissemination, and by metastasis.

Direct extension takes place sometimes to the *stomach and pharynx by continuity.* Invasion of the stomach is not rare when the cancer reaches the cardiac extremity, but it occurs to so slight an extent that the implication of the stomach has little signification in reference to the general form of the disease. The continuation to the pharynx, by reason of the infrequency of cancer in the upper part of the œsophagus, is very rare.

The excellent engravings by Baillie—A Series of Engravings, etc. London, 1812. p. 51 (copied in Froriep's Surgical Plates. No. 172. Figs. 1 and 2)—show two examples of this rare continuation to the pharynx from preparations in the Hunterian Museum.

Much more important and various are the extensions *by contiguity.* Such extension is found chiefly in the connective tissue of the posterior mediastinum and neck, which has previously become inflamed, and usually thickened to a moderate extent; this thickness is materially increased by the consolidation of this tissue with the œsophageal wall. This may develop into very large, compact masses, which compress the trachea or push it aside. Other structures in the mediastinum, especially the left vagus and recurrent nerves, may be involved in the cancerous degeneration, or affected by pressure and ulceration (Petri, Case I.). In one case (Petri, No. 21) there was found a cancroidal node on the external surface of the dura mater spinalis in the region of the ninth and tenth vertebræ, after perforation into the mediastinum posticum, which, inasmuch as the vertebræ were intact, had apparently crawled through the intervertebral foramina, and by pressure on the spinal cord had caused paralysis of the lower extremities.

Furthermore, all the organs directly connected with the œsophagus or mediastinum may, by the extension of the cancer, first become firmly adherent to them, after which the cancer grows rapidly into their interior, or by breaking down leads to the establishment of a perforation in them. In this way the cancer extends to the walls of the *trachea* and *bronchi*, and makes its appearance on their internal surface, as it has been found on the posterior wall of the trachea, in the form of a hilly growth, occupying its entire length. It attacks the peritoneum in the region of the cardiac extremity, higher up the pericardium and pleura, and spreads itself over these membranes. It grows directly into the lung, although more rarely. The adventitia of the aorta is occasionally infiltrated by the cancer, but not the other coverings, which are only liable to rupture by ulceration or sloughing.

The cancer may extend directly to the *vertebræ*, to which the cancerous œsophagus is frequently firmly united, and cause total destruction of one or more of these ; it may then, by projecting into the vertebral canal, lead to fatal paralysis from pressure on the spinal cord.

Up to the present time only *one* instance of this interesting event is recorded by Aussant, Diss. inaug. sur les squirrhes de l'estomac. Paris. An. X. p. 12 (*vide* Mondière, Arch. génér. T. 30. p. 515).

We are able to add a second case, precisely similar, seen by ourselves (Zenker) ; we give it in abstract :

Aug. Holder, sixty-six years old, compass-smith, died January 20, 1852, in the Dresden Hospital, to which he was admitted four weeks previously with paralysis of the lower extremities and bladder. He had not complained of any considerable dysphagia, and no diagnosis of œsophageal disease had been made.

Autopsy, Jan. 21, 1852.—*Lesions : Carcinoma of the œsophagus. Extension of carcinoma to trachea and two vertebræ. Metastatic carcinoma of the tracheal and bronchial glands, lungs, liver, and kidneys. Serous cysts in the cerebellum, with hemorrhagic infiltration of neighboring parts. Gangrenous cystitis. Hydrocele on left side.*

Body small and emaciated; skin flabby and earth-colored; feet slightly œdematous. The skin over the sacrum, for a space as large as the palm of the hand, of a blackish green color, and the epidermis detached. Left half of the scrotum swollen to the size of a man's fist, and fluctuating (hydrocele).

Mucous membrane of *pharynx* normal. Exactly at the beginning of the *œsophagus*, corresponding to the lower border of the cricoid cartilage, a number of whitish gray nodules of medullary cancer (Markschwamm), about the size of the head of a pin, in the submucous cellular tissue, and on the anterior wall a larger tumor of the mucous membrane, from which on section a reddish gray pultaceous substance exudes. About an inch lower down begins a superficial ulcer, several inches long, including the entire circumference of the tube, the upper border of which is much undermined and projecting, its base very uneven, with deep sinuses, and covered by greasy, greenish, fetid débris. Above and below this ulcer, a number of round ulcers, size of a pea, with thickened, infiltrated edges. Below this follows a space, one and an half inches long, perfectly normal. Then begins a cancerous infiltration of the entire œsophageal wall, as far as the cardiac extremity, at which point it is about half an inch thick. The internal surface here with exception of a deep ulcer at the cardiac extremity, and a slight erosion higher up, intact. At the cardiac extremity the tube is so narrow that the index finger can only with difficulty be introduced. Below this contraction are two nodes of medullary cancer, size of a pea or bean, under the mucous membrane. The *arch of the aorta* firmly united to the œsophagus by cancerous infiltration which has forced its way into the adventitia; same in regard to trachea. The *tracheal* lymphatic glands show more or less cancerous infiltration, in the midst of melanotic tissue. Finally, the œsophagus, in several places, is firmly adherent to the spinal column. *Laryngeal* mucous membrane pale, normal. *Trachea:* beginning about one inch below the cricoid cartilage, the mucous membrane of the posterior wall is infiltrated by cancer, slightly swollen, the surface in the infiltrated region uneven, greenish gray. In the neighborhood of the infiltration above and on the sides, isolated, round, whitish gray nodules of medullary cancer about the size of a lentil; at the entrance to the left bronchus, a round cancerous ulcer, at the base of which, covered by a villous, whitish gray, soft mass, the cartilaginous rings are exposed. Immediately below, reaching into the bronchus itself, a wider, deeper and more sinuous ulcer, with infiltrated edges and base. Both lobes of *thyroid gland* swollen to the size of a hen's egg; left lobe contains numerous cysts, as large as a cherry, some filled with clots of blood, others with a colloid material; right lobe calcified throughout, with numerous large and small cavities. On opening the *spinal canal*, the second and eighth dorsal vertebræ are found to be softened, and the latter forms a soft tumor projecting into the canal. By sawing through the vertebræ, the two mentioned above appear completely destroyed, and their places occupied by medullary cancer, except at single spots, which still contain splinters of bone. The rest of the spine normal. The head of the seventh rib is also destroyed by cancer. Moderate quantity of serum under the spinal arachnoid membrane; on the posterior surface a thin, milky white cartilaginous layer, 2–3 lines in thickness. Pia mater somewhat pallid. Spinal cord softened in the region of the eighth dorsal vertebra, protrudes somewhat on section, elsewhere of normal consistence. The left lobe of the cerebellum contains, in its white substance, a serous cyst, size of the head of a pin, with a hemorrhagic circle, about one-third of a line wide, surrounding it. Rest of the brain normal.

Right *pleural cavity* contains a moderate quantity of serum. Both *lungs* consolidated at their apices; a large number of dull, whitish gray nodules, size of grains of gravel, scattered over all the lobes, partly isolated, partly arranged in groups. In the posterior portion of the lower lobes, small, lobular, pneumonic infiltrations. In the *pericardium*, a large quantity of serum. Heart small; muscular substance softened. In the *aorta*, some atheromatous spots. *Liver* rather small; on its upper surface a number of round, yellowish, slightly projecting nodules, from the size of a pinhead to a bean, the largest of which are distinctly umbilicated. On section, these appear as round, whitish gray nodules of soft cancer, the largest of which contain a central cavity, quite well defined, about the size of a cherry-stone. *Spleen* very small; substance pale. *Kidneys* present on their surface numerous gray nodules, size of a millet-seed, partly isolated and partly arranged in groups, which, on being cut into, appear as round nodules or as vertical stripes extending into the pyramids. Mucous membrane of *pelvis of kidney* covered with a loose exudation, darkly injected, and much ecchymosed. *Bladder* contains a large quantity of thick, pale red, highly albuminous urine; its wall very thick ; mucous membrane of a dark red and greenish marble color, in part gangrenous, and has a very bad odor. Mucous membrane of *stomach*, with exception of dark congestion and slaty color near the pylorus, normal. *Small intestine* contracted, normal. *Large intestine* also contracted ; mucous membrane at the ileo-cæcal valve ulcerated, but no infiltration of the vicinity.

Extension of carcinoma by *dissemination*, as discrete nodules developed in the vicinity of the original cancer, but distinctly separated from it, occurs very rarely in the mucous, as in the serous membranes. In order to explain this form of extension, it must be conceded that cells of the original cancer, capable of proliferation, are carried by the currents into the tissues, or by their own movements into neighboring parts, and that possibly, as far as serous membranes are concerned, whole fragments of cancer are mechanically pushed along and implanted in other places. In this way can we best explain the nodules found on the pleuræ, sometimes in places quite far removed, which can scarcely be regarded as true metastases, since nothing of the kind is found in other parts. As a rule, however, these disseminated nodules are situated in the immediate vicinity of the original cancer, in the pleural and peritoneal coverings of the œsophagus and cardiac portion of the stomach, and at the apex of the pericardium, from which point we have seen the disease extend to distant portions of the same membrane. In the mucous membrane they appear as large nodules, size of a lentil or still larger, confined to the œsophagus, or extending beyond the cardiac extremity, into the stomach. By junction with one another and with the original cancer, they contribute very much to the enlargement of the latter.

Metastatic extension of œsophageal cancer, by means of the lymphatic and capillary circulation, has, strange to say, been described by the earlier authors as extremely unfrequent compared with other forms. To the degree insisted upon by them, this statement is certainly not correct.

On close examination, some of the *lymphatic glands* will generally be found infiltrated by the cancer, and that to a considerable extent, as for instance, the glands lying on the œsophagus itself, the tracheal or bronchial glands at the bifurcation and at the root of the lung, and, when the cancer is situated in the lowest portion, the epigastric glands. When, as happens in rare cases, these enlarged glands are actually wanting, their absence can probably be accounted for by the fact that the lymphatic vessels of the œsophagus sometimes open directly into the thoracic duct, without previously passing through these glands.

Metastases in other organs, most frequently the *liver*, and next the *lung*, are by no means rare. With reference to the frequency of such metastases in the liver, Petri insists, and very justly, that when the disease involves the lower portion of the tube, the cancerous elements may be carried directly to the liver, through the inferior œsophageal veins, which empty into the portal vein. Such metastases have been found in the *kidneys*, *supra-renal capsules*, *pancreas*, in the *bones*, and even in the *brain*. In these different organs, notably in the liver, they were sometimes very considerable both in number and size.

Petri, who was the first to describe minutely the metastases following œsophageal cancer, found such in twenty-five out of forty-two cases (59.5 per cent.)!—a very large number, as great as that observed in many other cancers. In our fifteen cases we found metastasis occurring nine times (nearly equal to the 60 per cent. given by Petri), partly in the glands only, partly (six times) in other organs (liver, lung, kidneys)—some of considerable size.

The following report of a post-mortem examination will serve as an example of abundant secondary development of cancer in all three forms of extension :

Karl H., forty-eight, mechanic (autopsy July 4, 1861—Zenker).

Carcinoma of the œsophagus. Continued carcinoma of trachea and adjacent connective tissue in the neck and mediastinum. Disseminated carcinoma of the pericardium. Metastatic carcinoma of the lungs and liver. Displacement of the trachea. Purulent bronchitis and broncho-pneumonia of right lower lobe. Degenerative atrophy of the kidneys. True diverticulum in small intestine.

Body much emaciated. Skin flabby, of an earthy hue. Thighs slightly curved by rachitis. Brown cicatricial spots on the lower portion of the right thigh. Nothing worthy of mention in the *cranial cavity. Neck :* thyroid gland of normal size ; substance pale brown, with small, soft, goitrous nodes. Mucous membrane of *pharynx* somewhat pale, normal. *Œsophagus* much narrowed, from immediately below the pharynx, for the distance of 11 ctms. ; only pervious above to the sound, but somewhat wider below. The wall, in its whole extent, much thickened (to the extent of 1 ctm.) ; muscular coat hypertrophied (2–3 mm.). Mucous membrane and submucous cellular tissue converted into one layer, pale gray on section, and pouring out abundant gray fluid; this layer projects into the canal, and presents throughout a granular, irregularly hilly surface. In the middle of the narrowed portion is a depression 3 ctms. in length, the base of which is quite smooth, and partly formed by the wall of the trachea, which at this point is almost entirely exposed. Lower portion of œsophagus normal.

On the left of the trachea and œsophagus, in the jugular fossa, a very compact oblong tumor, 2½ ctms. thick, surrounding the vessels, with whitish gray and rather dry cut surface, which gives exit to sausage-like plugs from small openings. In the posterior mediastinum, especially on the right side, a uniform, hard, scirrhous tumor, which partially encloses the right bronchus.

Thorax : in the *pleural* cavities, a slight amount of serum ; pleuræ, especially the left, covered by a soapy material. *Lungs :* except at one point in the right, free from adhesions, emphysematous at their borders ; below, slight pleuritic blush ; tissue of lungs in great part inflated, moderately congested, studded on both sides with numerous white or pale gray round nodules of soft cancerous tissue, from size of a pea to that of a cherry-stone, lying partly below the surface and partly on the periphery, and mostly umbilicated; right lower lobe almost collapsed and flabby ; on section the tissue is of a dirty grayish red color, with fine gray points, giving exit to a dark gray fluid; the bronchi somewhat dilated, filled with yellow pus. *Pericardium* contains a moderate amount of serum ; on the visceral portion numerous tendinous spots ; the parietal portion on the right side, where it joins the root of the lung, studded with hard, scirrhous nodules. *Heart* small, flabby ; valves thin.

Peritoneal cavity contains a few drops of serum. *Liver* somewhat small, flabby ;

on the anterior surface, to the right, a soft pale gray node of cancerous tissue, size of a hazel-nut; posteriorly, in the left lobe and in the lobus quadratus, a sharply defined node of cancer, with faint gray, pale yellow cut surface; the rest of parenchyma anæmic.

Gall-bladder contains greenish brown thin bile. *Spleen* small and soft. Both *kidneys* somewhat small; capsule adherent, surface very uneven, with deep cicatricial depressions and firm granulations on the surface; intermediate portions covered with coarse granules and numerous fine points of calcification. On section the cortical portion throughout dark, congested, thin, and shrunken in places; pyramids grayish red; in the papillæ some chalky infarction. *Bladder* empty, mucous membrane pale. Mucous membrane of *stomach* moderately congested. *Small intestine* contains scarcely anything but masses of mucus; mucous membrane moderately congested, with slight pigmentation of the tufts in its upper portion. 96 ctms. above the ileo-cæcal valve is a true intestinal diverticulum, 4 ctms. long, in the form of the thumb of a glove, which goes off at an acute angle from the side of the intestinal wall, and at its point shows numerous hernia-like projections about the size of a pea. Large intestine narrowed, mucous membrane pale.

As *causes of death* in cases of œsophageal cancer, the autopsy frequently reveals merely the most advanced degree of inanition caused by the stricture; very often, however, the various consequences of the different perforations sooner or later lead to a fatal termination. Among these the most important are the perforations into the air-passages, causing death from inflammation, ulceration, and gangrene of the lungs, or from pleurisy and pneumo-thorax; again, in cases of perforation of the pericardium, death results from pericarditis and pneumo-pericardium; the less frequent perforations of large blood-vessels carry off the patient suddenly by hæmatemesis, or with symptoms of internal hemorrhage. It has been seen above that paraplegia with its consequences may result from the extension of the cancer, and terminate the scene. On the other hand, there are certain diseases, only very indirectly or not at all related to the œsophageal cancer, which occasionally cause death, and this applies particularly to the small insular cancers, which have never as yet been recognized during life.

The *etiology* of œsophageal cancer, as of all cancers, is enveloped in the deepest obscurity. Several circumstances, however, connected with the etiology appear very definite.

The *predisposition* to this, as to other cancers, is very materially influenced by the *age*, but, unlike many other cancers, it is influenced very decidedly by the *sex*. On this point the earlier writers and all statistics agree in stating that the male sex is immeasurably more exposed to the disease, and this is so much the more remarkable since cancer of the stomach, coming next to this in point of space, manifests no distinction whatever between the two sexes (*vide* Vol. VII., p. 237).

Of Petri's forty-four cases, only three occurred in women. In our fifteen cases the proportion of men was not so overwhelming, but still very decided (eleven men, four women). Combining these figures, there results a percentage of 88.1 men and 11.8 women, or a predisposition seven to eight times as strong in men as in women.

Inasmuch as it is impossible to make out any difference in the construction of the œsophagus in the two sexes (neither is any such difference probable), the reason for this striking disproportion must be looked for in the fact that the female is far less exposed to the probable exciting causes, presently to be described, than the male. The objection that the exciting causes, valid in œsophageal cancer, might apply *mutatis mutandis* to cancer of the stomach, may be met by the answer that the more sensitive mucous membrane of the stomach requires less irritation, and is more frequently affected by diseases in general, than that of the much better protected œsophagus, which is able, for a short time at least, to ward off such irritations.

As regards *age*, it is generally acknowledged that in this, as in all cancers, the disease makes its appearance in persons more advanced in years, and that œsophageal cancers are very rare before the age of forty. The majority occur between the ages of forty-one and seventy (about eighty per cent.). The age of fifty supplies the greatest number of all.

Petri's cases and our own are divided as follows with reference to age:

	21–30.	31–40.	41–50.	51–60.	61–70.	71–80.	81–90.	
Petri,	3	1	7	18	6	3	0	= 38 cases.
Zenker,	0	1	5	4	3	1	1	= 15 "
	3	2	12	22	9	4	1	53 "

We suppose, in conformity with Thiersch's ingenious hypothesis, that the explanation of this predisposition in advanced age is to be found in the fact that the continuous proliferation of the epithelium (as is sufficiently verified by its rapid restoration after removal) diminishes the power of resistance in the connective tissue, already undergoing retrograde changes, and when the exciting causes are brought into action the production of epithelium exceeds that of the connective tissue. From this point of view it is neither a question of total non-resistance on the part of the connective tissue, nor of an absolute increase of the epithelium.

Whether *heredity* has any share in the predisposition to this, as it has to other cancers, is not fully established, although it is not improbable. Single cases have been published which favor this view (*e. g.*, case by J. Frank,[1] taken from an English publication). However, these cases are entirely too scarce to establish this point.

Some observers would regard the existence of tuberculosis or the tubercular diathesis as a disposing cause of œsophageal cancer (Lebert, Hamburger, Fritsche). But, although tuberculosis occurs not very unfrequently with œsophageal cancer (the two diseases certainly do not exclude each other), yet their combination is by no means so frequent (according to Petri, only four times in forty-four cases) that any etiological relation can be deduced from it. Finally, as regards arterial sclerosis, which has also been adduced as a cause of œsophageal cancer, its appearance at these periods of life is so common that we can draw no conclusions from their comparatively frequent combination. We found no trace of aortic sclerosis in patients of somewhat younger age (thirty-seven and forty-one years).

Finally, the question, often raised, whether cicatrices of the œsophagus are disposed to undergo a cancerous transformation remains to be considered. This question is a very proper one in view of the undoubted relations which many cancers of the stomach bear to round cicatrizing ulcers of the same organ. In point of fact, so far as the œsophagus is concerned, several cases have been observed which admit of no other construction, and especially in one case, carefully described by E. Neumann,[2] where the

---

[1] Vide quotation in *Fritsche's* dissertation. pp. 4 and 16.
[2] Virchow's Archiv. Bd. 20. p. 142.

post-mortem pnenomena could scarcely be explained in any other way than that a simple cicatrix (the cause of which unfortunately could not be ascertained from the history of the case) was subsequently converted into a cancer. A similar case of our own (very remarkably, the youngest patient, thirty-seven years old) admits of this construction, although it does not directly demonstrate the correctness of it. The subject is worthy of careful investigation.

On general principles, we must look for the *exciting causes* chiefly in the mechanical, thermal, and chemical irritants which are strong enough to induce proliferation in the mucous membrane. The substances which pass through the canal as food and drink, under certain circumstances, become such irritants, sufficient in number and strength to produce this assumed action in tissue already disposed thereto. Experience, derived from various sources, demonstrates in a remarkable manner that the most important exciting causes are really included among these substances. In this connection belongs the theory, insisted upon by many, that frequent tipplers are especially liable to œsophageal cancer, inasmuch as such an individual exacts so much more from his œsophagus than others. If we regard drinking as producing a direct effect in these cases, the rule will apply only to the strongest liquors, brandy in particular, while the ordinary beers and wines, in their rapid passage, can scarcely produce irritation sufficiently intense to injure the well-protected œsophagus. Much more importance, it seems to us, should be attached to the intemperance which attends the love of drink; to overloading of the stomach, with the eructation and vomiting which follow it; to eating hastily, by which food in large pieces and too hot, or containing foreign bodies, is swallowed; to the use of highly seasoned, sharp viands, since all these expose the œsophagus to the most varied diseases.[1] The same causes may be accused in the case of many a patient obliged to live well, whom it would be very unjust to designate as a "tippler." Since all the vices men-

---

[1] Moreover, *Fritsche* insists very correctly that the condition of the tippler may act as a predisposing cause, for the reason that his ability to resist the disease is much reduced by this habit. In this respect he places himself, by his own act, in the condition of persons more advanced in years and more disposed to cancer.

tioned are, to such an overwhelming extent, peculiar to the male, the very striking predisposition of that sex to cancer is easily explained.

In point of fact, however, some cases have been published in detail where the patients themselves traced with great clearness the very beginning of their trouble to some injurious influence, of which they were immediately conscious ; as in an interesting case described by Henoch,' where a lump of hot food lodged in the throat of a man forty-eight years old, who was eating rapidly ; he began immediately to complain of pain on swallowing, which steadily increased ; symptoms of stenosis supervened, and the patient died exactly one year after the accident, from œsophageal cancer, as the autopsy showed. In Deininger's case (*vide* his dissertation), a healthy farmer, forty years old, attributed his trouble to a large piece of smoked meat, after eating which he immediately felt ill.. Very soon after there was marked dysphagia, which increased more and more, and after thirteen months he died from epithelial cancer of the œsophagus, as was verified by post-mortem examination. The case described by Fritsche (loc. cit., p. 74) speaks loudly in favor of this view ; a healthy woman, fifty-two years old, took one swallow of very hot tea, which immediately produced a burning sensation in the throat. Two or three weeks afterwards she complained of an oppression in the pharynx on swallowing, with which were subsequently associated marked symptoms of stenosis. Then follows the long history of suffering from cancer of the œsophagus, which was clearly diagnosticated during life by the fragments of cancer thrown off, and after death, which followed in thirteen months, was confirmed by the autopsy. In every such case the evidence may be rejected on the ground that probably at that time the cancer existed in a latent form, and that the attention of the patient had been called to it for the first time when the accident occurred. This is not impossible. Yet nothing favors this view, and it certainly seems more natural to assume that the injury so distinctly felt was really the cause of the trouble, which commenced at once, and continued more and more to develop itself.

---

[1] Casper's Wochenschrift f. d. gesammte Heilk. 1847. No. 30.

In former times the only thing that militated against this latter view was the preconceived idea that every form of cancer repre-sented an effort on the part of Nature to rid the blood of some pernicious element. Since this opinion has, fortunately, been set aside, such scepticism has no firm foundation on which to rest when opposed by cases which have been carefully observed and not hastily sketched. Moreover, it loses authority as more of these cases come to light.

That foreign bodies actually lodged in the œsophagus can bring on this whole process, is proved by positive instances in which such substances as fish-bones and cherry-stones (Lebert) have been found imbedded in the cancerous ulcer. Such cases as these are really much more entitled to the suspicion that the foreign body found a lodgment after the growth had already made some headway.

As a more remote proof of this theory of mechanical irritation as an exciting cause of cancer, reference has been made—and very justly—to the fact that the lower and middle thirds of the œsophagus are the parts affected by preference. In the lower third, the narrow cardiac extremity easily obstructs the passage of the food, while in the middle third the œsophagus is pressed by solid food against the rigid wall of the left bronchus at the point of intersection ; these constitute the causes which chiefly favor mechanical injuries in these sections of the canal.[1]

Secondary carcinoma of the œsophagus, inasmuch as a metas-tatic variety has in point of fact not been observed, occurs only in the disseminated form and in that which owes its existence to an extension of the disease from other parts ; both forms almost invariably being derived from the stomach, in cancer affecting the cardiac extremity of that organ ; in extremely rare cases, the

---

[1] In a long, creditable article, which has just appeared concerning the localization of diseased action in the œsophagus (Philadelphia Med. Times, Oct 13, 1877), *Harrison Allen* lays particular emphasis upon the very frequent occurrence of disease at the point of intersection with the left bronchus, and, referring to English surgical authors, says that this fact has hitherto been entirely overlooked. This remark certainly does not apply to German authors, for they, especially *Klebs, Rindfleisch, Koenig,* have made this very prominent in speaking of cancer of the œsophagus. In these pages, also, it has been repeatedly pointed out.

primary disease is in the pharynx, although cancer in this organ is, as a rule, very infrequent. The cancers extending from the cardiac extremity of the stomach are not so very infrequent (we have seen six such against thirteen primary cancers). But they generally advance only a short distance beyond the orifice, not more than a few centimetres. When stenosis has taken place in consequence of cancer at the cardiac extremity, the secondary growths in the œsophagus are always so slow in making their appearance, and so little liable to deep ulceration, that the general course of the disease is scarcely modified in any way by their presence. Consequently very little pathological interest is attached to this secondary form of cancer.

According to Rokitansky, mediastinal carcinomata, in rare cases, extend to the œsophagus.

Whether *tubercle* and *tubercular ulcers* occur in the œsophagus has not as yet been clearly demonstrated. Oppolzer alone asserts their existence in a positive manner. In the absence of all detailed statements, however, this assertion can only be received with restrictions, notwithstanding the positiveness with which the author makes it. An ulcer described by Paulicki[1] as "probably tubercular," was certainly not such. So also the tubercular nature of the ulcers described by Chvostek[2] and Kraus (quoted by Birch-Hirschfeld) cannot be regarded as fully demonstrated. We have seen only two ulcers, after close attention to this subject, which we believe could be called tubercular: once, in a tuberculous child, a single, small, round ulcer, with very finely pointed nodules by the side of it; the second time, in the case briefly described above (p. 116), of extensive perforation of the œsophagus caused by caseous glands. Microscopical examination in both cases revealed nothing which could justify their designation as tubercular. The question is still an open one. It is certain, however, after all these negative results, that the œsophagus is highly exempt from tuberculosis, in which respect again it coincides with the integument.

---

[1] Virchow's Archiv. Bd. 44. p. 373.

[2] Oesterr. Zeitschr. f. prakt. Heilk. 1868. XIV. 27, 28. Schmidt's Jahrb. Bd. 141, p. 293.

Symptomatology and Diagnosis.

The *symptoms* of *œsophageal cancer* are those of a slowly increasing stenosis, frequently accompanied by pain and spasm of the œsophagus, and by emaciation and loss of strength, which are observed early in the disease. The dysphagia occasionally exists for months without any intimation of pain or cachexia. Such cases are observed in younger individuals particularly, and then on account of the age give rise to doubts as to the diagnosis. The sound generally decides the question, as it reveals a narrowing, moderate at first, but gradually increasing, at some fixed point in the œsophagus, and a pain that is always referred to the same spot when the point of the instrument enters the contracted portion. As the disease advances, the pain is seldom absent. The dysphagia increases slowly, and is associated with regurgitation of a portion of the food, at least of solid food, until finally the canal is completely closed, and not even fluids can pass through. According as the cancer is situated in the upper or lower portions of the œsophagus, the regurgitation of the food follows at an earlier or later date. In the first stage, the food will be mixed only with large quantities of mucus; subsequently, however, when the cancer ulcerates, the food comes up covered with blood and mucus, or with foul, cancerous ichor. Cancers situated high up, when ulceration occurs impart a fetid odor to the breath, and frequently at an early stage, by secondary hyperplasia of the peri-œsophageal connective tissue, cause a constriction and paralysis of the inferior laryngeal nerve of one, and more rarely of both sides (compare p. 38).

With the beginning of ulceration, the stricture occasionally becomes considerably dilated, so that the patient is able to swallow even solid food tolerably well. In this stage, small particles of the cancerous growth may sometimes be extracted from the fenestra of the sound.

In one of the cases observed by ourselves (Ziemssen), when the coincidence of several circumstances (less advanced age, supposed injury of the œsophagus from swallowing a bone, absence of cachexia, etc.) made the diagnosis more difficult, the extraction of a fragment of cancroid finally established the nature of the stenosis.

The *diagnosis* presents, for the most part, no difficulties. Special importance is to be attached to the more advanced age, male sex, absence of traumatic or other cause, slow increase of the stenosis, pain independent of any pressure, the result of ex. amination by the sound, and the cachexia.

The large proportion in the male sex has already been demonstrated by figures which are indisputable, because founded on anatomical investigations. We will state, however, that we (Ziemssen) find our clinical observations in complete accord with them. Unfortunately, an autopsy could not be made in every case, so that our figures cannot claim that absolute certainty which those given by Petri and Zenker possess.

In the 18 cases of œsophageal cancer which we (Ziemssen) observed and treated, 17 were males and 1 female. Of these 18 cases, there were found between the ages of

30-40	41-50	51-60	61-70
2	4	7	5

In 13 of these 18 cases the cancer was situated in the lower third, which harmonizes exactly with the figures given above.

The pain, although not always present, is a very valuable aid to diagnosis when it does occur, especially when we notice that it is not simply elicited by mechanical irritation (introduction of the sound, etc.), but exists spontaneously, shooting through the chest and radiating in other directions. The occurrence of pain *at night* sufficient to keep the patient awake, when preceded by no mechanical injuries, makes the existence of cancer probable.

The location of the pain, as well as its extent, will vary according to the higher or lower situation of the cancer, the greater or lesser extent of the morbid growth, and the neighboring organs involved (spine, pleura, pericardium, etc.).

The *duration* of the cancer very rarely exceeds one year. Cases of two years' duration, and longer, are sometimes observed, although in such cases it is supposed that a new growth has sprung from a cicatricial stricture. In many cases death occurs after a few months.

The *result* is always fatal, and this termination is either caused directly by perforations of neighboring organs, and consequent inflammations and ulcerations, by extension of the cancer by contiguity or metastasis, by gangrene of the lung, etc., or by simple inanition as the result of obstruction in the alimentary canal.

Treatment.

The treatment of carcinoma of the œsophagus is merely palliative and purely symptomatic. In those cases only where the cancer is situated in the upper portion, and is accessible to the knife, will the attempt at a radical cure by extirpation of the cancerous portion be possible. Whether the attempts of Billroth and others in this direction will have any result, remains to be seen.

The most important question in the palliative treatment is the mode of feeding the patient, which includes the *admissibility of mechanical dilatation of the cancerous stricture by the use of the sound.* In reference to this point, there is found in most manuals a warning against the use of the sound in the later stages of cancer, on account of the danger of producing perforation by the point of the instrument.

From our experience, we (Ziemssen) are compelled to believe that these warnings are founded more upon theoretical reasoning than upon actual observation of any bad results. At least, in the seventeen cases which we treated methodically by the introduction of the sound, perforation of the lung was observed in one case, and this perforation seemed to have no causal relation with the use of the sound. (This was the case described on p. 122.) In our eighteen cases perforation of the pericardium was found once, but in this case the sound was not used.

On the other hand, the introduction of the sound is followed by such excellent results in the way of palliation, that we are compelled to recommend its use (daily, or every other day).

In several cases we have seen life prolonged for several months, although when this treatment was commenced the canal was completely closed, to the extent even of not allowing fluids to pass. It is not improbable that the mechanical pressure may produce shrinkage of the morbid growth, or even cicatrization of its base, when the cancerous mass has been cleared away ; at all

events, in some cases (case given on p. 123 belongs to these) a condition very much like cicatrization has been found after death,
by the side of recent appearances of cancer, and slaty discoloration of the narrowed portion (a condition which certainly admits
of another construction as well, compare p. 188). Whether,
under these circumstances, such very rare cases terminate in a
radical cure, as Rokitansky (p. 178) supposes, must be left undecided.

The improvement in swallowing resulting from the introduction of even the smallest sound is very striking, and, so far as
concerns the nutrition of the patient, is very important. Two or
three days after the permeability of the stricture is established,
the patient is able to swallow meat, and for the next few weeks
his bodily weight increases rapidly and considerably. Unfortunately, this favorable effect only continues as long as the use
of the sound is kept up. When, as frequently happens, the
patient becomes tired of this mechanical treatment, and discon-
tinues its use, he generally returns after a few weeks to the same
condition as before, for the reason that a few days after it is
given up his ability to swallow is reduced to a minimum.

It is scarcely necessary to mention that the sound must be
made to feel its way, and that it must be used with the greatest
caution, especially at first, when the stricture is not thoroughly
permeable. It is advisable to begin with the smallest size ; it
will be found that rapid progress can be made to the largest
size. The conical bougies of Bouchard have proved very suitable in cancerous strictures, as in those resulting from cicatrization.

As for other treatment, the well-known rules for the artificial
feeding of patients find their application here. Narcotics, as a
matter of course, are not to be omitted.

Concerning the symptomatology and treatment of other
morbid growths, there is scarcely anything to be added to what
was said when speaking of their pathology, since most of them
are without symptoms, and neither diagnosis nor treatment is
satisfactory. When they attain such a size as to produce stenosis, we can recognize the latter, although ignorant of the nature

of the morbid growth which produces it. The protracted course of the tumor justifies the suspicion of its non-malignant character. In the certainly very rare cases of a stenosis due to the presence of a sarcoma (see Chapman's case, p. 169), it would be impossible to distinguish during life between such a tumor and carcinoma. The treatment of all such cases must be conducted on general principles. In regard to the treatment of polypus, as this is purely surgical, we refer the reader to the surgical text-books (particularly Koenig, l. c.).

VEGETABLE AND ANIMAL PARASITES.

The narrow œsophageal tube, with its smooth surface constantly bathed by the fluids which pass over it, presents a soil but little favorable to the settlement of parasites. Accordingly, we find here but very few parasitic diseases. The most frequent by far, and most important, is *thrush*, which appears in the œsophagus under the same form as in the mouth, and always as an extension from that cavity.[1] It occurs most frequently in children, but, although somewhat more rarely, it is found at all other periods of life, equally divided, and that without distinction as to sex. In children it occurs chiefly in connection with intestinal catarrh, with the acute exanthemata (measles, smallpox), and with phthisis. In adults we have found it most frequently in phthisical persons, next in protracted cases of typhus fever ; occasionally it occurs in pyæmia and puerperal fever, and always in very exhaustive diseases, whether acute or chronic, which are much prolonged.

The thrush-masses in the œsophagus present themselves partly as small, soft lumps or shreds, which are loosely adherent to the mucous membrane; partly, and more frequently, as very soft, gray, grayish white or yellowish gray adherent membranes, 1 mm. or more in thickness, sometimes presenting various colors, derived from the fluids which pass through the canal. These hang on the wall of the œsophagus throughout its entire length, or in spots, and for the most part adhere so loosely to the mucous membrane that a strong jet of water washes them away,

---

[1] Further particulars concerning thrush, with its bibliography, will be found under Diseases of the Mouth.

while in some places they are often more firmly attached. The internal surface of the membrane generally presents numerous shallow longitudinal fissures, corresponding to the folds in the mucous membrane, when the tube is contracted. These fissures occasionally extend through the entire thickness of the membrane, and divide it into single longitudinal stripes. The subjacent mucous membrane is generally normal, sometimes markedly congested, and very rarely studded with superficial (catarrhal) ulcers.

The microscopical examination of thrush in the œsophagus, very carefully prosecuted by E. Wagner, has shown that the fungus masses, here as in the mouth, consist of a very thick net-work of filaments, with numerous spores interposed, and abundant masses of very uniformly fine granules, developed chiefly in the middle layers of the thick epithelial covering, while the deepest layers remain as a thin superficial covering. Wagner discovered, furthermore, that single filaments penetrated the deeper epithelial layers into the tissue itself of the mucous membrane, even as far as into the blood-vessels, a fact which was confirmed by A. Vogel after examination of a case of thrush in the mouth, and which is of the greatest importance in explaining the metastasis of thrush, as we (Zenker) found it beautifully shown in the brain.[1]

With the appearance of thrush in the œsophagus, the fungus is commonly developed to the same or a less extent in the pha-

---

[1] Jahresber. d. Ges. f. Natur- u. Heilkunde in Dresden pro 1861-62. Dresden, 1863. p. 51. The theory recently advanced by *Grawitz*, at a meeting of the Berlin Medical Society (Berliner klin. Wochenschr. 1877. No. 41), that in our case it might have been masses of thrush, which "had grown in the vascular system, and afterwards had been torn off and transported to the brain, but did not develop there" (since *Grawitz* was never able, by repeated attempts at injection, to produce a growth of thrush in the circulation), is not tenable. In that case it was a nodule, easily seen with the naked eye, consisting of a dense filamentous net-work, the circumference of which far exceeded that of the largest blood-vessel in the interior of the brain-substance. Moreover, as it is not to be supposed that the fungi grow directly in the arteries leading to the brain, but in the blood-vessels supplying the mucous membrane of the mouth, throat, and œsophagus, the fungus masses would have to pass through the capillary net-work of the lung before they could be deposited in the brain. Hence, it can be seen that merely the *fungous spores* are conveyed to that organ. The development of the filamentous net-work could only have taken place in the brain-substance.

rynx, and even in the mouth, where it appears mostly in the form of islands on the tongue, cheeks, and lips. It is sometimes wanting, however, in all these parts, in which case the fungus masses may have been previously removed.

In very rare cases the fungus may extend from the œsophagus to the *mucous membrane of the stomach*, so little disposed to thrush, as Klebs found in a case described by Plaskuda,[1] where it existed in very large masses.

Small patches of thrush are occasionally found growing exuberantly in the larynx itself, rather firmly adherent to the mucous membrane, and the same are found on the vocal cords and on the epiglottis. They may extend still farther, over the *trachea* and *bronchi* (compare Virchow's case, given below in detail).

We have twice seen such deposits in the larynx, which the microscope showed to be thrush, with the same fungus in the œsophagus (a child, five weeks old, which died from intestinal catarrh; and a woman, thirty-three years old, dead from puerperal fever).

Small portions of the thrush-fungus will frequently be thrown off by the patient. Gerhardt,[2] however, in the case of a child, saw the whole mass thrown off at one time in the form of a cylinder, corresponding to the form of the œsophagus, after the administration of an emetic.

On the other hand, the fungous growth may be so considerable that the œsophagus is not only lined, but its cavity completely filled by it, so that food can no longer be swallowed. Such a case was first observed by Virchow[3] in a boy, seven weeks old, whose death was apparently caused by it, and in whose larynx, trachea, and bronchi were found large masses of the fungus. A similar fatal case has recently been published by Buhl.[4] Such complete stuffing of the œsophagus by the thrush-fungus has been observed several times by Virchow (l. c.), Liebermeister, and Hoffmann,[5] in convalescent typhus fever patients.

[1] Berlin. klin. Wochenschr. 1864. 52.

[2] Deutsche Klinik. 1858. 9.

[3] Verhandl. der physik.-med. Ges. in Würzburg. III. Bd. 1852. p. 364.

[4] Intelligenzblatt der bay. Aerzte. 1875. No. 15. p. 146.

[5] Vol. I. of this Cyclopædia, and *C. E. E. Hoffmann*, Veränd. d. Organe beim Abdominaltyphus. Leipzig, 1869. p. 170.

Letzerich [1] has lately published a case, under the title "Mycosis œsophagi," which he describes as a genuine mycotic disease, well marked and never before observed: a girl, fifteen months old, was taken ill with symptoms of dysphagia, to which were added certain gastric disturbances (eructation, marked distention and pain in the region of the stomach). The food, which was swallowed with great difficulty, was immediately thrown off, and after several days the child became much reduced. Muco-purulent masses, streaked with blood, were vomited on several occasions, in which the microscope detected, in addition to epithelial, pus and mucus-cells, larger or smaller colonies of micrococci. Besides large balls of micrococci there were seen "isolated cocci in motion, bacteria, and large masses of cocci arranged close together in the form of a string of pearls, varying much in length, and coiled in a serpentine form, together with large and small blood-globules." As characteristic of these colonies, Letzerich shows that they are rolled into long coiled threads, in the form of a string of pearls, by which this micrococcus is distinguished from all other known pathogenetic fungi (Schistomyceten). Having proved the mycotic nature of the affection, Letzerich ordered salicylic acid, first in solution, afterwards in substance, and recovery took place in the course of a few days. In looking about for the source of the infection, he noticed large wet spots on the wall-paper of the room, and the mother stated that the child had torn off little pieces of the same. Microscopical examination of these offensive bits of paper showed "the characteristic strings of pearls, very much isolated, and a quantity of bacteria, varying in length, moving about in a lively manner," together with more fully developed mould-fungus. By allowing these to breed in gelatine capsules, Letzerich obtained the same structures that he found in the masses vomited. "From this it was proved beyond all question that the infection of the œsophagus was caused by swallowing small pieces of dirty wall-paper." The micrococci may have penetrated the epithelium of the œsophagus, and, by their further development there, may have raised the epithelial flakes and given rise to slight inflammatory swelling of the mucous membrane. Letzerich traces the distention of the stomach to the processes of fermentation, which these low organisms, passing from the œsophagus into the stomach, had produced.

This case presents great interest, so far as its etiology is concerned (its correct observation and explanation being presupposed), and careful investigation in the same direction is strongly to be recommended in analogous cases. In the meantime, we hesitate to accept this new mycosis as an established form of disease, on the authority of a single case.

Of the *animal parasites* there is only one which builds its nest in the œsophagus, viz., the *trichina*. The muscular coat of the œsophagus, in its upper portion, consists of transverse muscular fibres, which in any part of the body where they occur are

---

[1] Archiv f. experimentelle Pathologie und Pharmakologie. Bd. VII. p. 233. 1877.

liable to become studded with trichinæ; so we find this muscular coat, in so far as its transverse fibres are concerned, studded with trichinæ, but in less abundant masses.

' There can be no doubt that, in the course of the trichinous disease, frequent and sometimes very considerable dysphagia is caused by the œsophagus becoming involved in addition to the muscular structure of the pharynx (Vol. III. p. 633). The œsophagi of persons who have recovered from severe trichinosis, when thickly studded, present capsules easily recognized by the naked eye (at least when calcification has taken place), a fact which assists very much in distinguishing the transverse fibres from the smooth muscular substance, since the latter always remains free from trichinæ. When thus enclosed in capsules, the trichinæ give rise to no further disturbance of any kind.

In post-mortem examinations there are found very rarely one or more *round worms* (ascaris lumbricoides) simply lying in the œsophagus. We found, in one case, three such worms lying close together. Apparently they make their way out of the stomach shortly before death, and would be without pathological interest, were it not for the fact that occasionally one end of the worm enters the larynx and causes danger from suffocation, as in the case of a child, reported by Delasiauve,[1] which was found lying in a comatose condition with symptoms of laryngeal constriction, and was saved by the speedy removal of a round worm which was astride the septum, between the œsophagus and trachea. But that a round worm found after death in the œsophagus of an imbecile patient had been the cause of an acute delirium, as Laurens[2] supposes, seems more than doubtful.

In conclusion, it may be mentioned that, in rare cases, *leeches* when swallowed have made their way into the œsophagus and caused hemorrhage by their sucking, but they soon died.[3]

---

[1] Schmidt's Jahrb. Bd. 144. p. 77.   [2] Ibidem.
[3] *Hager,* Die fremden Körper im Menschen. 1844.

NEUROSES OF THE ŒSOPHAGUS.

Bibliography.

Friedr. Hoffmann, De morbis œsophagi spasmodicis. Opera omnia. Edit. Genev. Tom. III. p. 130, and De spasmo gulæ inferioris. Halæ, 1733.—*Van Swieten's* Commentaria in *Boerhaave* Aphorismos, etc. Lovanii, 1773. Tom. III. p. 530. —*Richerand*, Nosographie chirurg. Edit. II. Tom. III. p. 816.—*Courant*, De nonnullis morbis convulsivis œsophagi. Montpellier, 1778.—*Bleuland*, De sana et morbosa œsophagi structura. Lugd. Batav. 1780. p. 56.—*A. Monro*, De dysphagia. Diss. Edinburgh, 1797, and The Morbid Anatomy of the Human Gullet, etc. Edinb. 1811. p. 223.—*Smyth*, Carmichael, quoted by Monro, loc. cit. p. 231.—*Mondière*, Recherches sur l'œsophagisme. Archiv. génér. de Méd. Sér. II. Tom. I. 1833.—*Oppolzer*, Wiener med. Wochenschrift. 1851.—*Follin*, Des rétrécissements de l'œsophage. Thèse de concours. Paris, 1853.—*Romberg*, Lehrbuch der Nervenkrankheiten. III. Aufl. 1853. Bd. I. p. 461.—*Gendron*, Sur la dysphagie, ses variétés et son traitement. Archiv. génér. de Méd. 1858.— *W. Brinton*, On Spasmodic Stricture of the Œsophagus. The Lancet. 1866. I. p. 2. —*H. Power*, On a Case of Spasmodic Stricture of the Œsophagus terminating fatally. The Lancet, 1866. I. p. 252.—*Broca*, Rétrécissement spasmodique de l'œs. Guérison par la dilatation forcée. Gaz. des Hôp. Août 7, 1869.—*Vigla*, Rétrécissement spasmod. de l'œs. Gaz. des Hôp. Sept. 25, 1869.—*Handfield Jones*, Studies of Functional Nervous Disorders. London, 1870.—*Eaton*, Case of Spasmodic Stricture of the Œsophagus. The Lancet. Jan. 13, 1872.—*Seney*, Sur l'œsophagisme chronique. Archives génér. de Méd. Juillet, 1873. p. 95. —*T. Curtis Smith*, A Case of Spasmodic Stricture of the Œs. Philad. Med. and Surg. Reporter. XXX. Feb. 21, 1874.—*Foot*, Cases of Œsophagismus. Dublin Quart. Jour. of Med. Science. Apr. 1874.—*Peter*, Rétréc. spasmod. de l'œs. Pronostic fatal à propos d'une pneumonie de mauvaise nature. Gaz. des Hôpit. 85. 1875.—*Sommerbrodt*, Berl. klin. Wochenschrift. 1875. Nos. 24 and 25.—*F. Ganghofner*, Zur Lehre von der nervösen Dysphagie. Vortrag. Prager med. Wochenschrift. 1876. Nos. 5 and 6.—*M. Mackenzie*, Spasmod. Stricture of the

Œs. Med. Times and Gazette. Oct. 21, 1876.—Paralysis of the Œs. Ibidem. Nov. 18, 1876.—*S. Jaccoud,* Traité de pathologie interne. V. Edit. Tom. II. p. 118. 1877.

Concerning functional diseases of the œsophagus in general, very little is known. The motor disturbances have been more closely investigated, and among these the phenomena of spasm of the œsophagus are best understood. No explanation is given in the literature of this subject concerning the disturbances of sensation. Yet such disturbances do undoubtedly occur; at least we believe that, according to our observations (Ziemssen), anæsthesia of the œsophagus can be shown to occur not very unfrequently in connection with anæsthesia of the pharynx and larynx in diphtheritic paralysis. That they occur as well in other disturbances of the vagus nerve, both in its peripheral course and in its central origin, is probable, although not yet demonstrated.

In the cases of diphtheritic paralysis of the pharynx and larynx, when the food could only be introduced through the œsophageal tube, owing to the imperfect closure of the larynx, it seemed to us (Ziemssen) that the tolerance with which the tube was borne, and the absence of all sensitive reaction on the part of the œsophageal mucous membrane, were very strong arguments in favor of diminished sensibility. In view of this observation and of the fact that in such cases the anæsthesia of the pharyngeal mucous membrane is known to extend as far as the entrance to the œsophagus, it may be regarded as probable that the same disturbance extends to the œsophageal branch of the vagus. Direct proof of the sensibility of the œsophagus might be furnished by the œsophageal electrode in cases favorably disposed to such treatment.

Hyperæsthesia of the œsophageal mucous membrane probably exists in connection with many cases of hysteria and hypochondriasis, although it cannot be directly proved. In many cases of primary spasm of the œsophagus a hyperæsthesia of the mucous membrane might exist, either as the cause of the spasm, or as another effect of one and the same exciting cause. The analogous conditions of hyperæsthesia and spasm in the mucous membrane of the pharynx and larynx on the one hand, and the favorable action of bromide of potassium and mechanical dilatation in the treatment of œsophagismus on the other hand, favor this view. Clinical observations, such as those published by

Foot, Seney, and Sommerbrodt, favor the opinion that hyperæsthesia is a frequent cause of œsophageal spasm.

Of the motor disturbances, spasm of the muscular coat of the œsophagus, although a rare occurrence, seems to be much more frequent than paralysis.

Spasm of the Œsophagus—Spasmus Œsophagi—Œsophagismus.

Spasm of the œsophagus was the occasion of considerable research at the beginning of the eighteenth century, and accordingly we find it variously described as Dysphagia spasmodica (F. Hofmann), Angina convulsiva (Van Swieten), Œsophagospasmus (Vogel), Œsophagisme (Mondière), Rétrécissement spasmodique (Broca), Stenosis spastica fixa et migrans (Hamburger).

We shall first consider the physiological facts which are important for a thorough understanding of the pathogenesis of œsophageal spasm.

The act of swallowing, so far as the œsophagus is concerned, is essentially reflex in its nature; the irritation of the terminal branches of the sensitive nerves in the mucous membrane, by inosculation with the ganglionic plexus supplying the wall of the œsophagus, causes a contraction in the irritated portion, and this proceeds by continuance of the irritation in a peristaltic manner to the lower portions of the tube. For the continuance of this peristaltic wave of contraction, the motion itself is to be regarded as the irritation, by which the successive portions of the tube are made to contract by reflex action (Wild [1]), or, as seems more probable from the recent investigations of Goltz,[2] by irritation of the ganglionic plexuses in the wall of the œsophagus, which have been demonstrated by Meissner, Auerbach, and others. These ganglionic plexuses of the œsophagus are connected with the medulla oblongata by nerve-fibres, and, as it appears, exclusively by the fibres of the vagus nerve.

While direct irritation of the œsophageal wall, as well as of the branches of the vagus nerve, produces contraction of the tube with peristaltic action. Goltz has demonstrated by experiments on frogs that disturbance of the brain and spinal cord, precisely as section of the pneumogastric, causes long-continued, firm contractions of the œsophagus and stomach. The same phenomenon may be produced by violent irritation of other centripetal nerves, not connected in any way with the œsophagus and stomach, e. g., the sciatic and mesenteric nerves, etc. The medulla ob-

---

[1] Ueber die peristaltischen Bewegungen des Œsophagus u. s. w. *Henle* und *Pfeufer's* Zeitschr. f. rat. Med. 1846. Bd. V. p. 76.

[2] Studien über die Bewegungen der Speiseröhre und des Magens des Frosches. Pflueger's Archiv. 1872. VI. p. 616.

longata seems to restrain or arrest reflex action in the muscular substance of the œsophagus, without which the ganglionic plexuses of the latter become so sensitive that the slightest causes, which escape our observation, produce tetanic contraction of its muscular coat.

Goltz regards the effect of peripheral irritation of other centripetal nerves on the œsophagus and stomach not as a reflex contraction in the ordinary acceptation of that term, but as a movement called forth by diminished energy on the part of the medulla oblongata, a kind of stupor of the same. During this apparent death of the medulla oblongata it remains inactive, and, as a result of this, there is developed the same unlimited increase of the ganglionic irritability in the œsophagus as follows extirpation of the medulla oblongata. When the cause of this stupor in the medulla oblongata is merely transitory, its effects in the œsophagus soon pass off, to return again with the renewal of the irritation.

The fact is not to be overlooked that many contradictions exist between the results of Goltz's experiments on frogs and those of earlier authors on warm-blooded animals (Schiff, Chauveau), for which reason other experiments on the larger warm-blooded animals are much to be desired.

For clinical purposes these experimental facts are of great value. They harmonize completely with clinical experience, that persistent spasm of the œsophagus may result from direct irritation of its wall, from the manifold lesions of innervation in the roots and branches of the vagus nerve and medulla oblongata, and finally, from severe irritations which affect other peripheral sensitive regions. In like manner the source of œsophageal spasm might be traced to powerful psychical affections, and as the result of hysteria and the psychoses it might, like the functional disturbances of the respiratory organs, be referred to lesions in the gray matter of the medulla oblongata—which, according to Goltz, must have a depressing influence, somewhat like paralysis.

Finally, as a possible factor of this increased excitability, must be mentioned a disturbance of innervation in the vaso-motor nerves of the œsophagus and its resultant ischæmia. This factor, however, according to Goltz's experiments, is entirely excluded.

Whether the preference shown by spasm for the upper portions of the œsophagus is related in any way to the transverse muscular fibres well represented here in the midst of the smooth muscular fibres, has not been determined, since no reliable statistics of its frequency in the different portions of the œsophagus have as yet been furnished us.

The customary division of œsophageal spasm into idiopathic and symptomatic cannot strictly be carried out.

Those spasms of the œsophagus are to be regarded as *symptomatic* which are produced by inflammation, corrosion, ulceration, morbid growths and foreign bodies in the wall of the œsophagus, as well as of the pharynx ; in addition to these may be mentioned those spasms which are caused by disease of the cervical vertebræ, retro-pharyngeal abscess, diseases of the brain, spinal cord, and pneumogastric nerve. Finally, may be included the spasms which occur in consequence of hysteria, epilepsy, hydrophobia, and tetanus.

The so-called *idiopathic* spasm includes all those cases in which no definite anatomical cause can be demonstrated. If this idiopathic spasm is admitted to be a true neurosis of the œsophagus, it will be necessary to include under this form all those cases which result from reflex action and from irritation of the terminal branches of the vagus nerve, external to the œsophagus, as well as irritation of other centripetal nerves.

In this way, as experience has proved, the reflex spasm may start not only from the stomach and intestines (carcinoma, intestinal worms), but also from the uterus (pregnancy, metritis, flexion, morbid growths), and may subsequently become, to a certain extent, an independent disease.

The origin of spasm is especially interesting when referred to psychical disturbances, as anger, fright, and particularly the dread of hydrophobia, even in cases where the bite came from a dog not at all suspected of being mad. The individuals most disposed to such disturbances are nervous, hysterical, hypochondriacal persons, and pregnant women.

Hamburger distinctly classes the so-called *globus hystericus* with spasm of the œsophagus, although in the former the most important symptoms of spasm—namely, pain, dysphagia, and regurgitation of the ingesta—are wanting ; moreover, the sound encounters no obstruction. Hamburger explains the appearance of the globus as the first (slightest) stage of œsophagismus, distinguished by antiperistaltic tonic contraction of the muscular structure of the œsophagus, with its auscultatory phenomena. There is heard very distinctly, at the moment when the patient complains of the rising globus, a sound as though the œsophagus "is contracting very rapidly at some point low down, in such a manner as to form a funnel turned upward, while the contraction gradually extends up the tube."

These reasons might not suffice to prove the spasmodic nature of globus, but least of all would they justify Hamburger in giving an affirmative answer to the question whether anti-peri-staltic contractions occur in the œsophagus.

In individuals much disposed to this affection, especially when they have once been afflicted, the dread of a recurrence of the attack, or the simple idea of swallowing, suffices to bring on a relapse.

As regards *age* and *sex*, spasm of the œsophagus occurs in women, and in middle life, much more frequently than in men, and during childhood and old age.

Symptomatology and Diagnosis.

The beginning of œsophagismus is marked by a sudden dys-phagia, of greater or less severity, commonly associated with a painful sensation of lacing and burning in the neck or chest. Occasionally, and especially in severe cases, are combined with these, spasms in the muscular structure of the pharynx, larynx, neck, and chest.

Interference with deglutition is complete in a small num-ber of cases only. In such rare cases, the ingesta, even in a fluid form, do not pass through the stricture. At every attempt to swallow, when the spasm is situated in the upper portion of the œsophagus, the food is immediately thrown off. When the spasm involves the lower portion, the ingesta are regurgitated after a short interval, mixed with quantities of mucus and gas.

In the majority of cases there exists simply a difficulty in swallowing, so that the food, after considerable exertion on the part of the patient, and repeated eructation, finally makes its way entirely, or in great part, into the stomach. In most of these cases, fluids are swallowed more easily than solid food; in rare instances the reverse of this obtains. Many of these cases swallow warm fluids more easily, others again cold fluids. The œsophageal sound, introduced during the attack, encounters a stricture at the spot where the spasmodic contraction is located. If stronger pressure is brought to bear upon this stricture with the instrument, or if the point is allowed to remain in the stric-ture for a few minutes, the muscular coat is suddenly or gradu-ally relaxed, and the sound passes down to the stomach without further resistance. Sometimes it is sufficient merely to introduce the sound into the pharynx, when the spasm of the œsophagus disappears at once.

Auscultation furnishes evidence of bubbles of air rising toward the pharynx; in the more advanced degrees of contrac·tion the audible signs of regurgitation of the ingesta are present.

The spasmodic attack returns after a longer or shorter inter-val, and is commonly produced by the act of swallowing or by some psychical emotion, *e. g.*, anger, dread of a relapse, etc.

The *duration* of a single attack varies considerably; it may continue for minutes, hours, days; indeed, the spasm has been known to persist for weeks and months. This "stenosis spastica fixa continua" of Hamburger runs its course without pain, and shows fluctuations of intensity, without at any time complete disappearance of the spasm. In this rare form, even though the ability to swallow has never been abolished, deglutition suffers, and with it, very perceptibly, the nutrition of the patient.

The total duration of the intermittent form, in troublesome cases, may extend over many years (Seney saw a case of fifteen years' duration; Lasègue relates a case in which the spasm existed about thirty years; and finally, Aird mentions a case where the spasm existed during the whole course of a long life);[1] recovery, however, generally takes place much earlier.

No *anatomical lesions* have been found in the few cases which have been examined after death.

One of the oldest cases on record is that of Dr. Rutherford, which is quoted by Monro. It occurred in a girl, twenty years old, who, on account of persistent spasm of the œsophagus, was fed for two years and eight months by means of the œsopha-geal tube. She then recovered so far as to be able to swallow food, although not entirely free from the convulsive disturbance. She died of pneumonia three years after the artificial feeding was discontinued. The most careful examination could detect no lesion of the œsophagus.

The second case published by Monro, but observed by his father, occurred in a woman, forty-five years old, who was suffering from carcinoma of the stomach and consequent dysphagia spastica. The stricture was located about the middle of the œsophagus, was at times so firm that the finest bougie would not pass through, and was, from its very beginning, associated with pain beneath the sternum, extending

---

[1] Edinb. Med. Essays. Vol. I.; and *Monro*, Morbid Anatomy, etc. p. 224.

to the clavicular regions, and considerably increased by a deep inspiration. These symptoms continued from October 10th until May 26th of the following year, when death occurred. The autopsy showed a cancer of the stomach; not the slightest lesion was observed in the œsophagus.

Equally negative were the results in other cases of reflex spasm of the œsophagus.

The only instance in which a purely idiopathic spasm of the œsophagus resulted fatally was published by Mr. Henry Power in 1866, but was observed by him in 1857, and has since been repeatedly quoted (compare bibliography). Power's report of the disease, however, is so brief, and so much has been omitted in the examination of the case, both before and after death, that by a critical observer it must be rejected as of no value.

It is difficult to understand how this doubtful case could be reproduced in the text-books and manuals of all nations for a period of ten years—generally under the name of Pomer or Pomes—as a proof of the possible fatal termination of idiopathic œsophagismus.

The case occurred in a farmer, forty-eight years old, of nervous temperament, but otherwise healthy and strong up to the time the disease appeared. It began with hoarseness and attacks of coughing when he used his voice. Then was added difficulty in swallowing, by reason of the explosive attacks of coughing which followed every such attempt. He was able to swallow fluids in very small quantities; large quantities brought on these attacks of coughing. Solid food was swallowed more easily. The sound at first would not pass through the œsophagus, but subsequently it did so by using some force. The patient was much annoyed by the tenacious mucus and saliva which he could not swallow. An abscess over the thyroid cartilage was opened by Power. Extreme emaciation, hoarseness, and alternations of heat and cold were present. The respiration and the functions of the sympathetic nerve were undisturbed, and the muscular strength unimpaired. Speech was unintelligible towards the end, on account of defective articulation.

The autopsy revealed a normal condition of the pharynx, larynx, œsophagus, pneumogastric nerves, and other organs—in a word, the result of the examination was negative throughout.

What renders this case so doubtful is the fact that there were symptoms of imperfect closure of the larynx during the act of swallowing, especially in the form of explosive attacks of coughing, which occurred during this act, so that the patient consulted several physicians on account of his " cough." Paralysis of articulation occurred ultimately, as it appears, and, taking this in connection with the symptoms of imperfect closure of the larynx and the troublesome collection of mucus, we are involuntarily forced to believe that it was a case of bulbar paralysis. Unfortunately, nothing is said of the anatomical condition of the medulla oblongata.

The *diagnosis* presents very considerable difficulties, and is possible only when, by long-continued observation, the most important diagnostic symptoms are recognized, or when, on the other hand, all those disturbances which produce secondary spasm or feign a resemblance to it can be excluded. In the differential diagnosis, special value is to be placed on a known predisposition to spasms in general, on the coincidence of the dysphagia with spasm of the glottis, neuralgia, palpitation of the heart, and mental disturbances; but, above all, on the intermittent character of the dysphagia, the occurrence between the paroxysms (due to swallowing, eructations, etc.) of longer or shorter intervals of complete or almost complete ability to swallow ; and finally, on the result of examination with the sound.

Among the disturbances which occasion confusion in the diagnosis of œsophageal spasm, and on that account must be excluded, deserve to be mentioned inflammatory narrowing, morbid growths in the wall of the tube, general and partial dilatation, foreign bodies impacted, and well-developed bronchocele.

A careful review of the foregoing observations will aid in the diagnosis ; thus, the rapid disappearance of the spasm after the introduction of the sound, after the administration of antispasmodics, and, in doubtful cases, after the use of the galvanic current, all favor the convulsive nature of the contraction.

In this connection the cases published by Ganghofner are very instructive, both of which occurred in women, aged respectively thirty-nine and forty-four years. In both patients there was a bronchocele of medium size, although no special signification could be attached to this fact in the etiology of the spasm ; in both patients there occurred spasm of the glottis, particularly on introduction of the sound, although the laryngoscope revealed no anatomical changes in the organ. It was impossible at first to pass the pharyngeal sound through the spasmodic stricture, as every attempt to do so brought on paroxysms of suffocation. Galvanization of the neck, in both patients, produced a wonderfully favorable result, and, by its further use, this result was rendered apparently permanent. After the application of the galvanic current, the sound could be passed without difficulty as far as the stomach. In one case there existed abnormal sensations in the track of the auricular branch of the pneumogastric nerve.

Prognosis.

The *prognosis* of the *purely neurotic form* may be designated as favorable, since the majority of such cases recover quite rapidly, and the most obstinate cases, notwithstanding their many years' duration and visible effect on the nutrition of the body, do not cause death. Power's case, quoted hitherto by many authors as proof of the possible fatal result of the spasm, cannot for reasons stated above be regarded as convincing. In regard to the *duration* of this affection, all predictions must be made with great caution, for the reason that the spasm, as the preceding observations show, may extend over a number of years, with continual remissions and exacerbations—indeed, with long intervals of complete freedom from the affection.

The prognosis of the *symptomatic* spasm depends of course on the nature of the primary disease, and on the possibility of producing a favorable influence on the same.

Treatment.

The treatment of the idiopathic, purely nervous form of spasm must, on the one hand, be directed to the general condition, the nervousness, hysteria, etc.; and on the other hand, must be almost entirely local. As regards the latter form of treatment, the greatest reliance is apparently to be placed on the reduction of reflex sensibility by repeated use of pharyngeal sounds of the largest possible calibre,[1] aided perhaps by the administration of bromide of potassium in large doses (the effect of which, in reducing the sensibility and reflex action of the upper portion of the alimentary canal, according to recent investigations by Krosz[2] and others, cannot be doubted), as well as by the application of the galvanic current. However, these agents must certainly be employed for a long time, and their use not discontinued too soon.

---

[1] In many cases a single introduction of the sound, which is allowed to remain for some time in the stricture, is sufficient for complete and permanent cure.

[2] Archiv für experim. Pathologie und Pharmakologie. 1876. Bd. VI.

Paralysis of the Œsophagus — Paralysis Œsophagi — Dysphagia Paralytica.

Etiology.

Our information concerning paralysis of the œsophagus, and of the causes which produce it, is exceedingly meagre. This is due in great part to the rare occurrence of isolated paralyses of the œsophagus. Paralysis of the œsophagus occurs frequently as part of the phenomena of extensive cerebral paralysis, but is never observed until a short time before death, and occurring in this way with severe apoplexy, bulbar paralysis, and multiple cerebro-spinal sclerosis, as a phenomenon of the death-agony, it is no longer susceptible of extended observation.

Limited to the œsophageal wall, with or without implication of the laryngeal and pharyngeal muscular structure, paralysis appears to occur in connection with disease of the central points of origin and branches of the pneumogastric nerve, as well as of its peripheral ramifications, and possibly of the spinal accessory nerve. Diphtheritic paralysis of the throat and larynx seems, in severe cases especially, to be attended by such a condition of the œsophagus. Moreover, syphilitic infection, as well as chronic plumbism and alcoholism, severe concussions of the whole body from falling or slipping, and finally, the inevitable catching cold, have all been accused of taking part in the etiology of this paralysis. The atrophy of the muscular layers, developed as a consequence of advanced general and partial dilatation, leads finally to a paralysis which is indeed of purely myopathic nature.

Symptomatology and Diagnosis.

The paralysis is developed suddenly or gradually. The chief symptom is the dysphagia, which may increase until the patient is no longer able to swallow solid food. The food remains lodged at some point in the upper or lower portion of the œsophagus, and is finally pushed along to the stomach by large quantities of fluids, not without painful sensations. In other cases the food is regurgitated after an interval, and that in spite of the most troublesome efforts on the part of the patient to prevent it. Large morsels of food can often be swallowed better than small ones. Fluids pass down to the stomach with a loud, rumbling noise, which is sometimes audible at a great distance from the patient (dysphagia sonora of the older writers). The erect position is much more favorable for deglutition than the supine. The sound passes downward without obstruction; if the instrument is stiff enough, the relaxed condition of the œsophageal wall can be made out by moving it from side to side.

The auscultatory phenomena are in general those of diffuse dilatation of the œsophagus; the noise produced by swallowing is slowly transmitted downward, and ceases at the spot—about midway—where the food is lodged. Fluids pass along with a loud, rumbling noise.

In the most advanced degrees of this affection, when anæsthesia of the mucous membrane exists in connection with motor paralysis, the solid food often remains for many hours in the œsophagus without giving rise to any other trouble than moderate oppression and palpitation of the heart, due to mechanical pressure on the lungs, pleura, and heart. If this alimentary thrombus (Speise-thrombus) is not removed by the succeeding meal, nothing remains but to push it into the stomach with the œsophageal tube.

The _diagnosis_ of œsophageal paralysis is always very difficult; according to the cases observed, it seems chiefly liable to be confounded with diffuse dilatation of the œsophagus. Whether an absolute distinction is possible in these two rare conditions must remain a question. As a matter of course, a sudden onset of the disturbance and simultaneous paralyses of the muscles of the pharynx and larynx favor very strongly the paralytic nature of the œsophageal affection. When the paralysis, however, develops slowly, without any discoverable cause, and is limited to the œsophagus, the differential. diagnosis may be opposed by insuperable difficulties.

The danger of mistaking it for spasm of the œsophagus can always be avoided by long-continued observation, and especially by objective examination frequently repeated.

Prognosis.

The prognosis of idiopathic paralysis, limited to the œsophagus, does not appear to be so unfavorable, although, on account of the obscurity of its etiology, it is rarely possible, in single cases, to predict with any certainty. At all events, cases of recovery have been recorded. The diphtheritic and the hysterical here, as in the pharynx and larynx, are the most favorable forms. The paralysis due to syphilis should be amenable to anti-syphilitic treatment (Wilson).

On the other hand, the paralyses which are part of the phenomena of diseases of the central nervous system invariably furnish an unfavorable prognosis.

Treatment.

Treatment directed to the cause will only be possible in the rare cases where such causes are clearly understood, and even then success will rarely be attained. Only in the syphilitic, hysterical, and diphtheritic paralyses, as well as in those resulting from alcoholic and lead-poisoning, will the indicatio causalis suffice for the indicatio morbi. In these latter forms strong general and local stimulants are mostly to be relied upon. Prominent among these stands the local application of electricity, in both forms, by means of the pharyngeal electrode, which acts at the same time as a mechanical irritant ; of benefit also are powerful hydrotherapeutic measures (cold affusions, douches to the chest and back), the subcutaneous injection of strychnine, and methodical exercise of the muscles of deglutition.

The treatment by derivatives, recommended in earlier times (fly-blisters, setons, actual cautery), is deserving of little confidence. It is scarcely necessary to mention that, in any considerable disturbance of deglutition, the use of the œsophageal tube is not to be omitted in feeding the patient.

THE

DISEASES OF THE PERITONEUM.

———

BAUER.

DISEASES OF THE PERITONEUM.

The malformations of the peritoneum present, for the most part, exceedingly little clinical interest ; some, however, are so far of importance, in that they may give rise to displacement and constriction of the intestines.

As these conditions have already been fully considered in this Cyclopædia (Vol. VII.) in discussing the displacements of the intestines, we must refer for information on this point to the chapter in question.

Inflammation of the Peritoneum.

Walther, De Morbis peritonæi. Berol. 1786.—*S. G. Vogel*, Handbuch. IV. 272. 1795.—*Bichat* (Beclard's printed manuscript of Bichat's Cours d'Anatomie path., published by Boisseau).—*Pinel*, in the second edition of his Nosographie. *Laënnec*, Histoire des inflammations du périt. 1804 ; and elsewhere.—*Gasc*, in Dictionnaire des sciences méd. p. 490. 1819.—*Portal*, in Rhein. Jahbücher, Bd. I. St. 2. S. 117.—*Broussais*, Hist. des phlegm. 2d ed. II. p. 391.—*Louis*, Recherch. anat.-path. 1826.—*Pemberton*, Pract. Treatise on the Diseases of the Abdom. Viscera. Transl. 1836.—*Abercrombie*, Diseases of the Stomach.—*Chomel*, in Dictionnaire de méd. Tom. XVI.—*Andral*, Clinique méd. Tom. IV.— *Gendrin*, Histoire anat. des inflammat. I. pp. 131 and 250.—*Bright*, Rep. of Med. Cases. London, 1827-31.—*Scoutetten*, Arch. gén. de méd. III. 497; IV. 386 ; V. 537.—*Hodgkin*, Lect. on the Morbid Anat. of Serous Membr. Vol. I.— *Corrigan*, Dublin Journal. 1836, July.—*Graves* and *Stokes*, Dublin Hosp. Rep. V. 110.—*Scuhr*, in Hannoeversche Annalen. N. F. III.— *Logérais*, Refl. sur quelques observ. de périt. aiguë. Thèse. 1840.—*Genest*, Gaz. méd. 1832. Nos. 107, 110, and 112.—*Beatty*, Dublin Journal. 1834, Sept.—*E. Thompson*, Trans. of Med. and Surg. Assoc. 1834. Vol. II.—*Badham*, Lond. Med. Gaz. 1835. Feb.—*Toulmouche*, Gaz. méd. 1842.—*Carswell*, Illust. fasc. 12. Pl. 3.—*Champouillon*, De la périt. simple spont. Gaz. des hôp. 1853.—*Fondeville*, Obs.

d'épanchement gélatineux dans la cavité périt. Ibid.—*Hughes*, Clinic. Lect. on the Nature and Treat. of Acute Traum. Perit., the Result of the Rupture or Perforation of one of the Hollow Viscera. Dublin Hospital Gaz. 1, 2, 3. 1856. —*C. Chandon*, Beitr. z. Lehre von d. Perit. 1856.—*Bonamy*, Note sur l'ulc. et la perf. du diaphrag. dans la périt. Journ. de la soc. acad. de la Loire-Inférieure. XXIV. 177.—*St. Ward*, Perit. Lancet. Sept., 1858.— *Herrmann*, Bemerkg. über d. Ther. d. acut. Perit. Med. Zeitung Russland's. 10. 1859.— *v. Dahl*, Perforationsperit. mit glückl. Ausg. Rigaer Beitr. Bd. IV.—*Foerster*, Ueber Perit. in Folge purul. Entzündung d. Eileiter. Wien. med. Wochenschrift. 44. 1859.—*Second-Feréol*, De la perf. de la paroi abd., etc. Thèse. Paris, 1859.—*Bourdon*, Calcul. biliaire, etc. Gaz. des hôp. 72. 1859.—*Habershon*, The Etiolog. and Treat. of Perit. Brit. Med. Journ. Dec., 1859.—*Fuhrmann*, Diss. de perit. e perf. subort. Vratisl. 1859.—*v. Plazer*, Ein Fall von Ulcerat. perf. der Gallenblase durch einen Gallenstein, etc. Wien. Spit. Zeitg. 1860. 14.—*Marten*, Zur operat. Behandlung der Perit. Virch. Arch. XX.— *Labalbary*, Cas remarqu. de tymp. périt. Gaz. des hôp. 104. 1861.— *Brizio Cocchi*, Amora sulla cura della perit. con l'appl. cont. de freddo. Gaz. Med. Ital. Lomb. 1862. 32.—*Patenotre*, De l'empl. du collod. ricin. contre la périt. aiguë. L'Union méd. 93. 1863.—*Habershon*, Path. and Pract. Observ. on Dis. of the Abdomen. London, 1862.—*Breslau*, Ein ausgezeichneter Fall freier Gasentwickelung aus eitriger Perit. Wiener med. Wochenschr. 1863.—*E. Chauffard*, Étud. clin. sur la const. méd. de l'an 1822. Arch. gén. 1863.—*Scoda*, Bemerkung. über Peritonit. Wien. allg. med. Ztg. 1864. 10 und 12.—*M. Prudhomme*, Observ. de péritonite et considérat. sur la diag. de cette mal. Journ. de méd. milit. 1865.—*E. Busch*, Ueber Behandlung der Perit. rheum. Wien. Wochenschr. 79. 1865.—*Lehmus*, De perit. Diss. Berol. 1867.—*Blachez*, Périt. spont. Gaz. des hôp. 1867. 109 ; and *Duparcque*, De la périt. aig., ess. ou spont. Ibid. 110. —*E. Wagner*, Perit. durch eitrigen Catarrh u. Perforat. d. rechten Tuba. Arch. d. Heilkunde. 1866.—*Schweiger* and *Dogiel*, Ueber die Peritonealhöhle und ihren Zusammenhang mit d. Lymph. Bericht d. sächs. Gesellsch. 1865 ; u. Arbeiten aus d. phys. Anstalt z. Leipzig. 1867.—*E. Cyon*, Ueber die Nerven des Peritonaeum. Sitzungsbericht d. sächs. Gesellsch. d. Wissensch. Bd. XX. 119.—*Charbonier*, Quelques consid. sur l'étiolog. de la périt. aiguë. Thèse. Strassburg, 1868.—*Sieveking*, A Case of Perit. Lancet. March 17, 1868.—*Th. Ballard*, Disease of the Perit. Transactions of the Path. Soc. XVIII. 99.— *Lesser*, Peritonitis diffus u. perit. circumscr. Diss. Berol. 1869.—*Leroy*, De la périt. spontanée. Paris. Thèse. 1869.—*Demarquay*, Arrêt du testicle droit dans le canal inguinal, où il reste fixé par une bride épiploïque derrière laquelle une anse intestinale est venue s'étrangler, d'où péritonite et mort. Gaz. des hôp. No. 89. 1869.—*Needon*, Perfor. des Zwerchfelles nach ausgebr. Perit. Wien. med. Presse. S. 990. 1869.—*Erc. Galvagni*, Sulla perit. ad essudato sieroso, etc. Rivista clinica di Bologna. 1869.—*Dutzmann*, Bubo, Peritonitis, Tod. Wien. med. Presse. No. 26. 1869.—*K. F. Walle*, Omorsakene tillinflam. i bukhinnan Akad. Afhandl. Helsingfors. 1869.—*Léon Labbée*, Adénite inguinale suppurée. Périt. par propag. Erysip. Mort. Gaz. des hôp. No. 111. 1869.—*G. Mancini*, Peritonite suppurat., complic. adocclus. intest. da coprost. Riv. clinic. di Bologna. 1870.—*A. Areus*, Ein merkwürdiger Verlauf von Perit. unter dem Einfl. der localen Anästh. Deutsche Klinik. 29. 1870.—*Wasastjerna*, Perf. vid perit. Notisblad for läkare och farmac. 1869.—*Lereboullet*, Note sur un cas de bubon iliaque suivi de périt. Gaz. hebd. de méd. et de chir. 1870.—*Heymann*, De la périt. spont. Gaz. des hôp. 62. 1866.—*G. F. Giles*, Gonorrhœa and Perit. Brit. Med. Journal. April. 29, 1871.—*N. Dobson*, Gonorrhœa and Perit. 76. May. Ibid.—*R. W. Egan*, Perit. meret. Ibid.—*Ménière*, Note sur un point d'anat. path. du tube digest. Bull. de l'Acad. XXXV. p. 854.—*Lange*, Eigenthüml. Verlauf einer Perit. Berl. kl. Wochenschr. 1871. 7.—*E. Winge*, Perit. behandlet med. Paracenth. Norsk Magaz. f. Lägevidensk. R. Bd. 1. 241.— *Loebel*, Zur Aetiologie u. Diagnostik des Perit. Wiener med. Presse. 1871. 2.— *Dessauer*, Perit. in Folge purul. Eutzündung der Eileiter. Monatsschr. f. Geburtskde. Bd. 27.—*Vogelsang*, Perit. suppurat. mit Perfor. des Nabels. Memorab. No. 3. 1872.—*H. Luce*, A Case of Peritonitis with Singular Complic. Boston Med. and Surg. Journ. July, 1872.—*A. Weil*, Péritonite par propag. à la suite d'un abscès périnéal. Gaz. des hôp. 89. 1872.— *Vidal*, Emploi de la térébinthine à l'extér. dans le trait. de la périt. Ibidem. No. 18.—*Stephanesco*, Quelques considerations sur le périt. au point de vue chir. Thèse. Strassburg, 1870.—*Julien*, Contribut. à l'étude du périt., ses nerfs et leurs termin. Lyon. Gaz. méd. 10. 1872.—*Heckford* and *Bathurst-Woodman*, Introd. of Irrit. Fluids within the Perit. Cavit. Med. Presse. June, 1872.—*Kundrat*, Ueber die krankh. Veränderungen der Endoth. Oest. med Jahrb. 2. 1871.—*E. Klein* and *Burdon Sanderson*, Zur Kenntniss der Anat. der serösen Häute im norm. und pathol. Zust. Med. Central-Bl. X. 1872.—*J. M. Bigelow*, Rheumatic Perit. Philad. Med. Tim. May, 1873.—*Julius Garbiel*, Enteroperit., etc. Wien. med. Presse. 9. 1873.—*Kobryner*, Périt. aiguë trait. avec succ. au moyen des merc. Bull. gén. de thérap. Sept. 1873.—*Morin*, Périt. rhumat. Gaz. des hôp. 52. 1873.— *H. Desplats*, De la périt. rhum. l'Union méd. 89. 1873.—*Traube*, Ges. Abbandlungen. Berlin. 1871.— *Wagner*, Fall einer eigenthüml. Affect. des Dünndarmes u. d. Mesenterialdrüsen, vielleicht durch Spulwürmer veranlasst. Wunderlich's Archiv d. Heilk. 1857. 4.—*Friedrich*, Die Paracent. des Unterleibs bei Darmperforation im Abdominaltyphus. Berlin. 1867.—*Canstatt*, Spec. Path. IV. 3. 1845.—*Bamberger*, in Virchow's Handb. der spec. Path. VI. 1.—*Henoch*, Krankheiten des Unterleibs.— *Wunderlich*, Spec. Pathologie. III. 3.

The symptoms attendant on inflammation of the peritoneum remained for a long time not understood. In accounting for the phenomena, an accidental and secondary part only was attributed to the serous membrane, the various cases of the disease being described as inflammations of the abdominal viscera, more especially of the intestinal canal, as the disturbance of the functions of this latter was what attracted most attention. The serous covering was believed to be necessarily involved in the processes occurring in the viscera themselves.

Although mention is made of peritonitis by the older writers, they still seem to consider an independent symptomatology impossible (for example, Cullen, in his First Lines) ; and even anatomical observations, by which the existence of peritonitis was demonstrated, were not sufficient at first to remove this idea.

Hence, Gasc, writing in the year 1809 in the Dictionnaire des Sciences Médicales, is right in ascribing to his own time—a period of scarcely twenty years—the first stage in the development of our knowledge of peritonitis. An attempt was made at the close of the last century by some medical men—Walther, P. Frank, and S. G. Vogel, in particular—to raise to the dignity of an independent disease inflammation attacking the serous membrane. The facts in question first received general recognition through Bichat. Actual fact could no longer be cried down by weighty opinions, such as Portal's, who, resting on Morgagni's authority and Haller's decision as to the non-irritability of the peritoneum, disputed the independence of peritoneal symptoms, and brought up as evidence the painlessness of the abdomen in chronic peritonitis.

A number of very careful observations on peritonitis were published by Laënnec, which added considerably to the elucidation of the subject. Corvisart, Bayle, Gasc, and others did important service in removing previously existing errors, and in separating anatomically peritonitis from inflammation of the abdominal viscera. The objections raised by M. Gastellier and others were no longer capable of producing any effect.

Owing to Broussais, the clinical aspect of peritonitis attained to a certain degree of completeness, as he took chronic peritonitis more fully into account. From his time the views then held have undergone a gradual transformation into those of the present day, owing to the light afforded by anatomical observation and the histological investigation of the serous membranes. The former clinical subdivision into enteritis substantialis and peritonitis enterica, as well as the arbitrary and subtle localization of peritoneal inflammation, has by degrees vanished from our hand-books.

The peritoneum is histologically analogous to the other serous membranes of the body. It represents a large lymph-space, into which the greater part of the abdominal viscera project. Thus, the splitting of the serous membrane into two layers affords the great requisite mobility to the viscera covered by it. Each of these layers is covered by endothelium ; and the spaces occurring in this—the so-called stomata—lead into the lymph-canalicular[1] system in the subjacent connective tissue.

This correspondence in morphological, and, in a great part also, functional relationship, in no way precludes the peritoneum from being much less frequently the seat of idiopathic inflammation than is the case with other serous membranes, as, for example, the pleura. The reasons why the serous membranes should exhibit so varied a behavior are not yet understood ; they may depend upon minor differences in the serous membranes themselves, or upon dissimilar influences in their local relations.

The peritoneum possesses a very great extent of surface ; it is the largest serous cavity in the body. Hence, as extent is a most important element in the significance of any process, diffuse peritonitis must ever be regarded as serious. To this must be added the tendency in the abdominal viscera to partake of any affection of the serous membrane—a state of things which for many a day stood in the way of a correct explanation of the symptoms.

Acute Diffuse Peritonitis.

Pathogenesis and Etiology.

Diseases of the peritoneum are of much more frequent occurrence in the female than in the male, and this is due to the manner in which the various parts of the sexual organs in the female are related to it, the uterus projecting partially into the abdominal cavity, and the Fallopian tubes opening freely into it.

---

[1] Saftkanälchen. I adopt Klein's translation as the most adequate.—TR.

Hence, in the several functions of these parts, menstruation, pregnancy, delivery, and the puerperal state, the peritoneum is very intimately concerned, and, consequently, is more liable to inflammation than is ever the case in the male.

Actually idiopathic inflammation of the peritoneum is, as has been already urged by Louis, a very rare disease. Most cases may be traced to pathological conditions in organs invested by peritoneum, and hence are secondary.

The greater the care in the anatomical examination, the smaller the number of those cases of peritonitis which may be looked upon as spontaneous; post-mortem examination generally points to a connection with some primary cause. From this circumstance, the very existence of idiopathic peritonitis has come to be doubted. An absolute denial of its existence is, however, so far in advance of actual demonstration, that isolated cases do now and then occur in which the most minute anatomical examination is unable to discover any connection with disease of the abdominal organs or neighboring parts. We are forced to regard cases of this kind, for the present at least, as idiopathic peritonitis.

As long as the question as to the occurrence of purely idiopathic peritonitis remains undecided, we must be very cautious in admitting as exciting causes all that is generally held accountable for producing it. Amongst these are to be found excesses in diet, and, most frequently of all, cold; and, in connection with this latter, spontaneous peritonitis is considered equivalent to rheumatic peritonitis. Taking all the cases into account, this mode of production is not rare, and the scanty data as to epidemics (Frank, also in Dict. des Sc. Méd.) suggest the probability of some mistake.

Those stray cases also which occur in the course of acute rheumatism are considered by many as rheumatic peritonitis, analogous to pleuritis and pericarditis. Cases of this kind were recorded by MacDowel and by Andral, and the more recent literature also contains notices of such cases.[1] It is undoubtedly an exceedingly rare complication of acute articular rheumatism, and cases of this kind do not strictly come under the category of idiopathic peritonitis, as, indeed, further, they are said to be distinguished from other forms of the disease by the favorable nature of the course they run.

---

[1] E. g., H. Desplats, L'Union méd. 1873. No. 89.

Similarly, peritonitis occurring as a sequence of some severe general morbific process cannot be considered spontaneous. Such occurs in particular in pyæmia, sometimes also in the acute exanthemata and other infectious diseases, and may be regarded as dependent on the general infection, or possibly they may be produced by a local infection in the course of lymphangitis.

In the course of some chronic diseases, also—chronic Bright's disease, for example, and, perhaps, also scurvy—peritonitis is comparatively frequently observed.

Whether this increased tendency to peritoneal inflammation in chronic degeneration of the kidneys is to be ascribed to the altered constitution of the blood—hydræmia, retention of the constituents of urine—or to the mechanical element of distention of abundant serous infiltration, and stagnation of blood, due to the pressure of the ascites, cannot yet be determined; for both views there exist reasons pro and contra. We generally find the peritoneum thickened and swollen after old-standing ascites; nevertheless a terminal peritonitis is more frequently met with in cases of Bright's disease than in dropsy from any other cause.

In 292 post-mortems collected by Frerichs, peritonitis, in connection with Bright's disease, occurred 33 times; in 114 cases in the Stadtlazareth, in Danzig, there were 13 of peritonitis. Those persons, however, in whom pregnancy and nephritis are combined, seem to be predisposed to peritonitis in a very special degree.

In the last-mentioned conditions, some special excitant from without is probably required for the production of inflammation, and hence we speak of an "increase in disposition." We may also set down the occurrence of an exalted tendency to inflammation in connection with other unimportant deviations from the normal condition of the serous membrane, or of individual abdominal viscera. Under this head may be enumerated, more particularly, menstruation, pregnancy, and the puerperal state, as well as the previous existence of peritonitis, perhaps also fæcal accumulations, the use of drastic cathartics, and the like.

In these cases, the existence of a contemporaneous cold must not be lost sight of. We meet with cases of menstrual peritonitis where this relationship can scarcely be doubted, so definitely and immediately did cause and effect follow on one another.

Injuries of various kinds may be followed directly or remotely by peritonitis. Anything further on this point belongs to the region of surgery.

Authorities are not agreed as to how far the peritoneum feels and resents injury and interference. The results obtained in the lower animals are not directly applicable to man; we find in many animals that the tendency to reaction is decidedly very slight. In the case of man, modern surgery has shown that most extensive interference with the peritoneum may be borne without reaction. Tapping of the abdomen, or puncture of the intestine with a fine trocar, to let out intestinal gas, is very seldom followed by peritonitis. Very different is the behavior in the case of foreign bodies, especially those substances which act as irritants of a chemical or infectious nature, which, if they but gain access to the peritoneum, rapidly induce diffuse inflammation.

The instances in which we meet with all the various predisposing causes already mentioned, are but few in number in comparison with those cases in which the peritonitis is secondary, brought about by various abnormal processes in the abdominal viscera. The reason why the peritoneal investment is so frequently involved may be readily understood if we bear in mind the real significance of the serous membrane. We must remember that the connective tissue stroma of the organs and the serous membrane form one continuous whole, and that therefore the two layers of peritoneum cannot be looked upon as independent structures.

The various pathological processes may give rise to local inflammation wherever they spread to the serous membrane. The circumscribed peritonitis thus set up may, in its further course, remain circumscribed, or it may extend and become diffuse.

The manner in which a previously localized inflammation extends may be understood by supposing that the primary irritant and the products of the inflammation are being continually moved onward by the motions of the serous layers, and that thus fresh portions of the serous membrane are continuously brought into contact therewith, and become to a certain extent impregnated. Or else the further extension may occur by the transport of irritant material by means of the lymphatic vessels. A simple extension of inflammation, *per continuitatem*, appears not to be thought of, as otherwise it would be difficult to understand the protective importance of general adhesions.

Accordingly, two principal conditions exist which materially influence the extension of inflammation. One of these is the element of time;—the more slowly any process attacks the peritoneum the more surely will a general protective adhesion be produced. Secondly, it is a matter of importance whether infecting substances are, or are not, disseminated through the lymphatic vessels.

In other cases of secondary peritonitis, where the action of the irritant is very intense and sudden, or occurs simultaneously in several places, the inflammation may be diffuse from the outset. This most frequently occurs when foreign bodies and substances which act chemically get into the peritoneal cavity. We may place in this category fæces and fæcal calculi, bile and gall-stones, intestinal gas, worms, urine and urinary calculi, material from the Fallopian tubes and the uterus, the contents of abscesses and cysts, and in a certain sense also blood. It seldom happens that irritating substances from without get into the peritoneal cavity.

As these cases occur as the result of ruptures and perforations of membranous canals they are described under the title of *Peritonitis from Perforation.*

The processes in the abdominal viscera and the neighboring organs, which are most frequently concerned with the production of peritonitis, are fully discussed under the pathology of the various organs in question; hence, I shall only enumerate briefly those of most frequent occurrence.

1. *Stomach and intestine.* In every case of occlusion of the intestine, whether from the twisting, bending, or compression of the gut, or from fæcal accumulation, as also in every case of incarceration and invagination, the serous membrane becomes inflamed, generally as the result of a disturbance or interruption of the circulation, which may lead to circumscribed gangrene. The amount of inflammation set up in the peritoneum in these cases is not always the same, but depends upon the extent of the occlusion and the extent of the disturbance in the circulation. Frequently a circumscribed peritonitis only is produced, and this, in particular, is more often the case in invagination and compression, and also in incarceration in a hernia sac, than the occurrence of diffuse peritonitis.

The various cases of ileus present a very varied aspect, according as the part taken by the peritoneum is more or less intense, the degree and extent of the secondary peritonitis being a very essential item in the symptoms in these cases. (The subject of displacement and constrictions of the intestine is fully discussed in Vol. VII. of this Cyclopædia, to which the reader is referred.)

Ulcerative processes in the stomach and intestine may, with or without perforation, lead to peritonitis. Complete oblitera- tion and adhesions from a previous circumscribed peritonitis are of much import, particularly in the case of ulceration, as in the first place they diminish the tendency to rupture by increasing the capability of resisting the pressure from within; and sec- ondly, when the rupture has actually taken place, they tend to prevent the contents from passing into the peritoneal cavity. The adhesions may doubtless subsequently be broken down and destroyed, and then rupture ensues.

The perforating gastric ulcer and the rare duodenal ulcer have the general tendency, owing to their origin in hemorrhagic infarctions, finally to break through the serous membrane. If a firm adhesion have been established with a neighboring hollow viscus, a *fistula bimucosa* will ensue as the result of further arro- sion from the digestive fluids, and even in the case of adhesion with a solid viscus, this last-mentioned process may ultimately eat through it.

The perforation of the circular ulcer generally occurs as a round, wide opening, and thus a great deal of material passes out. The same most frequently is the case in duodenal ulcers and in the ulcers of the anterior wall of the stomach, because the extensive mobility of this part tends to prevent adhesion.[1] Ulcerations in the stomach and duodenum which occur as the results of corroding and caustic substances, must at the outset have involved the tissue very deeply to perforate the serous membrane; the arroding influence of the secretion is decidedly less in this case than in hemorrhagic infarction.

The peritonitis which complicates the course of enteric fever (Vol. I.), is for the most part connected with typhoid ulcers, and in a few instances with other causes of irritation, exudation from the mesenteric glands, rupture and disintegration of the abdominal muscles, enlargement and rupture of the spleen, etc. The perforation of a typhoid ulcer is comparatively rare; these ulcers may, however, induce peritonitis by cell-proliferation ex- tending to the serous membrane without causing any perforation of it.

---

[1] *Rindfleisch*, Lehrb. der pathol. Gewebelehre. 3. Aufl. p. 226.

In the severe diphtheritic form of dysentery, a circumscribed inflammation of the serous covering of the part of the gut attacked is the rule, and from this general peritonitis may arise. Perforation seldom occurs as the result of the deep extension of the necrosis.

Phlegmonous inflammations of the stomach and intestine, on account of their rarity, do not call for much consideration; still they readily extend to the peritoneum. More important are the catarrhal and stercoraceous ulcers. These, after healing, may, from their great extent, lead to stenosis of the gut with its several consequences; and thus stasis above the stricture may, by exudation, produce peritonitis, similarly with syphilitic processes in the intestine.

It is not often that carcinoma of the stomach and intestines, as also tubercular and caseous ulceration, leads to a simple diffuse peritonitis. These processes very uniformly extend to the peritoneum. They may perforate or induce strictures, and thereby cause a rupture of the brittle tissue. Nevertheless these are comparatively rare causes, because these processes run a chronic course and tend to produce adhesions. (*Vide* Tubercular and Carcinomatous Peritonitis.)

Foreign bodies may pass out into the peritoneum at any spot of the digestive canal, according to circumstances, either with or without previous ulceration. The presence of a diverticulum or of anything that tends to produce stagnation is an important favoring circumstance. Intestinal calculi and parasites may act as foreign bodies.

In connection with perforation we sometimes find round worms in the peritoneum, either free or in depressions—the so-called worm abscesses. In the majority of these cases the state of affairs is, that perforation has occurred as the result of some other cause, and that subsequently the parasites have wandered out through the opening. The lumbrici can only cause perforation, either when an enormous mass of them is collected at any part of the intestinal tube (Mondière), or in the case of their wandering into some narrow canal. That, however, these worms should perforate the intestinal wall or separate the various layers from one another is at least very unlikely, and it is certainly not definitely proved by the records in point. Similarly improbable appear the statements that round worms were found free in the peritoneal cavity after death, without perforation and without peritonitis.

As regards vegetable parasites it may be mentioned that in mycosis intestinalis a considerable exudation may rapidly take place into the peritoneal cavity.

The region of the cæcum, together with the vermiform process, presents a favorite locality for the occurrence of general and circumscribed peritonitis; and to so great an extent is this the case, that experienced practitioners have laid it down as a maxim, that in every case of secondary peritonitis, especially in the male, we must first suspect hernia, and secondly, some affection of the vermiform process. The various inflammatory conditions of the cæcum and vermiform process, together with the exudation phenomena, are comprehended under the title Typhlitis. The inflammation of the areolar tissue in this region outside or behind the peritoneum,—perityphlitis,—may also, though less frequently than typhlitis, reach the peritoneum; and still less frequently, inflammations situated behind the fascia iliaca, as in the case of psoas abscess (compare the chapters on Typhlitis, Perityphlitis, and Cold Abscess). The rectum, in its lower portion at least, which possesses no peritoneal covering, has comparatively little to do with the production of peritonitis. As is well known, it is only the portion from the sigmoid flexure to Douglas's folds, where the rectum passes through the pelvic fascia, that it has any peritoneal investment, and this superiorly is complete and inferiorly is incomplete. Ulceration in the lower part of the rectum and inflammation in the posterior and lateral areolar tissue are principally concerned in the production of fistulæ (*vide* Pelvic Abscess). Strictures of the rectum—and of these most frequently the carcinomatous—may occur in the upper portion, and thus produce all the accompanying phenomena ; and further, peritonitis may occur as the result of operative interference and forcible distention.

2. The *spleen* may give rise to peritonitis either through infarctions which have become markedly fluid, through abscesses with or without rupture of the capsule, and by rupture of the spleen itself. In this last case, however, death generally supervenes very quickly, and even in instances which have run a more protracted course there is often no trace of peritonitis.[1]

[1] *Vigla*, Arch. gén. 1844. See also *Henoch* and *Bamberger*.

3. The *liver* frequently gives rise to peritonitis through the occurrence of hepatic abscess.

Frerichs mentions a collection of cases by Louis, including 162 fatal cases, in 14 of which perforation into the peritoneum had occurred. According to More-head perforation occurred only twice in 140 cases, whereas general peritonitis occurred fourteen times, and circumscribed seven times. In cases like these last the sacculation of the effusion and burrowing of the pus may take place as described by Cambay and Haspel.

The echinococcus tumor generally leads to peritonitis only when it bursts into the peritoneum, which most frequently occurs as the result of external violence, and seldom spontaneously. In the few cases of multilocular echinococcus which have been observed, a purulent effusion was several times found in the peritoneal cavity.

Chronic interstitial hepatitis leads constantly to a firm fibrous thickening of the covering of the liver (perihepatitis); this is rarely followed by a terminal peritonitis, although the ascites and the general disturbance of the nutritive functions may be regarded as predisposing to such a result. The same is true of the syphilitic liver and of amyloid degeneration.

The gall-ducts may give rise to peritonitis by occlusion of their lumen, particularly by concretions, with consequent ulcerations. Rupture, which may thus be produced by a foreign body, has also been observed to follow an ulceration of the gall-bladder independent of gall-stones; some few such observations, at least, are to be met with in the literature of the subject. Carcinoma, as in the case of other abdominal organs, may in the liver also spread to the serous membrane (less frequently in the case of small secondary cancerous nodules in the liver), but a diffuse sero-fibrinous peritonitis is not a frequent result, and a purulent, the exception (Frerichs).

4. The *kidneys* and *urinary passages* may give rise to peritonitis from suppuration, nephritis, and pyelitis, from calculi, from perforation of the ureters, and from perinephritis. The inflammation resulting from an escape of urine into the peritoneal cavity is, moreover, intensely violent. From the bladder phlegmonous inflammation, cystitis, and pericystitis may extend; and

further, cancer of the bladder may lead to peritonitis. On the
other hand, rupture of the bladder from the simple pressure
of the contained urine is not possible if the wall of the bladder
be healthy; it can only occur from traumatic causes, and
through destruction and gangrene of the wall of the bladder;
moreover, abscesses in and around the wall of the bladder may
burst into the peritoneal cavity. Abscesses of the vesiculi seminales have also been observed to give rise to peritonitis.[1]

5. The *pancreas* may very occasionally give rise to peritonitis
from abscesses and also perhaps from calculi in its ducts.
Hemorrhage, almost without exception, produces instantaneous
death.

6. From the *diaphragm* and *pleuræ* peritonitis may be set up
by the perforation of a pulmonary abscess or a purulent pleural
effusion. It is very hard to decide whether the peritonitis which
supervenes on pleuro-pneumonia or pleurisy, with an intact diaphragm, is to be regarded as an extension of the inflammation
through the diaphragm, or as an accidental coincidence. The
echinococcus of the lung may break into the peritoneum.

7. The *blood-vessels* of the abdomen (aneurisms of abdominal
aorta and of some of its branches[2]) have not the great tendency
to produce acute inflammation of the peritoneum, which might
to a certain extent be expected, *a priori*, from the way in which
the aneurismal sac affects the tissues in its neighborhood. Experience teaches us that, as a rule, they produce but circumscribed inflammation, thickening, and adhesion, as also circumscribed suppuration. The short space of time which, as a rule,
though not universally, intervenes between the patient's death
and the uplifting of the peritoneum by the rupture of the sac
into or behind the abdominal cavity, is opposed to the occurrence
of peritonitis. Embolism in branches of the abdominal aorta, if
the plug be of an infectious character, may be followed by peritonitis.[3] Phlebitis and periphlebitis are of moment in the
production of peritonitis principally as conducting paths of

---

[1] Med. Chirurg. Transact. Vol. XXXIII.

[2] *Lebert*, Ueber das Aneurysma der Bauchaorta und ihrer Zweige. Berlin, 1865.

[3] *Virchow*, Gesammelte Abh. pp. 420 and 450; and *Cohnheim*, Emb. Proc. Berlin,
1872.

inflammatory processes ; this occurs most frequently in the case of the spermatic veins and the umbilical vein. Calley's case, in which there occurred rupture of the thoracic duct from obstruction and peritonitis, is such as has certainly been very seldom observed since.[1]

8. The *reproductive organs*, especially in the female, where the processes connected with menstruation, delivery, and the puerperal state are frequent predisposing causes, may give rise to peritonitis. Menstrual congestion, if complicated by injurious influences—amongst which cold must be regarded as important—may lead either directly to inflammation of the serous covering of the uterus and general peritonitis, or indirectly by the development of metritis and endometritis.

In connection with premature delivery we have to remark that the individual is, after this event, so far as her chance of peritonitis is concerned, similar to a lying-in woman ; that, further, if the ovum has not been completely cast off, and if a part remains to undergo decomposition in the uterus, the endometritis connected with this readily extends to the peritoneum. The expulsion of the embryo by mechanical means is not unfrequently followed by peritonitis. The peritonitis which occurs in connection with the puerperal state presents anatomically several forms ; these will be specially discussed in one of the following sections. The behavior of the peritoneum in connection with extra-uterine pregnancy belongs to the region of midwifery. Pelvic peritonitis, parametritis, retro-uterine hæmatocele, as also tumors of the uterus and ovaries (even in the case of exceedingly small cysts and ruptures), inflammation of the ovaries, inflammation, ulceration, and tuberculosis of the Fallopian tubes—all these processes may take part in the production of diffuse peritonitis. For further information see Vol. X. of this Cyclopædia. Further, gonorrheal infection is of some moment in the production of peritonitis, and by some observers the frequent peritoneal affections in prostitutes have been considered to depend on virulent gonorrhœa. (Egan believes that one of the causes of *peritonitis meretricum* lies in the fact that they often suppress menstruation

---

[1] Trans. of the Path. Soc. XVII. 163.

by the application of cold, or conceal it by the use of sponges.)
The phenomena attendant on injections into the uterus and the
possibility of the production of peritonitis thereby are discussed
under the head of Gynæcology, Vol. X.

9. Those parts which surround the peritoneum, or lie in contact with it—inflammation and abscess of the abdominal parietes
—may set up peritonitis. Attention has been already specially
called to these forms of inflammation by Rembert Dodeus and
P. Frank. The contents of these abscesses in the abdominal
parietes may take on a feculent smell without there being any
communication with the intestine, as was first observed by Dance.
Similarly with psoas and lumbar abscesses and the abscesses in
the retroperitoneal areolar tissue of the pelvis, the peritoneum
may also become attacked in caries of the vertebræ, ribs, and
bones of the pelvis. The mesenteric glands, and also more distant lymphatic glands, as, for example, those in the inguinal
region, may, by degeneration and suppuration, induce peritonitis.[1]

Pathological Anatomy.

The anatomical changes which acute peritonitis bring about
present great varieties with regard to the amount and character
of the effusion ; and these are, in part at least, dependent upon
the primary exciting cause.

Generally enormous quantities of gas are present throughout
the entire intestines, so that the latter, when the abdomen is
opened, actually burst forth *en masse.* The distention is apt to
occur most intensely in occlusion of the intestine, above the
stenosis, but in peritonitis from other causes it is the rule, and
a small quantity of gas in the intestine is the exception. The
stomach is completely covered by the distended colon and the
small intestines ; and it generally is found small and contracted,
rarely distended with gas.

The serous membrane is found in various degrees of injection,

---

[1] *Lereboullet*, for example, describes a case of bubo in the right groin, in which extension of the inflammation to the deep glands, and from these to the retroperitoneal
glands, induced a fatal peritonitis. Gaz. hébd. de méd. et chir. No. 3. 1870.

the capillaries are dilated and elongated, extravasations of blood are seen, sometimes in great number, in the form of hemorrhagic spots. The hyperæmia is apt not to be equally well marked in all parts of the peritoneum ; in different places we see various gradations without any sharp margin. The injection is most distinct at the spot where originally the exciting cause acted. This is apt to be particularly intense in incarceration, as in this case the stasis tends to increase the hyperæmia.

The effusion forms in the first place a thin, fine covering upon the serous membrane, of a grayish yellow color, which may be readily detached, and which loosely connects the various organs together ; simultaneously a somewhat reddish fluid is poured into the abdominal cavity. The further course assumes a very different aspect, according as the effusion proceeds in the manner just indicated, thus leading to intensely firm products—adhesive peritonitis,—or as a more or less copious fluid effusion is produced—exudative peritonitis.

The deposition of fibrin occurs before the endothelium presents any changes. This fibrinous effusion encloses primarily hardly any cellular elements, and only a few cast-off endothelial cells are to be found in it. The endothelium itself is swollen and turbid ; the cell-body is increased in size ; the contents are granular ; multiplication of the nuclei is apparent ; the cells are, in fact, in active division. In the tissue of the serous membrane itself, soon after the deposition of fibrin on the surface, an accumulation of indifferent cells takes place, especially around the vessels, so that the spaces between the vessels are thus completely filled up. The fixed connective-tissue corpuscles also take part in the inflammatory process.

If the process goes no further than a dry, fibrinous exudation, and ends as adhesive peritonitis, the cell-proliferation is soon at an end, and then the cells do not preponderate over the ground substance. In the further course there is formed directly out of this mass, which is to bind the different organs together, a fine, delicate connective tissue, the newly formed offsprings of the endothelium and the wandering cells developing themselves into spindle-cells. A formation of blood-vessels also takes place. The fibrin takes no active part in this metamorphosis; it undergoes fatty degeneration, and thus becomes absorbed.

If a more extensive sero-fibrinous effusion into the cavity of the peritoneum have taken place, the deposition of fibrin is apt to be more considerable on the surface of the serous membrane, and the process of the change into connective tissue assumes a somewhat more complicated form. In this case the connective tissue of the serous membrane is found in more intense proliferation ; vascularized granulations are produced, and these newly formed vessels are, later on, of great importance in absorbing the fluid effusion, when, owing to the considerable deposition of fibrin on the free surface, the absorbing capability of the lymphatic vessels has been interfered with. As soon as two surfaces of the serous membrane come into contact, the connective-tissue adhesion may ensue, and the fibrin splits up, with a development of fat when the rich blood-supply is cut off.

In the purulent condition of the effusion also, matting together occurs primarily for a short time, but the cell-proliferation so completely outweighs everything else, that the cellular elements get the better of the ground substance, namely, the fibrin, and there remains no longer any firm intercellular substance. The yellowish-green spots, also, in purulent effusion, consist only of masses of cells rolled together. The connective tissue of the serous membrane is thickly beset with young cells. The endothelium is thus raised up from its basis substance, and we see considerable areas of the serous membrane denuded of its endothelial covering, and masses of newly formed cells piled over it instead. In these cases especially we find fat-granules in the endothelium and in the connective-tissue corpuscles, and, in the further course of the disease, we see larger and smaller cells metamorphosed into granular balls, and fat-granules free in the tissue. That the pus-corpuscles of the peritoneal effusion are not exclusively cells which have wandered out of the blood-vessels in the serous membrane, and have thus reached the free surface, but that there takes place a new development of pus-cells from the endothelium, can, it appears from the foregoing observations, scarcely be doubted.

If resorption of the pus takes place, it occurs through fatty degeneration, and the serous surfaces adhere by granulations.

In the septic and unhealthy forms of peritonitis, the processes of proliferation just mentioned are less marked in the endothelium; the cells are simply cast off, and we find them in a state of fatty degeneration and commencing decomposition.[1]

As the effusion increases, the injection of the serous membrane becomes less or becomes obscured, and owing to the alternating pressure of the abdominal organs against one another and the parietes, the impressed surfaces tend to remain freer from deposit. If we tear the pseudo-membranous deposit from the serous membrane we find the latter everywhere raw, dull, flabby, with frequent small hemorrhages, the result of diapedesis. The peritoneal tissue is œdematous, and similarly the subserous tissue. The other layers in the intestine also are intensely œdematous, soft, and readily torn. The serous layer, as well as the mucous, may be very readily torn off. There seldom occurs in the tissue of the serous membrane an accumulation of pus-corpuscles of such a kind as to produce purulent infiltration and

---

[1] *Vide Cohnheim*, Virch. Arch. XXII. 516 ; *Buhl*, Das Faserstoffexsudat ; *Kundrat*, Ueber die krankh. Veränderung. der Endoth, etc.

abscesses in the peritoneum. The collection of pus between the matted knuckles of intestine is often exceedingly like an abscess, but on examination the pus is found lying on the serous membrane.

The abdominal muscles underneath the inflamed peritoneum are somewhat pale, discolored, and soft; the surfaces of the liver and spleen similarly present an absence of their normal color, to the depth of a centimetre.

Actual gangrene of the peritoneum occurs in circumscribed spots in incarceration and twisting of the gut, in abscesses, and also in urinary and fæcal infiltration; further, in infants as the result of gangrenous death of the umbilical cord. The discoloration of the corpse and decomposition, which so rapidly sets in, must not be mistaken for actual gangrene.

Besides the various degrees of hyperæmia and the modifications occasioned by the primary local cause, it is the effusion pre-eminently which, in the recent state, presents such a great diversity, both as regards quantity and quality,—a diversity which, partly at least, depends upon the nature of the exciting cause.

The quantity of the effusion varies within very wide limits; it ranges from a small quantity in the true pelvis, or in the spaces between the intestines, to a quantity which is sufficient to press up the abdominal viscera far into the thorax. The diaphragm may be pushed up to the third rib, and thus the liver becomes placed on its edge; the heart is displaced, with its apex outward and upward, and the posterior inferior portions of the lungs may be compressed to an airless condition.

As regards the quality of the effusion we may distinguish some few principal forms depending on physical and histological characters, with, of course, wide limits as regards quantity.

1. *Fibrinous effusion*, with an exceedingly slight quantity of fluid, hence dry or adhesive peritonitis. This forms a continuous false membrane, which invests the abdominal viscera in various thicknesses, but is specially prone to form a thick covering on the liver, spleen, and uterus. Sometimes the effusion does not form any continuous membrane, but merely occurs in isolated patches.

In the further course of the disease adhesive connective tissue, with newly formed vessels, is produced out of the inflammatory proliferation products. The newly formed connective tissue may appear as a slight thickening of the serous membrane, or it may be deposited as a firm, thick membrane on the abdominal viscera, and thus cover them. An important consequence arises out of the manifold adhesions to which the connective-tissue metamorphosis leads. The adhesions of the abdominal viscera with one another, with the parietes, with the omentum, or with the mesentery, are either loose, effected by means of a delicate tissue, or they are firm and callous, and give rise to retraction as in the case of cicatricial tissue. It may be regarded as established that the adhesions may, as the result of the extensive motion, be partially freed or even made to vanish altogether, and thus the firm tissue produced may remain merely as cord-like fibrous ligaments. The adhesions become the means of producing permanent displacements, of fixing organs, of causing constrictions in organs, namely, when they are included in the firm retraction of the new formation, and they may further produce a whole series of disturbances in function, or later they may give rise to incarceration, twistings, constrictions, and a fresh inflammation of the peritoneum. Rokitansky records a case in which, as a result of delivery, a fatal hemorrhage occurred in the great omentum and its neighborhood. The omentum was fixed by a kind of brooch in the right inguinal canal, and was during the act of delivery stretched so as to cause a tearing of its vessels.

The observations of Ménière record the occurrence of remarkable results ; for, according to these, by retraction of the mesentery the small intestine may be reduced to one-half its normal length, with shrivelling of the serous membrane and of the longitudinal muscular layer, while the mucous membrane is folded transversely and its layers are readily torn.

In some few cases the new production of connective tissue may occur to so great an extent, and at the same time be of such a firm consistence, that the entire viscera are united together into a ball. I saw a case of the kind in which the viscera presented the appearance of a large fibroid of the uterus beset with canals.

We may give the form the title of *peritonitis deformans*, after Klebs, but the author's explanation, namely, venous stasis in connection with valvular disease of the heart, does not appear adequate in all cases.

The layers of the false membrane often include fluid. They are also frequently pigmented. Occasionally concretions occur embedded in thick connective tissue, the result of calcification of the effusion.

2. *Serous and sero-fibrinous effusions.* Occasionally the effusion approaches in its characteristics pure ascitic fluid ; it is yellowish green or milky white, turbid, and flakes and separated pieces of false membrane are suspended in it.

These free flakes behave themselves similarly to the adherent false membrane. The quantity of fluid poured out into the abdominal cavity may be very large ; it may run up to twenty litres and even more. These enormous fluid effusions, often with but scanty deposition of fibrine, are seen most frequently in terminal peritonitis supervening on ascites. In other cases the fluid part is apt to be less considerable. As soon as the fluid has become absorbed, all further alterations proceed in the manner already detailed in connection with connective-tissue metamorphoses.

3. *Purulent effusion.* Even in a well-marked instance of purulent effusion, the quantities of the solid, fluid, and formed elements vary so much that we may have either a creamy, thickly fluid pus, or a very mobile, purulently turbid fluid. The masses of pus are often very considerable. As is the case in all the forms of effusion into the abdominal cavity, pus gravitates to the lowest spot, namely, to the pelvis, unless it be prevented from doing so by matting and adhesions. It generally happens that the principal mass of the effusion is found to have sunk downward, while smaller quantities remain pent up between the matted viscera.

The formation of pus may be associated with suppuration of the peritoneum, *peritonitis ulcerosa*, owing to an early purulent dissolution of the serous tissue. More frequent is the secondary dissolution after long contact with masses of pus, as is the case, for example, with encysted collections, which are characterized by the occurrence of numerous ruptures of the effusion into the viscera, and occasionally also outward, through the parietes, into the bladder, through the diaphragm, etc. Where the intestine has thus become perforated, its contents may subsequently escape into the encysted pouch of the peritoneum, or even into the free peritoneal cavity. In this way, also, fistulæ bimucosæ may be produced.

Purulent effusions are more frequently met with in point of number than any other; they occur almost without exception in the case of chemical and infectious irritants, as also often enough under other etiological conditions. By admixture with gastro-intestinal contents the pus may present a foul, discolored appearance, and feculent smell, and gases may be found occupying the free abdominal cavity (*vide* Perforative Peritonitis). In the case of septic (puerperal) processes, the effusion is also discolored and like unhealthy fluid pus. A slight admixture of blood, and even more copious extravasation, occurs as well in the purulent as in other conditions of the effusion, likewise, as well in the case of any special disposition to hemorrhage, as in scorbutus and severe acute general diseases, as when this disposition does not exist; hemorrhagic effusion occurs with great regularity in chronic tubercular peritonitis.

If, in the case of purulent peritonitis, death does not early ensue, the acute inflammation gives place to a chronic one, often very protracted in its course, which is characterized by the formation of adhesions and sacculations, and repeated exacerbations of the inflammation. The pus may find its way by perforation outward in very various directions, and this occurs either after complete sacculation or else relatively early and then generally through the umbilicus.

The view was formerly advanced that the way in which this form of perforation occurred was definite and readily understood, the determining conditions specially mentioned being the division into layers of the parietes, and the position and inclination of the pelvis. According to another view, perforative peritonitis is to be regarded as a particular form of the disease, with special symptoms and a special course. Observation does not confirm these views.

The encysted collections of pus may break through the false membrane, and thus be the means of setting up a fresh diffuse peritonitis. If the fluid in these sacs becomes absorbed, the pus becomes gradually thicker and undergoes caseous degeneration and, more rarely, calcification. These caseous masses harbor within them the danger of a subsequent tuberculosis.

5. A rare form of effusion possesses a colloid consistence.

A chemical analysis of the various effusions has doubtless frequently been made, but on account of the necessarily varied composition the results obtained are but of little value, except where in a particular case special questions arise in connection with the analysis.

Such analyses are to be found, amongst other places, in Scherer's " Chemische und microscopische Untersuchungen zur Pathologie," 1843, and in Kiwisch, "Krankheiten der Wöchnerinnen." Prag, 1840.

Pathology.

General Description of the Disease.

The etiologically various forms of peritonitis present in their symptoms and course numerous variations and deviations from what may be laid down as the general type. Two forms of disease may be combined, as, for example, enteric fever and peritonitis, the respective symptoms of which may thus be considerably modified. The symptoms of a primary disease may tend to disappear on the access of peritonitis, and even occlusions of the intestine present very various phenomena, according as the portion of serous membrane attacked is extensive or not.

Those forms of peritonitis which do not stand in any direct connection with a local cause generally begin acutely, sometimes even with an initial rigor. Phenomena which could be regarded: as prodromal are rare. Pain in the abdomen sets in at the outset, and this may from the start be distributed over the entire belly, or at first be confined to a circumscribed spot.

In secondary peritonitis the symptoms of the primary disease may have already disappeared ; or, if it should happen that the condition which induces the peritonitis had remained hitherto without symptoms, or that the peritoneum became simultane-.

ously affected, pain may set in suddenly, and increase more or less quickly.

Pain is a symptom that is always present, and presents, moreover, some characteristic features,—if not actually at the commencement, at least in the course of the disease. It is exceedingly severe, sometimes intolerable, and leads to excessive tenderness of the abdomen, as a result of which the very lightest touch or any change of position causes it to be most intensely increased. Patients lie generally, therefore, on their back, with their legs drawn up and their knees bent, tossing their head and arms restlessly to and fro. The respiration becomes shallow and rapid, and assumes altogether the costal type. Every cough, and every full respiratory movement, is most anxiously avoided. The aspect of the countenance soon becomes altered in a remarkable manner ; the eyeballs retreat within their sockets, and are surrounded with a bluish black ring ; the face assumes a hollow, withered expression, the nose becomes pinched, the cheeks fall in, the lips become thin and bluish, and the expression of pain and anxiety is vividly depicted. The voice becomes weak and loses its ring. These phenomena of collapsé are generally connected with the quantity of the effusion and the severity of the vomiting. Vomiting may often be the first symptom, or it may set in early and become a very prominent feature of the illness ; it is seldom altogether absent. At first the material vomited consists of mucus and the contents of the stomach, but later on it assumes a grass green color, and, in cases of occlusion of the intestine, feculent masses, often in enormous quantities, are vomited. Whatever is taken, even in the fluid form, often comes up again instantly, and in the intervals the tendency to vomit is almost constant. In many cases, also, there is a tormenting hiccough.

The desire for fluid already existing is increased by the vomiting to a tormenting thirst, while the taste in the mouth becomes bitter and bilious, or actually disgusting. The tongue is usually coated.

As regards the bowels, continual constipation is the rule, with numerous exceptions, even in the case of intestinal occlusion, while, in direct opposition to this rule, profuse diarrhœa is sometimes present. The passing of the urine is often accompanied with scalding pain, while in other cases there is complete retention. The quantity of urine passed is small, and often throws down, on cooling, deposits of urates.

The abdomen becomes more or less quickly distended ; still, in connection with this symptom, great variation is observed. The distention attains its greatest dimensions if the abdominal muscles have been previously very lax, and if extensive masses of effusion are deposited in the peritoneal cavity, and also in most cases of constriction and occlusion of the intestine. The individual knuckles of distended gut may become recognizable externally, and present the well-known futile peristaltic motions which generally end in a rumbling, gurgling sound (*vide* Intestinal Occlusion). The distention of the abdomen may, further, be symmetrical or not. It leads to the pressing upwards of the diaphragm as far as the third rib, and to compression of the lungs. Coinciding with the collapsed appearance of the patient is the condition of the pulse ; the wave is generally small, and the artery narrow ; the pulse is very rapid—as a rule, 120. In the further course of the disease, the pulse becomes thready, even to vanishing, and may rise to 140. With this state of things, the prominences have a frog-like, cold feel, and are intensely cyanotic. The skin is covered with cold perspiration. The withered expression of countenance, the livid color, the vanishing pulse, and the noiseless voice remind one forcibly of the collapse of cholera.

The temperature is generally very considerably raised, and those places which are protected from cooling, as, for example, the axilla, produce an actually burning sensation.

More or less effusion is developed in every case, which, when small in amount, is very difficult of demonstration. If the amount be more considerable, the fluid collects in the most dependent parts of the abdomen, compresses the viscera, and gives rise to dulness on percussion over an area which is found generally to be bounded by a distinctly horizontal line, corresponding with the height of the fluid. By altering the position of the patient, the fluid is generally found to be easily movable.

With the increase in the effusion there sometimes occurs a

remarkable feeling of improvement, which forms a striking contrast to the objective condition of the patient.

Consciousness, in the majority of cases, remains perfectly clear, and instances have been observed in which a previously existing delirium has disappeared on the occurrence of peritonitis. Consciousness may remain perfectly unclouded up to the very last, or slight delirium may set in immediately before death.

As the disease gains ground, which occurs generally in a very rapid manner, the symptoms of collapse continuously increase, and, in conjunction with the insufficiency of respiration, tend to bring about a fatal issue.

Acute diffuse peritonitis is a severe and dangerous disease, in which the danger and the rapidity of its course are dependent, within certain limits, upon the character and quantity of the effusion. The fatal termination occurs generally in the course of a few days, or may be delayed until the middle of the second week. Again, death may occur after a longer interval, with symptoms of chronic peritonitis. Recovery occurs most frequently in cases of plastic fibrinous effusion.

Analysis of the Individual Symptoms.

Meteorism and effusion—the physical phenomena. At the very outset of the disease, the abdominal muscles are tensely contracted, and consequently the abdomen appears to be retracted within the level of the arch of the ribs, while every touch causes the muscles to contract still more firmly. Soon, however, the abdomen becomes distended, and all the more so, if the parietes had been in a lax condition previously; the statement made by Broussais that peritonitis may run its course in muscular individuals without apparent distention is thus far authorized.

In the commencement both the abdominal muscles and the muscular coat of the intestines are in a state of strong reflex contraction from the excitation of the sentient nerves, but soon paralysis of the muscular layer of the intestine sets in, whereupon distention from gas and fluid contents ensues. Gradually the activity of the abdominal muscles becomes impaired, and then the abdomen arches forward, the normal flattening under the ribs and epigastrium becomes convex, and finally the height of the abdomen considerably exceeds that of the thorax.

If the abdominal parietes offer any resistance to distention, the diaphragm is pressed upward. This may occur to so great an extent in cases of great meteorism and copious effusion that the anterior margin of the diaphragm is found to lie at the level of the third rib. The apex of the heart is thus frequently dislocated upward, and the inferior posterior parts of the lung are so compressed that a large portion of the lower lobe is rendered completely airless. Hence we find, on examining the back of the thorax, that in the inferior portion there is considerable dulness, which extends high up, and that the respiratory sounds are either diminished or loudly bronchial. If there be simultaneously effusion into the pleural cavities, this compression will, of course, thereby be increased. It is often exceedingly difficult to diagnose whether, in addition to the high position of the diaphragm and the compression of the lung, pleural effusion also exists, as in both cases the dulness descends somewhat regularly in a straight line from behind forward through the axilla, and vocal fremitus cannot always be turned to account.

The liver also is, of course, pushed upward and backward, and thus, owing to its rotation and its being placed on its edge, the normal dulness is decreased. The anterior hepatic dulness may actually completely disappear without any escape of gas having taken place into the peritoneum, owing to the distended transverse colon or the small intestines inserting themselves between the liver and the wall of the thorax. The same holds good for the spleen.

That hepatic dulness may completely vanish from the anterior wall of the thorax without perforation and entrance of air is shown by the record of a case in point from von Ziemssen's clinique in Munich. A man, seventy-three years of age, taken ill eight days previously with severe pain in the abdomen and frequent vomiting. Aspect that of collapse, great distention of the abdomen, and the epigastrium markedly projecting. On percussion the high pulmonary tone changes to the deep intestinal tone on both sides in front at the level of the fourth rib, in the position of hepatic dulness on both sides of the median line there is an amphoric sound, and not until we come to the line of the right axilla is a somewhat sharply-defined dulness met with. Percussion sounds are not the same all over the abdomen; the tone is lowest in the region of the liver on either side of the middle line, corresponding to the course of the transverse colon; highest in the left umbilical region.

On post-mortem no perforation was found (nor was such believed during life to exist), but the liver was completely separated from the wall of the thorax by the interposition of the greatly distended transverse colon and some coils of intestine. The cause of the peritonitis was found to be a deeply eroding, sloughing ulcer in the ascending colon, and another in the cæcum, the former approaching to perforation.

A similar state of things had been previously several times observed, as also recently by Leuhe.[1] (See also Perforative Peritonitis.)

Owing to the great accumulation of gas, the lower outlet of the thorax becomes widened, and the intercostal spaces appear narrowed, and are not drawn inward in consequence of the firm pressure exerted from within. A transverse sulcus, running across the epigastrium, may frequently be seen.

We sometimes see the contour of certain distended knuckles of intestine very distinctly mapped out, and if there be an obstruction in a portion of the gut which does not lie very deeply, the distention may be unsymmetrical, and occasionally we are able to trace the distended coils of intestine in their course from some definite point. This arrangement, however, in reality, cannot be so simply made out, as the knuckles of intestine become coiled up together into an inflated ball. In cases of stenosis we may often observe very distinctly externally the occurrence of the peristaltic action, and when it has passed on as far as the obstruction, we hear a loud gurgling murmur. These visible futile motions of the intestine cease when, as the result of inflammation, its muscular coat becomes paralyzed.

The percussion sound is very clear and unusually deep over the inflated portions of intestine, but the tone is higher or lower according to the size of the vibrating column of air in the various portions of the gut; thus the sound may be tympanitic or not tympanitic, according as the stretching of the intestinal walls and the possibility of sonorous vibration vary.

According to the statement of Gerhardt, in cases of intestinal stenosis, it may be observed that the coils of intestine lying in contact with the abdominal parietes

---

[1] W. Leube and Fr. Penzoldt, Klinische Berichte. Erlangen. 1875.

produce a uniformly high tympanitic sound, and that this is to be explained by the fact that these coils are uniformly filled with a kind of frothy admixture of air and fæces.

As soon as a large quantity of fluid has collected in the abdominal cavity, the sound on percussion is found to be dull wherever the fluid lies, and as this is always in the most dependent parts the dulness, as the patient lies on his back, is found on the posterior portions of both sides and over the symphysis pubis. The line of demarcation is a straight line, and corresponds to the line of section of a horizontal plane. If we change the position of the patient and turn him over on his side, we find that the dulness disappears on the elevated side, while it correspondingly increases on the other. A similar state of things takes place in a change from the horizontal to the upright position, the dulness over the pubis rising to a higher level, but this test is only practically applicable where the effusion is considerable. The dulness in the dependent parts and its rapid shifting when the position of the patient is changed, are the only definite criteria for the presence of fluid in the peritoneal cavity.

The line of demarcation of the area of dulness is found, on mapping it out very accurately, to be zigzag, corresponding with the wedging in of the fluid between the loops of intestine (Breslau, Gerhardt). These irregularities in the line may become more fully marked in the case of solid matting together and adhesions. But we find, in spite of adhesions and a purulent character of the effusion, that the mobility is neither soon nor frequently interfered with. Unlike pleural effusion, spaces and channels generally remain open between the various loops of intestine which permit the motion of the fluid. It is only when the fluid becomes actually encysted that its mobility ceases.

On tapping the parietes at a spot with which the fluid is in contact a wave is propagated through the fluid and strikes against the parietes at other parts of the abdomen, where it may be felt by the hand, giving the sensation of fluctuation. Where the amount of effusion is small, fluctuation may be rendered more distinct by placing the patient on his side and allowing the fluid to gravitate. A sharp tap is made by the hand and the other is placed flatly at a spot not too far off. Fluctuation is of no very important diagnostic value as to the existence of fluid effusion, and there are a number of conditions which may give rise to fallacy, as, for example, œdema of the parietes, these latter being very soft and fat, or fluid in the intestines, etc., etc.

The abdomen feels hard and tense, and gives one the idea of a fully distended india-rubber air-cushion, the hardness and amount of swelling being in inverse ratio to one another. As a result of distention the normal irregularities and furrows in the epidermis become obliterated, and the skin, reflecting the light in an altered manner, becomes shining.

On auscultation of the abdomen we generally hear numerous gurglings and rumblings — coarse, loudly sounding bubbling which may occur spontaneously or may be produced artificially by pressure on the intestines ; in the latter case a fine bubbling fluid murmur more frequently is produced. On succussion distinct splashing may sometimes be heard, owing to the fact that the stomach and distended intestines fulfil the necessary conditions of being smooth inflated spaces containing movable fluid. Hence this symptom is no proof of the existence of free air in the peritoneal sac.

Under certain circumstances also we may perceive friction sounds, generally in connection with the respiratory movements, or produced artificially by pressure, which present the characters of something between the crepitation of emphysema and the leather-creak (Bright). The occurrence of friction sounds is not so frequent as one might be induced to expect, *a priori*, from the rough fibrinous deposit on the serous membrane. The movements, however, are too slight, and they are interfered with by the matting of the parts together, and the parts themselves are too yielding to allow of attrition occurring with sufficient force. Hence these sounds are most readily heard over the liver, perhaps also over the spleen, the uterus, or over abdominal tumors, if such should chance to be present.

The friction phenomena were first observed by Beatty in a case of oöphoritis, and were perceived both by the stethoscope and by the hand during inspiration. Beatty believed that the occurrence of solid tumors was necessary for their production. Desprey, Wright and Corrigan, similarly observed peritoneal friction phenomena, and explained them as dependent on the movement of the effusion and false membranes.[1]

---

[1] Compare *Gerhardt*, Arch. der Heilk. 1861 ; and *G. Terfloth*, Diss. Greifswald. 1868.

Vomiting and fæcal evacuations.—Gastro-intestinal symptoms occur generally early, the tongue becomes coated and the taste impaired. Vomiting is one of the most frequent symptoms of peritonitis, and it often sets in both spontaneously and after the taking of fluids, or medicine, and even in intervals between the attacks of actual vomiting the nausea remains constant, and flatus comes up with a choking sensation (ructus). At first the remains of food are vomited, later on masses of mucus or grass green material—*vomitus aeruginosus seu herbaceus.* In some few cases no vomiting occurs, or it may cease in the course of the disease. The occurrence of a grass green vomit is not characteristic of peritonitis. We must admit that in the production of this frequent vomiting several factors concur. The vomiting is a reflex act, but the excitants to its production may be sought for in irritation of the sentient fibres supplied to the inflamed serous membrane, and of the gastric branches of the vagus, in the upward pressure of the effusion and inflated intestines, and in the extreme distention of the intestines ; and lastly, there exists an excessively irritable condition of the gastric nerves themselves, every drop of fluid or anything of the kind that enters the stomach causing instantaneously an attack of vomiting.

Frequently distressing singultus is at the same time present. As regards the activity of the intestine, complete constipation is the rule. If the disease be associated with intestinal stenosis— especially when this condition is situated low down,—as in cases of incarceration, twisting, and fæcal accumulation, we have, of course, the element of mechanical obstruction to account for the constipation. Constipation is, however, frequently present under other conditions, and is then no doubt dependent on paralysis of the muscular coat of the intestine, which in its turn may be adequately explained by the inflammation of the serous membrane involving the other layers of the gut. In this way, previously existing diarrhœa may give way or be replaced by constipation.

The occurrence of constipation is, however, by no means a necessity, and some few forms of the disease, as, for example, puerperal peritonitis, are characterized by frequent diarrhœa (vomitus sympathicus in gravi malo vix unquam deest, alvi tamen constipatio minus constans, Hildebrand).

There is no difficulty in discovering a reason in well-known facts to account for the diverse phenomena met with in connection with the evacuations. In the first place, it is not necessary to assume that the excitability of the intestine is in all cases reduced to zero ; and if its activity be only diminished, the resorption from the intestine will be less, and this will tend to promote a fluid condition of the contents. Further, the paralysis need not be equally distributed over the entire intestine. We find, as a matter of fact, that the intensity of the inflammation is not equally well marked in all parts of the serous membrane.

The fact observed that peritonitis may give rise to stercoraceous vomiting without mechanical obstruction accords with this view. This phenomenon is evidently to be explained by assuming that lower portions of the intestine are unable, owing to total paralysis, to pass their contents downwards, and thus the power of the muscular coat above the obstruction is unable to take effect downwards, and hence sends its contents upwards. A short time ago a patient in v. Ziemssen's clinique, in whose case this symptom existed, died of tubercular peritonitis, and on post-mortem examination not the slightest trace of mechanical obstruction was discovered. Bamberger has also observed this.

Further, in connection with the character of the dejecta, we must bear in mind the part sustained by the mucous membrane of the stomach, whether, for instance, nothing whatever be absorbed or whether a fluid even be exuded, a circumstance which in the lower portion of the intestine is of moment for the occurrence of diarrhœa.

Pain.—The pain of the abdomen sets in at the very commencement, or it may have existed before the occurrence of the other peritonitic symptoms at a circumscribed spot of the abdomen, as, for example, in ulcerative processes in the intestine when they attack the serous membrane.

The character of the pain is not easily described, for in any definition of painful sensations, we have to make use of illustrations and comparisons with the more commonly experienced forms of pain, such being generally described as boring and cutting. The intensity of the pain is distinctly dependent upon the quickness with which the inflammation and effusion extend, in accordance with the well-known maxim that the more sudden the change the more intense will be the irritation of the nerves. The intense severity of the pain in peritonitis is further connected with the great extent of surface of the peritoneum and consequently with the enormous number of nerve-terminations which are thus affected by the inflammation.[1]

The intensity of the pain, which is equalled in but few other diseases, gradually gives way after some time ; but, as an older writer expresses it, it only becomes, as it were, dull, while the patient is impressed with the feeling that it will very readily recur. There are occasionally colicky exacerbations on any motion of the intestine and its contents, this being associated with a change in the position of the gut, and an increased pressure on the nerve-terminations. The increase of pain occurs further in every movement of the body, even in the movements of the diaphragm and viscera in respiration.

It is characteristic of the pain in peritonitis that the slightest pressure increases it intensely, hence the guarded movements of the patient, and the anxiety evinced at the examination of the abdomen. Even the pressure of the lightest covering is often unbearable.

This sensibility to pressure must not be mistaken for hyperæsthesia of the parietes, in which pain is produced by a simple touch, but not by firm pressure.

In those cases where a local process leads to diffuse peritonitis, the primary seat of sensibility is often of diagnostic value. These spots often remain, during the further course of the dis-

---

[1] The question as to the mode of termination of nerve-fibres in the peritoneum is not yet definitely decided. As *E. Cyon* was unable to discover any specific terminal organ, he believes a free nerve ending in part possible. The fibres form numerous plexuses and present an irregular network.

Julien described a peculiar mode of termination of the nerves in the peritoneum. According to him the fibres are transformed into pale, non-medullated fibrillæ, and these pass into peculiarly formed capsules. From the other end of these capsules passes a pencil of radiating terminal fibrillæ which end in small heads. This statement requires confirmation.

Under normal conditions the nerve-fibres of the peritoneum convey no impressions, they possess no tactile capability, and we have no sensation of these parts. Their excitation occurs only from painful irritants.

ease, the most sensitive. It happens also in idiopathic peritonitis that certain spots of the abdomen are particularly painful—for example, the neighborhood of the umbilicus; and this exalted sensitiveness may, in fact, be connected with a more intense degree of inflammation at the spots in question. The character of the effusion has no influence on the intensity of the pain.

Circulation — Temperature. — Numerous variations in the pulse are observed in the various cases. It may, at least at the beginning, show but little deviation from the normal; the rule is, however, that it at once becomes considerably increased in frequency. The wave at the same time is small, and the artery contracted. According as the other symptoms of the disease increase, the pulse becomes smaller, and almost vanishes completely, while its frequency increases to 140, or even to 160. This great rapidity of the pulse results, doubtless, from several concomitant circumstances; it is certainly not occasioned by the high temperature alone, to which it is in no way correlated.

Peritonitis. Cause unknown. Death.

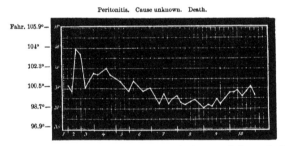

The temperature presents great variations and irregularities, which, up to the present, we are unable to account for. The character and extent of the effusion have, undoubtedly, some effect upon them, but still the temperature is not solely dependent upon these conditions alone. The rule is that the temperature rises considerably in the commencement of a case of acute diffuse peritonitis—up to 40° C. in the axilla—and during the further course of the disease retains this height either pretty continuously or with more or less well-marked remissions. Later on the temperature may sink below the normal—collapse temperature. Death may ensue while the temperature still remains at its height, or after it has become normal or subnormal (compare the curve in peritonitis with fatal issue). Recovery takes place, as a rule, by means of lysis, with the gradual decline of the exacerbation. In more protracted cases, particularly on their transition into a chronic stage, we not unfrequently see considerable variations both up and down, which probably are connected with the changes which are taking place in the serous membrane. The second curve shows these variations.

Many cases run their course from the outset without any rise in temperature. Intestinal occlusion, for example, may lead to considerable effusion into the peritoneal cavity with a normal or subnormal temperature.

Respiration. — The number of the respirations is increased threefold or even more; they are of a purely costal type and are shallow. These alterations in the respiration are primarily dependent on the tenderness of the abdomen, the pain being increased by the movement of the abdominal viscera on the descent of the diaphragm, and hence this latter is kept as quiet as possible, and the patient breathes as superficially as he can with the upper part of his thorax. Every attack of coughing is most anxiously suppressed, and when the irritation can be no longer overcome the patient coughs gently, so as to avoid, as far as possible, any pressure on the abdomen.

As the respirations are not so ample, their frequency must be increased. The increase is, however, further dependent on the encroachment on the space of the thorax and on the inadequate circulation, and lastly on the rise in temperature. Further, it happens by no means unfrequently that peritonitis is associated with pleuritis, or even with pericarditis, such being particularly the case in the infectious forms of the disease.

Outward Condition, Sensorium.—Patients lie, as a rule, on their back, and in order to relax the abdominal muscles as much as possible the legs are drawn up. Every change of position is most studiously avoided on account of the pain it produces; the arms alone are tossed to and fro, an evidence of restlessness and anguish.

The changes in the countenance are in part due to the pain, and in part to the general collapse in which it participates; this collapse is partly brought about by the frequent vomiting, and partly by the effusion into the abdomen and the great excess of blood in the abdominal vessels; but the excitation of such a number of nerve-terminations may also have something to do with it by producing the effect of shock. The coldness of the prominences and the cyanosis result from the imperfect filling of the arteries, due to weakened vis a tergo, whereby the blood accumulates in the veins, and thus, as the result of an inadequate supply of warmth with arterial blood, a well-marked cooling takes place. The insufficiency of respiration is naturally of importance in accounting for the cyanosis.

The intense excitation from the pain has probably something to do with the clear condition of the sensorium, which usually persists throughout, even to the very death-struggle; we may at least account for the disappearance of previously existing disturbances of consciousness on the supervention of peritonitis in this way (Traube).

Delirium occurs before death, and may be regarded as an indication of commencing paralysis or as the result of cerebral œdema; complete loss of consciousness occurring soon after the commencement of the disease is a most rare exception. In such a case all manifestation of pain may be absent, but even then pressure on the abdomen calls forth distinct indication of pain and reflex movements.

The condition occasionally observed, in which the patient, after the lapse of some time, and when effusion has taken place, feels better and more comfortable, is due to the decrease in sensibility of the sentient nerves.

The evacuation of urine frequently cannot be effected by natural means, the detrusor vesicæ becoming paralyzed by the extension to it of the inflammatory process. Patients often feel a painful urgency to pass water, and when a little urine flows away, it is accompanied by pain along the urethra.

The quantity of urine passed is very small, and correspondingly concentrated; hence generally a brick-dust sediment is thrown down on cooling. The reduction in the quantity of urine depends upon the losses of water from the vomiting and the effusion, upon the low arterial pressure, as well as upon the effects of compression of the tightly distended abdomen on the renal arteries.

Albumen is by no means constantly found in the urine; if albumen be found in the urine, and if there be no actual complication of nephritis, it is to be regarded as the result of the feverishness and stasis.

The occurrence of pleuritis and pericarditis has already been referred to; in addition to these we must mention jaundice, which, however, is an exceedingly rare concomitant of simple peritonitis. As regards other complications, suffice it to say that peritonitis is itself a much more frequent complication of previously existing disease; and in this way the aspect of the symptoms which it presents is liable to numerous modifications.

Course, Duration, Results. Prognosis.

The course of acute diffuse peritonitis is generally a rapid one, and a fatal issue is moreover very frequent. It would be difficult to adduce any statistics which would accurately show the rate of mortality, since cases of peritoneal inflammation, etiologically distinct, can scarcely be compared one with another.

Death occurs in many instances within five or six days, or in any case it results within the first few weeks under conditions of

increasing collapse and imperfect respiration.   Meanwhile, there
are changes for better and worse.

The more rapid and sudden the extension of the inflammation
and the occurrence of the effusion, particularly if this latter be
of a purulent character, the more likely is death to occur early.
In the case of internal incarcerations and twistings it is the primary lesion which is, as a rule, the cause of death ; the intensity
of the accompanying peritonitis tends only to modify the symptoms, and to hasten the fatal issue.

The most unfavorable cases are those of a septic nature, and
those in which substances which act as chemical irritants are
poured into the cavity of the peritoneum, as is often the case in
perforation.   Those forms are most favorable in which a dry
effusion preponderates, such as may occur in the extension of a
simple inflammatory process to the peritoneum, or in connection
with menstruation, etc.   Cases of sero-fibrinous effusion terminate comparatively often in recovery.

The symptoms which indicate a change for the better are a
uniform decrease in the tenderness, meteorism, and fever, the
cessation of vomiting, the regulation of the fæcal evacuations,
and the return of sleep.   The fluid portion of the effusion is
absorbed, and if this takes place rapidly we may observe an increase in the quantity of urine and sweating.

The further metamorphoses of the solid elements of the effusion are important.   The new connective-tissue products—the
false membranes and adhesions—may be of little moment, so far
as the future life of the individual is concerned, or may be the
means of engendering a vast number of dangers and functional
disturbances, according as they assume a loose or a firm retractile character, and according to their extent and the manner in
which they are arranged.

Owing to the fixation and retraction of the intestines and
mesentery, as also owing to the shortening of the former, the
mobility of the gut may be greatly interfered with, and thus
continous disturbances of the digestive functions and impairment of nutrition may result.   Similarly, in the cases of adhesions affecting the uterus, ovaries, and Fallopian tubes, the
course of pregnancy and delivery may be seriously complicated.

A number of nervous phenomena also met with in the female may have their origin in such conditions. The intestines may become contorted and have some of their coats ruptured, owing to the shrinking of the mesentery ; and firm ligamentous bands, as well as more slender cords, may produce compression and constriction, and further may give rise to pouches and dilatations, which may be the means of producing incarcerations. The fixation of the intestine is further of moment in the production of invagination.

The richer the effusion be in cellular elements, the greater is the difficulty of its complete absorption ; after the acute stage has passed off such cases may pass into a chronic condition. The effusion may become encysted in several places, and the further history of these masses is associated with new dangers. Under favorable circumstances they become inspissated and ultimately become fibrous, caseous, or calcareous, or else the pus finds its way outward in some way or other. Perforations of the intestine, of the diaphragm, of the abdominal parietes, of the uterus, and of the bladder or vagina may arise, with occasionally the formation of chronic abscesses and fistulæ. In this way the encysted portions may become converted into fæcal cavities, and communications may become established between two portions of intestine, or else the newly formed false membrane may be broken down, and a fresh attack of peritonitis and death may be the result. The encapsuled hardened masses may frequently be perceived on examination long after as tumors and indurations.

The liver and spleen are occasionally invested by a dense coating of connective tissue, and varying degrees of atrophy are developed as a result of compression, especially if the vena portæ be implicated. A permanent jaundice may further arise from compression of the ductus choledochus. The encysted portions of the effusion may produce deep furrows in the liver from atrophy.

These remains of effusion may give rise to further danger in the form of pyæmia and septicæmia. Such encysted effusions may also lead to general disturbance of nutrition, anæmia, and actual marasmus.

From all this it will appear that the prognosis must throughout be serious, and in many cases absolutely fatal. For even
when the acute stage has passed off we must keep in view the
possibility of the effects of resulting conditions.

Diagnosis.

We have to decide whether a case be one of peritonitis or not,
and if it be, we must make out, as far as possible, with what
primary affection it may be connected. The latter part of the
question is by no means equal in importance to the first, either
as regards our opinion of the case or the treatment. The diagnosis of peritonitis is, in the majority of cases, not difficult; it
rests upon the intense painfulness of the abdomen, the vomiting,
the constipation, the quickening of the pulse, and the collapse,
as well as on the concomitant rise in temperature and distention
of the abdomen. The demonstration of freely movable fluid in
the abdomen is a very important item.

In the commencement, so long as there is only tenderness,
excitement of the pulse, and vomiting, no differential diagnosis
can be definitely established from many other painful affections
of the abdomen, more especially from such as cardialgia, enter-
algia, colicky affections of the kidney, gall-bladder, and uterus,
also rheumatism of the abdominal muscles and inflammation and
hyperæsthesia of the abdominal walls.

The pain in peritonitis is characterized by being greatly intensified on pressure and motion; in colicky conditions and neuralgia, the pain often does not present this peculiarity, and firm
pressure may even give relief. This characteristic is, however,
not invariable, more particularly as frequently processes lie at
the root of these various painful conditions which may induce
inflammation of the organ in question, together with participation of the serous membrane, and immediately pass on into peritonitis. In these cases we must have recourse to the history
which may be obtained as to the manner in which the various
functions of the entire abdominal viscera have been performed
(character of menstruation, whether such attacks had occurred
previously, whether there had been jaundice, or abnormities in

the urine, or whether there had been symptoms of gastric ulcer, etc.). A definite diagnosis rests upon the demonstration of free fluid in the abdominal cavity. Here mistakes may most easily arise, if there be a simple serous effusion from any cause, disease of the kidneys, for example, and if pain in the abdomen occur simultaneously; under such circumstances, the diagnosis may be difficult, and all the more so as the general sensibility of the abdomen is not always present in its fully characteristic form.

Mistakes may further arise owing to tumors in the abdomen, the enlarged uterus, ovarian tumors, echinococcus cysts, even the distended bladder, all of which on altering the position of the patient present a certain mobility, being mistaken for effusion. The emptying of the bladder and an accurate examination preclude mistakes of this kind.

As far as the diagnosis of the primary affection is concerned, it is not always possible to clear the matter up completely; we must take into account the entire pathology of the abdominal viscera, but, as in the category of these affections some few stand prominently forward in point of frequency, these must especially be borne in mind. In coming to a diagnosis, everything which tends to disclose symptoms of a previously existent abdominal disease is very important. Too much weight must not be attached to the starting-point and primary seat of the tenderness.

I saw a case in which the starting-point of the pains was always referred to the right iliac fossa, and their intensity in this place was particularly complained of. On post-mortem examination a fibrinous peritonitis was found without any primary disease in this locality. In another case, where the patient came into hospital with perforation, the epigastrium was always described as the seat of the pain that had previously existed; perforation had been caused by a corrosive ulcer in the cæcum. The localization of the pain is thus often deceptive.

After the various affections of the uterus we must constantly bear in mind the possibility of incarceration, and, therefore, carefully examine the hernial openings (in this case, as well as in the case of internal constrictions, strictures from cicatrices, etc.; see Intestinal Diseases). Next after this we must think of the right iliac fossa, with the inflammatory processes which occur in it, and, further, simple fæcal accumulation, then ulceration in the stomach and intestine.

The majority of other diseased conditions can only be had recourse to when we have independent positive data for their existence.[1]

Treatment.

The treatment of peritonitis can and must be, in many cases, aimed at its exciting cause. This is more particularly the case in all forms of intestinal occlusion and constriction. The prospect of success is certainly never great, but in fæcal accumulation, for example, systematic and rational treatment may be the means of saving life. We cannot here repeat in extenso what has been already said on the subject in "Intestinal Diseases;" we shall only refer again to the value of large enemata.

But even in other cases of peritonitis which are not dependent on ileus, we must not leave altogether out of sight the primary disease and starting-point of the inflammation, so far as we have been able to determine it.

In the symptomatic treatment of peritonitis the objects to be attained—so far as the means at our disposal in the present day will allow—are to prevent the further extension of the disease and the intensity and extensiveness of the effusion, to lessen the pain, to control as far as possible the vomiting and hiccough, and ultimately to remove the constipation.

Further, we know that direct danger to life may accrue from excessive distention of the abdomen, and from the pressure thereby induced on the thoracic organs. We have, therefore, to contend against this as well as against the menacing collapse.

The first question is as to how we are to carry out these indications, and whether we may expect to succeed in checking the intensity and extent of the inflammation by the use of antiphlogistic remedies in general, or by any special ones. Under this head, the remedies most frequently employed are depletion—general in the earlier stages, and local by means of leeches in the later,—inunction of mercurial ointment, under some circumstances

---

[1] *L. M. Waton* observed a rare occurrence, namely, intermittent attacks of pain in the abdomen, vomiting, the type of countenance that of tertian ague; which disappeared on the exhibition of quinine.

so as to produce salivation, and the exhibition of calomel. I must state that I have not been able to recognize any distinct benefit from such treatment, but, on the contrary, that extensive depletion by means of fifty leeches or more on the abdomen must produce subsequently a prejudicial influence on the circulation. The application of a smaller number of leeches (10–15) may with safety be recommended as a means of improving the subjective condition of the patient without producing any subsequent bad effect. I believe, however, that in most cases we may dispense with local depletion without in any way being guilty of neglect.

On the other hand, the use of the ice-bladder at the outset of peritonitis is most strongly to be recommended on various grounds. First, as a means of withdrawing heat—we abstain from other antipyretic means in acute peritonitis for obvious reasons—then, as an antiphlogistic remedy, and lastly, as a means of influencing the peristaltic motion and allaying the pain.[1]

The ice-bladder and ice-compresses must not be too heavy on the abdomen, or they will increase the discomfort of the patient and cause more upward pressure than is otherwise the case. By a well-adjusted use the cold is generally well borne, and with evident alleviation of the symptoms. We must, however, in practice, place considerable reliance on the patient's own opinion as to whether the cold ought to be continued or not.

I believe that by the application of cold we may lessen the hyperæmia by causing contraction of the vessels, reduce the nervous irritability, and effect the spasmodic peristaltic action. Hence, the beneficial effect met with at the outset of peritonitis which is no longer attainable when once the abdominal vessels and the intestines have become paralyzed. At this period the application of warmth, on the other hand, is indicated. As, however, we cannot from without accurately inspect the processes which are going on, we shall find the subjective condition of the patient a very important guide.

---

[1] According to an apparently accurate and plausible statement, the use of cold is called for on account of the meteorism, to condense the gas in the intestine; we have only to refer to the well-known formula to estimate how much the volume of intestinal gas may be reduced by actually reducing the temperature several degrees, and thus to see how important it is to attain such a result.

Since Graves and Stokes set us the example, the use of large doses of opium in the treatment of peritonitis has ever been the universal practice. The mode of action of the opium was explained by its narcotic properties, and by the property it was supposed to have of arresting peristaltic action. If opium did arrest peristaltic action, the practical results which, as a matter of fact, follow its administration in the treatment of peritonitis, would not be attributable to it. The action of opium and morphia is much more readily understood if we accept the view that they tend to excite peristaltic action, but at the same time to diminish reflex excitation. On this latter property depends a farther useful effect of opium, namely, its action in allaying vomiting and hiccough. If we, then, regard the action of opium in its entirety, we must conclude that in scarcely a single case of peritonitis can it properly be withheld. The great tolerance of this medicine evinced by patients is enough to excite wonder. The phenomenon depends doubtless on the fact that the preparations are but to a very small extent absorbed. This tolerance does not exist in the case of subcutaneous injections, and hence, if there be great painfulness, we may combine this method with internal administration, as the latter has the advantage of acting directly upon the stomach and intestines. It is doubtful whether any essential difference exists between the results of opium and those of morphia.

Complete rest and complete abstinence are demanded throughout the entire disease. Even small quantities of fluid are often quickly vomited. We should recommend, therefore, to give the patient small pieces of ice (also fruit-ices), which in itself lessens the vomiting by allaying the irritability. A series of other means of allaying the vomiting has come into use, such as drinks containing carbonic acid, alkaline carbonates, lime-water, and others.

The violent hiccough often does not yield to opium and morphia, and the whole series of narcotic remedies have been applied in such cases, and, in addition, sinapisms, blisters, and similar counter-irritant treatment. In exceedingly urgent cases the use of chloroform may produce the wished-for result.

The use of cathartics for the meteorism and constipation has been completely given up ; we have generally learned to recognize the fact that drastic cathartics must in many cases of peritonitis increase the symptoms. The simple symptomatic constipation in peritonitis requires no special treatment. A few doses of calomel may be of use under certain circumstances in overcoming the meteorism ; in addition to this, amongst the various internal remedies which have been tried, we should choose calcined magnesia, lime-water, vegetable charcoal, etc. They will not bring about any wonderful effect. The introduction of the rectal bougie has not, unfortunately, the effect which we might expect ; gas, no doubt, passes down, but frequently fluid or solid fæcal matter stops the way, and, as a rule, but little wind is passed. This method ought always to be given a trial. In urgent cases there is nothing left but to puncture the intestine with a fine trocar, to let out the flatus. We must, however, puncture in several places. The danger of the exit of fæcal matter through the puncture is not great ; still, I lately saw gas pass in this way into the peritoneal cavity.

As soon as the collapse appears to threaten life, those stimulants must be employed which the circumstances of the case appear to permit. The best are subcutaneous injection of camphorated oil, and, internally, ether, musk, wine, cool champagne, etc.

In cases of excessive purulent effusion, the question arises as to whether we ought not to give an exit to the effusion by operative means, namely, puncture, or even incision. During the acute stage of the disease such an interference must be rejected. After this stage has passed away, however, if the effusion be excessive, and is not becoming absorbed, this proceeding may be justifiable and productive of good results, especially in the case of threatening rupture. In the case of a favorable turn, it is necessary to pay the greatest attention to bodily rest and nourishment.

To assist the absorption of the remains of the effusion, baths, derivations to the skin, and painting with tincture of iodine may be of use in connection with good nutrition.

Special Forms of Diffuse Peritonitis.

a. Perforative Peritonitis.

All those cases must be included under the term Perforative Peritonitis which are associated with rupture of the peritoneum at any place, whether this occur from suppuration and ulceration or from mechanical violence.

The serous membrane is most frequently perforated, owing to suppuration and ulceration in the abdominal viscera. Its mode of occurrence is such that perforation takes place into the abdominal cavity from the viscera, and thus the peritoneum is the last to give way. The reverse process occurs more rarely, namely, the pus in contact with the serous membrane gradually breaks it down, and thus makes its way outward. In the latter case the perforation is widest at its peritoneal end If peritonitis had occurred as the result of perforation, the resulting effusion might further produce a second perforation, and thus both varieties may be combined in the same case.[1]

If we regard the cases of acute diffuse peritonitis in their etiological aspect, and compare them with one another, we shall find that a considerable portion of the whole are those resulting from perforation.[2] Those cases only, however, are characterized by special symptoms in which the perforation is associated with the exit of gas from the stomach or intestines; no other symptoms can be relied on as indicating the presence of perforation.

The examination is therefore not immediately directed to the existence of a perforation, but merely to the presence of free gas in the peritoneal cavity. Hence the question has to be answered whether or not in some other manner, owing to decomposition of a peritoneal effusion, free gas may not be developed in the peritoneal cavity, thus causing pneumoperitonitis. The statements on this point are very contradictory, many observers entirely denying the occurrence of this phenomenon. This much, at any rate, may be regarded as definite, that the development of free gas in the peritoneum is an exceedingly rare occurrence. That, however, large quantities of gas may be developed in individual cases, even during life, owing to

---

[1] *Buhl*, Bericht über 280 Leichenöffuungen. Zeitschr. für rat. Med. N. F. VII. 1.

[2] *Willigk* found perforation 32 times in 365 cases of peritonitis, hence 8.8 per cent. Prag. Vierteljahrschrift. 1853. X. II.

processes of decomposition, cannot be doubted with the record of observations which we have before us. I shall here only refer to the testimony of O. Bamberger and to a case accurately observed by Breslau. We may remark, *a priori*, that the conditions for the decomposition of effusion occur much more frequently and readily in the peritoneum than in any other serous cavity, in that nowhere else does there appear to exist such an opportunity of taking up septic material in a state of decomposition ; still it is a rare phenomenon during life, and hence the path by which the excitant to decomposition reaches the peritoneum must be a difficult one. In Breslau's case, this probably took place in connection with the puncture which had previously been made.

Small quantities of gas may rapidly disappear owing to absorption, but greater quantities require undoubtedly a longer time, as has been established from the histories of the few cases of cure recorded after the occurrence of perforation (Traube's case).

That gas may get into the abdominal cavity by means of diffusion from the intestine cannot be contended, and is supported by the fact that odorous gases can be communicated through the intestinal wall to masses of fluid (abscesses) in contact with it. But according as the diffusion of gases takes place, absorption proceeds at an equal rate, so that a pneumoperitoneum is certainly never produced in this way.[1]

The rupture of the wall of the stomach or intestine may take place traumatically, owing to a blow, fall, etc., if the viscera be very full. By far the most frequent inducing cause for perforation is to be found in the various ulcerative processes in the stomach and intestine, and in the vermiform process. The ulcers extend gradually more and more deeply, until, at last, the thin serous membrane is all that remains. This also may finally become necrosed, and thus give way, or some other cause may arise which produces the rupture of the serous membrane, namely, a concussion or a blow, strong peristaltic action, filling of the intestines with excessive quantities of fæces, or with ingesta, which tend to produce direct mechanical violence.

Anatomy.—The distention of the abdomen is generally exceedingly great, the parietes more quickly assume a greenish discoloration than is the case in non-perforative peritonitis. As soon as the peritoneal cavity is opened pus gushes out, generally with considerable force. The gases, which have exuded and become collected, vary according to the place where the perfora-

---

[1] Compare *Catani* and *Dressler*, Prager Vierteljahr. 1865. I. p. 115, in which also analyses of these gases are given.

tion has been produced; in the majority of cases they have a strongly feculent odor.

The coils of intestine are matted together, of a dirty green color, and beset with a deposition of fibrin. The effusion is apt to be very great, generally of a dirty purulent character, rarely healthy pus.

It may contain the contents of the stomach or intestine mixed up with it, in which case triple phosphate or fæcal concretions and even worms may be found to have passed out through the perforation. The fact that such masses have passed out requires the opening to be of a certain circumference, as it may easily become covered over or secluded. Gas permeates through exceedingly small openings, but even the passage of gas itself may be prevented by occlusion, by fæces, etc. Furthermore, the quantity of material which passes out depends upon the degree of fulness and distention of the intestines at the time.

In some few cases the opening of the perforation is so great and death supervenes so rapidly that we find in the abdomen only exuded fluid contents, but no inflammatory processes and no effusion. I saw a case of the kind where the patient was brought in a dying condition to the hospital. The perforation had taken place a few hours previously. The contents of the stomach had been almost entirely poured out into the peritoneal sac through a large ulcer which had perforated, but there was not a trace of inflammation to be seen.

Still rarer are those cases in which a greater space of time intervenes between the perforation and death, but where still the evidences of inflammation are wanting. Such cases have been communicated by Bardeleben and Siebert. The attempt was made to explain this circumstance by the fact that the peritoneum had lost its normal structure as the result of previously existing inflammation, and had become metamorphosed into a firm fibrous membrane.

It is often easy to discover the opening of the perforation if gas and the contents of the intestine still pass through it. Occasionally it is very difficult if it have subsequently become closed up, and if the rupture be very small. We must in these cases guard against mistakes arising from subsequent artificial tears, which may very readily occur in the brittle intestines in cases of ulceration. The abdominal organs present a more or less advanced discoloration, and this is frequently most evident on the surface of the liver on either side of the falciform ligament, often simultaneously with a slight depression of its convex surface and a drying up of its peritoneal investment (Traube). This gray discoloration is probably the result of chemical action, and the presence of sulphuretted hydrogen in the gas, even as a mere trace, may have something to do with it.

Symptoms.—The phenomena which may precede the occurrence of perforation are referable to gastric and intestinal ulceration, fæcal accumulation, intestinal catarrh, typhlitis, enteric fever, etc. Before the occurrence of the perforation there may have existed at a circumscribed spot pain and tenderness on pressure. But these preliminary phenomena are by no means necessary, and the perforation may take place quite suddenly.

The occurrence of perforation is sometimes connected with a severe momentary pain, and with a feeling as if something in the abdomen had burst.

This severe pain depends upon the tearing itself and not on the subsequent peritonitis, for it occurs at the actual moment of the accident; furthermore, it does not depend on the contact of masses of the detruded material with the serous membrane, for it has been observed in cases where no such material has escaped.

The pain extends rapidly with great intensity over the whole abdomen, and simultaneously there often sets in a sudden and intense state of collapse. The countenance becomes drawn, the extremities cold and damp, the pulse small and frequent, and immediately the symptoms of the most acute peritonitis set in.

This is the form of peritonitis which is apt to follow perforation; perforation may, however, occur far less virulently and under circumstances of almost complete latency. This particularly is the case if peritonitis had previously existed, or if the perforation occur in the course of a severe illness, for example, a severe case of enteric fever. Further, the state of things assumes a different aspect if universal adhesions had been established prior to the rupture. In this case the rupture frequently occurs without symptoms, and is unattended subsequently by such serious phenomena.

The question as to what is the exact cause of the state of collapse which is apt to set in on perforation, cannot be definitely answered. Probably several factors combine, amongst which must be taken into account the shock of the perforation itself and the sudden occurrence of the peritonitis. The attempt has been made to explain this phenomenon by poisoning with sulphuretted hydrogen, but this mode of explanation falls to the ground, owing to the small quantity of this gas which can get into the peritoneum from the intestine, and, further, owing to the circumstance that perforation without the exit of sulphuretted hydrogen—as, for example, in the case of the stomach—is accompanied by the same set of phenomena. In those cases, also, in which, owing to decomposition of purulent effusion, considerable quantities of sulphuretted hydrogen might become developed out of the albuminous substances, poisoning by it is very improbable.

One might conclude from Emminghaus's[1] cases (in which the urine showed a sulphuretted hydrogen reaction—that is, it colored lead paper black) that under such circumstances considerable quantities of sulphuretted hydrogen may pass into the blood. The development of sulphuretted hydrogen in the urine does not, however, prove a previous absorption of the gas into the blood and its subsequent elimination in the urine. It is, in fact, not a rare occurrence that sulphuretted hydrogen is developed out of the sulphur compounds in the urine. It is, on the contrary, exceedingly unlikely that hæmoglobin should give up chemically united sulphuretted hydrogen as such to the urine; it is much more likely that there would be a decomposition into sulphuric acid and water by means of oxidation, a state of things which might be decided by experiment.

The entrance of air into the peritoneal cavity—the *tympanites peritonei*—is accompanied by a series of physical signs. Air and fluid occur freely movable in a smooth-walled cavity. The air has the lower specific gravity, and hence occupies the uppermost position in the abdomen. Necessarily connected with this is a dislocation of the viscera. As a rule, the abdomen is very markedly and uniformly distended and stretched, and no prominence of coils of intestine is visible. As when the patient is lying on his back, in the horizontal position, the epigastric region is the highest part of the abdomen, the gas collects here and presses it forward. We find, then, in addition to the high position of the diaphragm, a disappearance of the anterior hepatic dulness[2] from the thorax into the axillary region, where the dul-

[1] Berl. klin. Wochenschrift. 1872. X. 40, 41.
[2] *Schuh*, Mediz. Zeitschr. für Oesterr. 1842.

ness is often sharply marked off from the resonant portion. The liver is thus pressed upward and backward from the anterior wall of the thorax, and this occurs uniformly if not prevented by adhesions. The same is true of the spleen. On percussion the abdomen gives a remarkably clear, deep note, generally tympanitic or metallic in character; this characteristic of the percussion note is generally to be found over a large extent of the abdomen, and passes in the dependent portions into the dull note of the effusion.

Notwithstanding the accumulation of air in the peritoneum, we naturally meet with a change in pitch of the percussion note in various places where coils of intestine lie against the parietes. This will especially be the case when the quantity of air is not very considerable—only, in fact, a few bubbles. In this case the clear, deep note will only be heard of a uniform pitch in the epigastric region; in other places variations will occur. But as a tensely distended knuckle of intestine may dislocate the liver, and give a very full and deep note, the diagnosis in these cases becomes all the more difficult. The prominence of the intestinal convolution, the limits of the deep, full tone being confined to the course of the transverse colon, and the persistence of this character of tone in this position when the position of the patient is altered, are decisive evidences against the gas being free in the peritoneal cavity; in this latter case a bubble of air, being readily movable, will be found to shift about with the various changes in position of the patient.

Traube has several times observed, in cases of entrance of air into the peritoneal sac, a peculiar, easily pitted condition of the epigastric region, with a feeling of doughy fluctuation. This phenomenon must depend upon the great softening of the parietes at this spot, and upon the small resistance of the mobile bubble of air.

On shaking the patient we obtain succussion sounds. This phenomenon occurs also in a flatulent stomach and in distended portions of intestines; it is apt, however, to be louder in *tympanites peritonei*, and is moreover heard uniformly over a greater area. The same is true for the metallic character of the aortic sounds.

The other symptoms are those of acute peritonitis, and are but little altered by the occurrence of perforation, save only that they are generally intensified. Thus the vomiting is likely to be very intense unless the stomach be the seat of a large perforation ; in this case the contents of the stomach are emptied in the direction of least resistance, namely, through the perforation (Traube). This circumstance is of diagnostic value in the case of perforation of the stomach. The constipation is very obstinate, still it is not always present ; the meteorism is very intense.

The *course* of diffuse perforative peritonitis is very rapid ; death occurs with an increase in the symptoms of collapse, and frequently with a simultaneous fall in the temperature ; the fatal issue may result within a few hours or in the course of a couple of days. It may, however, be postponed for a longer time, disintegration taking place in various regions with fresh perforations, etc. Loebel has described a case of the kind in which subcutaneous emphysema occurred.

Recovery is a very rare issue, but its occurrence has been established beyond all doubt (Traube).

The *diagnosis* can only be based upon the physical signs ; hence, it is impossible to recognize a case of perforation with any certainty if the exit of air have not taken place.

The development of gas from the decomposition of an effusion cannot be distinguished from air which has escaped through a perforation ; but on account of the rarity of such an occurrence it does not demand much consideration.

As the occurrence of peritoneal symptoms is of primary moment in the diagnosis, there is no danger of mistaking for a case of the kind one of simple distention of the intestines or of acute yellow atrophy of the liver, even if the anterior hepatic dulness disappear. The only difficult question is whether the peritonitis be with or without perforation. To decide this point we ought not to rely on any one single well-established physical sign, but make an accurate digest of the entire group of phenomena. Notwithstanding, the diagnosis in some cases must remain undecided.

The *treatment* in perforative peritonitis can only be directed against the symptoms, essentially the same principles holding good in this case as in the uncomplicated form of the disease. Absolute rest and absolute abstinence, the use of large doses of opium, and the application of the ice-bladder are demanded, the diminution of the vomiting and the pain, and finally, the energetic contest with the collapse, being the principal indications for treatment. Under certain conditions it may appear right to let out the gas by puncture, with a view of diminishing the symptoms of compression.

b. Puerperal Peritonitis.

A. C. Baudelocque, Traité de la périt. puerp., etc. Paris, 1829.—*Robert Lee*, Res. on the Path. and Treatment of Some of the Most Important Dis. of Women. London. 1833.—*G. Eisenmann*, Das Kindbettfieber. Erlangen, 1834.—*R. Ferguson*, Essay on the Most Imp. Dis. of Women. 1839.—*T. Helm*, Monographie der Puerperalkrankh. Wien, 1845.—*Fr. Kiwisch*, Die Krankh. der Wöchnerinnen. Prag, 1840.—*C. T. Litzmann*, Das Kindbettfieber. Halle, 1844.—*H. Meckel*, Das bösartige Wochenfieber. Annalen der Charité. V.—*Veit*, Krankh. der weiblichen Geschlechtsorgane, in Virchow's Handb. der Pathol. VI. 2. 1856–1865. *Klob*, Path. Anatomie der weibl. Sex. Wien, 1864.—*Hecker* and *Buhl*, Klinik der Geburtskunde. Leipzig, 1861; and *Hecker*, Klinik der Geburtskunde. 2. Bd. Leipzig, 1864.—*Scanzoni*, Beitr. zur Geburtsk., Lehrb. der Geburtsh., etc. —*F. Winckel*, Die Path. und Therapie des Wochenb. 1869.—*Hirsch*, Handb. der historisch.- geograph. Path.—*O. Spiegelberg*, Volkmann's Sammlung klin. Vorträge. 3; und Monatsschr. für Geburtsk. XXVIII. u. a. O.—*Semmelweis*, Die Aetiologie der Begriff und die Prophylaxis des Kindbettfiebers. 1861.— *Oppolzer*, Allg. Wiener medic. Zeitung. 1862.—*C. Braun*, Die Puerperalfieberepidemie im Wien. Gebärh. Oesterreich. Zeitschr. für prakt. Heilk. 1861; und Monatsschr. für Geburtsk. 1862.—*E. Hervieux*, In various articles, principally in Union méd. and Traité clinique des maladies puerp., etc. Paris, 1870, 1871. —*L. Le Fort*, Des maternités. Étude sur les mat., etc. Paris, 1866.—*C. Schroeder*, Schwangerschaft, Geburt und Wochenbett. Bonn, 1867.—*Virchow*, dessen Archiv. Bd. 23.—*R. H. Ferber*, Die Aetiologie, Prophylaxis und Therapie des Puerperalfiebers. Schmidt's Jahrb. 139.—*Boehr*, Ueber die Infectionsth. des Puerperalf. Monatsschr. für Geburtsk. Bd. 32.—*Gruenewaldt*, Ueber Begriffsbestimmung und Benennung der sog. Puerperalp. Petersb. med. Zeitschr. XIV. 6. Heft XV.—*Graily Hewitt*, On Puerperal Fever in the British Lying-in Hosp., with Remarks on the Treatment of Puerp. Fever. Trans. of the Obst. Society of London. 1869.—*A. Braxton Hicks*, Lond. Obst. Transact. XII.— *Martin*, Ueber das Kindbettfieber. Berl. klin. Wochenschr. 1871. 32.—*R. Birnbaum*, De périt. puerp. phlégmon. Bresl. Diss. 1866.—*Waldeyer*, Ueber das

Vorkommen von Bacterien bei der diphth. Form des Puerperalsfiebers. Arch. für Gynäkologic. Bd. III. 2. Heft.—*B. J. Krauss*, Beitrag zur mögl. Entstehung und Verbreitung des Puerperalfiebers. Arch. für Gynäkologic. V.—*Breisky*, Zur Behandlung des Puerperalfiebers. Correspondenzbl. für Schweizer Aerzte. 1873.

The inflammation of the peritoneum in connection with the puerperal state may in itself be the entire expression of disease, or it may be but the local participation of a general process, namely, pyæmia.

These diseases are described under the general name of *puerperal fever*, which so far at least is justifiable, as these processes, one and all, in spite of anatomical and clinical varieties, have their origin in an injured condition of the genital canal and its surroundings, occasioned by delivery. The starting-point of the disease is to be found in the inner coat of the genital canal, and the morbid processes which underlie the affection in question are: endometritis and the ulcerative processes on the cervix uteri and in the vagina, and inflammation in the neighborhood of the uterus.

A subdivision of the entire group into forms which are anatomically somewhat sharply defined is made according to the various paths along which these morbid processes spread from their point of origin. Following the precedent of Buhl, we may distinguish three several paths by which the disease extends: first, directly through the Fallopian tubes, or through the substance of the uterus itself; secondly, through the medium of the blood-vessels; and thirdly, through the lymphatics. In the first of these the disease produced is peritonitis; the two latter connecting paths lead to pyæmic and septicæmic forms of disease; and these latter pre-eminently are what lead to the simultaneous occurrence of a number of mutually connected diseases of lying-in women—the so-called epidemics of puerperal fever.

The history of puerperal diseases extends back to the very earliest medical literature. It is doubtful, however, how far the older descriptions were identical with what we now call puerperal fever.

At any rate, long before the relations which exist between other forms of peritonitis had been elucidated, it was known that in many cases of puerperal fever the peritoneum became attacked by inflammation.,

The first definite notices of diseases affecting large numbers of lying-in women, in which the peritoneum was involved, are from the pens of French authors in the beginning and middle of the eighteenth century, viz., Delamotte,[1] and afterwards Malouin,[2] who described an epidemic of puerperal fever in the Hôtel-Dieu in Paris during the year 1746. On post-mortem examination the intestines were found coated by a coagulated material, and there was a milky effusion in the abdominal cavity, and sometimes also in the thorax. From the lungs also exuded a milky fluid; the uterus appeared inflamed; and in some cases there was suppuration of the ovaries. Since then the subject of puerperal fever has had an unusually large number of investigators, who generally have devoted themselves to the etiological relations of the general disease. The various opinions on this point have led to sharp controversies, the contending parties arranging themselves, some on the side of contagion, and others on that of miasma, some again on that of local, and others on that of general infection.

If we consider Buhl's three principal forms, based upon the anatomical mode of extension of the process :

1. Puerperal peritonitis without pyæmia;
2. Puerperal pyæmia without peritonitis;
3. Puerperal pyæmia with peritonitis;

we find that hardly any difference of opinion exists as regards the first form. This disease is to be regarded as a purely local inflammation of the peritoneum proceeding from the uterus and its appendages, such as may take place independently of the puerperal state. The questions as to the pyæmic and septicæmic forms assume a more difficult aspect. As, however, in these cases we have to do with pyæmic diseases, peritonitis being at most an important item in the phenomena presented, and as this is not the place to enter into an exhaustive discussion on these subjects, we can only cursorily touch upon them. Peritonitis is

---

[1] Traité compl. des accouch. Leyden. 1729.

[2] Hist des malad. épid. de 1746, obs. à Paris. Mém. de l'acad. royale des sciences de l'an. 1746. Amsterdam. 1755.

given this prominent importance in Buhl's third class, while his
second comprises those cases which, by means of metrophlebitis
and thrombosis of the spermatic veins, etc., lead to general embolic pyæmia by the breaking down of the thrombi.   Peritonitis is
not necessarily associated with this form.

As far as clinical observation is concerned, the distinction between these anatomical divisions is not always so evident ; the various forms may be combined ;
and partly from this cause arose the numerous attempts to lay down a useful and
comprehensive scheme from a clinical standpoint.   In doing so, however, the anatomical basis ought not to be disregarded.   Spiegelberg has given us a classification
which lays special stress on the inflammatory processes in the neighborhood of the
uterus.

This classification is the following :

1. Inflammation of the genital mucous membrane : endocolpitis and endometritis.
      a. Superficial.
      b. Ulcerative (diphtheritic).
2. Inflammation of the serous membrane of the uterus and its appendages :
   pelvic peritonitis and peritonitis diffusa traumatica.
3. Inflammation of the parenchyma of the uterus, of the subserous tissue,
   and the pelvic areolar tissue : metritis and parametritis.
      a. Exudative, circumscribed.
      b. Phlegmonous diffuse, with lymphangitis and pyæmia : peritonitis
      lymphatica.
4. Phlebothrombosis and phlebitis uterina and parauterina : embolic
   pyæmia.
5. Simple septicæmia : putrid absorption.

Another classification is the following, by Hugenberger :

A. Puerperal inflammatory conditions of the genital organs.
   1. Ulceratio puerperalis vulvæ, vaginæ et orificii colli.
   2. Colpitis and endometritis levior or catarrhalis.
   3. Perimetritis and peritonitis puerperalis.
         a. Levior or subacuta.
         b. Gravior or acuta and acutissima.
   4. Phlegmone puerperalis.
         a. Metritis, parametritis, and phlegmone pelvis levior.
         b. Colpitis, endometritis diphtheritica, parametritis, phlegmone abdo-
         minis diffusa gravior.
B. Puerperal venous thrombosis.
   1. Metrophlebothrombosis.
   2. Phlebitis cruralis.
C. Puerperal ichorrhæmia and septicæmia.

Metroperitonitis—Peritonitis without Pyæmia.

As the circumscribed inflammatory processes in the areolar tissue of the pelvis and in the serous appendages of the uterus, viz., parametritis and perimetritis, as well as the relation they bear to diffuse peritonitis, have been discussed in the Tenth Volume of this Cyclopædia, we have only to consider the diffuse peritonitis which is developed from the uterus in the puerperal state.

This disease is to be regarded as a purely local inflammation of the peritoneum, such as may arise independently of the puerperal state. The intra-uterine process extends through the Fallopian tubes to the peritoneum, just as it does in the case of menstrual peritonitis, as was first observed by Foerster ; or else an originally circumscribed peritonitis (perimetritis) spreads into a diffuse inflammation.

The traumatic element arising during delivery is of immediate importance in the production of this form, which occurs most frequently as isolated cases, having no connection one with another—thus unlike puerperal pyæmia, which generally attacks a number of parturient women at the same time, in lying-in institutions.

Anatomically, this form is characterized by the symptoms of peritonitis. The abdomen is, as a rule, markedly distended ; the effusion is fibrinous or fibrino-purulent, with the abdominal organs matted together in many places.[1] The effusion is apt to be copious in the true pelvis, particularly in Douglas's space, and the uterus and Fallopian tubes are completely invested by it. In the openings of the Fallopian tubes a purulent secretion may exist ; their lumen is widened, and their tissue loose and injected. In the uterus there is evidence of endometritis ; but we do not find either venous thrombosis or lymphangitis.

The effusion may be encysted, particularly if the disease runs a chronic course, or if the inflammation was originally circumscribed.

Symptoms and Course.—While puerperal oöphoritis and sal-

---

[1] For the analysis of an effusion of the kind, see *Kiwisch*, l. c. I. p. 77.

pingitis do not give rise to peritonitis for some time after delivery, metroperitonitis generally develops itself within from three to five days. It frequently begins with a single rigor, or with the less striking initial symptoms of pelvic peritonitis, which may extend more or less quickly. Corresponding with this, the course of the disease assumes various aspects, and we may distinguish a peritonitis acutissima from cases which run a more chronic course.

The symptoms of metroperitonitis differ but little from those of ordinary peritonitis. The abdomen becomes quickly distended, the softness due to the relaxed condition of the abdominal parietes after delivery is lost, and the abdominal wall becomes like a drum ; it is exceptional for the distention to be confined to the large intestine. In the very acute course of the disease the tenderness rapidly extends from the uterus over the entire abdomen. In the gradual extension of a perimetritis the tenderness of the uterus may be primarily very insignificant, so as only to be discoverable on firm pressure.

It is worthy of note that profuse diarrhœa occurs with great regularity in the course of metroperitonitis ; the occurrence of the diarrhœa has been rightly connected with the fact that in this form of peritonitis post-mortem examination very uniformly reveals the evidence of severe intestinal catarrh (Rokitansky). Obstinate constipation occurs now and then, and may even induce ileus.

As a rule, the general aspect of the patient is serious in the extreme ; there is great anxiety, a feeling of intense illness, and great prostration, and collapse sets in rapidly. The sensorium is but seldom affected. Headache is generally present. The fever is always very considerable in cases which begin acutely, the temperature in the initial rigor reaching 40-41 C., and even higher, and then it either remains continuously high or presents those irregular ups and downs which are observed in other forms of peritonitis. The pulse, as in other forms of peritonitis, is greatly quickened—120 to 130 beats per minute being the rule— and with the increase in the symptoms it becomes still more frequent, reaching 150. A decrease in the frequency of the pulse may be regarded as a favorable prognostic symptom.

On the occurrence of changes on the inner surface of the uterus, the character of the lochia becomes altered, and, in cases of excessive effusion into the abdomen, the secretion becomes scanty or ceases altogether.

A peculiar complication in these cases is a condition of the skin which, especially in lying-in institutions, is a frequent accompaniment of puerperal diseases. This condition consists in a transient erythema, often of considerable extent,—rarely in erysipelas. These inflammatory conditions of the skin have been described by English authors under the title of puerperal scarlatina.

In the more chronic course of the disease the phenomena primarily are those of circumscribed peritonitis with slight tenderness, considerable fever, and without excessive distention of the abdomen. These symptoms spread gradually and increase in intensity. This last mode of occurrence of the disease is especially apt to lead to the effusion becoming encysted, and to peritoneal and pelvic abscesses, with a protracted course of resulting illness.

The *course* of acute metroperitonitis is, as a rule, virulent; and if we regard those cases collectively in which a fibrino-purulent effusion occurs, we find that the issue is exceedingly unfavorable. If recovery be the result, it occurs by absorption, and by the effusion becoming encapsuled, together with all the consequences of this process. Further, the involution of the uterus takes place slowly, and there remains a tendency to sequelæ.

If the effusion be slight (fibrinous), and the course not virulent, recovery, more or less complete, occurs rather frequently, so that the cases of metroperitonitis, taken as a whole, show, when compared with other forms of peritonitis, a favorable death-rate.

With reference to the *treatment* of metroperitonitis, we have but little to add to the general principle laid down in connection with acute peritonitis.

Locally, the most careful cleanliness is required, so as to prevent the occurrence of bed-sores.

As regards the antiphlogistic remedies at our disposal, all agree that for this form of inflammation general bloodletting is to be discarded, and that the local form by means of leeches tends only to relieve the subjective condition of the patient, and hence ought only to be used cautiously (from ten to fifteen leeches). Mercury has always had its advocates in this particular form of peritonitis, and in point of fact many observations are confirmatory of its beneficial use (Kehrer). Whether, however, the favorable results are to be unconditionally ascribed to the influence of the mercurial treatment is certainly very doubtful; but new investigations on this point are being undertaken every day. Large doses of calomel, and inunction with mercurial ointment (the latter upon the abdomen and thigh) are the best modes of administering the remedy.

The use of cathartics must be regarded as dangerous and irrational in the treatment of peritonitis in general. In the treatment of puerperal peritonitis, on the contrary, drastic cathartics have been praised as exceedingly useful by much respected observers (Seiffert, Breslau, and others). It cannot be denied that interference of this kind is more authorized in puerperal peritonitis than in any other form of the disease. If the connection between inflammation of the peritoneum and the processes in the uterus in certain cases is once clear, we are no longer in danger of doing harm owing to a doubtful diagnosis. Hence the accumulation of the intestinal contents during pregnancy may require that energetic means should be taken to remove it. The intestinal catarrh which occurs is intensified by the stasis and decomposition of the contents. From this point of view it appears exceedingly important to clear out the intestine in those cases in which there is considerable accumulation, and this is best done by a few large doses of calomel. The other advantages which have been ascribed to an extended course of purging do not appear to have been definitely proved, nor to justify the consequences which this treatment may entail. One such consequence is that after the use of drastic purgatives a profuse diarrhœa not unfrequently spontaneously sets in, which may induce collapse.

The use of opium and morphia in the treatment of the symptoms is perhaps less useful in this than in other forms of peritonitis, but still in many aspects it is very valuable. In cases of profuse diarrhœa especially we may administer opium in the form of enemata, in combination with tannin and starch.

It is unnecessary to mention specially that the application of cold is exceedingly useful in the puerperal form of peritonitis; the ice-bladder and cold compresses are generally very well borne.

As regards the use of oil of turpentine, which has been recommended in various quarters, I have no personal experience.

Many considerations are opposed to the similarly recommended painting of the abdomen with collodion, more especially the excoriations and ulcerations of the skin which result from it.

Peritonitis Lymphatica. Pyæmia with Peritonitis.

In peritonitis lymphatica also we are in all probability concerned with a primarily local process, the act of delivery being the actual starting-point. From this the process extends, as may be traced anatomically, through the lymphatics, which convey the material they take up to the blood, and on their way excite inflammatory processes in the large lymph-spaces, more particularly the peritoneum.

This form of puerperal fever constitutes the greatest proportion of the cases in puerperal epidemics; it occurs, however, also, as indeed every form of puerperal fever may, spontaneously in sporadic cases. Further, it is not connected as anything specific with delivery, for the same process may result independently of the puerperal state from injuries to the female genital organs, for example, from operative interference (Buhl, Virchow, and others).

The majority of the puerperal epidemics which have been observed had their origin in lying-in institutions; and hence the fact of a number of lying-in women being collected in an institution of the kind must have something to do in increasing the tendency to puerperal disease, but not in producing anything specific, as is proved by the occurrence of spontaneous sporadic cases, and by the doubtless rarer occurrence of epidemics independently of lying-in institutions.

If the first statement, that there is always a primarily local process—a local infection due to the puerperal trauma—were incontestably established, our knowledge as to the mode of occurrence of puerperal fever would be placed on a very broad basis. The facts adduced may be readily brought up in support of this first statement, and shown to tally with the view which would place the essence of puerperal fever within narrow limits, and thus point to a definite end to be attained by future investigation.

But opposed to this view is another and older one, according to which, in all these puerperal diseases, there is primarily a general infection of the blood, which is the origin of the various local phenomena.

The defenders of the theory of a primary infection of the blood rely most prominently upon the fact of illness manifesting itself in puerperal women by febrile symptoms before the occurrence of any discoverable local lesion, even before and during delivery. Further, puerperal epidemics are said to become developed in places and districts, to explain which it is necessary to have recourse to the influence of miasmata. It would be difficult to refute these views altogether, but still many objections may be urged against them.

On going into the question further, it is important to observe that those groups of cases which occur outside lying-in institutions may sometimes be traced directly to a medical man or a nurse, who may have been the means of bringing the infection from a primary case or from a hospital. Instances are known in which the occurrence of the disease was strictly confined to the practice of one individual medical man or nurse. The morbific poison, therefore, is capable of being conveyed from place to place.

In the case of every disease which may be traced to the reception of an infectious material into the body old-established custom requires in each case an answer to the question as to whether the extension takes place through contagion or through miasma. The investigation in the case of puerperal fever has often the same requirement imposed upon it. As, however, the views only contain a part of the possible ways in which the disease may originate and extend, we are often enough forced by facts to a compromise, and are obliged to accept a miasmatico-contagious origin for the disease. So also in the case of puerperal fever.

If we put the question in this way, whether morbific poison may be actually developed and may proliferate within the person of the individual, we must, with the facts we have before us, answer in the affirmative.[1] On the other hand, it is not likely

---

[1] We cannot altogether discard the possibility that a parturient woman may beget the infectious material without becoming herself infected with puerperal disease, whereas others may take the infection from her, and develop the most severe forms of it.

that a similar materia peccans originates, and becomes developed externally to the human body, in the atmosphere and in rooms. We cannot here enter into a full discussion on the subject, but if we only observe the manner in which such epidemics arise, and the narrow circle in which all subsequent cases of the disease group themselves around the first case, we shall be unable to support the idea of an atmospheric origin for the infectious material.

Any conclusion like this, which has merely probability in its favor, in no way entails as a necessary consequence that the disease can only be communicated by personal agency, through the medium of the attendants and their utensils. This mode of communication is certain, but there are also facts which tend to prove an extension by means of other media, namely, the atmosphere. The very circumstance that the phenomena of the disease are often sharply defined, and are found to be confined to particular wards, while physicians and nurses do their duties throughout the entire house, supports this view, and is opposed to the teaching of Semmelweiss in its too strict limitation. Further, the puerperal diseases of newly born children ought not to be ignored, and these cannot be easily explained in any other way.

According to this idea, the more frequent occurrence of puerperal diseases in lying-in institutions, as compared with the general experience in private practice, does not altogether result from the increased tendency to communicate the disease through the medium of those who examine and attend the cases. Pyæmia in surgical stations also is not always communicated by the hands of the dressers,—washing the hands in carbolic acid does not put a stop to its spread. We may press the comparison between a surgical station and a lying-in institution still further without danger of any great mistake. In both cases the primary condition—the wound—may in itself be bad ; in the parturient woman, for example, a labor with great tearing and bruising, together with loss of blood, perhaps the previous occurrence of depression or the existence at the time of some disease (fever), may produce an unhealthy and infecting condition of wound. In addition to this, however, there is a hospital influence, and a good wound is in danger of infection, owing to the possibility that a bad one may communicate its deleterious, infectious material through the atmosphere.

The effects of an unhealthy state of the puerperal wound—diphtheritis—together with the putrid changes that are associated with it—are, owing to the local conditions, pernicious to a degree which is hardly met with in any other form of injury. The soft uterus just emptied of its contents, with its dilated veins and lymph-vessels, and its close proximity to the peritoneum, is the source of this specially great danger (Spiegelberg).

Peritonitis lymphatica is therefore probably to be regarded as an accidental disease of a wound—a pyæmic disease,—in which the septic matter is first taken up by the lymphatic vessels, and conveyed onward by them. On the blood taking up the putrid material from the lymph-vessels, there arises a general infection—an actual septicæmia.

A number of facts bear out the view that peritonitis lymphatica occurs as the result of absorption of the products of decomposition,—that it is the result of putrid infection.

Septic plugs do not readily pass from the lymph-vessels into the current of the blood, although fluid putrid effusion may, possibly on account of the low pressure under which the lymph moves. The principal and most obvious results are for the most part local, namely, the septic peritonitis and pleuritis, and the diffuse pelvic cellulitis.

The opinion has been repeatedly advanced, that the infection of the puerperal wound is due to the presence of lower organisms, and practically we are compelled in our conclusions to have recourse to such an hypothesis. The actual conditions observed authorize this view in so far that on the inner surface of the uterus, in the contents of the lymph-vessels, in the effusion, and in the pus-corpuscles bacteria abound in great quantities—the contents of the lymph-vessels consisting of pus and bacteria (Waldeyer).

But it still remains doubtful what exact rôle ought to be ascribed to these organisms; whether, owing to their enormous development, organic material becomes changed into poisonous compounds, or whether they are only to be regarded as the evidences of processes of decomposition, in that they thereby find a sphere for their existence, or lastly, whether their presence be necessary for the occurrence of septic processes, etc. All these questions delay the solution of the general inquiry.

Pathological Anatomy.[1]—The condition found in the genital

---

[1] See in particular *Buhl*, loc. cit.

canal and the neighboring tissues is generally the following:
We find on the inner surface of the uterus a brownish red or
greenish pap of gangrenous odor, and on the spots where there
are lacerations, especially in the cervix, and also in the vagina,
yellow or green diphtheritic ulceration. The uterus is large, its
tissue œdematous and easily broken down; on its surface distinct depressions produced by the superimposed coils of intestine; sometimes it is found engorged with blood, with the characters of rapid decomposition, and frequently in its substance
may be found wedge-shaped diphtheritic sloughs.

A very characteristic form is assumed by the changes which
take place in the areolar tissue of the pelvis, and in the appendages of the uterus, which during pregnancy had taken a part in
the general hyperplasia, and are traversed by dilated lymph-vessels. These abnormal conditions in the parametrium are described by various authors under different names, which, however,
all mean the same thing: for example, phlegmon of the pelvis
(Erichsen), parametritis phlegmonosa (Virchow), and purulent
œdema (Pirogoff [1]). We see in the subperitoneal connective tissue varicose, dilated, beaded lymph-vessels with yellow, friable,
or purulent contents — lymph-thrombosis, metrolymphangitis.
The connective tissue presents a jelly-like appearance. These
lymph-vessels, filled with pus, may be traced for a considerable
distance from the uterus into the retroperitoneal connective tissues; they are then lost, and the only indication of the process
remaining is the turbidly serous, fat-like infiltration of the connective tissue. Lymph-vessels filled with pus may sometimes
be traced from organs covered by peritoneum into the mesentery, as, for example, from the ovaries. The lymph-glands
lying in their course are swollen and sometimes contain masses
of pus.

The fluid of the parenchyma of the uterus, the broken-down
lymph-thrombi, are rich in granular masses; they consist partly
of bacteria, which are also found in masses in the pus-corpuscles,
and similarly in the effusion, in the serous cavities, and on the
pericardium.

---

[1] *Spiegelberg,* loc. cit.

The effusion into the peritoneal sac varies not only in quantity, but in character; it may be fibrino-purulent with matting together of the intestines and with but little fluid, or it may be of an unhealthy, discolored character, or even hemorrhagic, with a few flakes of lymph and no adhesions. The pelvic organs are sometimes actually covered up in masses of effusion. We seldom find pus in the Fallopian tubes, but their free extremities are reddened and covered with effusion.

The intestines are, as a rule, markedly distended with flatus, their walls œdematous, the mucous membrane in a state of catarrh, with the epithelium falling off, or with actual diphtheritic changes.

The spleen is enlarged, its tissue friable, the Malpighian corpuscles enlarged.

The liver is either of a large size and injected with blood, or, more frequently, reduced in size, pale, of a yellow color, and its parenchyma readily broken down. Microscopically, we find the characters of fatty degeneration and an increased amount of pigment, with which the general icteric hue of the body coincides. These changes in the liver are, according to Buhl, to be regarded as stages of acute atrophy, and are connected locally with the lymphangitis as well as with the general infection, owing to the imbibition of putrid material.

The degenerative changes in the muscular tissue of the heart, and in certain other muscles, seem indicative of the occurrence of a general infection; on the other hand, pyæmic abscesses exist only as the result of ulcerative endocarditis. Next to the peritoneum, the pleura is most frequently affected, as a result of lymphatic infection; the lungs also may be attacked by the same process—lymphangitic interlobular pneumonia of Buhl. Inflammation of the pericardium is of rarer occurrence.

Symptoms.—The disease begins, as a rule, soon after delivery, seldom later than the fifth or sixth day, and, according to Kiwisch, a woman who continues well during the first ten to fourteen days after delivery is safe from an attack of puerperal fever. The invasion is often indicated by a rigor, but this symptom may be absent. On the occurrence of the rigor the temperature in the axilla rises to 40–41 C. (104°–105.8° Fahr.), and then continues constantly high, with irregular remissions; the fever is subject to several kinds of variations, according to the intensity of the disease and the nature of the complications.

In its further course, the general aspect of peritonitis lymphatica assumes at once a characteristic form which has little in common with simple peritonitis, and which is due to the prominence which the symptoms of general infection and septicæmia assume.

With the rise in temperature, the pulse becomes considerably quickened—120 to 150 beats per minute, with but slight fluctuations, being generally met with; the character is moreover weak, the wave low and compressible, and the artery but imperfectly filled. The elevation of the temperature does not pursue at all a similar course to that of the pulse,—the temperature may fall, but the frequency of the pulse increases.

In the abdomen distention soon sets in; meteorism is a very constant symptom, and may attain to a very excessive degree. Nevertheless the patient complains but little of pain, the abdomen may be quite free from pain, and there is often complete tolerance, even of firm pressure. The absence of tenderness, the occurrence of which is so characteristic of peritonitis, is remarkable, and is pathognomonic of this form of the disease. Inflammation of the peritoneum and effusion occur invariably, and hence some cause must exist why the pain is not felt. Conduction and perception of painful excitations must be regarded as intact in the majority of cases, and hence we must conclude that a rapid destruction of the excitability of the nerve-terminations in the peritoneum takes place. The very great tendency to breaking down of the serous membrane may perhaps suggest the explanation of this phenomenon.

The effusion is not always, although very frequently, so considerable as to allow of its being diagnosed during life.

The uterus is always found to be large and not properly involuted. The lochia often assume a bad smell, and under certain circumstances we find diphtheritic ulceration in the vagina.

Vomiting is a constant symptom, and considerable quantities of green material are brought up. Diarrhœa is apt to make its appearance early, sometimes accompanied by tenesmus and pain in the abdomen ; sometimes the diarrhœa reaches such a pitch that a continuous involuntary evacuation takes place. The stools present a varied character : they may be dark, bilious, intensely stinking, or they may be watery, mucous, or like beaten-up eggs, rarely containing blood, and rarely also shreds and false membranes. Anatomically, conditions are found in the intestinal mucous membrane corresponding to various stages of intensity in the diarrhœa.

The tongue is frequently moist and seldom much coated ; the thirst is considerable, and the desire for nourishment greatly diminished.

Respiration is uniformly quickened as a consequence of the diminished space of the thorax from the pressure of the flatulent intestines, and also owing to the weakened state of the circulation. If effusion takes place simultaneously into the pleural cavities or pericardium, the breathing will become still more difficult. In this case patients suffer considerably from the "besoin de respirer."

The state of consciousness varies considerably. Delirium may be present, with a character varying from excitement to maniacal fury ; as a rule, however, consciousness remains clear up to the last moment of the patient's life. The head is somewhat affected ; patients complain of giddiness, of over-sensitiveness, and of sleeplessness. The absence of any subjective feeling of illness which exists in the case of many patients is remarkable and in striking contrast to their actual condition. They hardly ever complain of anything beyond great weakness and the difficulty of respiration. Sometimes, doubtless, this is due to a state of apathy, with indifference to all impressions, and a tendency to frequent light slumbers.

The general impression which patients convey is tha of intense weakness with great prostration ; the countenance is drawn, the face is of a sallow hue, the voice is altered, and the speech indistinct, the eyes have a weary look, the pupils are not unfrequently dilated (Litzmann), the face and the extremities are cold, and are covered with a clammy sweat, the skin of the trunk also perspires freely. Sometimes epistaxis is observed (Hecker).

The skin is not unfrequently the seat of inflammation ; we

meet with simple erythema, erysipelas, and even extensive phleg-mon. A further change has been described as hemorrhagic imbibition in the neighborhood of the cutaneous veins.

The lymphatic glands in the inguinal region are sometimes found enlarged ; the secretion of milk, as a rule, ceases, and the breasts become wrinkled and soft.

Course, Results, Prognosis.—The disease runs a course of great rapidity, unchecked, to a fatal issue ; and it is highly ques-tionable whether recovery be actually possible or not. Death may occur within the first twenty-four hours, and in the majority of cases it results within the first six or eight days.

In a hospital epidemic observed by Hecker, twenty-eight[1] women took ill with peritonitis lymphatica, all of whom died.

2 on the	1st	day of illness.	
4 "	2d	"	"
3 "	3d	"	"
5 "	4th	"	"
2 "	5th	"	"
3 "	6th	"	"
4 "	7th	"	"
2 "	8th	"	"
2 "	9th	"	"
1 "	11th	"	"

Death takes place either quite quietly, with increasing debil-ity and insufficient respiration and circulation, or in a more violent manner, with the supervention of convulsions. As the end draws nigh the vomiting ceases, fæces are passed involun-tarily, subsultus tendinum sets in, and the patient picks at the bed-clothes.

An absolutely fatal prognosis must, therefore, be made. The treatment of peritonitis lymphatica is of course somewhat pur-poseless, still it is possible to discover indications on which rational treatment may be based.

The perniciousness of this puerperal disease obviously con-sists in the inflammation of the serous membranes, especially the peritoneum, and in the septic infection of the blood ; hence we must treat the peritonitis on general principles, symptomatically,

---

Hecker, l. c. I. Bd.

and, as a means of combating the general septic infection, have
recourse to the various antiseptics—salicylic acid being the
favorite latterly,—in both cases doubtless with but slight prospect of success.

If we look more closely at the phenomena which the disease
presents, we shall find that, amongst the more serious and dangerous symptoms, that of weakness of the heart, in connection
with degenerative processes in other organs, stands prominently
forth. The application of those remedies which are adapted to
combat collapse, and in particular the weakness of the heart,
appear to be strenuously demanded, among which may be
mentioned wine, ether, camphor, and musk. The weight of the
fever tends to act as an incentive to the degenerative processes,
and the influence of a strenuous antipyretic treatment must, *a
priori*, be regarded as useful, although too much is not to be
expected from it. We must, therefore, reduce the temperature
of these patients by means of cold baths and the application
of the ice-bladder, and combat the high temperature and rapid
pulse by means of large doses of quinine.

Other empirical remedies have been repeatedly tried, but I do
not believe that an incontestable result can be ascribed to the
action of any.

Sanitary measures for preventing the spread of puerperal infection offer a wide field for activity, and are capable of application in the construction of lying-in institutions in an especial
degree. The principal point required, theoretically, is to take
care that institutions of this kind shall be as airy as possible,
that there shall be no overcrowding of the individual wards or of
the entire house, and that the most scrupulous cleanliness shall
prevail, the practical realization of which devolves upon technical and special art.

By merely reasoning as to the mode of origin of infection, we
deduce as a necessary conclusion that the utmost care in the
management of delivery, and the most stringent measures for
avoiding the ways and means by which the disease is propagated,
are essential.

c. Infantile Peritonitis.

Gregory, Med.-chirurg. Trans. XI. 258.—*Billard*, Malad. des enf.—*Dugès*, Dict. en XV. XII. 587.—*Romberg*, Caspar's Wochenschr. 1833. 329.—*Simpson*, Edinb. Med. and Surg. Journ. Oct. 1838.—*Rilliet* u. *Barthez*, Handbuch d. Kinderkrankh. übers. Leipzig. 1855.—*Thore*, Arch. gén.. Août. 1846.—*Heyfelder*, Stud. im Gebiete der Heilwissensch. Bd. II. S. 190.—*Duparcque*, Annales d'obstetr. Bd. I.—*F. Weber*, Beitr. z. path. Anatomie der Neugeb. Kiel. 1851. III. S. 59.—*Bednar*, Krankheiten der Neugeb. Wien. 1850.—*W. A. Hunt*, Fœtal Peritonitis. Trans. of the Obst. Soc. IX. p. 15.—*Dohrn*, Zwei Beobachtungen von Stenose des Darmes und fötaler Perit. Jahrb. für Kinderheilk. 1868. S. 216.—*Lange*, Perit. mit Periorchitis bei einem 3 Woch. alten Knaben. Berl. klin. Wochenschr. 1871. 7.—*C. Gerhardt*, Lehrb. der Kinderkrankh. 1871.—Consult also the text-books on Diseases of Children.

Pathogenesis and Etiology.—Peritonitis occurs even during intra-uterine life, and must be regarded as a frequent cause of the death of the fœtus. The first observations on the subject were made by Sir James Simpson. The disease appears frequently to arise during the latter months of fœtal life, and in some cases is to be referred to syphilis; it may, however, be associated with other abdominal affections, and Breslau has even observed intra-uterine perforative peritonitis. In other cases the cause of its occurrence is not cleared up.

Peritonitis occurs with comparative frequency shortly after birth, processes in the umbilicus—for example, gangrene and inflammation of the umbilical vessels, as well as umbilical hernia —especially tending to produce this frequent occurrence. Under the influence of puerperal infection, newly born children may become affected with peritonitis lymphatica by a lymphangitis being set up from the umbilicus, in a manner analogous to that which obtains in the case of the uterus of the mother. The subserous connective tissue on both sides of the umbilicus, as far as the vertebræ, as well as that in the mesentery and in Glisson's capsule, is found in a state of turbidly serous infiltration. This form of peritonitis occurs more especially in lying-in institutions, contemporaneously with an epidemic among the women. This, however, is but one form of disease which puerperal infection may produce in newly born children.

In the subsequent periods of child-life, inflammation of the peritoneum is much more rarely met with than in infancy,[1] and even more rarely than in adults. The causes of its occurrence are found to correspond more closely with those met with in the case of adults, the older the child is. The idiopathic form is certainly very rare ; in the generality of cases the disease is secondary. General infection plays an important part as an exciting cause, as, for example, pyæmia, scarlatina, and small-pox. Bednar has repeatedly observed that within from two to thirteen days after vaccination peritonitis supervened ; then also diseased conditions of the intestines, as invagination and incarceration, diseases of the liver and of the mesenteric glands. Peritonitis has also been observed to arise from the testicle, in cases of incomplete descent. Amongst traumatic causes may be mentioned the rough use of the enema syringe.

Symptoms.—In some cases in which peritonitis intrauterina was discovered as cause of the death of the fœtus, an unusual increase in the movements of the child and then their sudden cessation had been observed. This is not, however, uniformly the case. Sometimes the child comes into the world alive in a state of the most extreme marasmus, possibly with an intensely distended, painful abdomen, with œdema of the lower limbs, and with jaundice—symptoms which immediately suggest a diseased condition of the peritoneum. Frequently peritonitis is not discovered until the post-mortem examination reveals it. In cases where the children are born alive, death speedily ensues.

Many cases of congenital intestinal stenosis are dependent on a fœtal peritonitis, and thus may leave ascites behind it (Virchow).

Dohrn has described a case of the kind. A child, eight days old, had died of recent peritonitis; adhesions occurring in utero had obstructed the escape of the meconium.

The clinical phenomena of peritonitis in the child present some deviations from those usually met with in peritonitis of the adult.

---

[1] In 186 cases of peritonitis in children which Bednar observed, 102 occurred within the first fortnight, 63 in the third and fourth weeks; 15 children were over a month old, 4 over two months, 1 over four months, and 1 over five months.

The commencement of peritonitis is more or less distinctly marked, according as the pain from the outset is distributed over the entire abdomen, or primarily occurs only at a circumscribed spot. Pain, however, constitutes one of the most constant symptoms, and is never absent or uncharacteristic, except in the case of children but a few days old. The gentlest pressure increases the tenderness, which the child indicates, as a rule, by a short interrupted cry or a doleful whine. A continuous loud cry is prevented by the increase in pain caused by the contraction of the abdominal muscles.

The abdomen, as a rule, is early distended with flatus, and tightly stretched, especially in the epigastric region, and sometimes we see blue, dilated veins faintly showing through the abdominal parietes. In the last stage of the disease the tenseness of the abdomen gradually decreases. In some instances we may recognize externally the tumor formed by individual knuckles of intestine.

As the quantity of the fluid effusion in the abdomen is often very inconsiderable, it is frequently difficult to discover it even when we place the children on their side. We may further attempt to demonstrate the existence of free fluid by having the children held with their back upward and percussing the umbilical region, which thus becomes the most dependent point of the abdomen. In excessive effusion in the case of newly born children, some of it may descend into the still patent sac of the tunica vaginalis testis, and may even, in this way, rupture outward.

The tenderness in the abdomen causes the patients to remain quiet and motionless, generally lying on their back, with their legs either extended or else flexed and crossed. The expression of the face indicates pain, but otherwise is not specially characteristic, and soon shows signs of collapse.

The fever runs a different course in various cases ; in general, the temperature is considerably raised in the beginning, and falls to the temperature of collapse in the subsequent course of the disease. The prominences feel cold. Active sweating is rare. The pulse is uniformly very much quickened, varying from 150 to 200 beats, and even to uncountable frequency.

The color of the skin is, as a rule, dirty yellow, and becomes in the last stage cyanotic; more intense jaundice also is by no means uncommon.

The respiration assumes the costal type, with fixing of the diaphragm, and lessening of the movements; in other words, the inspirations are short. Corresponding to this, the number of the respirations increases up to 30–60. Rilliet and Barthez only observed considerable changes in respiration where there were complications of the thoracic organs.

Vomiting does not occur with the uniformity which characterizes the peritonitis of adults; and even in older children it would appear from the observations of Rilliet and Barthez to be often absent. In those cases in which this symptom is present the vomited material consists in the remains of food, and in a mucous or green mass; stercoraceous vomiting has also been observed without any mechanical intestinal obstruction.

Infants, at the very beginning of the disease, reject the breast, as the act of sucking increases the pain in the abdomen.

The evacuations also present a somewhat different character from that which is the rule in adult life. A watery diarrhœa is more frequent than constipation.

The urine is scanty and is voided with pain; frequently also complete retention exists.

Sleep is always affected, delirium is rather rare, and still rarer are general convulsions. Further, Bednar gives as rare nervous symptoms tremulousness in the eyes, which either converge or are turned to one side, and a jerking of the abdominal muscles in the beginning of the disease.

Apart from those abnormal conditions which depend either directly upon the peritonitis or upon one common cause, as in the case of general diseases, there are but few complications.

The disease may assume a very rapid course, and within twenty-four hours terminate in death. This is especially the case in the earlier months of life, in which the disease seldom lasts more than from two to three days. In the later periods of childhood the course is less acute, and children die generally between the fifth and ninth days—cases of perforation excepted. In a few cases, however, a somewhat chronic course has been observed. Peritonitis, whatever the exciting cause may be, is, with but rare exceptions, uniformly fatal; in the case of newly born children the prognosis must be absolutely fatal.

The *diagnosis* rests principally upon the distention and tenderness on pressure of the abdomen, taken in connection with fever and quickening of the pulse, upon the evidence of effusion, the quickly supervening collapse, the exciting cause under certain circumstances affording us important assistance. Mistakes may arise with simple tympanites of the intestines, with attacks of colic, with inflammation of the gastro-intestinal mucous membrane, with invagination, and with ascites. As regards the discovery of the cause, what is true in the peritonitis of adults holds good here also.

In the *treatment* absolute rest and restriction in the amount of nourishment are especially important. It stands to reason that the considerations already adduced against considerable depletion are of more weight in the case of children, and amount to absolute contraindication in the case of infants. On the other hand, the application of cold to the abdomen in the early stages of the disease is decidedly useful, and not until later on may they be replaced by warm poultices.

A mercurial treatment in the form of inunction with mercurial ointment and small doses of calomel has been greatly extolled by Duparcque amongst others. There is no serious objection to this proceeding, provided that it be not continued too long, beyond three to four days. Sometimes calomel produces vomiting, and then it must be given up. From the nature of the case, however, we cannot hope for great results from any therapeutic interference.

The same considerations may be adduced in favor of the administration of opium, as in the case of peritonitis in the adult. The doses, however, must be made to suit the age of the patient, and their action should be most carefully watched.

In cases which run a favorable course, warm baths and suitable diet may tend to promote the absorption of the effusion. Operative interference in the case of a purulent effusion has been successfully attempted by Martin.

Chronic Diffuse Peritonitis.

Stray observations on chronic peritonitis—principally referring to the pathological conditions—are to be found in the earlier
literature. Broussais was the first to investigate this disease
more thoroughly. Thereupon followed the works of Scoutetten
and Gendrin, and Andral also has recorded an example of chronic
peritonitis. A good deal of work has been done in connection
with this subject by English authors, amongst whom we may
name Gregory, MacAdam, and E. Thompson. Louis, notwithstanding his valuable work, has brought a certain amount of
confusion into the subject by making the statement that every
case of chronic peritonitis is tubercular. Up to the present day
the effect of the statement has not been altogether eradicated,
and hence the existence of a primarily chronic simple peritonitis
is by some observers entirely called in question.

Toulmouche wrote a paper on chronic peritonitis well worthy
of perusal, in the Gaz. méd., 1842, X., and recently Galvagni
(Rivista clinica di Bologna, 1869) has communicated a comparatively large number of very valuable observations on the subject.

On looking closely into the question it will be found convenient to distinguish several forms of diffuse chronic peritonitis.

1. *A chronic stage supervening on an attack of general acute
peritonitis.* This form is best known, and no special difficulty
is encountered in its elucidation. This issue of acute inflammation is not frequent. An originally circumscribed inflammation also may, by degrees, and in a chronic manner, extend
over the entire peritoneum; encysted masses of effusion most
frequently give rise to this form of slow extension.

When an acute inflammation of the peritoneum passes into a
chronic stage the more virulent phenomena decrease, but the
effusion in the peritoneal cavity persists either in whole or in
part. Sacculations are formed with dense membranes, which
cause considerable opposition to the absorption of the inclosed
effusion, while, on the other hand, there exist continually incentives to new inflammation in the intervening spaces. In this way,
we have a complex form of disease, the symptoms of which are

partly those of existing effusion and its metamorphoses, and partly those of fresh inflammatory irritation, with the occurrence of fresh effusion.

The intense sensibility of the abdomen decreases, without actually disappearing, a dull tenderness remains, together with the feeling of fulness and tightness, and firm pressure and the movements of the body may give rise to sharp pain. In some cases at times the tenderness again increases; attacks of colic also make their appearance, and not rarely are occasioned every time that nourishment is taken. The appetite remains either exceedingly bad, or is very variable. Copious vomiting has doubtless ceased, but now and then the patient again vomits, or each act of taking nourishment may induce vomiting. The meteorism and the tenseness of the abdomen decrease, particularly if the effusion becomes partially absorbed, but the intestines do not return to their normal condition, and the taking of nourishment may be regularly followed by renewed distention. In other cases, if, while absorption ceases, fresh effusion is constantly taking place, the distention of the abdomen may attain to an enormous degree. In connection with the evacuations, also, it is shown that the functions of the intestine have not returned to their normal condition; as a rule, obstinate constipation alternates with profuse diarrhœa, which latter sometimes assumes a dysenteric character.

If large quantities of effusion persist, the daily quantity of urine passed is uniformly very small, but if the effusion comes to be absorbed, great quantities of urine may be passed, and this polyuria may persist for a long time.

The temperature of the body is subject to many variations, apyrexial periods alternate with pyrexial, or there may be regular and considerable evening exacerbations, with a normal temperature in the morning. The pulse remains quick, and sometimes attains a very great frequency.

Respiration remains in the majority of cases normal, but as the wasting and anæmia increase, the call made upon this function lessens.

The abdominal integuments frequently present a peculiar, inflexible character, and often contain dark pigment after a pro-

longed application of poultices (Bamberger). Under certain circumstances more or less considerable fluid may be demonstrated
in the abdomen, seldom freely movable,—as a rule, completely
or partially encysted.

By the continuous falling in of the abdomen in cases where
absorption takes place and there is a decrease in the meteorism,
isolated or even numerous encysted masses become observable
owing to the irregularities which they present. On percussion
these give forth a dull sound; to the hand they present the
characters of more or less uneven tumors, rarely with fluctuation, and around their margin there is a feeling of still greater
resistance than in the tumor itself. In this way the entire abdomen may sound alternately tympanitic and dull. These encysted
effusions are, as a rule, distinguishable from abdominal tumors
by their less sharply defined margin, their lesser resistance, and
their less nodulated surface.

If firm adhesions with the parietal peritoneum exist, it will not
be possible for the two serous surfaces to move on one another at
this spot. This may be recognized, if we press on the parietes in
the neighborhood, by the fact that a fold will be formed at the
point of the adhesion, at some distance, therefore, from the point
where the pressure is applied. Cases of this form of the disease
are, as a rule, unusually protracted; the ever-recurring fever, impaired nutrition, vomiting, and diarrhœa, and finally the effusion
itself, cause a wasting of the body which ultimately reaches a degree of extreme emaciation and anæmia. The effusion and adhesions may produce constricting influences on nerves and vessels,
and hence may arise pain in the lower extremities, œdema, throm-
boses from enfeebled circulation (marantische Thrombosen), and
albuminuria. Patients also may die of pyæmia. On account of
the difficulty of moving, the tendency to bed-sores is very great.

If an opening be established in any direction it may lead to
recovery by getting rid of the pus, but, on the other hand, it is
fraught with new dangers—prolonged wasting, suppuration, the
production of fistulæ and irregular communications, and the
burrowing of the matter. Occasionally attacks of dysentery
may cause death.

In this way the majority of cases of the kind terminate, after a protracted course, fatally. Recovery may take place either by means of thickening and absorption, or by perforation and evacuation of the effusion (outward). Universal adhesions of the abdominal viscera naturally are accompanied by various forms of inconvenience and impaired nutrition, still they may be comparatively well borne, and the danger of constriction and twisting is probably less than in the case of partial adhesions; it is, however, really very hard to understand how the muscular actions of the intestine can be performed.

The following is a good example of a case of protracted peritonitis:

S. K., aged thirty, came into Lindwurm's clinique on the 29th of March, 1872. The patient had had a difficult forceps delivery some years previously, which was followed by an illness of about nine weeks' duration. Subsequently she became tolerably well; menstruation was regular, but the abdomen remained distended and the bowels irregular. For from three to four weeks she has been feeling unwell, has had loss of appetite and cough, and for a few days severe pain in the abdomen. Abdomen is distended and tender, the diaphragm is displaced upward; below the umbilicus a somewhat movable tumor with irregular surface, which on percussion is alternately dull and tympanitic; no fluid in abdomen. Bowels confined.

The tenderness increased, there was repeated vomiting and difficulty in pass-

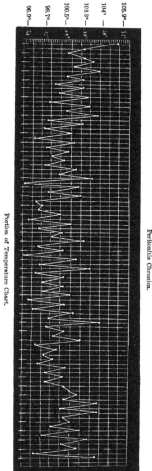

ing water, and the meteorism also increased. The great tenderness of the abdomen decreased again after a few days, without, however, actually disappearing, and with frequent exacerbations. Within the next few days fluid could be demonstrated in the abdomen, and this slowly increased in quantity. The course of the fever during forty-six days may be seen from the accompanying curve; the further course of the disease presented essential differences. The pulse varied between 112 and 136.

There was almost complete loss of appetite, vomiting returned every now and then. The course of the disease was one of continual change; at one time the pain in the abdomen was very severe, and at another very slight; constipation alternated with diarrhœa. By degrees several uneven tumors became discoverable in the lower part of the abdomen.

There was intense emaciation, and anæmia and œdema of the lower extremities. Ultimately an exhausting diarrhœa set in, mixed with blood and exceedingly stinking. Increasing exhaustion, and death on the 23d July, 1872. On post-mortem examination there was found a rather considerable, thinly fluid, purulent effusion in the peritoneal cavity, together with numerous adhesions between the abdominal viscera, partly loose and partly firm, producing tumors and encysted masses. An ovarian cyst about the size of a child's head. In the large intestine evidence of dysentery.

2. *Chronic peritonitis sometimes arises in the course of old-standing ascites,* particularly if this latter be dependent on stasis in the portal vein, and hence, in cases of disease of the liver and heart, and more especially when an atrophic nutmeg-liver is developed as the result of the stasis.

The symptoms which characterize this chronic inflammation are neither very well defined nor severe. Occasional pain in the abdomen, tenderness on pressure, vomiting now and then, impaired nutrition, and meteorism, may be all that is occasioned by the changes set up in the peritoneum. The anatomical changes are not considerable; they consist, as a rule, in thickening of the serous membrane with a slight deposit of fibrin, slight turbidity of the ascitic fluid, and a few flakes of fibrin suspended in it.

As the primary disease itself may frequently present the above-mentioned symptoms, it is evident that in the majority of these cases we are not able to recognize the inflamed condition of the peritoneum. The state of affairs is very different if acute peritonitis supervene in the course of ascites.

The interesting observations of Friedreich have reference also to this. A patient with disease of the heart was tapped sixteen times in the space of a year and a half.

The quantity of fluid removed on the several occasions varied from 3300 to 10700 c.c. It was uniformly of a greenish yellow color, except in the last instance, when it presented a well-marked hemorrhagic character. After each paracentesis an intense tenderness of the abdomen became developed, which was greatly increased on the slightest touch, and which lasted several days.

On post-mortem examination, both visceral and parietal layers of the peritoneum were found covered with a continuous membrane, which exhibited diffuse pigmentation, more intensely marked in some places than in others, and here and there was beset by hemorrhagic spots. This membrane was most fully developed on the anterior aspect of the abdomen, where it consisted of several separable layers, between which numerous larger and smaller tumors were embedded. These latter were of tolerably firm consistence, and on section presented a blackish red color, and proved to be accumulations of coagulated blood between the layers of the newly formed membrane.

Everywhere this pigmented membrane, and also the hemorrhagic nodules situated in it, could, without any special difficulty, be removed, *en masse*, from the subjacent peritoneum, which latter was rather intensely vascularized, but appeared otherwise normal. Nowhere were adhesions found between the intestines, which were covered by this pigmented layer. Of the several layers those which were next to the serous membrane were most fully organized, while those bounding the cavity proved to be the most recent. Hence, the production of new layers proceeded from those already formed. From the most recent layers also resulted the numerous hemorrhages, and these occurred partly into the newly formed membrane, and partly into the fluid effusion.

Friedreich described this form of inflammation as chronic hemorrhagic peritonitis, with the production of hæmatoma.

Etiologically, Friedreich laid great stress upon the tapping and the consequent diminution, in each instance, of the pressure which had previously been exerted upon the abdominal vessels, as causing a determination of blood with its further consequences.[1] A state of things which somewhat resembles that which has just been described, was observed by Baeumler in a case of chronic renal disease, also after repeated tapping. On post-mortem examination, on cutting through the abdominal wall, a sac, filled with purulent effusion, was opened into. The viscera lay entirely behind this sac. The posterior surface of this sac was intensely pigmented.[2]

3. A further group of cases is characterized by the fact that a more or less copious effusion becomes developed in the peritoneal cavity without there being any distinctly marked commencement of the attack. We may describe these cases as *latent*

[1] Ueber eine bes. Form chron. hämorrhag. Peritonitis und über das Hämatom. des Bauchfelles. Virchow's Archiv. Bd. 58.

[2] Chronische pseudomembranöse Peritonitis nach wiederholter Paracentesis abdominis. Virch. Arch. Bd. 59.

general peritonitis. It is, further, peculiar that in many of these cases no primary affection can definitely be made answerable for the occurrence of the effusion. Finally, the effusion itself is, in the majority of cases, completely serous, and approaches in its nature ascitic fluid; it very rarely possesses a purulent character. I have twice, however, seen, in the convalescent stage of fever, considerable purulent effusion take place exceedingly slowly, and run a chronic course, in which there was no distinct distress except in connection with the distention of the abdomen. In many cases the disease corresponds with the idiopathic dropsy of the older writers.[1]

This form of chronic peritonitis is so very rare that even its existence has been called in question, or even altogether denied, by most experienced medical men.

The following case, from Lindwurm's clinique, may be taken as an example:

A woman, aged thirty-three, had observed an increasing distention of the abdomen for about three months; pain was sometimes present, but was slight; she, however, complained greatly of the fulness and tenseness of the abdomen. Sometimes there was obstinate constipation, sometimes diarrhœa, rarely vomiting. Menstruation has ceased latterly. No fever; abdomen uniformly distended, with a considerable quantity of very movable fluid; slight tenderness on pressure. Nothing abnormal in the thoracic organs and liver, beyond their displacement. Uterus placed low, the vaginal portion swollen. On examination through the rectum, a stricture of firm consistence was met with, but the sensation conveyed to the finger was not that which is apt to exist in cancer. No symptoms of consumption, no elevation of temperature. After a short stay in hospital, the patient took small-pox, from a patient who had been in the house for some time, and quickly died. On post-mortem examination, there was found a great quantity of rather clear serum in the abdominal cavity; the liver presented numerous abnormal adhesions (there was no compression of the portal vein); the gall-bladder was firmly adherent by its under surface to the intestines; it was uniformly hypertrophied, and contained two gall-stones. The liver presented a furrow, the result of tight lacing. The intestines were greatly distended with flatus, and on their surface were numerous small connective-tissue appendages, especially in the case of the stomach. Intense catarrh of the stomach; a cicatrix, and consequent stricture of considerable extent, in the rectum; otherwise no considerable abnormity throughout the body.

---

[1] The existence of idiopathic dropsy is uniformly maintained by some, but I believe we ought to describe such cases as chronic peritonitis.

As already mentioned, the etiological conditions remain in many cases undiscovered. Galvagni, whose work is based on twelve cases, regards wetting and catching cold a frequent mode of occurrence of peritonitis, particularly of this serous, latent form.

The symptoms which are present in the beginning of the disease are, as a rule, very trivial ; anything the patient complains of is general and undefined. Dull pains occur in the abdomen, which are increased on pressure and on bending the body. The patient's general health is out of order ; he feels tired, and his appetite is bad. Going upstairs, especially, is frequently the source of an unpleasant sensation in the abdomen. Months may intervene between these primary, scarcely heeded symptoms and the complete development of the disease ; in other cases this stage, which Galvagni describes as prodromal, is shorter. We may consider the disease as fully developed from the time when effusion into the abdomen becomes evident.

The quantity of fluid effused may be limited to a small amount ; it may, however, also be such as to produce the greatest amount of distention and stretching of which the abdomen is capable.

Even in this stage of the disease the phenomena are in no way very urgent, and are such as might, for the most part, be quite as fully produced in simple mechanical ascites. The symptom which in other forms is the most important indication of an inflammatory irritation of the abdominal serous membrane, namely, the tenderness on pressure, is in many cases present to a greater or lesser degree, but by no means unexceptionally so. If we consider the excessive tenderness of the abdomen in acute peritonitis, there is something remarkable in the insignificance of the pain in many, and the complete absence of it in some few cases of chronic peritonitis. The temperature is often found to be quite normal ; in other cases there occur evening exacerbations of a moderate degree. The pulse, on the other hand, is almost always quickened. Increased frequency of respiration, and, under certain circumstances, actual dyspnœa, are specially dependent on the distention of the abdomen by the effusion, and by the constantly present meteorism. In cases of excessive effusion, we may sometimes remark that in the upright position the tenseness and pain in the abdomen increase, and hence the patients assume a bent posture ; going upstairs, also, is beset with much difficulty.

Constipation is frequently observed. Vomiting occurs occasionally. The quantity of urine passed daily falls below the normal average. The skin is generally dry and hard, and nutrition is greatly impaired.

This condition may persist for a long time, even for months ; or, now and then, changes for better or for worse may arise.

The more the effusion partakes of a serous character, and the less the peritoneum itself is altered, the greater is the chance of absorption. Absorption is indicated by considerable increase in the quantity of urine passed, over and above what would correspond with the quantity drunk ; the skin becomes, at the same time, moist, the bowels regular, and the patient feels well again. The more fibrinous the effusion, the more likely is absorption to be delayed, and to result in numerous adhesions, which are particularly apt to attack the colon and omentum. A well-marked tendency to fresh attacks has been observed.

If the effusion be purulent, the further course of the disease assumes essentially the same form as the chronic purulent peritonitis which supervenes on an acute attack.

The *diagnosis* of chronic non-tubercular peritonitis is very difficult. In order to distinguish it from ascites it is necessary to be able definitely to exclude stasis in the region of the portal vein resulting from disease in any organs whatever. The differential diagnosis requires special regard to be paid to this condition resulting from diseases of the liver. This, at times, becomes all the more difficult, as this organ may become atrophied in chronic peritonitis.[1]

The absence of jaundice may sometimes be of assistance in the diagnosis of chronic peritonitis. As, however, in the majority of cases, cirrhosis of the liver is what we want to exclude, we may find more stress is to be laid on the following considerations : in addition to the data which the external appearance,

---

[1] *Frerichs*, Klinik der Leberkrankh. I. p. 260.

the recollection of the patient, and the history of the development of the disease afford, the spleen, in the majority of cases of cirrhosis of the liver, is enlarged; the abdomen is free from pain; the stools, as a rule, are yellowish and clay-like; there is no elevation of temperature or quickening of the pulse; the urine is, as a rule, dark-colored, and occasionally dilated veins in the neighborhood of the umbilicus are visible. In chronic peritonitis, on the other hand, enlargement of the spleen is rare, although, according to Galvagni's observations, it occasionally occurs; the abdomen is more frequently painful; the pulse is uniformly quickened, and there are evening exacerbations of temperature; the color of the stools is, as a rule, dark; and enlargement of the veins, to a slight extent, exists uniformly over the whole abdomen. As regards the condition of the liver itself, the shrivelling in cirrhosis especially affects the left lobe, which must not be mistaken for dislocation of the organ toward the axilla, such as occurs from the pressure of the fluid from below, even in chronic peritonitis. If the liver be atrophied from chronic peritonitis, the diminution affects both lobes alike. In cirrhosis of the liver, ascites, as a rule, uniformly increases—the cases without ascites do not come into consideration; in peritonitis the effusion not unfrequently undergoes considerable variations in the course of the disease.

Aran has already laid great stress upon the difficulties in making a differential *diagnosis* between simple chronic peritonitis and the tubercular form, and, in point of fact, no trustworthy criterion can be laid down. The demonstration of tubercular or caseous diseases in other organs, especially in the lungs and in the testicle, is doubtless very important, but is not pathognomonic for either one form or the other; according to Aran's testimony, simple chronic peritonitis may occur in tubercular individuals, and, on the other hand, it is impossible to ascertain the existence of every caseous mass during life. The cord-like retraction of the omentum, and other indurated products perceptible to the touch, occur more frequently in tubercular inflammation, and the same is true of the circumscribed inflammation in the neighborhood of the umbilicus, but these data are not distinctive.

As we may regard a simple puncture with an exploring needle

as not dangerous, we may avail ourselves of the evidence afforded by the character of the effusion; this, in the tubercular form, showing a more or less considerable hemorrhagic admixture.

As regards *prognosis*, according to Galvagni, it is rather favorable in the case of serous effusion, particularly in children. It is less favorable in the more fibrinous forms, and in the purulent form it is bad. The course, under all the circumstances, is very protracted, and, in the fibrinous effusions, adhesions, etc., may arise. The fate and dangers of purulent effusion have been already alluded to.

In the *treatment*, according to Galvagni's experience, puncture is to be avoided, and he also warns us against the excessive use of drastic purgatives. He especially recommends an expectant treatment, rest in bed, and quinine and opium as they may be indicated.

In the stage of resorption, painting with iodine, the use of diuretics and the regulation of diaphoresis by means of Turkish baths (Schwitzbädern), are the proper measures to use.

In the treatment of purulent effusion strong nourishment must, as far as is practicable, be given as a means of meeting the waste. If absorption is actually not taking place, operative treatment may, under certain circumstances, bring about the wished-for end, especially if there be already a tendency to rupture.

Circumscribed Peritonitis.

Acute and Chronic Form.

Muench, Zur Aetiologie des Icterus nebst Bemerkungen über part. Perit. Deutsche Klinik. 1858.—*Albers*, Ueber Perit. circumscr. Deutsche Klinik. 1862.—*Eulenberg*, Ueber Abscesse in der Bauchhöhle. Preuss. Vereinsztg. 1858.—*Dressler*, Ueber Gasentwickelung aus einem abges. eitrigen Peritonealexsudate. Prager Vierteljahrschr. 1863.—*Oppolzer*, Ein Fall von Tympanit. abd. Allg. Wien. mediz. Zeitung. 1862; und Luft u. Flüssigkeit in einem abges. Raume der Bauchhöhle, Perf. des Darms von Aussen nach Innen. Weiner Spitalzeitung. 1862.—*J. Fayrer*, Local Perit. and Death Result. from a Kick in the Epig. Med. Tim. and Gaz. July, 1868.—*Habershon*, Local Perit. in the Neighborhood of the Gall-bladder, Adhesions, Gastric Symptoms, Fix. Pain; Irrit. Mucous

Membr., Fatal Hemorrh. Guy's Hosp. Rep. XVI.; and Gall-stones, Abscess, Calculi Discharged through the Abdom. Pariet., Subseq. Abd. Pains. Guy's Hosp. Rep. XVI.

Circumscribed inflammation of the peritoneum presents all possible degrees of intensity in its symptoms, and the course of individual cases, likewise, varies very greatly. Circumscribed peritonitis may induce very intense local and general symptoms, or it may run its course in an almost or completely latent manner; it sometimes begins very acutely with an attack of shivering, while in many other cases the symptoms make their appearance gradually.

These forms of inflammation present great varieties, also, as regards their issues and consequences. For, although circumscribed peritonitis in itself is not likely to produce symptoms which threaten life, the resulting encysted peritoneal effusions on the one hand, and the adhesions and alterations in position of the viscera on the other, may induce dangerous consequences or protracted illness. In many other cases, however, a uniform thickening of the serous investment of an abdominal organ is the only result of circumscribed peritonitis.

In circumscribed peritonitis, also, we may distinguish acute and chronic forms, but the line of demarcation between these is less sharply defined than in diffuse inflammation, as from the nature of the case many instances which begin acutely tend to assume a chronic course when once the process becomes one of merely the development of circumscribed fluid effusion.

Acute circumscribed inflammation of the peritoneum arises almost always (traumatic cases excepted) from locally acting irritants—which induce secondary changes in the peritoneum. These irritative causes have their origin in all the various diseases of those abdominal viscera which are invested by peritoneum, and are due essentially to the same process as was referred to in the etiology of diffuse peritonitis. The particular cause, also, which must be regarded as tending to prevent the further extension of the inflammatory process, was there mentioned.

The nature and aspect, also, of the primary disease has an important influence upon the character and course of circumscribed peritonitis. On the other hand, accidental inflammation of the peritoneum may, by means of general adhesions, put a stop to the extension and deleterious influences of the primary disease ; this is true particularly in ulceration and suppuration of the abdominal viscera. These circumscribed inflammations of the peritoneum arise most frequently in the cavity of the pelvis in connection with the serous investment of the female genital organs, namely, the uterus, the ends of the Fallopian tubes, or the ovaries (perimetritis, colica scortorum, etc.). These processes have been discussed in the tenth volume of this work.

Circumscribed peritonitis, further, very frequently arises in the region of the cæcum, and in connection with ulceration of the vermiform process.

Circumscribed peritonitis occurs on the surface of the stomach and intestinal canal, especially over the seat of ulcerations extending from within—perigastritis, perienteritis, and enteritis serosa ; also on the omentum and mesentery, and even on the parietal layer, especially in hernial sacs—peritonitis sacci herniosi ; and, lastly, peritonitis diaphragmatica may result from pleuritis.

The serous investment of the liver plays a very constant part in chronic inflammation and suppuration, similarly also in the case of the spleen—perihepatitis and perisplenitis. Inflammatory and destructive processes in the urinary bladder and in the gall-bladder may extend to the peritoneum, and perinephritis also may result by extension from the areolar tissue.

All forms of tumor which occur in the region of the peritoneum have a great tendency to excite peritonitis, either acute or chronic, and hence without any severe symptoms.

Virchow[1] has called special attention to chronic partial peritonitis, and has fully discussed its occurrence and signification. These forms of inflammation present clinically great difficulties on account of the absence of well-marked symptoms, and we may lawfully describe them as latent circumscribed peritonitis. The absence of symptoms in the majority of these cases does not, however, prevent our taking account clinically of the symptoms

---

[1] Historisches, Kritisches und Positives zur Lehre der Unterleibsaffect. Virch. Arch. Bd. 5.

which may result therefrom. These consecutive alterations are, under certain circumstances, of the greatest possible importance; it is doubtless, as a rule, exceedingly difficult rightly to interpret these during life, and to refer them to their anatomical basis. These chronic inflammatory conditions may occur at any one of the accustomed spots of the peritoneum, or at several simultaneously. Some few spots are, however, especially apt to be attacked, or assume, at least special importance in connection with this form of inflammation. Virchow has described a perimetritis chronica, and further a peritonitis chronica mesenterialis and omentalis, as well as a partial peritonitis of the hypochondrium.

This form of circumscribed inflammation of the peritoneum may occur even during intra-uterine life. In the majority of such cases it is difficult to prove how it arose, as, post-mortem, we only find the fully developed conditions without any remnant of the originating processes themselves, and without our having been afforded any data during life or any assistance from the history of the case. Virchow refers the mode of occurrence principally to mechanical causes; in particular, the development of connective tissue occurring on the omentum and mesentery must, according · to him, be referred to a mechanical cause operating from without. Another category of mechanical irritants is conveyed to the peritoneum by the abdominal organs, especially the intestinal canal, in the first row of which may be mentioned fæcal accumulations. The changes in point, due to this cause, are by far most frequently met with in the large intestine at the flexure of the colon ; and the inflammation arises all the earlier if along with this other causes combine, as, for example, pressure, a blow, or intense peristaltic action. The inflammation excited in this way may become diffuse, but it will remain circumscribed if the noxious influences exist only in a moderate degree.

In connection with this point, Virchow has raised the question as to whether these changes in the peritoneum can occur without the other layers of the intestine, namely, the muscular and mucous, having previously undergone palpable alterations. This question is answered by Virchow in the affirmative, and I do not believe that anything can be advanced against his reasoning. The serous membrane may be the most intensely affected by an irritant which simultaneously attacks all three layers, even though the irritant in point may be in immediate contact with the other layers. The changes set up in the serous membrane also lead to permanent connective-tissue products, while they may completely disappear from the other layers.

In addition to these mechanical irritants, there are, doubtless, numerous circumstances associated with every trivial disturbance in the abdominal viscera and the abdominal parietes, which, by frequent recurrence at the same spot, induce the described effects.

Pathological Anatomy.—In acute adhesive inflammation, we find fibrinous effusion more or less richly deposited on a circumscribed spot, by means of which the primarily affected organ may have become attached to a neighboring healthy one. The zone of inflammation is generally somewhat sharply defined from the healthy peritoneum. Connective-tissue new growths are immediately developed out of the effusion, and more or less firm adhesions, or the callous thickening in the investment of an organ (as, for example, the spleen), are very quickly completed. The chronic form does not always lead to adhesions. Without any matting together, flat, fibrinous layers of effusion are formed on the mesentery, most frequently on the left side, at a point corresponding with the sigmoid flexure, which immediately lead to the production of connective tissue, and finally result in a stellate, retracted cicatrix. The mesentery becomes thereby shortened and thrown into folds, and the intestine must, to a certain extent, participate. In many other cases, numerous adhesions arise in a chronic manner. Thus, the flexura coli dextra may become adherent to the liver and gall-bladder, or to the stomach and duodenum, or the omentum, and the left flexure to the spleen and omentum. The omentum, on the other hand, may become fixed in hernial sacs, to the abdominal parietes, or in the pelvis, or it may be driven upward and become attached to the surface of the liver or to the intestines, etc. By means of these adhesions, numerous abnormities in the position of the viscera may arise (Virchow).

While this last-named chronic process does not readily lead to suppuration, the latter not unfrequently occurs in circumscribed acute peritonitis. As soon as the primary limiting adhesion has become established, the inclosed effusion undergoes a continual increase in its cellular elements, until it actually becomes fluid, and then there arises an encysted purulent effusion.

This encysted purulent peritoneal effusion may for a long time increase in size, and may often be associated with the occurrence of fresh attacks of inflammation, and with the production of new adhesions. These encysted effusions, in their further course, undergo various metamorphoses, which not unfrequently afford more clinical interest than the primary process itself. The effusion may remain as such for a long time, in which case we find the pus-corpuscles altered, and quantities of fat-crystals, the result of the splitting up of their contents. This form of effusion, which remains a long time stationary, is very apt to lead, by means of purulent erosion, to perforation in various directions. By opening a way for itself into the intestine, the pus may escape with the stools, and, on the other hand, the intestinal contents and gas may pass into the cavity. The pus may find its way in various other directions, and thus pass into other cavities or reach the outer world ; even rupture into the larger blood-vessels has been observed. If the pus has been discharged outward in any way, subsequent recovery may take place. Caseous degeneration of the effusion, with partial absorption of its fluid elements, is an unfavorable result, as by absorption from the caseous mass, subsequently, tuberculosis may be readily set up. In favorable cases recovery takes place by the formation of concretions or a firm, callous mass, after the pus has become more or less absorbed.

Owing to adhesions, it sometimes comes to pass that ulcerative processes of the stomach or intestine, or of the gall-bladder, may extend to other organs, and thus irregular communications, arrosions of the liver, abdominal parietes, etc., result.

Symptoms.—The symptoms of a primary disease may precede those of acute circumscribed peritonitis, but the primary disease may, however, remain latent up to the occurrence of the peritoneal symptoms. These latter, in some few instances, begin with a rigor ; pain generally becomes established at a circumscribed spot in the abdomen, without any primary implication of the general health ; the pain either may set in with considerable severity, or at first it may be but slight, and only become distinct on firm pressure, and afterwards gradually increase.   The degree of the tenderness depends considerably on the extent and rapidity of the inflammation.   It is not rare for the pain, after a short time, to extend over the entire abdomen, and subsequently again to localize itself in the original spot.   After a longer time, the tenderness considerably decreases, without, however, being entirely lost as long as any effusion exists.

The majority of the symptoms which are characteristic of diffuse peritonitis may arise in the case of circumscribed inflammation, but they do not, as a whole, reach at all the same degree of intensity as is usual in the diffuse form.   Many of these symptoms also may be absent.   Thus vomiting and meteorism rarely occur in so intense a manner.   The pulse, as a rule, does not present the characteristic quickening and smallness of wave, and a rise in temperature may be entirely wanting; quite high temperatures may nevertheless occur, but, as a rule, they quickly fall again.   If encysted masses of pus are formed, the fever may persist for a long time with irregular variations, which probably are associated with changes taking place in the centre of inflammation.

On examination we find the tenderness generally confined to the seat of the inflammation; at first it is considerable, but subsequently it becomes slighter, and then, particularly if the mass be deeply placed, it may require a somewhat firm pressure to call it forth.   Varying with the size of the cavity and the quantity of the effusion there may occur an arching forward of the abdomen at a spot corresponding with the seat of the inflammation, which to the touch is resistant and gives a weak note on percussion.   Fluctuation can only be observed, as a rule, in these tumors when they are preparing to burst outward; in which case the skin over them is reddened.   It has been already mentioned that the contents of an encysted mass, if it have lain for a long time in contact with the intestine, may take up intestinal gas by osmosis and thus get a fæcal smell.   If several such masses of effusion exist, the abdomen presents a most irregular surface.

Even where no apparent arching forward exists we often find

an increased resistance over the position of the inflammation, and a more or less defined tumor and dull percussion note. It is, however, not always easy to determine the existence of these conditions, as firm contraction of the abdominal walls, fæcal accumulation, etc., may give rise to error.

In many other cases the inflammatory mass is so deeply placed and so imperfectly circumscribed that we are unable to discover any abnormity on examination.

The following is a case of the kind from v. Ziemssen's clinique, which illustrates both the changes which may possibly result and the frequently protracted course:

E. F., aged twenty, came on the 31st of March to the institution with intermittent fever in the ninth month of pregnancy. After the occurrence of a premature delivery on April 6th, she became ill successively with phlegmonous angina, otitis externa, and erysipelas of the face; the last ran its course with high fever and with diarrhœa, which occasioned some abdominal pain. Diarrhœa and abdominal pain continued and became worse. On 20th of April the region of the right ovary was somewhat tender on percussion; no meteorism; no vomiting; nothing to be felt in the tender spot. In the period which ensued the diarrhœa remained constant, the pain was at one time less and at another more intense, the tenderness on pressure, however, persisted, and from April 30th vomiting occasionally occurred. In connection with this the evening temperatures were constantly 39° C. and upward, while the morning temperatures were normal, and the pulse varied between 90 and 116. This condition continued during the whole of May; the patient coughed a good deal during the latter period, and brought up a great deal of frothy sputa; the appetite was completely lost during the whole time and the emaciation became very marked. The patient died within the first few days of June.

On opening the abdomen some turbid fluid was found in the abdominal cavity, the cæcum and some small intestines were adherent to the right ovary, between which was a small encysted mass of pus. At the point of adhesion the outer wall of the intestine was ulcerated, and the loss of substance in some of the ulcers reached the mucous membrane. The neighboring coils of intestine were adherent and matted together. The serous membrane, especially that of the intestine, contained numerous scattered nodules lying in it, surrounded in some places by hemorrhagic tissue. The intestine everywhere else was very pale, also the stomach; toward the pylorus only there existed small hemorrhages in the mucous membrane. The mesenteric glands, in parts, intensely injected; the spleen enlarged, its capsule clouded, numerous scattered miliary tubercles in its dark-colored parenchyma.

All the consecutive changes which may arise from this kind of encysted effusion cannot possibly be included in any general description, the possibilities being so very multifarious. Perforations are very important, as they give rise to irregular communications, to entrance of flatus from the intestine into the sacculated space, to emptying of the effusion outward through the intestine, etc.

The physical phenomena of the entrance of gas are not of such a kind as to allow of our definitely diagnosing such an occurrence. The most distinct indication is the presence of an air cavity in the position previously occupied by the effusion (the behavior of this latter having been previously established), which gives a tympanitic, very frequently metallic percussion note, which undergoes no change for a long time, and which, moreover, in a circumscribed spot, pushes forward the abdominal parietes like a tumor. The occurrence of such perforation into a circumscribed cavity is often characterized by an entire absence of subjective symptoms.

Spontaneous development of gas has been observed in cases of encysted effusion.

In a case of circumscribed peritonitis in the region of the cæcum that came under observation in Lindwurm's clinique, the ascending colon was completely embedded in effusion, and firmly adherent to the liver. Similarly there existed abnormal adhesions between liver and diaphragm. On the occurrence of perforation gas streamed upward through an open canal, and collected posteriorly above the liver, and pressed the lungs upward. This air space behaved similarly to a circumscribed pneumothorax, except that the phenomena of succussion did not exist.

The following case, communicated by Buhl, demonstrates the occurrence of cavities which, by perforation from without upward, communicate with the intestine. The peritoneal surfaces of such spaces often assume, according to Lambl, a peculiar velvety appearance, and are beset with fine villi, but are never provided with a coating of intestinal epithelium.[1]

Communication by perforation between two intestinal cavities, a fistula existing between colon and stomach simultaneously with a stercoraceous recto-vaginal fistula. A woman aged fifty-one, greatly emaciated, and with a yellowish brown skin. Is said to have suffered from cramps in the stomach three or four years previously, which, however, quickly—once and for all—vanished. For two or three

---

[1] *Klebs*, Handbuch der path. Anat. p. 268.

years she has had pain in the abdomen, with insatiable appetite, and pain over the sacrum. Latterly the abdominal pains have become concentrated in the left hypochondrium; there is frequent slimy vomiting, with persistent constipation and loss of energy. On her admission the region of the left false ribs was found distended, and two or three inches in front of them was a defined tumor, with smooth, tense surface. The dull, toneless percussion note of the spleen passed without interruption into this tumor; that is, upward as far as the tenth rib, and forward toward the umbilicus. The patient vomited material, which, from its firm consistence, its dark brown color, its smell, and its similarity to fæcal evacuations, could be recognized as coming from the large intestine. After every act of vomiting the tumor decreased in size. In the absence of any symptoms of ileus the diagnosis of a fistula between the stomach and colon was made. Three days before death fæcal particles were observed in the urine, which was passed with burning pain. On post-mortem examination perforative peritonitis was found. The left flexure of the colon was adherent to the parietes, to the great curvature of the cul-de-sac of the stomach, and to some knuckles of small intestine. The place where these adhesions existed formed the inner wall of a fæcal cavity, which was bounded externally and anteriorly by the parietes. The peritoneum on the latter, and a part of the muscular structure, were destroyed. After stomach and colon had been opened, a communication about the size of half a crown, with gangrenous edges, was found to exist between the two, by means of which the fæces from the large intestine had got into the stomach. The communicating passage was not closed the whole way round, but opened into a wedge-shaped, common fæcal cavity; and it was this which finally perforated into the abdominal cavity, and was the immediate cause of the fatal peritonitis. In addition to this there was found, as the result of a similarly ruptured and widened rectum, a fæcal cavity between it and the vagina.[1]

Other important conditions arise as the result of encysted peritonitis, in that neighboring organs are dragged within the reach of the adhesions; further, pressure of the effusion may produce obliteration of contiguous solid organs or compression of the intestines.

Chronic, partial peritonitis adhesiva is, as a rule, not productive of any symptoms which are referable to the occurrence of this process. The cause of this want of symptoms depends less upon the trivial character of the changes themselves than upon their chronicity.

It is probable that trivial changes, such as hyperæmia of the peritoneum, if they occur acutely, are more likely to be accompanied with pain and tenderness than chronic processes with the production of cicatrices. This increased sensibility, re-

[1] Zeitschr. für rat. Medicin. N. F: Bd. 8. 1.

sulting from various diseases of the abdomen, we are apt, as a rule, to ascribe to peritoneal irritation.

This chronic adhesive peritonitis remains subsequently either completely latent, or there may ensue resulting conditions that sooner or later induce a set of symptoms which, according to the locality affected, must be very varied in their character.

Inflammatory Processes in the Right Iliac Fossa. Typhlitis and Perityphlitis.

Housson and *Dance*, in Repert. gén. Tom. IV. 3. 1827.—*Louyer-Villermay*, Arch. gén. Tom. V.—*Mélier*, Arch. gén. Tom. XVII.—*Menière*, Arch. gén. Tom. XII. — *Pouchelt*, Heidelberg. klin. Annalen. VIII. 524.—*Goldbeck*, Ueber eigenth. entzündl. Geschwülste in der rechten Hüftbeingegend. Worms, 1830.—*Duplay*, Journ. hebd. Tom. II.—*Roesch*, Württemb. Corresp.-Bl. 1834. No. 37.—*Merling*, Diss. sist. process. vermif. anat. path. Heidelberg, 1836.—*Wilhelmi*, Diss. de perityphl. Heidelberg, 1837.—*Posthuma*, Diss. de intest. coec. ejusque proc. vermif. path. Gronningen, 1837.—*Grisolle*, Arch. gén. 1839.—*Chomel*, Lancette franç. 1844.—*Marchall de Calvi*, Annal. de Chirurg. 1844.—*Volz*, Die durch Kothsteine bedingte Durchbohrung des Wurmforts. Carlsruhe, 1846.—*Rostan*, Lanc. franç. 1846.—*Battersby*, Dublin Quarterly Rev. 1847.—*Henry Hancock*, London Medical Gazette, New Series, Vol. VIII. (or VII. ?), p. 547. (Case of Perityphlitis, with operation.—*Szokalski*, Neue Zeitung für Medizin. 1849.— New England Med. Journ. 1843.—*Bamberger*, Wien. med. Wochenschr. 1853. —*Schnuerer*, Ueber die Perf. des wurmf. Fortsatz. Erlangen, 1854.—*Clauss*, Ueber spont. Darmperforation. Zürich, 1856.—*George Lewis*, Abscesses in the Appendix Vermiformis. New York Journal of Medicine, 1856. Third Series, Vol. I.—*Cless*, Württemb. Corresp.-Bl. 1857.—*Kottmann*, Tod durch Perf. des Proc. vermif. Schweizer Zeitschr. 1853.—*Forget*, De la périt. par la perf. de l'app. ileo-coec. Gaz. méd. de Strassb. 10. 1853.—*Henri Fabre*, Hist. des perf., etc. Thèse. Paris, 1851.—*Buhl*, Zeitschr. für rat. Mediz. IV. 1854.—*Sulzer* and *Reuling*, Deutsche Klinik. 1855. 38.—*Gurdon Buck*, Post-fascial Abscess, Originating in the Iliac Fossa, with a New Method of Treatment. New York Journal of Medicine. 1857.—*Stannus Hughes*, A Case of Fatal Perit. Dubl. Hosp. Gaz. 3. 1858.—*Ruetter*, De perityphl. Diss. Berol. 1858.—*Fraenkel*, Nonnulla de perityphl., etc. Diss. Berlin, 1859.—*Leudet*, Ric. anat. path. e clin. sull' ulz. e la perf., etc. Annali universali di Med. Ag. 1859; and Arch. de méd. 1859.—*van Holsbeck*, Abcès de la fosse iliaque dr., etc. Ann. de la soc. méd.-chir. de Bruges. Janv. et Févr. 1860.—*Lang*, Perityph. mit gl. Ausg. Würt. Corr.-Bl. 13. 1860.—*Muenchmeyer*, Unters. über Typhl. und Perityph. Deutsche Klinik. 1860.—*Keber*, Ueber Entz. u. Perf., etc. Diss. Bern, 1859.—

Riesenfeld, De intest. grasso, etc. Diss. Berol. 1860.—*Philip*, De proc. vermic. perf. Diss. Berol. 1860.—*Colin*, Observ. de tum. phleg. de la fosse iliaque dr. Rec. des mém. de méd. et chirurg. 24. 1861.—*Rouyer*, Mém. sur les tum. sterc. Gaz. hebd. 1862.—*Oppolzer*, Ueber Unterleibsgesch. mit bes. Rücks. auf deren Diagn. Wien. med. Wochenschr. 1862.— *Larret-Lamalignie*, Des perf. de l'append. iléo-coecal. Thèse. Strassb. 1862.—*Guarini*, Obs. sul tum. che si svilupp. nella reg. iliac. annal. univers. di med. Vol. 182. 1862.—*Herold*, De proc. vermic. perf., etc. Diss. Berol. 1862.— *Th. Matzal*, Typhl. supp. Oesterr. Zeitschr. für prakt. Heilkunde. 1864. 2.—*Tissier*, De la pérityph. Thèse. Paris, 1865.—*Ch. A. Crouzet*, Des perfor. spont. de l'app. ileo-coecal. Thèse. Paris, 1865.—*Prudhomme*, Périt. de la fosse iliaque dr. par perf. intest., périt., périhepat. Rec. de mém. de méd. mil. Juin. 1866.—*Petit*, Entérolith ayant perf. l'app. coec. Revue méd. Juin, 1866.—*A. D. Hall*, Fatal Perit. from Perf. of the Append. Vermif. Amer. Journ. of Med. Science. Octbr., 1866.—*J. K. Wardell*, Acute Perit. and Displacement of the Cæcum. Brit. Med. Journ. Oct., 1866.—*R. Bartholow*, On Typhlitis and Perityphlitis; on Disease of the Cæcum and Appendix Resulting in Absc. in the Right Iliac Foss. Amer. Journ. of Med. Science. Oct., 1866.—*Eisenschitz*, Perit. hervorgerufen durch Perforation des Proc. vermif. Wien. med. Presse. 11. 1866.— *Willard Parker*, Case of Perityphlitis, with Operation. New York Medical Record, March 15th, 1867; also June 15th, 1867.—*Blatin*, Rech. sur la typhlite et la pérityphl. conséc. Thèse. Paris, 1868.—*Hallete*, De l'app. coecal. Thèse. Paris, 1868.—*R. Farquharson*, Case of Pericæcal Absc. Caused by Perf. of the Vermif. Appendix and Proving Fatal by Rupture into the Perit. Cavity. Edinb. Med. Journ. June, 1868.—*G. H. Wynkoop*, An Acct. of the Post-mortem App. of an App. Vermiformis, which Two Years Previously had been the Seat of Absc., and had been Operated on, etc. New York Medical Record, 1868.—*S. Adler*, Typhlitissterc., Perit. circumscr. Zellgewebsabscess, etc. Allgem. Wiener med. Zeitung. No. 48. 1868.—*Moers*, Pylephlebitis, etc. Arch. für klin. Med. Bd. IV.—*Peacock*, Ulceration of the App. Vermif., etc. Trans. of the Path. Soc. XVIII. 87.—*Down, Langdon*, Ulc. of the App. Vermif. Ibid. 97.—*L. F. Toft*, Om Ulceration og Perfor. af proc. vermif. Diss. Kjöbenhavn, 1868. — *W. Duddenhausen*, Typhlitis sterc. Diss. Berl. 1869.—*J. Pouzet*, De la pérityphl. Thèse. Paris, 1869.—*R. Bossard*, Ueber die Verschwär. u. Durchbr. des Wurmf. Diss. Zürich, 1869. — *Behm*, Vereiterung des wurmf. Forts. Deutsche Klinik. 29. 1869.—*E. Aufrecht*, Entzündung des Proc. vermif. Perityphl., Phlebitis u. Thrombose der Vena mesent. magna, Pylephlebitis. Berl. klin. Wochenschr. No. 29. 1869.—*A. Briess*, Leberabscess unter d. Krankheitsbilde einer acuten Leberatrophie verlaufend. Wien. med. Presse. 1869.—*Earl Cushman*, Dis. of the Ileo-cæcal Region. Phil. Med. and Surg. Rep. July, 1869.— *Duguet*, Note sur un cas de typhlite phlegmoneuse survenue dans le cours d'une entérite tuberc., etc. Gaz. méd. de Paris. No. 1. 1870.—*Cowdell*, Fatal Case of Typhlitis. Med. Times and Gaz. Oct., 1870.—*J. A. Campbell*, Case of Perityphlitic Absc., with Remarks. Brit. Med. Journ. Febr., March, April, 1870.—

L. Weber, Case of Perityphlitis, with Operation. New York Medical Journal,
Aug. 1871.—*O. Fromme*, Ueber perityphl. Abscesse. Diss. Göttingen, 1872.—
E. Putschkowski, Sechs Fälle von Perityphilitis. Diss. Berlin, 1872.—*A. Herr-
gott*, Ulcération de l'appendice iléo-coecale, péritonite conséc., mort. Gaz. méd.
de Strassb. 2. 1872.—*C. Th. Williams*, Ulceration of the Vermiform Append.
giving Rise to Limited Perit. Trans. of the Path. Soc. XXXIII. 106.—*Marsh
Howard*, Injury to Abd., Typhlitis, Perf. of the Vermif. App., Perit., Death.
Brit. Med. Journ. 9. 1872.—*S. E. Thompson*, Two Cases of Perityphlitis in
which Recov., etc. Lancet. May, 1873.—*J. W. Allan*, Case of Acute Typhl.
Lancet. May, 1873.—*Werner*, Perf. Peritonitis durch einen am Wurmforts.
steckengebl. Kirschkern. Württemb. med. Correspondenzbl. 10. 1873.—*Chan-
delux*, Note sur un cas de perityphl. avec épanch. stercoral consécut. Lyon
méd. 8. 1873.—*Henry B. Sands*, Case of Perityphlitis, with Operation. New
York Medical Journal, Aug. 1874.—*Gurdon Buck*, Perityphlitic Abscess in the
Ileo-cæcal Region. New York Medical Record. 1876; On Abscesses originating in the Right Iliac Fossa, with Table of Statistics. Transactions of the
Academy of Medicine of New York. 1876.

Occasional notices of inflammation and ulceration of the cæcum are to be found in the older writers, and fæcal accumulations were described even by Santorini. Any more definite
knowledge as to the nature of the processes in question belongs,
however, to recent times. P. Frank described perityphlitis as
peritonitis muscularis, and hence was in the dark as to the
actual seat of the disease. Husson and Dance further called
attention to the disease and described it as "engorgement inflam-
matoire qui se developpe dans la fosse iliaque droite." The
inflammatory conditions of the connective tissue in the iliac fossa
were described by Dupuytren and Velpeau, and in Germany
first by Puchelt, and Volz published some very interesting
observations on the vermiform process. Finally, Bamberger
subdivided the various processes in question according to their
pathological bearing, retaining at the same time their unity clinically.

The cæcum and vermiform process are often the seat of diseases which lead to circumscribed peritonitis. The connective
tissue also, which lies behind the cæcum over the iliac fascia, is
sometimes the seat of inflammation and abscess. The two first-
mentioned processes are from the outset intraperitoneal, while
phlegmonous inflammation in the areolar tissue behind the cæcum is first retroperitoneal, but frequently involves the peri-

toneum, and may secondarily extend to the intestinal wall. These inflammatory processes are therefore anatomically distinct in their position, and they also possess from the outset a different significance and importance; nevertheless they present in their symptoms so much uniformity that the clinical distinction between them is in the majority of cases impossible. We must frequently be satisfied with recognizing the inflammation in the right iliac fossa without distinguishing whether the cæcum, the vermiform process, or the retroperitoneal areolar tissue, be the starting-point. In many cases, furthermore, the distinction is impossible, it being at the same time, however, a matter of no practical importance, owing to the fact that the forms of inflammation mentioned pass into one another, so that by an ulceration of the vermiform process the cæcum becomes involved.

It may further happen that other retroperitoneal inflammations, lying behind the iliac fascia in the psoas and iliacus muscles, etc., extend to the peritoneum, but these processes induce an essentially different set of symptoms, so that we must separate these diseases from those now mentioned.

According to Luschka (Lage der Bauchorgane, 1873) the cæcum lies in such a manner on the right iliac muscle that its extremity corresponds nearly with the middle of Poupart's ligament. It lies just above the external half of this latter on the inner portion of the anterior abdominal wall. In exceptional cases the cæcum assumes a higher position, or is turned further round toward the entrance of the true pelvis, and may even extend across the middle line. The cæcum is not in immediate contact with the iliacus muscle, as it possesses a complete peritoneal investment, so that when it is distended it projects freely into the peritoneal cavity. This portion of intestine presents a wedge-shaped form with its end pointed or truncated, according as the vermiform process opens into its posterior aspect and thus represents its true end, or enters in such a way that the connection between the two is to all appearances lost.

The vermiform process has an average thickness of 7 mm. and is 7 to 8 ctms. long, but it may, however, exceed even 20 ctms. According to its length, it is either but slightly curved or considerably contorted. As a rule, it is very movable, so that it may assume various positions.

Circumscribed peritonitis, which attacks the serous coat of the cæcum and its neighborhood, is most frequently due to an accumulation of fæces (typhlitis stercoralis).

One of the physiological phenomena of this portion of intes-

tine is that its contents become more solid and remain a long
time in it. There are a number of circumstances which may
induce the contents to remain for a much longer period than
usual, and in connection with this to become very hard. Among
such circumstances may be mentioned want of exercise,[1] unsuitable diet, producing a great quantity of fæces; altered position of the intestine, especially of the colon, chronic intestinal
catarrh, impaired activity of the intestinal muscular coat. When
fæcal accumulations repeatedly occur, chronic catarrh ensues,
with thickening of the intestinal wall, dilatation of the tumor,
and finally ulceration. Independently of ulceration, pressure of
the hard fæcal masses may set up peritoneal inflammation, and
complete occlusion of the intestine may arise from the same
cause. Certain external influences may tend further to increase
the tendency to the occurrence of inflammation. Intestinal calculi or foreign bodies, which have been swallowed with the food,
such as fruit stones, etc., may produce the same effect as hard
fæcal masses.[2]

Other ulcerative processes also, if they extend deeply, produce similar symptoms.

In the vermiform process, as a rule, it is intestinal calculi
which cause inflammation, ulceration, and, comparatively frequently in this position, perforation. (For further information
on this point see Diseases of the Intestinal Canal.) It is more
rare for foreign bodies to get into the narrow lumen of the vermiform process and produce ulceration after varying intervals of
time. In addition to catarrhal and sloughing ulceration tubercular ulcers and the ulcers of enteric fever have been observed
as causes of the inflammatory process in question. If, owing
to the obliteration of the entrance, the secretion of the mucous
membrane in the vermiform process be retained, this latter becomes distended in a sacculated manner and assumes the characters of a cyst.

---

[1] According to *Luschka*, each time the thigh is bent a pressure is exerted by the
iliacus muscle on the upper portion of the cæcum, and thus the activity of this portion
of intestine is stimulated.

[2] In other cases it is known that such foreign bodies have remained for a very long
time in the intestine without doing any harm.

The inflammation of the retroperitoneal areolar tissue—perityphlitis—arises either in connection with the anomalies of the cæcum just mentioned simultaneously with circumscribed peritonitis, or else independently, owing to traumatic causes and catching cold, or finally, owing to the extension of an inflammatory process in the neighborhood. In the female perityphlitis occurs comparatively often in connection with the puerperal state.

The inflammatory conditions of the right iliac fossa occur much more frequently in the male than in the female; all observers who have collected statistics on this point have arrived at the same result. Bamberger found the ratio to be ·26 : 4. Further, according to this observer's statistics these diseases occur most frequently between the ages of sixteen and thirty-five.

The pathological changes present many varieties according to the duration of the disease. We find the evidence of catarrh of the cæcum ; we find, further, dilatation of its lumen, considerable thickening of all its coats, and often extensive ulceration. The serous membrane is inflamed, has a deposition of fibrine upon it, the parts in the neighborhood are matted together, and in the sacs formed by these we often find pus.

The vermiform process likewise presents a catarrhal and swollen condition, frequently with prominence of the follicles and with mucous or purulent secretion, and, as a rule, also with well-marked œdema of its walls. If an intestinal calculus have been the cause of the inflammation, we find ulceration and perforation at the seat of direct pressure, and the entire vermiform process may, in this way, become completely separated. The concretions may be packed in the lumen of the vermiform process, or they may have fallen out and be found lying in the mass of pus which surrounds and covers it. The pus may be mixed with particles of fæces, and always possesses a feculent odor. In rare instances the vermiform process becomes connected by circumscribed adhesive peritonitis to a neighboring portion of intestine in such a way that in the occurrence of perforation the concretion gets into the intestine, and thus the entire process may terminate without doing any harm. As a rule, the inflammation extends and leads to formation of pus. It is often difficult to find the vermiform process in these masses of pus. As a rule, it is not in its normal position, and is very often found attached to the cæcum.

These accumulations of pus may, as in other cases of circumscribed peritoneal effusion, end in recovery by absorption and the development of connective tissue, with, however, the residua of fixity and retractile cicatrices, and with arrosion of the vermiform process. It somewhat frequently passes on to general peritonitis. If perforation into the intestine takes place, a cure may be thus effected. The pus, however, in a few cases travels a long distance. If a secondary suppuration or breaking down of the retroperitoneal areolar tissue be established, we have perityphlitis arising out of typhlitis. Perityphlitis, whether secondary or primary, may result in cure by the production of a connective-tissue cicatrix. In cases of considerable production of pus, an abscess may be developed on the fascia iliaca behind the cæcum. If a mass of pus of this kind communicates with the cæcum and elements of fæces become mixed with it, a suppurative process of great dimensions, as a rule, is the result ; such an extensive destruction is seldom developed unless perforation exists.

The destructive suppuration attacks particularly the retroperitoneal areolar tissue of the pelvis, as far as the neighborhood of the rectum ; it extends towards Poupart's ligament, and even on to the anterior surface of the thigh, and passing upward, it reaches the region of the kidneys or even the pleural cavities, in all cases following the course of the retroperitoneal areolar tissue on the fascia iliaca. The external opening occurs, as a rule, in the bend of the groin, sometimes, however, with the formation of long fistulæ, or with extensive destruction of tissue. After bursting through the fascia iliaca, muscles and bones may be destroyed (rupture through the acetabulum has been observed by Aubry). It is obvious that the chances of pyæmia and septicæmia from such abscesses and purulent masses are very great. Serious consequences may also accrue to the liver from these conditions, as radicles of the portal vein (the ileo-cæcal vein) are involved in the inflammation, and thus there results pylephlebitis with metastatic abscesses in the liver (*vide* Diseases of the Liver).

Symptoms.—The phenomena presented in a case of inflammation in the right iliac fossa may naturally assume very different aspects. The primary seat of the process, the exciting cause, and the extent of the pathological changes, are of great importance as regards the subsequent course of the disease. The more rapidly and intensely the serous membrane is attacked, the more virulent will the course be; on the other hand, the entire process may remain just as latent as has been already stated to be the case in circumscribed peritonitis occurring in other parts of the abdomen. Further, the intestinal symptoms may, in certain cases, assume a more or less prominent importance. Lastly, the further alterations in the effusion may vary in many ways, as may also the dependent resulting phenomena.

The pathological changes in the cæcum and vermiform appendage, which ultimately lead to peritonitis, may, for a considerable period, have given rise to more or less distinct symptoms. Most frequently we meet with irregularities of the bowels; either constipation has existed for a long time, or this has alternated with diarrhœa, until finally obstinate constipation has become established. Sometimes digestion had been for a long time impaired; tenderness in the region of the cæcum, or even more active pain in the abdomen, had occasionally occurred (compare Diseases of the Intestinal Canal). In other cases, all premonitory intestinal symptoms have been absent, and the phenomena of inflammation in the region of the cæcum set in quite suddenly. In cases of this latter kind, particularly, various predisposing causes are mentioned which, under certain circumstances, may have a certain significance, such as straining of the body, overloading with food, or the eating of indigestible things. The sudden occurrence of pain may be accompanied with shivering, and a somewhat smart fever at the outset is the rule. Subsequently, the fever is regulated by the increase and decrease of the inflammatory symptoms and the suppuration, and may, like these, be subject to many variations.

The general symptoms behave like those of other forms of acute or subacute circumscribed peritonitis, and vary with the intensity and extent of the inflammation. Thus the pain in the region of the cæcum is generally very severe; it may, however,

allow the patient to go about as usual. Accumulation of fæces
in the cæcum is a very constant occurrence, due to the paralysis
of its muscular wall from pressure of the mass of effusion in the
neighborhood, and to certain abnormities of position, and further
promoted by the primary disease of the intestine itself. The
accumulation of fæces thus occurring may reach such an extent
as to induce ileus. As a rule, it occasions either complete suppression of the stools or diarrhœa may simultaneously exist.
This latter is the result of catarrh of the large intestine, and may
even arise in cases of complete intestinal occlusion. The stools
in this case contain for the most part nothing but mucous, watery
masses, which are to be regarded as the secretion of the mucous
membrane below the obstruction. In other cases, the passage
alongside the accumulated mass is not completely obliterated.

Stercoraceous vomiting is not frequent; ordinary gastric vomiting, on the other hand, is a common symptom. Meteorism may
be very intense; it is rarely absent, except in purely primary
perityphlitis, this form being characterized usually by the moderation of the symptoms.

The most important physical sign is the tumor in the right
iliac fossa, owing to which this region is visibly prominent.
This tumor corresponds with the position of the cæcum, and frequently also with the course of the ascending colon. It extends
downward, as a rule, to within a short distance of Poupart's
ligament. Internally, the margin of the tumor may occasionally
extend to the middle line; it almost constantly extends beyond
the normal limit of the cæcum, this being due to the fact that
the distended cæcum projects inward into the cavity of the peritoneum. The tumor generally feels comparatively superficial,
and is not movable, or only slightly so. It is more or less sharply
defined round the circumference, the surface is smooth, and the
resistance frequently very considerable. Fluctuation is but
rarely observable, and then only in those cases where the contents are about to burst outward. The sound on percussion is
either perfectly dull or dully tympanitic. It is only when the
inflammatory mass lies entirely behind the cæcum that this latter can retain its normal quantity of air.

In the formation of the tumor, the collection of fæces in the cæcum, the exudation upon the serous membrane, the adhesions, and, to a certain extent also, perhaps, the thickening of the walls of the intestine, all concur.

If the tumor attain to any considerable extent, or if it exist for a long time, œdema, and sometimes even thrombosis, may result from pressure on the veins. Similarly, pain and the feeling of numbness and weakness in the lower extremities—the latter particularly in perityphlitis—may arise from pressure on nerves. The tumor in many cases is formed very quickly—sometimes, however, gradually. Numerous residual processes arise in connection with it; the tumor alternately decreases and increases, and in this manner the process may take several months before there is any definite issue.

The symptoms that are induced by the occurrence of perforation have been already alluded to.

The *duration* of the disease may, according to circumstances, extend from a few days to many weeks, and even months. Simple cases of perityphlitis and of stercoraceous typhlitis may end in recovery in the course of from eight to fourteen days; this may be the case even if complicated with ileus. In cases of ulceration in the cæcum and in the vermiform appendage, this kind of favorable issue is no longer the rule; the formation of pus, with all its consequences, frequently ensues, and a favorable issue is protractedly postponed. An unfavorable issue may result from extension of the peritonitis, often in the course of a few days, from intestinal occlusion, from unfavorable processes which are set up by the suppuration, from pyæmia, or from general exhaustion resulting from protracted suppuration and impaired nutrition. Those cases in which perforation, whether primary or secondary, has taken place, run an unfavorable course.

In cases of recovery, protracted disturbances of the functions of the intestine, altered positions and narrowing of the intestinal tube, fistulæ, and even fæcal fistulæ, may remain for a long time, or as ultimate residua.

The *diagnosis* rests most prominently on the painful tumor in the region of the cæcum, and, further, on the previously existing symptoms, and the symptoms of circumscribed peritonitis which are subsequently developed in connection with the tumor. The

diagnosis in most cases is beset with no difficulties.   Mistakes
might arise with abscesses in the parietes ; but the absence of
motion of the parietes over the tumor, and the absence of intestinal symptoms, clear up the real state of affairs.   Tumors of the
kidney are distinguishable by their position, by abnormities in
the urine, and by the absence of characteristic intestinal symptoms ; on physical examination, they are found to lie much
more deeply.   Cancer of the cæcum is characterized by its chronic
course, by the cancerous cachexy of the individual, and by the
absence of inflammatory symptoms ; the resulting tumors, moreover, are nodulated and uneven.   Simple accumulation of fæces
in the cæcum doubtless causes a tumor ; but, on the other hand,
all the other symptoms, even pain, are wanting.   What the disease may be most readily mistaken for is a psoas abscess.   In
this case the movement of the right leg is, as a rule, greatly impaired ; it is drawn up against the pelvis and bent.   The inflammatory tumor lies more deeply and inferiorly, and is covered by
coils of intestine.   The process runs a very chronic course, and
presents no intestinal symptoms.

The question as to the starting-point of the inflammation
remains, as a rule, one of probability.   It is impossible to decide
from objective considerations whether abnormities have their
seat in the cæcum or in the vermiform process ; the latter are by
far the most frequent.   The sudden occurrence of peritoneal
symptoms, and the absence of long previously existing intestinal
phenomena, are indicative of the starting-point being in the vermiform process.

The inflammation of the areolar tissue behind the cæcum is,
in the majority of instances, connected with a primary typhlitis.
In other cases it is doubtless idiopathic, but it immediately
involves the cæcum.   Under these circumstances, any more definite recognition of the series of pathological changes is impossible during life.   It is only in the rare cases in which perityphlitis
occurs as an isolated process, and remains as such, that the seat
of the disease becomes probable, owing to the insignificance of
the symptoms, to the absence of meteorism, to the less obstinate
constipation, to the deep position of the tumor, and to its being
partially covered by the cæcum.

The *prognosis* is, in cases of pure perityphlitis and stercoraceous typhlitis, rather favorable; but here it is uncertain whether the true pathological condition can be absolutely recognized; a case where primarily the symptoms are very insignificant may subsequently assume a very grave aspect. All cases of perforation must be regarded as unfavorable.

Statistics show a very varying rate of mortality; Volz had thirty-nine deaths in forty-nine cases, and Bamberger, on the other hand, in thirty cases had only ten deaths. This difference depends obviously on the dissimilarity of the cases met with, and partly also on the different treatment employed; Volz treating the greater number of his patients according to the old principle—antiphlogistically,—while in cases where he adopted the opium treatment he saw very good results.

The plan of *treatment* which is often very beneficial in this form of disease must consist in first attempting to relieve the accumulation of fæces, whether this be the sole *causa mali*, or whether it only occur symptomatically. This is to be effected by injections, repeated one after the other, and not by purgatives. The latter are not suitable until a later period, when, after the subsidence of the acute symptoms, inactivity of the bowels continues, as is frequently the case. Castor oil is then the best form to administer.

While we endeavor in this way to remove the accumulation from the cæcum, the simultaneous administration of opium is also indicated; this will in no way weaken the effect of the injections, and will be productive of the beneficial results described in connection with general peritonitis; furthermore, absolute rest, suitable diet, and the use of cold are indicated in the acute stage.

With a view to promoting absorption of the effusion we may try mercurial ointment, tincture of iodine, baths, etc.

If there be a tendency to burst outward, it will be promoted by warm fomentations. The maxim of many physicians—if possible, to allow the opening to occur spontaneously—is a good one, but it is possible that gradually, by means of improved antiseptic treatment, this precept may come to be reversed.[1]

---

[1] Since the publication of Prof. Willard Parker's paper in 1867, it has been the practice of American surgeons to cut down upon the tumor as soon as fluctuation can be distinguished.—EDITOR'S NOTE.

Tuberculosis of the Peritoneum and Tubercular Peritonitis.

Demon, Ess. sur la périt. tuberc. chez l'adulte. Thèse. Paris, 1848.—*A. Kyburg*, Ueber Perit. tub. bei Erwachs. Diss. Zurich, 1854.—*Buchanan*, A Case of Chronic Perit. Assoc. with Tub. Dis. of the Mes. Glands, and Mil. Tub. of the Lungs, etc. Med. and Surg. Rep. Febr. 15, 1868.—*Aran*, De la périt. chron. simple et tuberc., etc. L'Union méd. 93, 94. 1858.—*E. Vallin*, De l'inflamma- tion péri-ombilic. dans la tubercul. du péritoine. Arch. gén. de Mai, 1869. p. 558.—*Robert*, Périt. tuberc., infl. péri-ombil. et perfor. intest. Rec. de mém de méd. milit. Novbr. 1869. p. 419.—*Eug. Miran*, Quelq. mots sur la péritonite tuberc. chez l'adulte. Thèse. Montp. 1869.—*Albanus*, Zwölf Fälle von Tuber- kulose d. Bauchfelles. Petersb. med. Zeitschr. XVII. 313.—*Luc. Hemey*, De la périt. tuberc. Thèse. Paris, 1866.—*J. F. Clement*, De la périt chronique. Thèse. Paris, 1865.—*F. A. Hoffmann*, De la périt. tuberc. Thèse. Paris, 1866.—*Bier- baum*, Deutsche Klinik. 1870.—*Steinthal*, Ein Fall von Tuberculose des Bauch- felles. Berl. klin. Wochenschr. No. 20. 1866.—*Klebs*, Virchow's Archiv. 44. Bd.—*J. Kaulich*, Klinische Beiträge zur Lehre von der Perit. Tuberkulose. Prag. Viertelj. II. 36.—*J. F. Payne*, Two Cases of Fibrous Tuberc. Growth in the Perit. with Caseous Format. in the Other Org. Trans. of the Path. Soc. XXI. pp. 198 and 236.—*Barthez* and *Rilliet*, L. c. III. p. 933.

Acute miliary tuberculosis of the peritoneum, if only a part of a general eruption throughout the body, presents but little clinical interest, no essential influence being thereby exerted on the disease as a whole, for at most a slight serous effusion takes place into the abdominal cavity. The same is true of the localized production of tubercles, such as are prone to occur on the serous membrane in the neighborhood of caseous ulcers of the intes- tine; they produce no further consequences, although the oc- currence is frequently connected with circumscribed adhesive peritonitis—recognizable by tenderness on pressure.

In a number of cases, however, the development of tubercle of the peritoneum induces most striking symptoms, and either forms the exclusive aspect of the disease, or at least distinctly outweighs, in clinical importance, any simultaneous occurrence of tubercle in other organs.

These cases have been long known and described as tuber- culosis of the peritoneum and as tubercular peritonitis. A dis- tinction between tuberculosis of the peritoneum and tubercular peritonitis has been assumed by many authors, but such a separation is not authorized, inflammatory products being found in all these cases alongside the new formation, and the slight dif-ferences, as, for example, the nature of the tenderness, must be referred to other causes.

The form of disease in question has recently been most care-fully depicted by Kaulich.

Pathogenesis and Etiology.

The causes of peritoneal tuberculosis are for the most part identical with those of tuberculosis in general. It is not often that the peritoneum is primarily and exclusively attacked by tuberculosis ; this occurring, as a rule, only in connection with caseous masses in the region of the peritoneum, especially in the genito-urinary organs, and of these, caseous masses in the epi-didymis are specially important, as similarly caseous lymph-atic glands or encysted peritoneal effusion, and also suppuration of bone, may form the starting-point. In rare cases no starting-point whatever can be discovered. As a rule, tuberculosis of the peritoneum is but a part of a tuberculosis distributed throughout the body, and we find the lungs simultaneously dis-eased, the process in them being either of older date or actually in course of progress.

In the later periods of life tubercular peritonitis rarely oc-curs, and, according to the observations of Barthez and Rilliet, it is likewise rare before four years of age.

Pathological Anatomy.

In the majority of cases the extension of the process in the peritoneum occurs successively and in a chronic manner, and is accompanied by an extensive formation of connective tissue (the adhesive tubercular peritonitis of Klebs). In this way numerous adhesions and extensive false membranes are generally devel-oped, and in these again the tubercle may become deposited to an enormous extent. Owing to the fibrous proliferation and the caseous metamorphosis of the new growth, thick skin-like masses are formed, which are spread upon the surface of the peritoneum

or extend from the visceral to the parietal layer, and thus separate the abdominal cavity into several subdivisions. The omentum in this way may cover the entire intestines as a thick apron
beset with tubercles.

Owing to the rich fibrous proliferation important shrivellings
and retractions frequently arise, the omentum usually becomes
retracted into a thick, firm lump, which lies transversely across
the abdomen just above the umbilicus. The folds of the mesentery form into a thick mass and draw the mutually adherent
intestines upward. A more or less copious effusion occurs, as a
rule, simultaneously with the development of the new formation,
and it is quite the exception when effusion is altogether absent
at this stage of the process, and extensive adhesions and proliferation are alone present. The effusion is either greenish yellow
and turbid, or, as is the rule, it contains the coloring matter of
the blood in various stages of metamorphosis, more or less copiously mixed with it. The color of the fluid thus varies from
pale brownish to intensely dark brown. Along with the admixture of blood in the effusion we find numerous black petechiæ
on the surface of the peritoneum.

In rare cases the eruption of tubercle takes place rapidly and
simultaneously over the entire peritoneum, and is accompanied
by a serous or sero-sanguineous effusion. The development of
connective tissue then ensues.

The formation of tubercle in the peritoneum does not, as a rule, take place
simultaneously at every spot; we find the tubercles in every possible stage of
development, both formative and retrograde, at one and the same place; also caseous
tubercles may be found alongside recent ones.

According to Kundrat, if we examine a preparation from the omentum, the
miliary tubercles are principally found situated on the stronger, vascularized trabeculæ. We find them, however, also on the finest trabeculæ which contain no blood-
vessels, generally at a nodal point, and extending into the spaces of the net-work.
Kundrat also found the following conditions in the omentum, namely, the cells enlarged, projecting considerably into the spaces of the net-work, and their nuclei
generally multiplied. Occasionally giant-cells are found with 40–50 nuclei. These
latter are often placed thickly crowded together, with the margin of the mass extending a considerable distance beyond the delicate trabeculæ, so that thereby the
space is sometimes almost completely filled up. In addition to this, small cells
also occur, generally in the neighborhood and on the borders of the masses of larger

cells, and also in the interior of the smallest nodules of these latter. Between them we may discover the fine dark granules which characterize caseous metamorphosis.

According to Sanderson, we see beautifully arranged endothelial cells over the tubercular nodule, which is contradictory to Kundrat's observations, according to which the tubercle probably owes its origin to a new formation of endothelium.

According to Kundrat, we are not to look for the origin of the tubercle-cells exclusively in endothelium; around the vessels an infiltration takes place of cells which resemble the so-called lymphoid cells.

Sometimes we find the process at a standstill, the newly formed products are everywhere in the condition of caseous metamorphosis without fresh eruption, and, corresponding with this state of things, the effusion is absorbed. This standstill, however, ends, as a rule, by the process breaking out afresh in other organs, thereby causing death, or a fresh outburst occurs in the peritoneum.

Owing to the adhesions, distortions and bendings of the intestine occur, and at these bends the mucous membrane may ulcerate and induce intestinal hemorrhage, and even perforation.

In addition to tuberculosis of the peritoneum, similar conditions are often simultaneously found in the lungs, pleura, and pericardium; and furthermore, amyloid degeneration of the spleen, kidneys, and, more rarely, of the liver, are also found. The spleen is often somewhat enlarged. The liver is normal in size, or it is sometimes enlarged, owing to amyloid degeneration, or as a result of the deposition of fat (chronic fatty liver). I have repeatedly seen it in a condition of simple atrophy.

General Form of the Disease.

The symptoms and course of tubercular peritonitis assume a very different aspect according as the course of the disease is of a more or less chronic nature, according as intermissions and remissions occur, and according as there is simultaneous disease of other organs. A symptom may in one case attain a very considerable intensity, while in another it may be completely absent.

In order to make it possible to get a certain general view of the features presented by the disease notwithstanding all this multifariousness, Kaulich has distinguished three groups of cases, which may, however, in many ways pass into one another. Those of the first group begin acutely with fever, and pain in the abdomen, either at a circumscribed spot or over a larger area. Along with this, we have repeated vomiting, constipation, and meteorism, and the indications of circumscribed peritonitis are discoverable. After a short time all these phenomena disappear, but the resistance at the circumscribed spot remains. The same state of things is repeated in various places until finally almost the entire abdomen has been attacked. The parietes are drawn in, flatulent knuckles of intestine may be here and there recognized, and between these we find cord-like fibrous thickenings with no fluid effusion; the diaphragm is pressed upward. After these individual attacks a stage ensues in which the process remains rather stationary, save that the symptoms of wasting, which had already set in, continue unchecked, and the disturbances in the function of digestion, the constipation, and the vomiting continue. Death may ultimately ensue in various ways, more particularly by the occurrence of tuberculosis in other organs.

The peculiarity of these cases is the acute way in which they begin, the fitful manner in which the process proceeds, and the absence of fluid effusion. But by no means all the cases which begin acutely present the characters just described; a well-marked effusion may become rapidly developed after a rigor, with considerable disturbance of the general health, and with or without tenderness of the abdomen; and this may be followed by a chronic stage.

The cases which form Kaulich's second group constitute the most general form in which abdominal tuberculosis occurs.

The commencement of the disease remains almost latent, the primary disturbances are so indistinct and trivial that the patients, as a rule, do not come under observation until they seek relief owing to increasing weakness or to the progressive distention of the abdomen. Pain in the abdomen is, as a rule, present, but only in a moderate degree, or it may be entirely absent, the principal complaint being a feeling of fulness and tenseness in the abdomen. Slight fever, occasional vomiting, and digestive disturbances exist, and constipation alternates with diarrhœa.

On. examination, the ascites is found to be the most prominent symptom ; the abdomen is considerably distended, in which the almost invariably coexisting meteorism plays an important part. We often see the tumors formed by the coils of intestine projecting in the upper part of the abdomen. Owing to the effusion and to the distention of the intestines, a dislocation of the thoracic organs and of the liver ensues, œdema of the lower extremities becomes developed, the veins of the abdominal parietes become distended, and the urinary secretion is but small. Tumors in the abdomen are sometimes perceived, but this is not always the case. The aspect of the patient becomes rapidly worse, if he have not been pale and emaciated from the outset; the cachectic aspect, however, is absent. On closer examination, we find, as a rule, that changes have already taken place in the apices of the lungs, which may increase with the further course of the disease, and may become associated with pleurisy and pericarditis. Night-sweats are sometimes present ; the pulse, as a rule, is small and rapid.

Sometimes considerable effusions of blood may take place into the peritoneal cavity, which may be indicated by symptoms of collapse.

Some of these cases are characterized by the fact that in the course of the disease a temporary subsidence of the general symptoms, with decrease of the effusion and an improvement in the general health, sets in for a longer or a shorter period. These cases form Kaulich's group No. 3.

A few examples of cases may suffice to illustrate the views deduced from many observations.

1. A girl, aged sixteen and one-half years, parents healthy, well nourished, gracefully formed; had previously had no disease but measles. In June, 1865, during menstruation, a sharp pain occurred in the abdomen, which quickly became diffused ; rigor, repeated vomiting, collapse. On examination shortly afterwards, there was found, in addition to the quickly disapppearing symptoms of collapse, general meteorism, great tenderness in the right inguinal region, with a circumscribed resistance without any definite dulness on percussion. In the course of a few days the patient had somewhat revived, the meteorism subsided, and a circumscribed peritonitis remained in the right inguinal region. The fever was moderate, and in the course of a week the local symptoms had considerably decreased. Then fever returned and the inflammatory affection lit up again, and quickly extended to the

level of the umbilicus. ·Periods of this kind, consisting in remission and relapse, were repeated several times, and the disease of the peritoneum extended gradually over the whole abdomen. In connection with this, no further distention of the abdomen occurred; the parietes remained tense, and place was afforded to the distended portions of intestine by the retraction of the lungs. After the course of two months the development of the process seemed to have come to an end, the feverish symptoms disappeared entirely, no spontaneous pain occurred, and the abdomen remained somewhat tender on pressure in some few resisting spots. A gradually increasing retraction of the parietes was then observed, while the position of the diaphragm remained the same; the abdominal parietes took scarcely any part in the respiratory movements. From the history just given, as well as from the almost completely unaltered position of the inflated coils of intestine observable through the attenuated parietes, the conclusion was drawn that a progressive gluing together and shrivelling of the peritoneal layers was taking place. Difficulty of defecation continued, with intercurrent attacks of vomiting and other disturbances of the digestive organs. In the course of November considerable fever set in afresh, and pleurisy, first of the left side and subsequently of the right, was discovered. There was cough with mucous expectoration and crepitating râles. In the beginning of December small quantities of tarry blood were passed, and this recurred in nearly every motion. Along with this there was pain at a circumscribed spot in the left hypogastrium, and after a short time it became possible to demonstrate an encysted collection of gas here, owing to a circumscribed, very elastic arching forward of the parietes, with a clear tympanic percussion sound. In the middle of December, the patient died after a second attack of rigor. On post-mortem examination there were found recent tuberculosis of the lungs, diffuse tuberculosis of the pleura, and a few tubercles in the pericardium. The parietal and visceral layers of the peritoneum were everywhere matted together, thickened, slaty gray, pigmented, and beset by countless firm miliary tubercles. The intestines formed a single, firmly united convolution, over which the omentum, considerably thickened and beset with numerous tubercles, was extended. A knuckle of small intestine had ulcerated on its mucous surface, at a point of bending, and its wall was perforated to the extent of the size of a pea, through which masses of fæces and intestinal gas had found exit and made a way through the adhesions and formed a mass larger than a closed fist. (Observed by Kaulich.)

2. A man aged thirty-four, previously healthy, with the exception of a skin eruption—parents healthy—took ill in the first week in May with a febrile rigor, after several days' feeling of weariness. Soon afterwards whitish, fluid stools occurred, and along with this eructation and loss of appetite. In the course of a few days the abdomen had become considerably swollen, without becoming painful. Œdema of the lower extremities came on quickly after this, and subsequently disappeared. This condition induced considerable emaciation within six weeks. On his admission into hospital on the 10th of June, anæmia, emaciation, and a palish brown discoloration of the face were observable. Tongue white and coated; dryness of the mouth and great thirst; bad appetite; no motions from the bowels

for two days; fever only occasionally present. Abdomen 85 ctms. in circumference at the level of the umbilicus; evident fluctuation on both sides; on the whole, soft; a somewhat resisting spot in the epigastrium; nowhere painful, either spontaneously or on pressure. Dull sound on percussion everywhere; for the space of four fingers' breadths below the umbilicus, there was a tympanitic note. Thoracic organs pressed upward. Urine normal; no albumen and no bile-pigment. Pulse 92—not very strong. The skin brownish, dry, wrinkled. In the course of the following six weeks, up to the time of patient's death, the subjective conditions, as also the diarrhœa, the distention of the abdomen, etc., were liable to variations. The resisting spot became more distinct and painful on pressure. During the last fourteen days there was frequent vomiting. On post-mortem examination, there were found tuberculosis of the pleuræ; caseous bronchial glands; and in the abdominal cavity a considerable quantity of clear, yellow serum. The entire peritoneum was marbled black and white. The great omentum formed a hard, knotty, rolled-up tumor along the course of the transverse colon, and, on section, it was found to be beset with masses of tubercle. All the intestines were united together, and formed a single, marbled mass. The peritoneal covering of the spleen was metamorphosed into a thick mass of effusion; this was true also of the investment of the liver; the liver itself was very small and atrophic; the kidneys were normal (Kyburg, l. c.).

3. A man, aged fifty-seven, came into the institution on the 22d of April, but had previously been under medical treatment, because he had felt so great weariness and want of energy; this debilitated condition had developed in the course of the previous winter. Two years previously the patient had been operated upon for a rectal fistula. He had suffered for a considerable time rather severely from cough; no hereditary history; the patient had always been in good circumstances.

The patient lies on his back; costal type of respiration; aspect of countenance not indicative of pain, but wrinkled; voice weak; face anæmic, pale gray; no jaundice; great emaciation; loss of substance of muscle; finger-nails pale, presenting a deep groove about ¼ ctm. from the quick. Sterno-cleido-mastoids somewhat prominent; the intervening depression very deep; the jugulars swell somewhat on expiration. The abdomen intensely distended, especially in the epigastric region; the umbilicus prominent and convex. On the left-hand side, a high position of the diaphragm; on the right, pleural effusion. The left lobe of the liver extends but slightly across the middle line. The apex of the right lung is more deeply placed than the left, sounds duller on percussion, and gives a weak bronchial expiration. On the left, a reducible hernia; testicle free; moderate œdema of the lower extremities. Abdomen hardly at all sensitive; when the patient lies on his back, the dependent parts are dull on percussion; when he lies on his right side, the fluid extends up to the umbilicus. Nothing can be definitely made out about the spleen; it does not appear to be particularly enlarged. No tumor, etc., to be felt in the abdomen. Small heart; weak, clear sounds; pulse 120—very small. Quantity of urine very small—about 200 c.c. in the twenty-four hours; sp. gr., 1022; dark, brownish red; neither albumen nor bile-pigment, but rich in indican. Stools frequent, thin, and clay-like. Appetite completely lost; repeated vomiting. Temperature slightly raised. Death after a few days.

On post-mortem examination the apex of the right lung was found adherent as far down as the third rib; below, an encysted pleural effusion; hide-like thickening of the pleura over the lower lobe; tissue of the lung itself somewhat cirrhotic. Left lung, in the actual apex only, somewhat cirrhotic. In the peritoneal cavity about four litres of yellowish brown, slightly turbid fluid. Omentum thickened, stretched, adherent to the anterior wall of the abdomen, and beset with hemorrhages; the same was true of the parietal peritoneum; between the hemorrhages whitish yellow and entirely white tubercles occur, varying in size from the head of a pin to a lentil. The intestinal serous membrane was similarly marbled. The intestine intensely inflated; a number of tubercular ulcers on the mucous membrane, one approaching to perforation. Spleen 14 by 9 ctms., rather firm. Covering of liver thickened with fibrinous deposition; substance of liver pale and fatty (Ziemssen's clinique).

By comparing a large number of cases many other variations in the form of the disease will be found, but the deviations, which actually occur from what may be laid down as the general forms, cannot be completely enumerated.

Amongst the various symptoms but a few require any further consideration.

The tenderness of the abdomen is in the majority of cases inconsiderable; occasionally it is completely absent, so that even firm pressure produces no sensation of pain. In other cases, particularly if the commencement be acute, the pain is sharp, either at a circumscribed spot, or diffused over the whole abdomen; sometimes pressure on any tumors that may be present, as, for example, the thickened omentum, gives pain; frequently there is a feeling of fulness and tenseness in the abdomen, particularly in cases where the course is very slow.

Effusion into the abdominal cavity is absent in but few cases; it generally occurs gradually, it often has a hemorrhagic admixture, and it may vary from a small to a very considerable amount. The tendency to hemorrhage is on the one hand dependent on an altered condition of the walls of the blood-vessels themselves, while, on the other, it is distinctly promoted by the stasis in individual vascular areas produced by the retraction of the connective tissue. During the course of the disease the quantity of the effusion may be subject to occasional increase and decrease, or it may, from first to last, continuously increase. A decrease of this kind in the effusion may arise in connection with a transient cessation of the process, or with an entirely different course of events, as, for example, as the result of profuse diarrhœa.

The fluid generally collects in the most dependent parts of the abdomen and is freely movable, while the intestines are either pushed upward or by the retraction of cicatrices are drawn upward and toward the vertebral column. Encysted masses of fluid, however, are sometimes found, and adhesions, particularly of the intestines with the anterior walls of the abdomen, may in many ways modify the condition of things just described. These adhesions to the anterior abdominal wall may sometimes be recognized, even in the presence of great quantities of effusion, while the thickening of the omentum and the callous membranes, being deeply placed, can with difficulty be discovered under these circumstances. On the other hand, when the quantity of the fluid is but trivial, we may feel the thickening and the new products just mentioned, and these, moreover, occur in every possible degree of development, from that of simply increased resistance to that of a nodulated tumor; the latter occurs more particularly in the epigastrium in a transverse direction, corresponding to the thickened, rolled-up omentum.

The meteorism is one of the most constant symptoms ; as a rule, it attains to a very considerable degree, and owing to the thinness and softness of the abdominal parietes, which so frequently coexist, the knuckles of intestine may be recognized externally. Owing to adhesions, the distensibility of particular portions of the intestine may be limited, and in cases of universal matting together of the visceral and parietal layers of the peritoneum, the distention of the abdominal walls may be prevented and the abdomen become retracted; in these cases the inflated intestines press the diaphragm upward.

Amongst the changes in the abdominal parietes which may be observed, considerable stress has been repeatedly laid on the inflammatory redness and œdema which is sometimes developed in the neighborhood of the umbilicus in the course of tuberculosis of the peritoneum. Vallin has particularly urged the importance of this symptom in peritoneal tuberculosis.[1] This inflammation may completely subside, or perforation may ensue as the result of suppuration, and the effusion empty outward. This symptom is not of any great importance, seeing that it is not frequent in tuberculosis of the peritoneum, and that it may occur not only in other forms of chronic peritonitis, but even in rare cases of simple ascites.

The fever during the entire course of the disease is in many cases very moderate, and periods occur during which the temperature remains perfectly normal. On this follows a series of greater and lesser exacerbations. In connection with this we may assume that the variations are partly connected with local processes of the peritoneum and the further extension of the disease. Occasionally excessive rises of temperature, even up to 40° C. (104° Fahr.), are observed, which, as a rule, are connected with the rapid development of complications—in particular, pleurisy and tuberculosis of the lungs. The pulse is uniformly quickened, but still not always very considerably so.

Course, Duration, Issue.—Tubercular peritonitis leads almost always to death, either through the progressive wasting incident to the disease itself, or owing to complications and resulting phenomena ; or lastly, tuberculosis of other organs, particularly of the lung, may be the actual cause of death. The cases which are recorded of recovery permit of a justifiable doubt as to the correctness of the diagnosis, and all the more so, as the existence of simple chronic peritonitis is disregarded by many. The course in the great majority of cases is chronic and extends to weeks and months.

The *prognosis* must be regarded as absolutely fatal.

The *diagnosis* of tubercular peritonitis is generally difficult, and must depend principally on the method of exclusion. As patients generally come under observation with ascites, and possibly also with œdema of the lower limbs, the first thing we have to determine is whether the effusion is not to be referred to simple stasis in the territory of the portal vein. As diseases of the heart,[2] lungs, and kidneys may, as a rule, be excluded with-

[1] Arch. gén. de méd. Mai. 1869.
[2] In a case of tuberculosis of the peritoneum (in Lindwurm's clinique) there was

out any difficulty, we have principally to deal with diseases of the liver, and most particularly cirrhosis. The phenomena which this disease presents are very similar to those of tuberculosis of the peritoneum, and if a secondary small size of the liver should be associated with this latter disease, they are almost identical. The following points may help to decide the question: in cirrhosis of the liver there is often a history of drink, while in tuberculosis some important etiological data may also be made out. In connection with this, great weight is to be attached to the occurrence of caseous masses, especially in the epididymis in the male, as well as in the lymphatic glands. The examination of the lungs is particularly important, as thereby simultaneous consolidation of the apices, progressive infiltration of the lungs, or pleural effusion may be discovered.

Further, in tuberculosis the abdomen is more frequently painful, particularly on pressure, than in cirrhosis; in the former we more frequently discover spots of increased resistance, or may recognize adhesions of the parietal and visceral layers of the serous membrane; a considerable enlargement of the spleen seldom occurs in tuberculosis, while it is frequent in cirrhosis. In patients suffering from cirrhosis of the liver there is no elevation of temperature, and seldom any quickening of the pulse, if we except transitory complications and the later stages of the disease. Both these symptoms are the rule in the course of tuberculosis. In tuberculosis vomiting occurs more frequently and more continuously than in cirrhosis. The stools, as well as the urine, present no distinctive characteristics between the two diseases; the stools in tuberculosis not unfrequently have a clay-like, yellow consistence. The appetite is generally much more affected in the peritoneal disease than in cirrhosis of the liver, and the wasting takes place more rapidly. As regards the appearance of the patient, in many cases some data may be afforded; in others, on the contrary, the difference is but slight. Finally, we must remember the collateral dilatation of the veins already mentioned, the occurrence of which is indicative of cir-

simultaneously tuberculosis of the pericardium and of the pleura, and during the entire course of the disease an intense cyanosis existed, which was a rare occurrence and rendered the diagnosis still more difficult.

rhosis of the liver. In doubtful cases we may have recourse to the exploring needle, the effusion in tubercular peritonitis being very often of a hemorrhagic character.

Thrombosis of the portal vein presents, as a rule, too distinct a form of disease to allow of its being readily mistaken for tubercular peritonitis. Stasis of the portal vein, on the other hand, from compression, may occasion difficulties; the marked jaundice which generally accompanies it must suggest the possibility of such an error. If tumors can be felt in the abdomen, as is the case if the effusion be either slight or absent, the question then is to distinguish the case from one of carcinoma of the peritoneum. The presence of a tumor in any other organ (for example, in the uterus) and the cancerous cachexy support the idea of carcinoma, as do also certain characters in the tumors themselves, the cancerous tumors being much more extensive and particularly rapid in their growth. The irritation phenomena in the peritoneum are, as a rule, but trivial in the case of carcinoma, and the course of the disease is almost altogether apyrexial.

The distinction between tubercular peritonitis and simple chronic peritonitis often cannot be made from the objective phenomena alone, and occasionally it cannot at all be established with certainty. In addition to the mode of origin and to the etiological conditions which favor the idea of tuberculosis, some distinctive points appear during the course of the disease. The absolute distinction between the two processes is all the more difficult, as, according to Aran's statement, a simple chronic peritonitis may occur in tubercular individuals.

In Kaulich's work a case is recorded in which the partial sacculation of fluid by means of firm membranes produced phenomena which gave rise to a similarity to an ovarian cyst.

The *treatment* can only be symptomatic; it should aim at making the condition of the patient as tolerable as possible, and preserving the strength in the most feasible manner. The proper nourishment of the patient, with the conditions which are generally present, is a matter of great difficulty, and it is scarcely possible to lay down general rules upon the subject.

The attempt to reduce the ascites by means of diuretics will scarcely have any effect, as, further, the majority of remedies will scarcely be borne on account of their producing disturb- ances of the stomach. It is more justifiable to attempt to reduce the effusion by means of diaphoresis, by warm baths, by Turkish baths, particularly when irritative symptoms of the serous mem- brane are absent. If the effusion become very excessive, and life be thereby threatened, puncture is the only means left. We must not, however, undertake this operation without very ur- gent cause, as the fluid frequently accumulates again, with renewal of the inflammatory irritation, and increased danger of considerable hemorrhage into the cavity of the peritoneum.

New Formations of the Peritoneum and Carcinomatous Peritonitis.

Morgagni, De sedibus et causis morh. Venet. 1761. Ep. XXXVIII.—*Sachtleben*, Klinik der Wassersucht. Danzig, 1795.—*Otto*, Selt. Beobacht. 1816. Bd. I.— *Bressler*, Krankh. des Unterleibs. 1836.—*Lebert*, Traité prat. des mal. canc. Paris, 1851.—*Koehler*, Krebs- u. Scheinkrebskrankh. des Menschen. 1853.— *Clar*, Oest. Zeitschr. für Kinderheilk. 1855.—*Demme*, Ueber Carcinosis acuta miliaris. Schweizer Monatsschr. III. S. 161. Jahrg. 1858.—*Bamberger*, Oesterr. Zeitsch. für prakt. Heilkunde. 1857. III.—*Seidel*, Ein frei in der Bauchhöhle gefundener Fremdkörper. Deutsche Klinik. 1863. 17.—*Joh. Erichsen*, Virchow's Archiv. XXI. S. 465.—*Habershon*, Med. chirurg. Transact. XLIII.—*Sanderson*, Canc. Tumor Compress. the Cœliac Axis and Simulating Aneur. Trans. of the Path. Soc. XVIII. 149.—*Colin*, Cancer encéph. du périt. à marche aiguë. Gaz. hebd. 45. 1868.—*P. Eve*, Case of Ext. Colloid Cancer Devel. in the Connect. Tissue of the Perit. New Orleans Journ. of Med. Oct. 712. 1868.—*Loomis*, Cancer of Mesent. Med. and Surg. Rep. 11. 1868.—*Ogle*, Cases of Abdominal Tumors. Med. Press and Circ. Sept. 9, 1868.—*Spencer Wells*, Fatty Tumor of Mesent. Remov. during Life. Trans. of the Path. Soc. XIX. p. 243.—*J. Cooper Forster*, Fibro-fatty Tum. of the Abdom., Weighing Fifty-Five Pounds. Ibid.— *H. Scherenberg*, Enormer Echinococcus des Netzes u. s. w. Virchow's Archiv. Bd. 46. 392.—*Cayley*, Cystic Colloid Dis. of the Ov. Assoc. with Colloid Dis- ease of the Perit. Trans. of the Path. Soc. Lond. XIX.—*E. Neumann*, Ein Fall von Retroperitonealabscess mit amyl. Deg. der Unterleibsorgane und secund. Sarkombildung in den Abscesswänden und im Perit. Arch. der Heilk. X. 221. —*G. Rippmann*, Eine seröse Cyste in der Bauchhöhle mit einem Inhalte von 50 Liter Flüssigkeit vom Urachus ausg. Deutsche Klinik. 1870. 29.—*Murchison*, Notes of Beds., Remarks on the Diag. and Treatment of an Abd. Tumor. Lan- cet. July, 1870.—*H. Barck*, Echinococcus-Cyste der Bauchwand. Deutsch. Arch. für klin. Mediz. VII. 614.—*Engel-Reimers*, Zwei Fälle von Krebs-

impfung in Punktionskanälen bei carcinomat. Perit. Arch. für pathol. Anat.
Bd. 51. H. 3.—*Dolbeau*, Tum. de l'abd., Ascite sympt. d'une périt. chronique.
Gaz. des hôp. No. 68. 1866.—*Chwostek*, Prim. Scirrhus des Bauchfelles. Oesterr.
Zeitschr. für prakt. Heilk. No. 39. 1866; und ein Fall von Echinococcus des
Perit. Ibid. No. 38.—*Ritter*, Myxom des Perit. mit Bildung von cyst. Hohl-
räumen und Gasentwicklung in denselben. Virch. Arch. Bd. 36. 591.—*Da
Costa*, Clinic. Lect. on Spurious or Phant. Tumors of the Abdom. Phil. Med.
Times. 1871. Sept.—*Garreau*, Tum. canc. du Més. Gaz. méd. de l'Algérie.
1871. No. 3.—*F. S. Bristowe*, Perit. Cancer. Trans. of the Path. Soc. XXI.
193.—*J. M. Duncan*, Cases of Malig. Perit. Med. Times and Gaz. Oct., 1872.—
Th. Petrina, Ueber Carcinoma Perit. Prager Viertelj. 1872. II. 41.

Many of the tumors occurring in the peritoneum are devoid
of much clinical interest, as, for example, the majority of lipomata; as, also, free bodies in the abdominal cavity, which, for the
most part, arise from the separation of fatty tumors by constriction.   The same is true of the smaller serous and colloid cysts.
In rare cases dermoid cysts and very extensive serous cysts have
been observed.

Echinococcus occurs independently in the peritoneum, in the
omentum, and in every part of the serous membrane, both parietal and visceral.   It may lead to enormous distention of the
abdomen.

Connective-tissue tumors are rare, still fibroids occur.   Myxoma of the peritoneum has further been observed.   Ritter has
described a case of myxoma cystoides with development of gas.

The abdomen was in all directions considerably distended, and in every position
retained the same round form, convex forward with uniformly smooth surface;
distinct fluctuation was present, but no tumor was to be felt.   On puncturing, 4900
c.c. of a thick reddish fluid were drawn off; this had an alkaline reaction, coagulated almost entirely, and had a specific gravity of 1018.   Moreover, white flakes
were floating in it.   On microscopical examination blood and pus-corpuscles, (?) numerous colloid granules, and coarsely granulated cells were found.   Tyrosin and leucin were found in it in great quantities.   After the tapping, physical examination
continued to give negative results.   Three weeks later a second puncture was made,
and 1700 c.c. of a very thickly fluid flocculent material were drawn off.   On post-
mortem examination a large sac, measuring about a foot in its long diameter, was
found attached to the parietes in front, which completely covered the other contents of the abdomen.   On opening this a great quantity of badly smelling air and
a grayish red turbid fluid gushed out.   The anterior wall of this cyst was about
1-1½ ctm. thick, and consisted principally of tense, firm connective tissue, and was

lined interiorly by a thin, whitish layer of detritus, which was readily torn off. The peritoneum was so firmly united to this wall that on section the border of each part could not be recognized. The entire intestines were drawn upward and backward, and were firmly adherent to the posterior wall of the abdominal cavity.

The cavity, which occupied the greater portion of the tumor, contained, in addition to the caseous and fluid materials which escaped on opening into it, a considerable quantity of colloid, partly light brown, partly transparent, partly light opaque masses, which on the upper wall formed a distinct large mass, and projected free into the cavity, but which for the most part was attached to the inner surface of the cyst as small beads, sometimes attaining the size of a bean; lastly, identically similar masses were found embedded in the walls of the cyst, and on section the cut surfaces swelled up into a semiglobular form over the surrounding connective tissue. The consistence was that of about half-fluid gelatine. These cavities lay generally very closely together, so that, as a general rule, there was an alveolar arrangement of the supporting connective tissue. The individual cavities were rarely found to communicate one with another.

The ground substance proved to be colorless, with but few fat-globules, and coagulated on the addition of acetic acid, but not on boiling; further, there were numerous elastic fibres.

Carcinoma of the peritoneum is in the majority of cases secondary, being either the extension of a new growth from one of the abdominal organs or from the retroperitoneal glands, or representing a metastasis from some other organ. Amongst the forty cases observed by Petrina fourteen were primary, and Bamberger saw but one instance amongst fourteen of primary carcinoma of the peritoneum.[1]

As regards etiological conditions no definitely established data exist. In cases of primary peritoneal cancer some previous injury is laid down as the cause of its occurrence, but we must accept all statements of the kind as very doubtful.

Carcinoma attacking the peritoneum is particularly apt to occur as secondary to cancer of the stomach and intestines, and also of the liver, the genital organs, and the retroperitoneal glands, in which case the disease may spread either by mere extension or by metastasis; and it may further arise by metastasis as secondary to cancer of the œsophagus and breast.

[1] On account of the absence of any true epithelium in the peritoneal cavity, *Klebs* considers it possible that an infection of the peritoneum may result from epithelial elements, without, however, carcinoma having been actually developed in those organs from which the epithelium is derived. *Vide* Kundrat, l. c.

Chronic peritonitis is thought by some to be a sufficient exciting cause for the development of peritoneal carcinoma, both where a new growth exists in some other organ, and even where no such growth exists. The former is possible, the latter, to say the least, is improbable; it is more natural to believe that in any case of the kind the first symptoms of irritation in the peritoneum are connected with the development of the new formation.

Peritoneal cancer is much more frequently met with as a disease of later life, between the ages forty and seventy ; still it has been known to occur in individual cases in childhood or even in fœtal life.

The forty cases reported by Petrina occurred as follows :

						Male.	Female.
Between 10 and 20 years of age						—	1
"	20	"	30	"		1	2
"	30	"	40	"		—	2
"	40	"	50	"		6	2
"	50	"	60	"		4	7
"	60	"	70	"		3	7
"	70	"	80	"		2	3
						16	24

This ratio between the numbers of males and females accords with the results of other collections of cases, and serves to show the generally established preponderance in the case of females.

In rare cases cancer of the peritoneum occurs acutely, as miliary carcinosis, but, as a rule, the new formation is developed slowly, and may occur as enormous masses, or it may metamorphose the peritoneum into a thick, hide-like structure—a mass of carcinomatous infiltration.

In miliary carcinosis the serous membrane is beset with numerous grayish yellow or white nodules, which much resemble tubercular deposits.

The usual form in the chronic course of the disease is carcinoma vulgare, sometimes melanotic cancer, occasionally also colloid cancer, which latter forms very considerable masses. In Eve's case the omentum weighed about 50 lbs., and a tumor has been described in the Boston Med. and Surg. Journ. which weighed 114 lbs. In cases where the new formation grows rapidly the serous membrane may remain without any evidence of reaction, so far as the naked eye can ascertain. In the more chronic course the individual nodules show a depression in the middle, and we may discover a cicatricial contraction of the peritoneum in the neighborhood. In slow development of the new formation, the peritoneum is always considerably thickened, there are general adhesions, and the mesentery, and more particularly the omentum, become shrivelled into hard, cord-like masses.

With the development of the new formation, there generally occurs a more or less considerable effusion into the abdominal cavity. This may present various characters, according to the varied intensity of the irritation and inflammation of the serous membrane, and according to the nature of the new formation; it may, moreover, be hemorrhagic. In addition to the peritoneal, hide-like structures, the new formation may attack the serous investment of an abdominal organ, whereby the organ may become completely encapsuled, and occasionally is destroyed. Jaundice and compression of the portal vein may arise in this manner (namely, by carcinoma of the glands in the porta of the liver).

The intestine may become bent and compressed; in addition to which, the mucous membrane may frequently be in a state of chronic catarrh, and its walls thickened and œdematous. By the breaking down of the cancerous masses, perforations in various directions may ensue.

Symptoms.—Acute miliary carcinosis may somewhat rapidly prove fatal under symptoms of moderate fever and disturbance of consciousness, together with slight effusion into the abdominal cavity. The actual significance of this set of symptoms is naturally a very difficult matter to ascertain during life, if the conditions do not occur as secondary to some previously recognized disease. When the development of the new formation in the serous membrane proceeds in a chronic manner, as when cancer of an abdominal organ extends to the peritoneum, the interpretation of the symptoms is often a matter of no great difficulty. When, also, deposits become developed metastatically, the existence of the primary carcinoma suggests the actual connection between the two. In these cases the phenomena of carcinoma of

the stomach or intestine, or even of the uterus or the breast, etc.,
will have existed for a long time, and then an effusion of fluid into
the abdominal cavity takes place; the abdomen may become
sensitive; not unfrequently severe colicky pains set in; there
occur disturbances in the function of the intestine; constipation
and vomiting either make their appearance, or increase; it may
be possible to recognize a certain hardness or an actual tumor in
various parts of the abdomen; the abdomen itself becomes distended, often unsymmetrically, and frequently an occasional
peritoneal friction may be heard or felt. In connection with this
there are well-marked evidences of cancerous cachexy and excessive anæmia, and these rapidly increase with the rapid development of peritoneal carcinosis. Occasionally the peritoneal effusion may diffuse itself more acutely, which may be indicated by
tenderness on pressure, slight fever, frequent vomiting, etc. The
patients die of wasting, or owing to the occurrence of complications.

It is, as a rule, a much more difficult thing to recognize the
state of affairs if the carcinoma in the peritoneum be primary, or
if the new formation extend from the retroperitoneal glands,
and if masses of cancer become early deposited in the peritoneum, before the lymphatic glands have developed into large
tumors. This state of things is, according to my experience,
very common. Cancer of the liver may also remain latent for a
very long time, owing to the position of the nodules, and thus
the secondary affection of the serous membrane may be the first
to produce any distinct symptoms.

Cases of this kind have a prodromal stage, which can in no
way be distinguished from that of tuberculosis of the peritoneum, or even from that of simple chronic peritonitis. Here
also, in most cases, the formation of ascites occurs in connection
with ill-defined symptoms. The examination of the abdomen by
no means universally affords unequivocal results, and even if
tumors be actually discovered, there is nothing definite to distinguish them from tubercular infiltration of the folds of serous
membrane or from inflammatory adhesions. Under such circumstances, the rapid wasting and the cancerous cachexy, and also
perhaps the swelling of the lymphatic glands, must suffice to

decide the question. The fluid effusion may, however, be so considerable that it is impossible to feel any tumor in the abdomen. In other cases the rapid growth and spread of the tumors, and the existence of numerous irregular bodies, afford definite data.

Pain of varying intensity is a frequent symptom in the course of the disease; it generally occurs in a paroxysmal manner, and may at times be altogether absent. It is partly dependent on the development of the carcinoma, and partly on the accompanying peritonitis, and finally, the alteration in the intestine and the obstruction to the motion of its contents connected therewith may have something to do with it. Pain in these cases occurs more frequently spontaneously, whereas tenderness on pressure may be entirely absent.

Vomiting is often observed, particularly in the later stages of the disease.

The effusion of free fluid into the peritoneal cavity is seldom absent; it is developed with varying rapidity, and is to be regarded partly as the product of peritoneal irritation, and partly as the result of stasis in the larger and smaller vessels, while it is further promoted by the hydræmia which occurs. The quantity of effusion may vary from a few ounces up to twenty pounds, the average quantity being from six to ten pounds (Petrina).

Meteorism and constipation are likewise frequent symptoms; diarrhœa not unfrequently appears in the later stages; if stenosis of the intestine occur, the symptoms of obstruction make their appearance.

Fever only occurs occasionally during the course of a chronic abdominal carcinosis, when an exacerbation of the peritonitis takes place, and also in cases of sudden, rapid extension of the new growth.

Hemorrhages into the abdominal cavity may in some cases be so considerable as to induce the most extreme anæmia and collapse.

The course of the slowly-growing peritoneal carcinoma extends, as a rule, over months; at any time, however, a fatal issue may be brought about by such complications as peritonitis, perforation, or hemorrhage. A fatal issue is the result in every case.

The diagnosis is seldom beset with any particular difficulty in secondary carcinoma of the peritoneum. In those cases, on the other hand, in which the primary carcinoma has remained latent, as well as where the peritoneal carcinoma is primary, the diagnosis may present considerable difficulties. As far as the distinction from simple stasis of the portal vein is concerned, everything that was mentioned in connection with tubercular peritonitis holds good here. The principal difficulty, however, consists in distinguishing it from tubercular peritonitis, so long as the cancerous masses do not assume the form of unequivocal tumors. Disease and retraction of the omentum occur in both instances. In such cases we must rely on the cancerous cachexy on the one hand, and on the presence of tuberculosis or caseous masses in other organs on the other, on the absence of remissions in the course of the cancerous disease, on the almost uniformly apyrexial course of carcinosis, and on the occasional swelling of the lymphatic glands. In addition to this, the urine in carcinoma is throughout very poor in coloring matter, being of a pale yellow color and of low specific gravity.

Such complications as intense jaundice or tuberculosis of the lungs may greatly increase the difficulty of the diagnosis.

The *treatment* can only be symptomatic. As regards puncture, it must be remarked that the fatal issue may be thereby considerably hastened; we must therefore have recourse to it only when it is urgently demanded.

Ascites.

Serous transudation into the peritoneal cavity occurs as a part of general dropsy, or it may result from stasis in the territories of abdominal vessels, particularly the portal vein. In children, also, slight serous effusions into the peritoneal cavity are rather common, and occur likewise in the course of acute diseases.

Formerly, in addition to these secondary effusions into the abdominal cavity, the existence of an idiopathic ascites was believed in, and even nowadays the possibility of such an occurrence is upheld by many observers. The fact is, that in very rare instances effusions into the abdominal cavity come under observation, for which no explanation can be discovered, either in their being a part of a general dropsy or occasioned by local stasis. The changes also in the serous membrane itself are so slight as to cause some hesitation in referring their genesis to inflammatory processes. The alterations which are discovered in cases of the kind consist in turbidity and thickening of the endothelium, thickening of the subserous tissue, and fatty degeneration of the endothelium. On the other hand, there are no new connective-tissue products and no deposition of fibrin. These alterations differ certainly but little from those which may become developed in secondary ascites as the result of stasis in the tissue of the serous membrane. The question is therefore this, whether the same alterations may not arise from chronic inflammatory processes in the serous membrane, which afterwards lead to a serous transudation through degeneration of the endothelium and the alteration in the lymphatic and bloodvessels.

I consider it more probable that these processes are inflammatory, as, amongst other things, the clinical phenomena are in favor of this view (*vide* Chronic Peritonitis).

As serous transudations into the abdominal cavity are always to be regarded as secondary processes, it is not practicable to give an exhaustive account of ascites here, and all the less so, as the effusions present quite important varieties according to the nature of their producing cause. Thus chemical and physical varieties in peritoneal transudations are observed. The color may be dark brown, as in cirrhosis of the liver, or light yellow, and even as clear as water, in chronic fatty degeneration of the kidneys. Between these all possible degrees exist. The quantity of solid constituents and the amount of albumen is from one to five per cent., and appears to increase with the length of time the effusion has existed. The fluid presents generally a somewhat viscid consistence, and frequently contains fibrinogen. All the constituents in it occur also in blood-serum, but in different proportions. Naunyn has found the ascitic fluid very poor in albumen in cases of amyloid degeneration of the abdominal glands, where the vessels of the serous membrane itself were in a state of amyloid degeneration.

The facts just alluded to, as well as the investigations made by Hoppe and C. Schmidt, tend to prove that in transudations in general the process is not one of simple filtration of serum out of the blood-vessels, that, in fact, the composition of the blood and the pressure in the venous radicles are not the sole determining factors. Hence, in the peritoneum, some part in the formation and composition of the transudation must be ascribed to the endothelium and to the lymphatic vessels, although we have been unable to discover the exact modus operandi.

DISEASES OF THE SPLEEN.

MOSLER.

DISEASES OF THE SPLEEN.

Introduction.

Recent general treatises: *C. F. Heusinger*, Betrachtungen und Erfahrungen über die Entzündung und Vergrösserung der Milz. Eisenach, 1820. Nachträge zu den Betrachtungen, etc. Eisenach, 1823. Ueber den Bau und die Verrichtungen der Milz. Eisenach, 1824.—*S. L. Steinheim*, Doctrina veterum de liene, etc. Hamburg, 1833.—*P. A. Piorry*, Mémoire sur l'état de la rate dans les fièvres intermittentes. Paris, 1833. Ueber die Krankheiten der Milz, die Wechselfieber u. s. w. Aus dem Franzos. von G. Krupp. Leipzig, 1847.—*Giesker*, Splenologie. I. Abth. Zürich, 1835.—*Naumann*, Medic. Klinik. Bd. V. S. 508.—*C. B. Heinrich*, Die Krankheiten der Milz. Leipzig, 1847.—*Virchow*, Medic. Zeitung. 1846. Nr. 34-36. Sein Archiv. 1853. V. S. 43. Krankhafte Geschwülste. II. Band. Berlin, 1864-1865.—*Wilhelm Mueller*, Ueber den feineren Bau der Milz. Leipzig u. Heidelberg, 1864.—*Billroth*, Virchow's Archiv. XX. XXIII.—*Bamberger*, in Virchow's Spec. Path. u. Therapie, Krankheiten des chylopoëtischen Systems. S. 597. Erlangen, 1864.—*Mosler*, Die Pathologie und Therapie der Leukämie. Berlin, 1872.

Physicians and naturalists have directed their attention to diseases of the spleen from the most ancient times; in the writings of the school of Hippocrates, Aretæus, Galen, Ætius of Amida, Alexander of Tralles, and others, numerous communications are to be found. The knowledge of the ancients upon this subject has been carefully collected by Steinheim and Naumann.

The old Grecian school has sketched a picture of splenopathy which even to-day one often encounters. It does not conform very accurately to the truth, since at that time any views which might be held as to the function of the spleen were entirely erroneous, and autopsies were undertaken very seldom and with preconceived ideas. The ignorance of physical diagnosis has

been the occasion of many errors. Diseases of the lungs and
heart were especially often confounded with those of the spleen ;
inflammation of the spleen, as well as of the liver, was preferably
diagnosticated, when one had to deal with pleurisy, pericarditis,
and other diseases of an entirely different character; besides this,
they did not know how to separate primary and secondary affections of the spleen from each other. Hippocrates, Celsus, Paulus
Aegineta, ascribed to the enlarged spleen, " lien magnus," bad-
smelling breath, spongy gums, bleeding from various parts, and
lax, badly healing ulcers.

The thorough investigation of diseases of the spleen was first
made possible by the powerful impulse which medical science
received from physiology and pathological anatomy, but for all
this, the questions relating to this subject still present special
difficulties. First of all, it is not easy to limit the field of the
pathology and therapeutics of diseases of the spleen ; so far as
the present position of medicine permits, I will endeavor to be
accurate in the task allotted to me.

Instead of a general historical introduction, I propose, with
each particular form of disease, to mention by name the contributions of earlier authors.

Anatomical and Pathological Remarks.

In order to understand the pathological processes of the
spleen, which, as is well known, represents a blood-gland without an excretory duct, an accurate knowledge of its anatomical
position, as well as of its finer structure, is requisite. With what
difficulty this organ is accessible to methods of physical examination is a matter of every-day experience. In a healthy condition,
it can be found only by means of percussion. In order to be able
to feel the spleen in front of the curvature of the ribs, it must be
considerably enlarged. It lies deep in the left hypochondrium,
behind the great cul-de-sac of the stomach, to which it is attached
by the gastro-splenic omentum. The cavity in which it is here
situated is formed above by the concavity of the diaphragm ;
backward and outward by the concave arch of the ninth, tenth,
and eleventh ribs ; inward by the convex arch of the cul-de-sac of

the stomach; downward and forward by an extension of the transverse mesocolon. These are all elastic, movable parts, and, as a consequence of this, considerable increase in the size of the spleen takes place with much greater ease. No parenchymatous organ of the human body is subject to such striking changes in size and weight as the spleen; it changes its volume several times a day.

In spite of the great zeal which has long been bestowed upon topographical anatomy, the more accurate relations of the normal position of the spleen remained somewhat obscure, until Von Luschka furnished us with trustworty results by means of the method lately employed by him, for which we owe him special thanks. The importance of the subject justifies me in repeating in this place the statements as to the size, weight and position of the spleen, contained in v. Luschka's excellent work on the Position of the Abdominal Organs, page 29.

The size and the weight of the spleen vary within no narrow limits, according to age, individuality, and manner of living. In childhood it is comparatively larger, and especially inclined to temporary enlargement. A reduction in size occurs normally in advanced age as atrophia senilis; in middle life, the healthy spleen is, on an average, not reckoning the curvatures, 12 ctms. long; at the widest part, 7$\frac{7}{10}$ ctms. wide, with a maximum thickness of 3 ctms. The absolute weight of the spleen amounts on the average to seven ounces, but may reach ten ounces without the occurrence of any abnormal condition, either of the organ itself, or of the system in general.

The spleen is situated entirely in the left hypochondrium, where it is so packed in between the diaphragm, the kidneys, and the posterior surface of the stomach, that it is not seen at all from the front until the stomach is pushed out of the way; it forms a part of the contents of the left vault of the diaphragm. The relation of the spleen to the left kidney is such that it surrounds it from its upper end to near the middle of its lateral border, and at the same time comes in contact with the supra-renal capsule and the tail of the pancreas, which passes along the lower border of the latter. In the normal condition the spleen takes up such an oblique position that it follows the course of the ninth, tenth, and eleventh ribs, and its upper end lies sometimes close by the body of the eleventh dorsal vertebra, or is sometimes 2 ctms. from it. The lower extremity of the spleen is distant from the point of the tenth rib 7.5 ctms., from that of the eleventh rib, on an average, 4 ctms., so that the organ, in its normal position and size, does not pass farther towards the median plane than the costo-articular line drawn from the left sterno-clavicular articulation to the point of the eleventh rib.

In describing the structure of the spleen, we will begin with its capsule. This is formed of a white, fibrous membrane, which receives a serous investment from the peritoneum, and sends very numerous processes into the interior of the proper tissue of the spleen. These branch in various directions, and are connected with each other, so that a close net-work is formed. In man the fibrous capsule, together with the trabeculæ just described, consists of connective tissue with elastic fibres. If hardened preparations are washed out with a fine brush, an exceedingly fine net-work may be demonstrated, consisting of fibres connecting with each other, which are to be looked upon as the finest ramifications of the trabeculæ, which are constantly becoming more and more delicate. These are formed of a network of connective-tissue corpuscles, in which the formation of lymph-cells takes place by division of the mother-cells.

The spaces of this beautiful net-work (reticulum, Billroth) are filled with the numerous vessels and nerves, as well as with the various cells of the spleen. The contents may be pressed out of the spleen as a paste, and are therefore called the splenic pulp.

The extraordinary development of the splenic artery (a branch of the cœliac axis) has a special interest for pathologists ; not only are its coats unusually thick, but it is remarkable that the calibre of this artery, in comparison with the size of the blood-gland which it supplies, is greater than in any other organ of the human body, except, perhaps, the thyroid gland. This unusual capacity explains the frequent occurrence of hemorrhagic infarctions of the spleen. The splenic vein is also remarkable for its uncommon size. It appears from the observations of Haller, Wintringham, and Giesker, that the calibre of the splenic vein increases in a striking degree with years—in adults up to five times the circumference of the artery. This fact may be explained on purely mechanical grounds, by the considerable dilatation which this fine and thin-walled vein undergoes whenever digestion is going on, and especially with every congestive condition of the spleen.

The interior of the spleen is separated by its blood-vessels into tolerably regular divisions. The pathological anatomist gets a clear view of this in certain peculiarly limited affections of the spleen.

The independence of the single vascular districts can be proved by injection after the manner of Billroth, since from one arterial branch only a corresponding part of the spleen can be filled. The last kind of distribution of the splenic arteries is formed by the so-called penicilli ; each penicillus, with the corresponding veins, forms a closed and independent vascular system. Thus the spleen is divided into a number of separate parts, or, so to speak, lobes and lobules. The lobular form becomes apparent chiefly when the spleen is enlarged.

In near relation to the finest arterial branches stand the splenic corpuscles, splenic vesicles, or Malpighian vesicles. On section of the spleen, these can generally be perceived, even with the naked eye, as round, white bodies. They have an average size of a sixth of a line. On a more careful examination, it can be seen that these are situated on the smallest arterial branches, like berries. They appear like a thickening of the connective-tissue coat of the arteries. In their interior they contain lymph-cells of various sizes, imbedded in a fine, fibrous net-work, and also, like the follicles of the lymph-gland, a delicate capillary net-work.

In order to understand many pathological processes of the spleen, these prominent points must be borne in mind : that the splenic arteries branch according to the anatomical arrangement just described ; that they support the berry-like appendages, the Malpighian corpuscles, and finally break up into tufts of very fine branches, the so-called penicilli, which then pass into the true capillaries. According to Billroth's investigations, the capillaries are in direct communication with the veins, and pass, usually at right angles, into the veins of the cavernus sinus. Billroth named the structure which Grobe, Beer, and Key call splenic canals, cavernous splenic vein-sinuses, in order to distinguish them from other splenic veins which possess a peculiar structure.

Wilhelm Mueller has arrived at other results from his investigations, which were made upon a large number of species from all classes of vertebrates. He separates two constituents of the splenic parenchyma—one whitish, connected with the various parts of the arterial system, which he calls the parenchyma of the arterial sheath ; and another, brownish red, rich in blood— the true pulp. The first parenchyma has the structure of the follicular apparatus of the intestine—in particular, the so-called conglomerate glandular substance. The pulp, on the contrary, which fills uniformly the interior of the capsule and the inter-spaces of the trabeculæ, is formed of cells which correspond with the lymph-corpuscles. Instead of the venous sinus of Billroth, Mueller supposes an " intermediate blood-channel " of the pulp —a system interposed between the capillary vessels and the com-mencement of the veins, in which the blood moves in channels without walls. From the intermediate channels the blood is again collected into the broken beginnings of the venous system, since the walls of the venous radicles proceed from the pulp-tissue, and thus the blood comes into many and close relations with the anatomical elements of the pulp.

On the basis of his anatomical investigations, Wilhelm Muel-ler ascribes to the spleen the function of constantly carrying on a new formation of colorless blood-corpuscles, and steadily supply-ing them to the current of blood. He compares the structure of the spleen to that of the lymphatic gland, in which the lymph-stream is replaced by the blood-stream, the vasa afferentia and efferentia by the arteries and veins.

An excellent authority, Max Schultze, after seeing, in Jena, Wilhelm Mueller's large collection of natural and artificial injec-tions of the spleens of various animals, has recognized Mueller's view as the correct one, that the blood in the red splenic pulp, instead of flowing in closed capillaries, finds its way in the spongy connective substance just as the lymph does in the lymph-glands.

Besides this anatomical foundation, the view that the spleen is a place for the formation of colorless blood-corpuscles is sup-ported by a great number of physiological experiments as well as pathological facts. Our knowledge of the influence of the spleen upon the constitution of the blood has been materially advanced by Virchow's discovery of splenic leucocythemia. It fully con-firms the changes which have been found in the normal blood of the splenic vein. It has been often proved that the blood of the splenic vein contains a great excess of colorless cells.

In order to understand the other functions of the spleen, the experiment of its extirpation has often been made upon animals by Dupuytren, A. S. Schultze, Bardeleben, Czermak, Hyrtl, Fuehrer and Ludwig, Gerlach, M. Schiff, Lusanna, and others, and the most various results have been observed. Lately I have turned my attention to the same subject, in my monograph upon leucocythemia; my numerous experiments are carefully described and all the earlier views considered. I will content myself with communicating the conclusions from my experiments in the following propositions:

I. The spleen is *not* absolutely necessary for the life of the animal.

II. After extirpation, as well as after artificially induced atrophy of the spleen, its function is assumed by the other lymphatic glands. The osseous marrow appears to have played an important rôle. Striking changes were found in it a long time after extirpation of the spleen, just as in leucocythemia.

III. The vicarious activity of these lymphatic organs, which appears to be dependent upon many external influences, is not always a complete one, since, especially in the first months after extirpation or artificially induced atrophy of the spleen, a changed constitution of the blood is found. An immediate influence of the spleen upon the formation of the blood may, therefore, be supposed, and in particular on the new formation of white as well as of red blood-corpuscles.

IV. The spleen exercises no influence upon gastric and pancreatic digestion ; the voracity of animals deprived of their spleen, which, together with chemical analysis, has been assumed as proof of such influence, does not exist as a constant symptom.

Etiology of Diseases of the Spleen in General.

It is desirable to be able to begin the etiology of diseases with accurate data in regard to their geographical distribution. The historico-geographical pathology of Prof. A. Hirsch testifies that we have as yet little information in this direction concerning diseases of the spleen. The geography of splenic diseases, as a whole, is there treated from three points of view ; the following data are chiefly taken from this work.

This distinguished observer correctly remarks that the geography of splenic diseases is only of interest so far as they occur in the form of acute or chronic tumor of the spleen as a concomitant or consecutive disease of malarial fever ; or, independently of this, are more or less widely distributed in the form of idiopathic malarial affections in all the regions where malarial fevers prevail to a great extent. The geographical distribution of this most frequent form of splenic affection coincides pretty accurately with the occurrence of malarial fevers. The severity and extent of the two classes of affection everywhere correspond, and therefore the interest which physicians take in diseases of the spleen usually varies with their place of residence.

In the great swampy regions of tropical and subtropical countries, especially in nearer and farther India, we find tumors of the spleen in their highest development. Similar reports in regard to its endemic occurrence come from the Indian Archipelago, from Arabia and Egypt, from the islands on the east coast of Africa, from the west coast of Africa, from Algiers, Brazil, Cayenne, Central America, etc. Tumors of the spleen arising from malaria form an important feature in the statistics of disease in regions with only a warm climate—as along the coast of Syria, in Turkey, in Greece, the Danubian lowlands of Hungary, in Moldavia, and in Italy. We know in particular of Italy, whose climate has undergone no essential variations in the course of time—where the same Lombard and Pontine Marshes, which long ago wrought destruction, still engender malaria and intermittent fever, that diseases of the spleen were frequently observed by the Roman physicians, perhaps even more frequently than at the present day. Plautus describes admirably the sufferings arising from hypertrophy of the spleen, Celsus and Scribonius Largus mention a large number of medicines and compounds "ad lienosos."

Even in higher degrees of latitude, especially in the marshy districts of France and the Netherlands—the low-lying plains of Germany and Russia, the occurrence of diseases of the spleen may fairly be called endemic. In order to form an opinion upon the extent of their distribution, we are here referred to the numerous reports upon the endemic and epidemic prevalence of malarial fever. In these, tumors of the spleen are everywhere referred to as more or less permanent remains of that fever, and as the source of the dropsies so frequent there.

Climate. Weather. Condition of the Soil.

The influence which climate, weather, and conditions of the soil exercise upon tumors of the spleen is partly explained by the close relations they bear to intermittent fever; more complete information cannot yet be given upon this point.

A certain immunity from malarial fever was formerly said by some observers to be enjoyed by indigenous populations, particularly the negro race, but Sigaud has found tumors of the spleen exceedingly frequent among the negroes brought from the west coast of Africa to South America. Henderson remarks that in some highly malarious regions of Hindostan every third person has a tumor of the spleen. Twining and others express themselves to the same effect.

Sex, Age, Diet, and Drink.

Observations up to the present time have shown that just as no distinctions of race exist in this point, so no age, neither sex, nor position is free from diseases of the spleen. They occur as well in the male as in the female sex, from the tenderest nursling to extreme old age, and in nearly all ranks, from the poorest day-laborer to the millionaire.

In regard to sex, the male appears to be more frequently affected than the female. Among the sixteen cases of splenic leucocythemia observed by me, four patients, or one-fourth, were of the female sex. And although diseases of the spleen, in consequence of endemic influences, may be almost equally frequent in the two sexes in many regions, yet at other times the disposing causes in man are very different from those in women. Disturbances of the sexual functions in the latter have an unmistakable influence upon the occurrence of diseases of the spleen. Ballonius[1] and Portal[2] have frequently observed enlargement of the spleen after suppression of the menses.

In diseases of the female sexual organs, if, in addition to a splenic tumor, a slight increase of the white blood-corpuscles is found, continued treatment is necessary to prevent actual leucocythemia.

In a girl of eighteen years I was successful in relieving a splenic tumor, occurring with amenorrhœa, as well as the leucocytosis, only by the long-continued use of quinine and iron.

Among the twenty-one cases of leucocythemia which have come under my observation, which were chiefly of the splenic form, there were in all sixteen in which anomalies in the function of the sexual organs were present.

Every age gives opportunity for observing affections of the spleen. Wrisberg mentions an enlargement of the spleen even in utero. Since the spleen in the fœtus has arrived at only a very low stage of development, such cases are very rare. In the first year of life, on the contrary, splenic derangements of various kinds occur much more frequently, as a consequence of scrofulosis, syphilis, rachitis, intermittent. We can speak of the inheritance of diseases of the spleen only so far as the diseases named above are hereditary.

The spleen, like the digestive organs in general, shows a specially great susceptibility to disease in the middle years of life. All kinds of splenic affections occur frequently at this period. Many causes are assigned for this, even the influence of particular articles of diet. Hippocrates[3] in one place charges the excessive use of fresh figs, of too much fruit, grapes, and new wine with causing dropsy; in another place, the free, abundant use of raw vegetables, with much water-drinking, with being a disposing cause of induration of the spleen. Such kinds of food as are coarse and tough, and consequently remained undigested a long time in the stomach, were said to dispose to splenic affections.

---

[1] De morbis mulier. et virgin. T. IV. p. 46. Cpp. ed. Venet. 1736.
[2] Sur la nature et le trait. de quelques maladies. p. 36. 192.
[3] De internis affectionibus. T. II. p. 473. Cpp. edit. Kuehn.

The connection of the spleen with the digestive organs is anatomically proved: disturbances of the digestion react upon it; congestive swellings occur in it in consequence of affections of the stomach and liver; hence, it may be supposed that articles of food hard to digest, or indigestible, cause affections of the spleen; no further influence is yet known—the same thing is true of drinks. In gluttons and drunkards the older physicians mention various diseases of the spleen.

Dobson usually found a considerable swelling of the spleen in persons who were in the habit of drinking ale or porter to excess. The drunkards' dyscrasia was said to be followed, according to the degree of its development, sometimes by simple swelling of the spleen, sometimes by swelling with softening, in other cases by atrophy or cancerous degeneration; we are not as yet acquainted with any irritating or relaxing influence of alcohol upon the spleen. Diseases of the spleen occur in drunkards secondarily to affections of the liver in the form of congestive swellings, or in consequence of the general cachexia in the form of amyloid degeneration.

Bad drinking water and water from the springs of swampy and marshy regions were looked upon as causes of swellings of the spleen even in the medical writings of Grecian antiquity, in the works of Hippocrates and Galen; modern times have confirmed this view. The formation of acute tumors of the spleen after the use of such water is directly proved.

Intermittent fever, with its specific enlargement of the spleen, has been frequently observed after the use of drinking water with which decomposed organic substances have been mingled. In August, 1872, a great part of the population of Lausen, a little village in the Canton of Basle, were attacked with abdominal typhus so suddenly and in so astonishingly short a time, that it was at once clear to every unprejudiced person that all these cases must have been produced by one and the same cause acting at the same time upon all. There had never been an epidemic of typhus in Lausen within the memory of man, and for many years not a single case of this disease had been observed, and thus neither the air nor the soil could be accepted as a carrier of the poison; but the drinking water was clearly proved to be such by Dr. A. A. Haegler, in Basle, in a way that is very instructive for the study of our question. Thus it was clearly shown that tumors of the spleen may arise from the use of polluted drinking water. The epidemic of abdominal typhus in Lausen was the consequence of infection of the drinking water by typhoid dejections, which mingled with manure; the drainings of privies and other decomposing organic matters had been admixed in Furlen with the brook which ran down the valley. Similar interesting observations in Zürich and Berne have been communicated by Biermer. These are important facts in regard to the origin of tumors of the spleen by infection from the gastro-intestinal mucous membrane.

Infectious Diseases.

In most of these the spleen appears to be the most interesting, if not the most important organ; the typical course of many fevers is perhaps explained by its behavior. It has been long known that many acute diseases are accompanied by enlargement of the spleen. Its relation to precise stages and to definite processes therein is to be determined by future inquiries; unfortunately, a more accurate insight into the minute anatomical changes of the acutely enlarged spleen is as yet wanting. Our knowledge of the manner of its development has been recently increased by experiments. Since Ponfick directly proved the retentive function of the spleen in relation to granular coloring matters—cinnabar, india ink—which were artificially introduced into the circulation, it is less mysterious why a large number of so-called dyscrasic diseases, acute as well as chronic, intermittent fever, typhous, puerperal, pyæmic processes, acute exanthemata, syphilis, tuberculosis, are accompanied by tumors in the spleen.

Birch-Hirschfeld has already demonstrated, in regard to the carriers of contagion, facts similar to those connected with the coloring matters. When he injected into the blood of a rabbit two to ten grammes of blood which had stood in a room for five days and had then been filtered, the white blood-corpuscles immediately took up the micrococci in great number; afterwards the spleen retained in its pulp-cells a part of the micrococci, and when a considerable number of the latter were present, a decided swelling of the spleen took place. Davaine has already stated that the bacteridia in malignant pustule were found in special abundance in the spleen. In a pyæmic enlargement of the spleen examined a short time after death, Birch-Hirschfeld found enlargement of the pulp-cells, and micrococci within them; in puerperal fever also he has found exactly the same thing, enlargement of the pulp-cells and micrococci within them. The condition described seems to speak in favor of the view that these spleen enlargements are dependent upon the presence of micrococci in the blood.

In typhoid it is probable, but not yet positively proved; the most interesting discovery which has been lately made in this direction is the demonstration by Obermeier, of the occurrence of spiral vibrio-like threads in the blood of patients with recurrent fever, and indeed only during the febrile access; whereas in the time between the attacks of fever, that is, in the non-febrile period, these organisms were entirely wanting.

As is known, Salisbury long ago expressed the view that intermittent fever also was caused by fungi. Now, since Ponfick has proved that the spleen is a filter for small corpuscular admixtures in the blood, filters from the blood the granules circulating in it, and retains them itself, it is not difficult to imagine that, since the spleen retains the fever-producing organisms also, the typical febrile attacks are produced by a periodical outstraining of these organisms or their germs from the spleen. A febrile attack would then always occur when the development of these organisms had exceeded the capacity of the spleen.

Since this path of inquiry has been marked out, we can certainly hope in the immediate future for further information on the interesting question of the connection of infectious diseases and enlargement of the spleen, especially the mode of origin of the latter. Is it not possible that other poisons, and medicinal substances also, which are received into the blood, are floated into the spleen and there retained?

Medicines. Poisons. Nervous Influence. Congestion.

Unfortunately, we are not in a position to mention the names of those substances after the use of which a permanent or temporary change of the spleen may be perceived.

According to the older statements, mercury is said to act injuriously on the spleen. "A great disposition to obstructions of the spleen was said to arise from the use of large quantities of mercury" (Heinrich).

Since Ponfick's discovery it is not in the least improbable that quicksilver also may be deposited from the blood in the spleen and retained therein. As is well known, Overbeck, in opposition to Donders and Baerensprung, has confirmed the fact discovered by Oesterlen, Voit, and others, that metallic mercury, either rubbed in, in the form of mercurial ointment, or from the intestinal canal, forces its way through the tissues, and is not simply absorbed as an oxide. He found it after inunctions upon animals in the corium, subcutaneous cellular tissue, in the liver, in the kidneys, in the intestinal canal. In man also mercury was demonstrated by the microscope, after a previous inunction treatment, in the secretions and excretions. A retention of the mercury in the spleen is not mentioned in these statements. So far I have not succeeded in finding special morbid changes in the spleen in chronic mercurialism. Nothing more precise is known about the morbific action of other drugs; unfortunately, no special attention has so far been directed to this point.

Since the volume of the spleen depends on its richness in blood, which is a consequence of the greater or less contraction of its vessels, and therefore stands in connection with the nervous system, it may be suspected that some drugs and poisons may in this way give rise to tumors of the spleen.

A direct paralyzing influence of certain substances on the vaso-motor nerves and on the vaso-motor centre, producing a dilatation of the peripheral vessels, has been frequently determined by the latest inquirers in this department.

In cases where, at the same time, the central organ of the vascular system is found in a condition of debility, so that the movement of the blood, and especially the blood-pressure, seem to be particularly affected, the dilatation of the peripheral vessels is still more clearly marked. The influence which these substances exert would probably have an indirect action upon the volume of the spleen. The latest experimental investigations in regard to the spleen give some ground for such a supposition. Observations at the bedside have shown that obstructions in the

portal circulation, by diseases of the portal vein itself, its surroundings, and its capillary distribution within the liver, anomalies of menstruation and the cessation of hemorrhoidal bleeding, act indirectly upon the spleen by overloading the portal
system. Obstructions to the circulation produced by diseases
of the heart, of the great vessels, and of the lungs, have less
influence.

I have often clearly convinced myself in numerous vivisections, how rapidly a pressure on the splenic vein distends the
spleen to an enormous extent. If it lies only for a short time in
front of the abdominal walls, the pressure exercised thereby soon
gives rise to a considerable congestive tumor.

The same appearance has been several times observed by me
after cutting the visible nerves of the spleen. Even during the
operation this organ enlarged to more than double its former
volume, and became of a dark bluish red color; it could no
longer be replaced through the original abdominal wound, which
had to be enlarged for this purpose.

In such cases the autopsy disclosed after several months a
tumor of the spleen, which was distinguished by a vessel running
the whole length of the parenchyma, enlarged to the size of a
goose-quill, having thickened walls and containing a thrombus.

By these experiments the influence of the nerves, which, in
medical practice is frequently not very manifest in the origin of
affections of the spleen, is placed in a clear light. Oehl[1] has
lately observed that, under the influence of irritation of the vagus, a contraction of the trabeculæ occurs, giving rise to a granulated appearance of the surface of the organ. Oehl suggests the
inquiry—which he is inclined to answer in the affirmative—
whether the enlargements of the spleen occurring in swampy
regions may not be referred to paralysis of the muscular elements, in consequence of frequently occurring and long enduring
deficiency in innervation.

Dr. von Tarchanoff has also communicated some interesting
experiments in regard to leucocythæmia (Vol. VIII. of Pflueger's
Archiv).

---

[1] Zur Physiologie der Milz von Prof. *E. Oehl* (Gazz. Lomb. 9, 10. 1868.)

By irritation of the central extremities of the nervus vagus with the induced current, a vigorous contraction of the spleen of about one to two ctms. could be produced. Irritation of the peripheral end gave rise to a scarcely perceptible contraction of the organ. The most decided action occurred after irritation of the medulla oblongata if the splanchnic nerves were completely intact: the spleen changed its color and density, and became slaty-gray, and very hard. The diminution of the size of the spleen proved to be an effect of the contraction of the splenic vessels, which depends on an immediate irritation of the vaso-motor centre, or upon its irritation through sensitive nerves.

After section of the splenic nerves Tarchanoff observed the same changes of the spleen which I have described above. On the second, third, and fourth days after this operation he determined a distinct increase in the white corpuscles in a specimen of blood taken from the ear of the animal; it was, however, only of short duration—so soon as the seventh day after the section of the nerves their number was normal. The changes in the dimension of the spleen went parallel with this appearance.

After the sections of the spleen-nerves which I observed and described in my monograph on leucæmia, I did not succeed in determining a distinct increase in the white blood-corpuscles.

Tarchanoff considers his observation as a new proof that the spleen is an organ which makes white blood-corpuscles, and also that leucæmia can originate as a consequence of a change of the nervous activity in the animal body.

In the special portion of this article I will treat more minutely the etiology of the separate diseases of the spleen, and show what processes in the spleen may be generated by diseases of the heart and of the vascular system, especially by endocarditis, and fibrinous coagulation in the arteries and veins, and also which diseases can occur from extension of inflammation from neighboring organs, or from serious traumatic injuries in the neighborhood of the spleen.

Symptomatology and General Diagnosis.

Every experienced physician knows that diseases of the spleen form a particularly dark and difficult region of pathology. Notwithstanding the immense impulse which medical science has received from physiology and pathological anatomy, striking abnormities of the spleen are still frequently observed for the first time on the post-mortem table, without any affection of the spleen having been suspected during life, or still less any special symptom for the particular kind of disease having been present. The older physicians have often fallen into the opposite error; with a sort of predilection they have diagnosticated diseases of the spleen, and directed their treatment towards them in cases where no organic disease of the spleen has existed. As a rule they were deceived by a group of symptoms which took their origin in the neighboring organs. Previous to a thorough knowledge of physical diagnosis the deficiency in pathognomonic symptoms of diseases of the spleen was so much the more perceptible, since a functional disturbance of the spleen is especially difficult to recognize as such; we need not, therefore, wonder that the array of symptoms from which the older physicians made the general diagnosis of the affections of the spleen was a very vague one. They were uncomfortable sensations of pain in the left hypochondrium; sympathetic pains in more distant parts; so-called positive results of local examination; prevailing affections of the left side; functional disturbances of the gastric, the respiratory, the circulatory, and the sexual organs; abnormal composition of the blood, making itself manifest by changes of the color of the skin; various forms of eruption; ulcerations; hemorrhoids; hemorrhages; melæna; anomalies of the urinary secretion; and finally, various reflex disturbances in the nervous system, and in particular a special mental disposition. After this it is easily conceivable that, previous to a thorough realization of the methods of physical examination, an accurate symptomatology of affections of the spleen was impossible.

I consider it even now by no means an easy task to state in their totality the symptoms occurring in diseases of the spleen, and fix the diagnostic value of the individual, local, and general signs.

Local Sensations in the Neighborhood of the Spleen.

It cannot be denied that affections of the spleen can be connected with morbid, more or less painful sensations; considerable clinical experience has, however, taught me that these phenomena are usually wanting. In hardly one-sixth of all the cases observed by me did any local abnormal sensations give rise to suspicion of the seat of the disease. The sensation so frequently spoken of as pain in the spleen, or stitch in the spleen, arises, as a rule, from affections of the pleura, of the peritoneum, from the diaphragm, from the heart, stomach, intestines, or other neighboring organs. One would be specially mistaken if he expected to find them with greater certainty in acute affections of the spleen than in chronic. The older pathology could at any rate make very precise rules: "the pains in acute splenitis are persistent, severe, and stabbing, less severe and dull in the chronic, lingering inflammation. An inflammation of the upper half, immediately pressed upon by the diaphragm, removes the painful sensation more upward, while an inflammation of the lower half has necessarily an opposite result" (Heinrich).

Although I have observed with particular attention a large number of persons suffering with diseases of the spleen, I have not succeeded in confirming the statements made above; this may be partly due to the fact that, since the diagnosis has become more accurate, diseases of the spleen in general, and inflammations in particular, are more seldom observed. Besides this, the latter usually occur only secondarily, as so-called metastatic forms, and give rise to no subjective symptom, except suppuration, and consequently to no abnormal sensations in the region of the spleen.

As Hamernik has already suggested in the Prager Vierteljahrschrift. 1846. II. S. 40, it is highly probable that the spleen, as an organ consisting almost entirely of vessels, possesses a low degree of sensibility. It is not, to be sure, wanting in nerves; these come from the splenic plexus surrounding the splenic artery in two or three main branches, and continue into the interior of the organ upon the arteries, with one or two here and there connecting branches. In animals they can be followed far into the spleen. Koelliker has frequently seen them, with the help of the microscope, upon the arteries which bear Malpighian corpuscles; hence it is explained why, after section of all the nerves visible in the hilus of the spleen, we observe as principal effect a decided increase in the volume of the spleen. During the section, the animals gave evidence of acute pain. The same thing happened when electrical irritation with the induced current was practised upon the surface of the spleen. From the pathological facts observed by me, I must consider it possible that the production of pain only occurs from irritation of the nerves of the serous covering; actual pain in diseases of the spleen happens only when the serous covering is affected.

In typhoid, as is well known, there is usually no sensitiveness of the spleen; on account of the meteorism, the organ cannot usually be felt. As a rare exception, I have observed disagreeable impressions on deep pressure upon the projecting surface of the spleen, when the capsule was much stretched by a high degree of swelling. The same thing is true of splenic tumors in malarial processes; even here a fixed pain in the spleen always points to some perisplenitic process. In recurrent fever an acute pain and sensibility are almost constantly perceived in the neighborhood of the spleen, which last even into convalescence. This symptom is very important for the diagnosis; it is produced by a peculiar inflammation of the splenic parenchyma, in which the serous covering takes part. Among sixteen leucæmic tumors I have only once observed intense painfulness; it occurred in a workman forty-four years old. The leucæmia had taken place in consequence of traumatic action upon an already enlarged spleen. The patient, while mounting a horse, had fallen with his left side upon the pommel. The autopsy showed a considerable tumor of the spleen, so strongly adherent to the abdominal wall for a considerable extent, that the serous covering, thickened by previous intense inflammation, could only be separated by the knife.

In Mayer's [1] case, a persistent, severe pain in the left hypochondrium, depended upon the burrowing of a large ascaris into the splenic substance, by which the serous covering had been torn. New formations and echinococci excite unpleasant sensations only when they have attained a certain size and begin to cause irritation by pressure. Large tumors of the spleen, when the abdomen is perfectly soft and painful neither spontaneously, nor upon pressure, may largely increase without causing trouble to the patient. Temporary filling of the stomach with food, distention of the colon by fæcal masses or gas, cause disagreeable tension and pressure on the tumor and its neighborhood. If meteorism and ascites be present the patients experience permanent pains in the region of the stomach and liver, for which they usually have to take to their beds. As long as they can walk and stand, they complain, on account of the stretching of the splenic ligaments, of troublesome sensations in the left hypochondrium.

I have treated patients with such voluminous tumors of the spleen that they could not walk without abdominal supporters. The neighboring organs suffered from pressure to a great extent. Heinrich saw one patient whose enlarged spleen

---

[1] Harless, Rheinisch-Westphälische Jahrbücher für Medicin und Chirurgie. Bd. I. H. 3. S. 321.

could be felt below the short ribs, in whom a strong pressure produced pain and breathlessness. Alibert treated a young man who was melancholy and complained of constant pains in the region of the spleen. He characterized them by the comparison that he felt as if drops of rain were constantly falling upon that spot.

Sympathetic Pains.

Still more mysterious are the statements of the earlier authors in regard to sympathetic pains in the region of the spleen, as well as in regard to sympathetic pains and other morbid sensations in other portions of the body which accompany troubles of the spleen. Pains in the spleen are said to occur sympathetically with inflammations of the liver when these have reached their height, under which condition the right hypochondrium can become perfectly painless, while the spleen itself is without the least organic change. I have often seen affections of the spleen occur secondarily to diseases of the liver in consequence of cirrhosis, amyloid degeneration, etc.

The kind of sympathetic pains in the spleen described above I have never observed.

Of sympathetic pains and other morbid sensations which are said to accompany affections of the spleen, I know but little.

Hippocrates speaks of severe pains which, originating in the spleen, shoot into the shoulder, into the neighborhood of the clavicle, of the nipple, and into the lower region of the ribs.

In a case described by Ayx, involving hypertrophy of the spleen, the sympathetic pains in the left scapular region were so severe, that the patient compared them to the shoulder's being forcibly torn asunder. According to Leue, frequent itching in the back, and a sensation as if cold water were running down the back; a dull feeling and frequent going to sleep of the limbs, were ascribed to chronic inflammation of the spleen; pains in the private parts, in the pubic region and more distant parts of the abdomen are described by other observers. According to Rademacher, sciatica occasionally depends, as a sympathetic affection of the sciatic nerve, upon an affection of the liver or spleen.

I have mentioned these statements without vouching for the facts. Purely sympathetic nervous affections may occur with diseases of the spleen, and, perhaps even more frequently, affect the left side of the body. For my own part, I accept the theory of sympathetic pains in diseases of the spleen with the more difficulty, since I have learned by experience how various are the anatomically demonstrable complications in numerous organs of the body. The other lymphatic organs—the lymphatic glands and the marrow of the bones—deserve special attention in this point of view. Who would have supposed a few years ago that we should to-day be in a condition to demonstrate an intense painfulness of the sternum occurring with.a leucæmic tumor of the spleen—an apparent neurosis—as a symptom of the myelogenous leucæmia described by Neumann, affecting this bone, as was done in the case described by me in the 25th Vol. of Virchow's Archiv? The same change has been already found in almost all the bones.

In consequence of lymphatic new formations, neuroses of the most various nerve-tracts can be observed with tumors of the spleen. Another possibility is given by a disturbed venous flow of the blood, in consequence of the pressure of glandular tumors. Frequently the neuroses are the consequence of diminution of the red or of increase of the colorless blood-corpuscles, which changes are known to be so frequent with tumors of the spleen. Thus may be explained headache, giddiness, disturbance of the head, a hypochondriac disposition, and especially dyspnœa, as well as disturbance of the respiration in general. These changes were unknown to the older physicians, and consequently could not be applied to the secondary appearances in diseases of the spleen ; they were, therefore, compelled to search for hypotheses. They attempted to explain the phenomena by spinal irritation, as well as by the nervous phenomena described by J. Mueller as sympathetic sensations, or as irradiation of sensations ; and, especially after De Bey, by the supposition that the morbidly swollen spleen pressed upon the cœliac plexus situated in its immediate neighborhood, and, by the intimate connection of this plexus with the other nerve-centres, set up reactions in various and distant parts of the body.

Disturbances of the Digestive Organs.

These occur in various forms in diseases of the spleen, but furnish nothing characteristic for diagnosis. Many cases have been observed in which the intestinal tract showed few or no anomalies.

Morgagni, Peter Frank, Marcus the elder, and others speak of increased thirst which has disturbed the patient. This is the most severe in acute febrile cases, as well as after profuse sweating. In chronic diseases of the spleen it is frequently entirely wanting. In a hundred cases of leucæmia it was increased only in fifteen cases. The statements in regard to hunger are still more various. In most cases the appetite was normal, or, more rarely, diminished. The older writers lay special weight upon an unappeasable hunger as a sign of disease of the spleen, since Dupuytren and Schultze saw great voraciousness set in shortly after extirpation of the spleen in animals. A connection of the function of the spleen with the digestive processes was supposed to be thus shown.

M. Schiff has carried out some thorough experiments in this direction. He sought to connect the loading of the pancreas with albumen-digesting ferment with the function of the spleen. According to Schiff, the loading of the pancreas with ferment for the digestion of albumen demands two conditions, namely, the presence of so-called peptogenous matter in the blood, and the occurrence of absorption from the stomach. According to Corvisart's and Schiff's observations, the pancreas begins to fill up in the fourth hour of digestion. Schiff, from his observations, determined a third condition for the loading of the pancreas, and believed that he had found in the spleen an organ in which the peptogens absorbed from the stomach were so changed that they were capable of forming the albumen-digesting matter of the pancreas. The spleen, as is known, enlarges during digestion. There occurs, as Schiff expresses it, an erection, which attains its maximum about the fifth hour of digestion. After the extirpation of the spleen, Schiff expected to find the infusion of the pancreas completely incapable of digesting albumen, and at the same time, in consequence of the excessive collection of peptogens in the blood then taking place, an increased functional activity of the gastric mucous membrane.

Schiff's experiments assured him that the albumen-digesting power of the pancreas, at every period of digestion, was dependent on the spleen and its increase in volume, and that absence or ligature of the spleen, or a mechanically induced insufficiency of the spleen, remaining in its diminished condition, hindered the filling of the pancreas, but so much the more increased that of the stomach.

Lusanna, as well as myself, in numerous and careful experiments upon the pancreas and gastric mucous membrane of animals deprived of their spleen, could not confirm the statements of Schiff. Extirpation of the spleen exercises no influence upon the stomach and pancreatic digestion; the voracity of animals deprived of their spleen, which, in addition to the chemical analysis, has been taken as a proof of such influence, does not, according to my experience, exist as a constant symptom; they usually ate as much as healthy animals; not unfrequently precisely the contrary was observed by me. The hypothesis was not a distant one that, in consequence of previous overloading of the stomach, a catarrh of the gastric mucous membrane, with loss of appetite, had set in; but I have never met with the signs of a catarrhal inflammation in animals deprived of their spleen.

In reference to this question, the comparative investigations which I have undertaken with dogs, with and without spleens, who received the same care and the same nourishment, seem to be not without importance; these have shown that in dogs without spleens, after they have for some time well recovered from the operation, the weight of the body increases and decreases in the same degree as in dogs with a spleen.

Real voracity I have but seldom observed in affections of the spleen. The appetite usually changes with the other symptoms, diminishes when they become worse, and returns to the normal or increases when the exacerbation passes off. The taste and the appearance of the tongue depend upon the condition of the mucous membrane of the throat and the stomach. Sometimes the patients complain of a sour taste and sour eructations. Some patients, said to have been affected with chronic inflammation of the spleen, had an extremely unpleasant salt or bitter taste (Heusinger); a whitish or yellow coating on the tongue is not seldom met with; a red and dry tongue belongs to a course of disease associated with fever.

Difficulties in swallowing often arise from secondary lymphatic hyperplasia of the tonsils and follicles of the pharyngeal mucous membrane. A stomatitis can also be produced in the same way, which has great similarity in its symptoms to stomatitis scorbutica. Loosening of the gums and offensive breath are, therefore, important signs of a splenic dyscrasia.

I have observed and carefully described such a stomatitis in a noticeable degree in leucæmia; on the other hand, I observed, in the summer of 1873, a very intense form of scorbutic affection of the mouth, without pharyngeal and tonsillar lymphoma, in a ship captain, who had returned from South America with a malignant malarial cachexia without leucæmia. All the splenic remedies applied by me had no permanent result—death occurred with the most distinctly marked appearances of scurvy.

An increased secretion of the salivary glands, ptyalism, some-

times occurs. In a young woman who had acquired an enlargement of the spleen from suppression of the menses, Schlegel[1] saw,
besides eructations and flatulence, ptyalism also. Wintringham
and Verga mention increased secretion of saliva as a symptom of
a scirrhous degeneration of the spleen.

Paulicki[2] reports a case of intermittent salivation, which lasted, every other day,
for many months, in an insane person thirty-eight years old. It began at 8 o'clock
in the morning and lasted till nearly 6 o'clock in the evening. The quantity was
from two and a half to three and a half kilogrammes; an enlargement of the spleen
could not be determined.

I have not myself observed salivation in patients with diseases of spleen, except after the use of mercury.

Pressure on the epigastrium, acid eructations, cramp in the
stomach, heartburn, nausea, vomiting, are functional disturbances which occur as complications of splenic affections as well
as of many other diseases; they are not characteristic, since they
are wanting in just as many cases. In the patient described by
Leue the irritability of the stomach, in the course of a "chronic
inflammation of the spleen," became so great that even the pressure of light articles of clothing could not be borne, and severe
cramp in the stomach, with pyrosis, frequently occurred. The
paroxysms which Portal[3] saw occur in chronic enlargement of
the spleen, regularly about two hours after eating, were truly
fearful, and threatened suffocation. In consequence of the pressure on the stomach produced by a tumor of the spleen, by which
the former was impeded in its dilatation, I have observed an uncomfortable feeling in the abdomen frequently produced after
taking food, and occasionally nausea and vomiting. Matters of
the most various character are discharged by vomiting; sometimes it is a clear and acidulous fluid, consisting for the most
part of saliva which has been swallowed. The vomiting usually
brings up the food and drink which has been taken. The longer
or shorter delay of the contents in the stomach; the greater or
less action of the gastric juice; the more or less abundant admixture of bile, which, when the vomiting is violent, is pressed back

---

[1] De scirrho lienis, page 12.   [2] Centralblatt. 1868. S. 596.
[3] Cours d'anatomie médicale. T. V. p. 339.

from the duodenum into the stomach according to mechanical laws; and finally, hemorrhage from the vessels of the stomach, are all factors which modify in various ways the vomiting according to the peculiarities of the individual case. The older physicians assign especial value thereto.

The intestinal evacuations are not alike in all cases of splenic disease; they are much more likely to be modified according to the kind of affection. The rule is, that larger tumors of the spleen, except in typhus and similar diseases, are attended by sluggish action of the bowels; hence the patients complain of obstinate constipation, and distention of the abdomen with gas. The fæces are usually dark, black, dry, and hard—so-called scybala, such as were considered by the older physicians as characteristic of abdominal plethora. These are occasionally, in consequence of compression of the intestines by the splenic tumor, more thinly formed than usual.

These changes in the activity of the intestinal canal may fairly be explained as symptoms of pressure; hypotheses, however, have not been wanting as to the influence of the spleen on the secretion of the intestinal mucous membrane. After its extirpation in animals, various experimenters have observed a sluggish movement of the bowels, together with symptoms of a disturbed action of the liver, and especially of the organs connected with the portal system. In the numerous extirpations of the spleen performed by me upon dogs, I have not seen these statements verified.

When chronic diseases of the spleen are complicated with diarrhœa, the evacuations are often from the beginning very thin and copious, and retain the same character during the whole of the disease. These phenomena of irritation of the intestinal mucous membrane are produced in leucocythæmia and its allied conditions, by the accompanying lymphoma; at other times it is a congestive catarrh of the intestinal mucous membrane. The stools contain large masses of mucus and pus, and are not unfrequently mixed with blood; dark, tarry blood is evacuated from the stomach as well as from the intestines (Melæna). The quantity varies. Two years ago I saw a patient with a leucæmic tumor of the spleen die with profuse vomiting of blood and bloody

stools.   The source of the hemorrhage was found in an ulcer of
the stomach produced by a lymphatic new formation.   At other
times the bleeding occurs simply from bursting of the walls of
the gastric and intestinal vessels, altered by the splenic cachexia.

The fatal termination of many splenic diseases is brought
about by colliquative diarrhœa.   Hippocrates[1] knew this symptom.   He considers the accession of a persistent dysentery as a
fatal complication.

For the sake of completeness, in order properly to represent
the earlier views, I will mention that the older physicians were
prone to assume a disposition to the generation of worms in the
intestinal canal, in consequence of splenic cachexia.

Heinrich mentions as a rarity the case of a girl affected with the principal
symptoms of a chronic enlargement of spleen, who several times passed considerable pieces of tapeworm.   "For a long time an acute observer had made the
observation that intermittent fevers in general favored the production of worms.
Wawruch has lately confirmed this observation by a considerable experience of his
own.   Tapeworm is an endemic affliction in regions where intermittent fevers
thrive.   In Vienna, intermittent fevers are endemic, particularly in damp years;
and in the lower suburbs lying on the Danube, scurvy is very frequent, and tapeworms so numerous, that they are said to occur among the poorer classes of the
population in the proportion of one to twenty."[2]

The helminthological experiments of Kuechenmeister and Leuckart have destroyed the belief in any such disposition.

Changes in the Liver and Mesenteric Glands.

The anatomico-physiological connection in which the liver
and spleen stand to each other leads us to expect a frequent
occurrence of changes of the liver in diseases of the spleen.   Tumors of the spleen are frequently accompanied by tumors of the
liver, but it is not always perfectly easy to determine with certainty the causal connection.   The same morbific influences frequently exist for each, as, for example, endocarditis, intermittent, and syphilis.   Both organs are not unfrequently affected
by the same causes of congestion in the venous circulation.   The
opening of the splenic vein into the portal vein shows us one

---

[1] Loc. cit. Sect. VI. 43.   [2] *Heinrich*, loc. cit. p. 105.

way in which affections of the spleen may originate secondarily from affections of the liver; and, *vice versa,* the liver can be affected by disease of the spleen.

In the latter point of view the leucæmic lymphoma of the liver has afforded very important explanations. Among ninety-two cases of leucæmia collected by Ehrlich the liver was diseased fifty-four times. Since we know that the walls of the smaller vessels, under certain circumstances, permit the passage of the colorless blood-cells, we can look upon the leucæmic new formation of lymphadenoid tissues in the liver as an infiltration produced by an emigration of colorless blood-corpuscles. In many cases they follow very closely the course of the vessels. In the liver this change occurs to so striking a degree because the colorless blood-corpuscles produced in excess by the spleen are carried, in the most direct manner, by the splenic vein into the vessels of the liver.

The same condition exists in melanæmia, where a washing-out of particles of pigment from the spleen into the liver can be observed. Abscesses, as well as new formations of the liver, often occur after primary affections in the spleen. It is therefore easy to explain why symptoms of disturbed action of the liver often complicate affections of the spleen.

Besides the liver, the other glands of the abdomen not unfrequently become diseased in affections of the spleen. When the walls of the abdomen are not too tense, the enlarged mesenteric glands can be felt as hard, movable knots. In the further course of the disease ascites sets in and makes the examination more difficult; the complication mentioned can then be suspected from the simultaneous swelling of the inguinal glands. The latter form painless, tolerably hard, knotty bunches, above which the skin is normal and movable. Exceptionally, redness and inflammation of the skin occur; the tumors then feel hot, soft, almost like fatty tumor, and fluctuating; their size varies, usually from that of a pea to that of a hazel-nut; in some cases glandular tumors as large as a child's head have been seen. In one of my patients with syphilis and leucæmia, large bunches made their appearance in the inguinal region on both sides, the single parts of which were larger than a dove's egg. From these, cords ran down the inner surface of the thigh to the knee, where again large tumors were met with; down the leg little knots could be felt.

Changes in the Respiration and Circulation.

The changes in the abdominal cavity are accompanied by a series of morbid appearances on the part of various other organs; very various symptomatic affections are produced in the thoracic organs by diseases of the spleen. A coincidence of the two leaves us often in doubt which has been the primary disease. As is known, inflammatory conditions of the lung react upon the spleen, which in pneumonia is usually, like the liver, distended with blood. We have been long aware of the very common increase of volume of the spleen in phthisis; pathological anatomy has taught us to recognize it as an amyloid degeneration. On the other hand, Morgagni[1] has called attention to the fact that certain diseases of the lungs must be dated from infarctions of the spleen and the disturbances of the circulation caused thereby.

Valsalva[2] describes two very severe cases of peripneumonia, both terminated by death on the seventh day of the disease: one in a mariner, fifty years old, the other in a young priest. Both patients had suffered some time before from obstinate intermittent, in consequence of which they had, as the autopsy proved, greatly enlarged spleens. In a third observation of Valsalva, a spleen, enormously enlarged by repeated attacks of fever, produced a secondary congestion of the lungs, and sudden death from hemorrhage.

Hence, the knowledge of secondary affections of the lung in diseases of the spleen dates from ancient times. The more intimate connection we have learned from the important progress of physiology and pathological anatomy. We now know very various causes from which difficulty of respiration arises in patients with diseases of the spleen. The mechanical pressure of the enlarged spleen upon the diaphragm, as well as the hydrothorax, which usually develops itself when the disease has existed for some time, produces compression of the lungs, diminution of the breathing surface, and short breath.

[1] De sedibus et causis morb. Epist. XX. 52. Tom. I. p. 419. ed. Tissot.
[2] Morgagni, l. c. Epist. XX. 2. 30. T. I. pp. 389, 399.

Dyspnœa in diseases of the spleen is often to be looked upon as a consequence of diminished respiratory capacity of the blood. Since the red blood-corpuscles are looked upon as the special respirators of the blood, it is not difficult to connect alterations in the exchange of the gases with the diminution of the red and the increase of the colorless blood-corpuscles, by which alterations in the blood, affections of the spleen are well known to be frequently followed.

The investigations of Pettenkofer and Voit on a leucæmic patient are of some importance in this point of view. These researches furnish a physiological explanation of the chief symptom of leucæmia—the dyspnœa,—since a leucæmic patient, on account of poverty in red corpuscles, is able to fix as much oxygen as a healthy person only while at rest, but not while taking exercise. The blood-corpuscles of a leucæmic patient cannot do any more than they can accomplish during rest, and the patient is therefore without strength and incapable of any exertion ; this symptom is of great importance, as many physicians know ; dyspnœa, occurring without apparently sufficient cause, is often the earliest symptom of leucæmia, and attains a considerable degree of severity before signs of emaciation and weakness occur.

It may be assumed that, in diseases of the spleen, every disturbance of the organs of respiration which diminishes the respiratory surface must have more serious consequences than in health ; disturbances in this function can probably occur with greater ease than we suppose.

Even during life, a stoppage of the vessels of the lungs by the colorless blood-corpuscles, present in excess, often takes place ; their greater diameter and their constant inclination to adhere to each other, favor this occurrence. A diminution of the respiratory surface is thus caused, which is of great importance in severe leucæmia. The occasional enormous glandular swellings of the mediastinum anticum, even when slowly developed, cause great difficulty of breathing. The volume of the lungs is diminished by them just as by a considerable exudation into the cavity of the pericardium, or by a well-marked enlargement of the heart itself. When all these causes act together they give rise to very great difficulty in breathing. I have noticed this most clearly in a case of leucæmia where a considerable tumor of the spleen, ascites, and enormous increase of size in the glands of the anterior and posterior mediastinum co-existed; the latter having increased the dyspnœa still more by the mechanical effect which they exercised upon the nerves of the thorax. When all these possibilities are remembered, it is easy to explain why transient difficulties—in respiration, at least—occur in the course of every well-developed leucæmia, or may even become one of the most important symptoms.

In uncomplicated cases of splenic tumor, the percussion and auscultation of the thorax vary very little from the normal; the lower portions of the left lung often give a duller sound, or their lower border is pushed higher up. We sometimes find catarrh, with cough, and mucous, purulent, or even bloody expectoration.

We owe to Boettcher our knowledge of the specific changes in the lungs which occur in leucæmia. They consist in groups of gray miliary granulations, as well as in larger and smaller caverns. The granulations are shown to be simple accumulations of lymphatic elements. Boettcher demonstrated in the wall of many of the smaller bronchi, infiltrations with lymph-cells, and also referred the formation of the small caverns to the rupture and ulceration of these bronchial infiltrated masses.

The leucæmic condition of the blood is not the only cause of respiratory troubles in patients with diseases of the spleen; the splenic tumors also, which occur in the so-called pseudo-leucæmia, in which the relative proportion of colorless and colored blood-cells is normal, but in which a diminution of the corpuscular elements of the blood may be suspected from the pale color of the skin and of the mucous membranes, often give rise to the same difficulty. Among eighteen cases collected by Mueller, dyspnœa was present fourteen times without any anatomical lesion of the organs of respiration; the average frequency of breathing was between 24 and 36 in a minute. The shortness of breath was probably dependent upon the diminution of the red corpuscles, which act as carriers of oxygen. Anæmia splenica is, as we shall afterwards see, present in most cases of splenic tumor. The frequency of respiratory trouble is in great part thus explained, since the heart and the vascular system show at the same time greater or lesser changes. Experience daily teaches us that blood rich in corpuscles acts to relieve and invigorate the action of the heart, but that, on the contrary, that condition of the blood in which the blood-corpuscles are diminished in number, but in which the proportion of water has increased, depresses its activity. We learn this from a diminished energy of the heart and of the arterial system. Hence, in patients with disease of the spleen we frequently find a weak impulse of the heart, palpitation, souffles in the heart and in the larger arteries, especially the carotid, and a frequent, empty, easily compressible, thrilling pulse. In connection with this, a peculiar condition of nervous and psychic irritability is developed, frequent fainting, and a melancholy and despondent disposition.

The more one observes diseases of the spleen, the more he will be convinced of the great variability of the pulse—the striking varieties in its frequency and character, according to the peculiarities of the individual case. In an inflammatory type of the disease the pulse is feverish; in a splenic affection without inflammation, this is not the case. The pulse is often intermittent, in consequence of weakness of the heart. I have found it retarded in complication with icterus. We can speak as little of a characteristic condition of the pulse in diseases of the spleen as of specific changes of the heart. The heart's dulness is often laterally enlarged, which is partly connected with a pushing-up of the heart in the thorax. The heart has a more horizontal position, and its impulse in then felt higher up.

Symptoms of Imperfect Formation of Blood.

In almost all cases of splenic disease, the symptoms of disturbed and imperfect formation of blood are among the most striking; how could it be otherwise? The anatomical structure of the spleen, as well as a large number of physiological experiments, clearly show that the spleen has an immediate influence upon the formation of blood, particularly in the new formation of the colorless blood-corpuscles, and probably of the red. Wilhelm Mueller, on the ground of his anatomical investigations, has assigned to the spleen only the function of continuous formation of colorless blood-corpuscles, and their constant introduction into the circulating blood. On the other hand, from not insignificant modifications of the peculiarities of the red corpuscles in the blood of the splenic vein, we may probably assume a transition of colorless cells into colored, as taking place in the spleen. Some physiological, as well as numerous pathological facts, add to the strength of this hypothesis.

Analyses of the blood of dogs, after extirpations of the spleen, which were carried out, at my suggestion, by Schwanert and Schindler, have given less specific gravity of the blood, smaller quantities of fibrine and albumen, and less iron. In the microscopical determinations of the relative proportion of the red and white corpuscles, which I have often carried on in connection with Penkert and Kolbe, we found in the first months after the extirpation of the spleen, the number of white corpuscles less than in dogs with a spleen. Welcker, in Halle, determined by means of his blood-stain measure in examining specimens of blood sent by me, that the blood of the dog without a spleen was paler than that of the dog with a spleen. By means of the method of settling the blood-corpuscles contrived by him, he found that the blood of the animal without a spleen contained twenty times fewer white globules than the blood of the animal with a spleen.

I have myself, with Penkert and Schindler, by means of the method of settling the blood-corpuscles in graduated tubes, invented by Welcker, examined the blood of a large number of dogs which were perfectly healthy, in contrast with others whose spleens had been removed a longer or shorter time before, as well as those who had contracted in some other way a lesion of the spleen or its vessels and nerves. In these experiments of mine, the white corpuscles have not settled so clearly that an accurately measured distinction could be marked out in the different kinds of blood. But this I can say with certainty: that after extirpation, as well as after other lesions of the spleen, no larger proportion of white corpuscles was observed by me. As to whether and how far they were diminished, my experiments have not given so distinct results as Welcker observed.

The results were otherwise in determining the amount of sediment of red corpuscles. I cannot consider it an accidental occurrence that the blood of all the animals whose spleen had been either removed, or injured, and consequently atrophied, deposited a distinctly smaller sediment of red corpuscles than the blood of all the dogs in which the spleen was still acting, but am rather inclined to connect it with the deficient action of the spleen and the insufficient vicarious activity of the other lymphatic organs.[1]

The importance of the spleen in the formation of blood makes

---

[1] *Mosler*, Pathologie der Leukämie. S. 44.

it easily understood why the symptoms of imperfect and altered composition of the blood belong to the most constant accompaniments of lasting extensive diseases of the spleen—a fact which has been known to physicians since Hippocrates. Chemistry has so far given us only meagre data in regard to the qualitative and quantitative changes of the composition of the blood in affections of the spleen. It may be correctly supposed that an entirely different composition of the blood occurs, not only in the various diseases of the spleen, but even in one and the same, at various periods. We are somewhat more accurately acquainted with the morphological changes of the blood than with the chemical. Various kinds of splenic cachexia may be separated, according to the presence of only a diminution of the red corpuscles without increase of the white—anæmia splenica; or, besides a diminution of the red corpuscles, a slight increase of the white—leucocytosis; or, a great increase of the latter—leucæmia; or, at the same time, a collection of pigment in the white corpuscles—melano-leucæmia.

In leucæmia we assume that the lymph-cells are generated in abnormally large quantities in their normal birthplace—especially the spleen—immediately pass into the blood, and here, as white blood-corpuscles, produce the leucæmic condition of the blood. The absence of the leucæmic composition of the blood, and the persistence of the relative proportion of the colored and uncolored corpuscles, in simple tumor of the spleen, allow us to suspect that a retention of the lymph-cells formed in the hyperplastic spleen has taken place. The distinction from leucæmia seems to consist only in this : that the lymph-cells generated in excess by the hyperplasia of the lymphatic elements, in cases of leucæmia, migrate from their birthplace; while, on the contrary, in the simple tumor of the spleen—the so-called pseudo-leucæmia—they remain at the place of their formation.

A case of melano-leucæmia, after intermittent, coming under my observation, gives further support to this theory of the passage into the blood of substances which have been deposited in the spleen. The pigment which was here proved to exist in the circulation is to be looked upon, just as in simple melanæmia, as a secondary product of the local changes which are excited in the spleen by the malarial process. The colorless cellular elements

which are carred into the blood in abnormal quantity, in consequence of the leucæmic processes of the spleen, were the carriers
of the pigment, and, in consequence of this, a complication of
melano-leucæmia had arisen, while in other cases we observe
only leucæmia or melanæmia.   In what way both these processes are developed out of the primary intermittent disease, we
can only guess.   Very probably the reason consists in a greater
or less intensity of the original fever.   Considerable disturbances
of nutrition in the vascular system are early produced by the
deep alteration of the blood in severe forms of intermittent,
which cause an inclination to capillary hemorrhages and to the
formation of pigment.   In the milder forms of intermittent, the
process of cell-formation in the spleen is intensified only in a
slight degree, and the only result is a simple hyperplasia of the
spleen, without exportation of white blood-corpuscles.   In the
severer grades, and after long duration of intermittent, the
activity of the glandular organ is increased in a more marked
degree.   The process of cell-formation in the spleen takes on a
permanently progressive character, so that the white blood-corpuscles which are formed are carried into the blood.

In the severest cases of intermittent, the nutritive changes in
the vascular apparatus result in a hyperplasia of the spleen,
with formation of pigment.

Besides the increase of the colorless blood-corpuscles, a very
considerable absolute diminution of the red corpuscles has been
clearly proved by Welcker, which corresponds with the decided
diminution of the iron contained in leucæmic blood.

Welcker had never before seen in human blood, either in the
extremest cases of chlorosis or in the last stages of tuberculosis,
so pale a color as in the two cases of leucæmia examined by him.

This is an important fact, which proves the influence of
chronic splenic tumors on the deficient formation of red corpuscles ; their number seems, to judge by numerous symptoms, to
be smaller than normal in almost all tumors of the spleen ;
hence, it is probable that, in consequence of important changes
which occur in the birthplace of the cells, the formation of the
red corpuscles is interrupted.   Besides the quantitative.relations
there are certain qualitative variations of the red corpuscles

which seem to favor this view. The observation of nucleated red corpuscles in this disease has great significance, and the peculiar contractility of the red corpuscles, which has been observed by Friedreich and myself in tumors of the spleen, is also important. In the case reported by Friedreich, where a splenic tumor of large size existed, together with swelling of the lymph glands, only a few red corpuscles displayed the normal condition ; most of them showed, at some point of their periphery, short, nipple-like processes, which were sometimes longer or were drawn out into threads ; others, from a circular constriction, assumed the shape of a biscuit, or, by a double constriction, were changed into three-parted forms ; but neither in color nor in refraction were these forms distinguishable from the normal red elements of the blood. The colorless were in no way changed ; even the leucocytosis occurring in anæmic persons was wanting. Friedreich has also found the same polymorphous forms of a great part of the red corpuscles, in a case of splenic leucæmia occurring after intermittent. I have myself seen, in a case of anæmia splenica, with a large splenic tumor, the red corpuscles marked by many caudal processes. Many had assumed the biscuit form. When I exhibited this patient in my clinic, in February, 1866, I described the condition of the blood by saying that these were not finished red corpuscles, but that they occupied a place between the red and the white ; I explained the condition as the earliest beginning of leucæmia. As is known, the place of transformation of the colorless into colored corpuscles is considered to be in part the whole course of the circulation, and in part the spleen.

According to Frey, cells may be found in the splenic blood of man and mammalia, of which one cannot say whether they are still lymph-cells, or whether they are already colored blood-cells. The spherical, colorless cell is probably metamorphosed to a smooth, circular disc, and, with the loss of the nucleus and of the protoplasm, the yellow-colored contents are produced therein. In the cases of splenic disease just mentioned, the change of form of the white corpuscles had already taken place and the nucleus been lost, but the protoplasm remained very contractile—indeed, more so than in the normal condition.

At all events, these interesting observations invite a more systematic examination than has been heretofore usual in diseases of the spleen, not only of the white, but also of the red blood-corpuscles.

The blood-changes caused by affections of the spleen are manifested externally by the symptoms of anæmia and by dropsical effusions, and later by symptoms of a hemorrhagic diathesis.

The anæmia occurs very gradually; its beginning is completely latent and can hardly be suspected, if an intumescence of the spleen has developed itself without previous loss of health.

The affection takes another form when it occurs as a sequel of intermittent or syphilis, or after irregular action of the sexual organs in the female, or after great mental excitement; then the previous loss of health usually passes immediately into the chronic splenic affections, betraying itself by anæmia. In the other case the patients become, without assignable cause, out of tune, irritable, or apathetic; weakness, depression, disinclination to work follow. More rarely it happens that the affection begins with a feeling of weight in the splenic region, or in the abdomen generally.

The symptoms on the part of the nervous system are mostly dependent upon the anæmia of the patient: they are headache, dizziness, buzzing in the ears, hardness of hearing, fainting; the patients are surly, irritable, sad; they become emaciated without apparent cause; increasing paleness and anæmia accompany the emaciation; the skin is very pale, frequently dry; the visible mucous membranes are pale red or completely bleached; over the heart and the great vessels of the neck souffles are heard; œdematous swellings of the skin, especially of the feet and legs, take place early, at first only in the evening or after long standing, but later all the time.

A mechanical cause of the dropsy from hinderances to the circulation is only to be found in rare cases. Preponderating ascites, as in liver diseases, connected with impaired circulation, does not occur in uncomplicated splenic affections. Collections of fluid in other serous cavities are seen more frequently. The most extreme degrees of dropsy follow in the not rare complications with diseases of the liver, of the kidneys, of the heart. The access, as well as the disappearance of the dropsy, takes place almost always very slowly.

Hemorrhagic Diathesis.

In many, but not in all cases, the symptoms of a hemorrhagic diathesis are added to those already described: the patients have repeated bleedings, which ensue usually from the nose; more rarely from the intestinal canal or the lungs, or into the tissues of the skin, or in many cases into the brain. The end is materially hastened by this complication. The patients either die suddenly, with apoplectic symptoms, or are so weakened by repeated and abundant losses of blood, that they die early with the symptoms of exhaustion and anæmia. If no hemorrhagic diathesis is developed, the disease takes, with few exceptions, a tedious course that may last for years; in such cases the swelling of the spleen and the lymphatic glands attains a high degree of development; the patients emaciate, and their pale, cachectic appearance becomes very striking.

The clinical importance of the hemorrhages may be seen from the frequency of their occurrence. In 69 cases of leucæmia collected by Ehrlich, hemorrhages were observed 57 times; among the 12 cases observed by me, 7 times; so that in 81 cases of leucæmia, hemorrhages took place 64 times. 35 times hemorrhages were observed from the nose; 13 times from the intestinal canal: 11 times into the tissues of the skin; 8 times from the gums; 6 times from the hemorrhoidal vessels; 5 times in the peri- and endocardium; 4 times each from the stomach and the lungs; 4 times profuse bleeding from wounds; 3 times from the uterus; 3 times each effusions of blood into the brain, the peritoneum, and the membranes of the gastro-intestinal canal; twice hemorrhages from the urinary passages; and as often effusions of blood into the conjunctiva bulbi and the choroid, into the tissue and capsule of the spleen, the kidneys, the walls of the urinary bladder, and the submucous and subserous connective tissue.

Nosebleed seems so far the most frequent and also the most profuse of these hemorrhages. In the summer of 1869 I observed in a patient with splenic leucæmia such profuse nosebleeding, in connection with moderate hæmoptysis, that all means of arresting it were at first without success; after several attempts, plugging the nostrils, together with the application of a solution of chloride of iron, stopped the bleeding. By this time the patient had become so anæmic that we were induced to try transfusion. This remedy proved of special use against the hemorrhagic diathesis. Whereas before, nosebleed occurred at short intervals, after the transfusion it was not repeated.

I am at present treating in my clinic a patient with considerable swelling of the liver and spleen after intermittent, without a leucæmic condition of the blood (pseudo-leucæmia lienalis). With her also a very profuse nosebleed occurred at intervals of from three to five weeks.

It has been often supposed that in diseases of the spleen in general, and especially in leucæmia, the bleeding occurs only out of the left nostril. I have known cases of chronic enlargement of the spleen where the nosebleed took place from both nostrils, or even from the right alone.

Occasionally the hemorrhages occur at regular intervals every twenty-four hours; every third, fourth or eighth day; or every three or four weeks; return again one or several times, or, in women, sometimes conform to the menstrual type; the duration of separate attacks varies, and the same is true of the quantity of the blood lost, which may range from a few drops to a quart. As a rule, the symptoms are observed to become strikingly worse after an attack, and occasionally lead to a very rapid end. Exceptionally, the subjective symptoms grow less, and a diminution of the splenic tumor takes place.

The causes which give rise to the hemorrhages in chronic tumors of the spleen are various. It might easily be supposed that in a blood so changed not only the white, but also the red blood-corpuscles, would have a tendency to leave the vessels more easily; but the more copious hemorrhages cannot be explained in this way. In such cases a solution of continuity of the vascular walls must be assumed; as an immediate cause, a weakness of the vascular walls may easily be supposed. Especially in leucæmia we are in a position to refer back the development of the so-called hemorrhagic diathesis, primarily, to an altered constitution of the blood. The latter gives rise to such a change of the walls of the vessels that they can no longer offer a sufficient resistance to the ordinary pressure of the blood—still less when it is locally increased. In consequence of the leucæmic condition of the blood, the nutrition of the vascular walls is permanently interfered with, and thereby a greater fragility produced.

Pathologico-anatomical investigation has not yet been sufficiently directed to the changes in the vascular walls, in chronic affections of the spleen; data are, however, often found which point to deficient nutrition of the vessels as a cause of hemorrhage. In the 49th Vol. of Virchow's Archiv, Roth reports fatty degenerations of the walls of the retinal arteries in leucæmia.

Febrile Symptoms.

These are almost always found in acute diseases of the spleen; their connection will be more minutely explained when the acute tumors of the spleen are treated of. In chronic splenic growths, fever occurs more rarely, but may arise either from the disease underlying the splenic affection, or from the complications and consequences. It usually has a material influence upon the course of the disease, whether it progresses with or without fever; when the disease, and with it the cachexia, which is never wanting in these cases, has attained a certain degree, its febrile character is manifested by the patients experiencing alternate feelings of chill and heat. The thermometer usually marks not over 39° C. (102.2° F.), and evening' exacerbation is often present. I once observed evening remissions in a case of splenic leucæmia.

The abdomen becomes more tense, and is sensitive in the region of the spleen and liver; the respiration is frequent, difficult, often accompanied by cough, with tough mucous or rarely bloody expectorations; headaches supervene, which are often limited to definite portions of the head, or are accompanied by various disturbances of the senses: giddiness, buzzing in the ears, or weakness of sight. On some days the fever with its accompaniments is less intense; the urine usually shows a copious deposit of urates and free uric acid. During the febrile exacerbation, dropsical accumulations, which may be already present, are increased, or new ones make their appearance in the

skin or serous cavities. Frequently movable painful œdemas
make their appearance on the lower extremities ; these can often
be referred to the formation of thrombi. Not unfrequently various eruptions occur : eczema, miliaria, boils, erysipelas, as well
as excoriations in places where moist surfaces rub together. As
a consequence of profuse perspiration, I saw in one patient the
skin of the head, neck, and trunk covered with eczematous
tubercles and vesicles, and even little ulcers.

The duration of the febrile condition is very various.

During two months I observed in a leucæmic patient a continuous fever, which
several times showed a remission of one or two days, only after profuse sweating or
nosebleed. The patient complained to a striking degree of stabbing pains in the
left hypochondrium, which shot upward to the shoulder and the back of the head.
Increase of the splenic growth was plainly determined at this time: the point of
the spleen was very painful to the touch, the intensity of the pains demanded two
subcutaneous injections of morphia daily, the fever on separate days corresponded
to the intensity of the pains. At the autopsy, extensive inflammatory processes were
demonstrated in the spleen.

It has also been stated by other observers that the enlargement of chronic tumors of the spleen and lymphatic glands,
taking place by starts, is accompanied by fever, and that often
in chronic diseases of the spleen new glandular growths come
into view during the febrile exacerbation. These facts explain
the origin of the febrile symptoms. It may be assumed that
these febrile symptoms are connected with irritative processes in
the spleen.

Change of the Urinary Secretions.

For a long time the attention of physicians has been directed
to the urinary excretion in diseases of the spleen. The older and
later writers agree upon this point, that its condition is very variable. In most cases the urine is normal in quantity, in many
cases even increased, but towards the end always diminished ;
more rarely during the whole disease a scanty secretion exists ;
the quality also is always strikingly different from the normal.
If one considers the importance which the spleen has as a lymphatic organ, and the influence which its diseases exercise upon

the fluids, it will appear reasonable that, according to the kind of disease and the composition of the blood depending thereon, the renal secretion derived from the altered blood should possess many peculiarities.

In his celebrated work upon the inflammation and enlargement of the spleen, Heusinger represents the urine in acute splenitis as dark yellow, at times scalding towards the end of the disease, with a yellow, firm sediment. This condition of the urine, as is well known, is generally caused by a deposition of uric acid and its combinations, and urinary coloring matters. Not only acute diseases of the spleen connected with fever, but chronic hypertrophies as well, often show the same sediment. When first passed, the urine is usually clear, of a yellow or yellowish red color, strongly acid reaction, and considerable specific gravity (1.020–1.025). After cooling it usually becomes turbid, deposits a clay-colored sediment of urate of soda and ammonia—sedimentum lateritium; often large rhombic plates of free uric acid, sometimes colored, and sometimes uncolored, are found, and during severe dyspnœa, also the well-known octahedra of oxalate of lime.

Heusinger observed these deposits to a striking degree in the person of a physician who, upon coming to consult him for enormous swelling of the spleen, brought with him a little package of very large uric acid crystals which he had obtained from his urine soon after its passage, which was very painful. In some regions—such as Holland, Pavia, Cremona, and India—according to Heusinger, endemic splenic affections are likely to occur with endemic uric acid calculus. Charlton, indeed, asserts that among 100 patients with stone hardly one can be found who has not trouble with his spleen.

Virchow first stated that the secretion of uric acid was increased in leucæmia. H. Ranke afterwards found the same thing. While he reckoned the average excretion in healthy persons at 0.648, he obtained from leucæmic patients on an average 0.915 grm. He drew from this the conclusion that uric acid, at least in great part, was formed in the spleen, in the juice of which Scherer has demonstrated uric acid as a normal constituent. Pettenkofer and Voit obtained the same result in examining the urine of a leucæmic patient. They were fortunate enough to be able to compare the amount of his uric acid excretion with that of two healthy persons who had taken exactly the same food; the increase of uric acid in the leucæmia was sixty-four per cent.

In the first case of splenic leucæmia which I observed, I had analyses made of the urine. In the proportion of the normal constituents, Dr. Koerner found no such important variations from the normal that any special condition peculiar to leucæmia could be fixed upon from them; large quantities of uric acid were found in the urine only when the fever was more intense. Our further observations also have shown an increase of uric acid and its salts as not constant in splenic leucæmia, for which reason I have assumed that, in this disease also, its presence is to be regarded as a consequence of incomplete oxidation—a relative deficiency in respiration; since, according to the investigations of Bartels, an increase of the uric acid above the normal, without simultaneous and proportionate increase of urea, is, under all circumstances, a consequence of an incomplete oxidation of the tissues of the body—that is, of a relative insufficiency of respiration.

Since Senator's experimental investigations upon the influence of respiratory disturbances upon the metamorphosis of tissue, as well as those of Naunyn and Riess, who found no increase of uric acid in a dog of eight kilos weight, from which, in four days, over 350 c.c. of blood had been drawn, one may have some doubt whether the increase of uric acid in the urine which occurs in leucæmia is really caused as explained by Bartels.

The hypothesis set up by Virchow, and later by Ranke, according to which the cause of the increase of uric acid is to be sought in the hypertrophy of the spleen, would, therefore, have to explain the increase of uric acid in the splenic leucæmia. In other tumors of the spleen, then, the urine must contain larger quantities of uric acid. This substance ought, then, to be demonstrated in every case of splenic leucæmia, even when the increase of white corpuscles is only moderate and the dyspnœa slight.

Salkowski, in one case, for thirty successive days made determinations of uric acid and urea; and in this long series the uric acid was constantly increased, both relatively and absolutely, especially in relation to the urea. In a second case which

Salkowski has recently observed, the uric acid was not increased to the same extent. A relative increase of the uric acid was, nevertheless, not to be overlooked, although it could not be considered marked. I have not recently had an opportunity to examine the constitution of the urine in a case of splenic leucæmia; but a case of simple splenic hypertrophy, after intermittent, entered my clinic, in which Dr. Schindler had studied the influence of the splenic tumor on the urinary secretion for thirty-five days, during which the patient took the same carefully weighed daily quantity of food. The uric acid was not increased either relatively or absolutely, nor in comparison to the urea.[1]

The variations which have been observed in the condition of the urinary secretion in chronic tumors of the spleen demand further investigation, until the question as to the increase of uric acid excretion is finally settled.

The qualitative analysis of the urine has also been made of value in the study of splenic diseases. After Scherer demonstrated in the blood of leucæmic patients substances which are known as derivatives of the spleen, it appeared interesting to study their passage into the secretions. In the urine of a patient treated by me, in whom well-marked splenic leucæmia was determined, Wilhelm Koerner found, by the method explained by him, hypoxanthin and lactic acid.

Carl Huber, who used the method given by Scherer, was not able to find hypoxanthin in the urine of a patient treated by me for syphilis and leucæmia. It was natural to connect this negative result with the peculiarity of the case, which was recognized as the lymphatic form of leucæmia. The material of my clinic in this place furnished opportunity for repeating this experiment.

Examinations of urine which Drs. Brasch, Diesterweg, Pfeil-Schneider, and Jakubasch have undertaken, at my suggestion, in the chemical laboratory at this place, showed that an increased formation of hypoxanthin in the spleen, and a consequent increase of hypoxanthin in the blood, occurs in splenic leucæmia, but that the increased formation of hypoxanthin does not belong exclusively to the leucæmic tumor of the spleen. The method given by Scherer, Salkowski considers inaccurate for the demonstration of hypoxanthin in the urine, and therefore believes that the presence of hypoxanthin in the urine is not suffi-

---

[1] *Mosler*, Die Pathologie und Therapie der Leukämie, S. 190.

ciently demonstrated by the earlier examinations, and that the conclusions drawn thence are unfounded, since, in a case at the Jena clinic, as well as in a case examined by him (Salkowski), hypoxanthin was not found in the urine of a patient who suffered from well-marked leucæmia. In a second case of leucæmia, Salkowski also found hypoxanthin in the urine by means of the method used by him, and its occurrence is no longer denied by him.

It is of interest to remark that after Salkowski had demonstrated hypoxanthin in leucæmic bone-marrow, it was very lately found by Heymann in the healthy marrow also.

As to whether the other substances which were found by Scherer in the splenic juice, especially lactic, formic and oxalic acids, pass into the urine when the spleen is hypertrophied, analyses have given varying results; further examinations must determine more accurately whether the presence, or, at least, the presence in increased quantity, of these bodies in the urine, in cases of tumor of the spleen, is to be considered a consequence of incomplete oxidation or of increased action of the spleen.

Physical Examination of the Spleen.

In acute as well as in chronic diseases of the spleen, the local changes demonstrable by physical examination deserve the preference. Previous to a thorough knowledge of physical diagnosis, the want of pathognomonic symptoms of diseases of the spleen was especially manifest, because a functional disturbance of the spleen can only be recognized with difficulty. Most of the symptoms mentioned above become of real value only when their relation to affections of the spleen is proved by the presence of a tumor. Since many physicians are not sufficiently practised in the physical examination of the spleen, the diagnosis of its diseases is made but rarely, or else too late.

Inspection.

In acute swelling of the spleen, as a rule, no visible change of the abdomen is present; chronic tumors often cause great distention.

This was so marked in a female patient with splenic leucæmia, whom I treated in Giessen, that it was very evident through her clothes. Even physicians, on superficial examination, thought of the possibility of a pregnancy in the last months, although upon more careful inspection one could easily be convinced that the growth was more plainly developed upon the left side.

A still more striking distention I observed in a boy of twelve years, who was treated a short time ago in my clinic for amyloid degeneration of the spleen, in consequence of hereditary syphilis.

The abdomen is usually tolerably soft, but often very tense. When the abdominal walls are lax, one can see the outlines of the tumor stretching from the left hypochondrium into the anterior regions of the belly.

Palpation.

The tumors of the spleen protruding from under the arch of the ribs can usually be more clearly felt than seen. The statement of Braune (Text to Plate XVI.) that the enlarged spleen can always be felt during deep inspiration is entirely correct, on the condition that the organ is not too soft, as in the different forms of typhus, where, in addition, the meteorism is often in the way. Leichtenstern [1] has lately called attention to an important source of error. If we allow the patient, lying upon the right side, with abdominal walls as lax as possible, to take a deep inspiration, and, with the hand laid flat upon the abdomen, press the surfaces of the fingers towards the spleen below the arch of the ninth to eleventh ribs, not unfrequently the costal serrations of the diaphragm, which here interlock with the serrations of the transversalis abdominis muscle, can be felt in their contracted condition. They may give the impression of a rounded point, which may be taken by the inexperienced for the anterior extremity of the spleen.

The enlarged spleen, in distinction from the normal, is thrust, upon inspiration, not only deeper, but also farther forward; it thus passes beyond the ligamentum pleuro-colicum, and therefore becomes, since it has lost an important point of support of the

---

[1] Physikalisch-diagnostische Bemerkung zur v. Luschka's Lage der Bauchorgane des Menschen. Separatabdruck aus Göschen's Deutscher Klinik. 1873.

normal spleen, generally more movable. One may often determine by palpation a large, resistant growth, which arises from the left hypochondrium, reaches forward to the navel, may be grasped in its anterior portion, and pushed somewhat outward. In my policlinic a patient is under treatment whose considerable splenic tumor has advanced from the arcus costalis to the navel, can be easily pushed back into the left hypochondrium, and in consequence of the thickening of the capsule exhibits a knobby surface.

One may often feel a crepitus, like that from pressing out the air in cutaneous emphysema (De Pury, Thierfelder, and Uhle). Uhle explains this appearance by the friction of peritoneal exudations. In the summer of 1869 I felt very clearly for five days a peritoneal friction over the leucæmic tumor in a patient in whom acute peritonitis had occurred after arterial transfusion.

The borders of chronic tumors of the spleen show at some distance from their anterior blunt end deep indentations, into which, when the abdominal walls are thin, a finger can be placed. The left lobe of the liver and the splenic tumor often touch. Under these circumstances the anterior end of the spleen is usually thrown a little downward, and we may hence follow the tumor in front of the navel in a curved line downward, so that at the level of the anterior superior spinous process of the ileum it sometimes reaches 5 to 8 ctms. beyond the median line. It often reaches into the pelvis. In the position upon the right side it sinks still more into the abdomen, and changes place to the extent of 4 to 6 ctms.

Percussion of the Spleen.

Notwithstanding many excellent works on the percussion of the spleen, it cannot be denied that it still presents many difficulties. This can scarcely be otherwise, when we consider that we have to do with an organ of only small volume in its normal condition, which is besides only half accessible to the percussion-hammer, and the limitation of which by percussion is rendered more difficult by the surrounding organs.

In relation to the normal position of the spleen, Luschka, as was mentioned upon page 351, has furnished trustworthy results. These data have been confirmed by the examinations of Pirogoff and Braune.[1] In his remarks upon the physical and diagnostic bearings of v. Luschka's[2] Lage der Bauchorgane des Menschen, Leichtenstern has materially promoted the practical application.

In connection with the excellent dissertation of Schuster upon percussion of the spleen, prepared in 1866 under Prof. E. Seitz's direction, this great work forms the basis of the description of this important method of examination, which has also been recently treated of in a meritorious manner in the Deutsches Archiv für klinische Medicin. XIII. 3. p. 322, by A. Weil. In a diagrammatic figure, which he has designed with the assistance of several drawings given in Leichtenstern's work, and which I have found suitable for the explanation of the present text, Weil has explained, for the purpose of percussion, the anatomical relations of the spleen in the following very clear manner :

The spleen lies in the left hypochondrium, between the ninth and eleventh ribs, with its longest diameter directed obliquely from backward and upward, in a direction forward and downward, following the course of these ribs. We can distinguish in this organ an upper end a, which lies at most 2 ctms. from the body of the tenth dorsal vertebra, and an anterior end c (or c'), which corresponds to the point lying nearest to the median line; when the spleen has an oval figure (a, b, c, d) we can mention, besides the upper and lower ends, only two borders, an anterior margo crenatus (a, b, c), and a posterior margo obtusus (a, d, c), which at the anterior extremity gradually round into each other. The anterior end in its normal condition does not pass the costo-articular line—that is, a line drawn from the left sterno-clavicular articulation to the point of the eleventh rib. The anterior border corresponds to the course of the ninth rib, and hence crosses over the lower border of the lung (k, l, m), at an angle which Leichtenstern calls the spleno-pulmonary angle; in this angle (l, b, c) are situated the stomach and the colon. The posterior border follows the eleventh rib, soon to meet with the outer border (e, f, g) of the left kidney. The posterior border of the spleen and the outer border of the left kidney meet at the so-called spleno-renal angle (d, h, g), in which the descending colon is placed. When the form of the spleen is more rhomboidal (a, b, c', d) its anterior border follows the course of the ninth rib farther forward than when its form is oval, and the lower border (c', d) then runs more obliquely backward and downward from the anterior to the posterior border. The position of the lower

---

[1] Topogr.-anat. Atlas. Leipzig, 1867–72. Tafel XVI. Text.
[2] Separat-Abdruck. aus Göschen's Deutscher Klinik 1873. Nos. 26–36.

border of the left lung is of great importance· in understanding the percussion of
the spleen. As appears from the statements of the various authors who have taken
the trouble to fix by percussion upon the living person the position of the lower
border of the left lung, this usually forms a line running around the thorax from
the vertebral column (M, M) to the anterior axillary line (C, C), horizontally or in
a slight curve, with a downward convexity (k, l). (Compare *Conradi*,[1] *Gerhardt*,[2]
and others in relation to this.) From the anterior line of the axilla the lower
border of the left lung passes inward and upward into an arc with its convexity
downward (l, m), to meet the border of the left lobe of the liver (n, m), and then

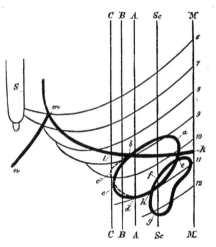

Fig. 1.—*S*, sternum : *M, M,* median line of the back : *Sc, Sc,* scapular line : *A, A,* posterior ; *B, B,* middle ; *C, C,* anterior axillary line ; 6, 12, sixth to twelfth rib ; *a, b, c, d,* oval form of the spleen : *a, b, c', d,*
rhomboidal form of the spleen ; *e, f, g,* outer convex border of the left kidney ; *l, b, c,* spleno-pulmonary
angle ; *d, h, g,* spleno-renal angle ; *k, l, m,* lower border of left lung : *n, m,* border of left lobe of the liver.

to pass into the anterior border of the lung. A glance at the diagram, Fig. I.,
makes evident two important circumstances for percussion : 1. About a third of
the spleen, namely, the upper end, and a part of the anterior and posterior border
are covered by the lungs. 2. The posterior border of the spleen is so placed against
the outer convex border of the left kidney, that, in the region of the greatest part of
the posterior border of the spleen, so far as it is not covered by the lung, the
spleen, and the kidney, two solid organs, meet each other.

[1] Lage and Grösse der Brustorgane u. s. w. Inauguraldissert. Giessen,. 1848.
[2] Lehrbuch der Auscultation und Perkussion.

The difficulties in percussing the spleen are materially increased by the fact that this organ is quite small, some 3 ctms. thick, and therefore by itself gives a much less dull sound than the much thicker liver. Hence, as a rule, strong percussion should be avoided, since the vibrations are immediately transmitted to the neighboring organs, lung, stomach, and intestine, and the dull sound of the spleen is almost entirely lost in the clear sound of the neighboring organs. In rare cases, in which slight percussion does not attain the object, the stronger must be used.

I use Wintrich's hammer and Seitz's double pleximeter of caoutchouc. The smaller portion of the latter is just small enough to be conveniently placed between the ribs of a thin person; others give the preference to immediate percussion by the fingers.

As to the posture of the body, the spleen has been percussed in the most various positions. Schuster had the objects of his examination take five different postures: back, right side, diagonal between the two last, on the face, and sitting. He prefers the diagonal position, which I almost invariably choose in my clinic. The patient lies upon the right shoulder-blade, in a position half-way between that upon the back and the right side; the region of the spleen thus becomes conveniently prominent. Like Schuster and Weil, I prefer to avoid the position upon the right side, since in this, even with the normal spleen, but still more when it is enlarged, the determination of its lower border in the axillary line is sometimes made more difficult or impossible by the lower ribs and the crest of the left ilium approaching each other so as almost to touch.

Von Ziemssen has called attention to the fact that the spleen can be very conveniently percussed while the patient stands. Weil considers the upright position and the diagonal position of the patient as equally justifiable. In a part of the cases we found, when the patient was standing, a clearer limitation of the dulness, especially in front and below, than when he was lying. In other cases, precisely the contrary.

In patients who can stand and sit upright, I have lately corrected the limits obtained in the diagonal position by the results when standing or sitting. In cases which make particular care in percussing the spleen desirable, I believe that such a compari‑son, which Weil also recommends, should be urgently advised.

The comprehension of the method of percussion and the results to be obtained thereby would be made much easier by a diagrammatic figure such as that represented in Fig. II., which Weil has constructed to correspond with the Fig. I. given above. In order to find the splenic dulness in the diagonal or right-sided position, I usually seek, while the patient is breathing quietly, in the left axillary line for the anterior border of the spleen (margo crenatus), which first becomes accessible to percussion in front of the posterior axillary line, since, in this place, the difference in resonance is most clearly marked, and it is conse‑quently advisable to begin the percussion here. Since the upper part of the spleen, covered by the lung, is not accessible to per‑cussion, even after strong expiration, no true upper border of the spleen can be made out on the posterior surface of the thorax; but the spleno-pulmonary boundary at the level of the tenth or eleventh rib can there be marked out by percussion.

Conradi[1] states that in a few cases one may learn by percussion how far the spleen is covered by the lung, while Piorry, on the other hand, says that this can almost always be determined.

Weil percusses first near the vertebral column (in M, M of his Fig. II.), then in the scapular line (Sc, Sc), then in the posterior (A, A), middle (B, B), and anterior (C, C) axillary line, vertically from above downward. He finds then in these lines the points (a, b, c, d, e) at which the clear, full sound of the lung passes into a dull or empty sound. These points may be connected by a line corresponding to the lower border of the left lung. Its course, near the vertebral column, lies on the tenth, in the scapular line on the ninth, in the middle axillary line on the eighth rib, or in the eighth intercostal space; it is generally horizontal, or at least slightly curved downward. It rises from the anterior axillary line in a slight curve (e, f) upward and forward, to pass into the anterior border of the lung at the sixth rib. This portion can only be clearly determined by percussion when the transition of

---

[1] Inauguraldissertation. Giessen. 1868.

the non-tympanitic pulmonary sound into the tympanitic gastric sound is not too indistinct.

After the lower border of the lung is determined, Weil percusses perpendicularly downward in the axillary line. We find in this line, below the border of the lung, an empty or dull sound, which, at *g*, *h*, *i*, passes into a clear tympanitic sound.

By percussion in the direction of several lines converging towards the axillary line (marked with dotted lines in the figure), the points *k*, *l*, *m* are determined at which the tympanitic passes into the dull sound. By connecting all these points, an oval (or three-sided) figure (*e*, *k*, *l*, *m*, *i*, *h*, *g*) is obtained, touching the lower border of the lung. The lower border of this figure can be followed only a short distance farther back to *n*, because beyond the line *n*, *o*, in which the tympanitic sound (of the colon) passes into the

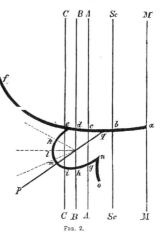

Fig. 2.

empty sound (of the kidneys and lumbar region), the sound from the border of the lung downward is everywhere alike dull. It is clear to the reader from this figure that there is thus obtained a region of dulness (*e*, *k*, *l*, *m*, *i*, *h*, *g*, *n*), open backward, which, as can be seen by comparison with Fig. I., corresponds exactly to that portion of the spleen not covered by the lungs, *i. e.*, to its anterior extremity, and to its posterior border, so far as it does not lie against the outer border of the left kidney. The line *n*, *o* is formed by the outer border of the left kidney. The spleno-pulmonary and spleno-renal angles are again found in Fig. II.

From this demonstration it is clear that only the anterior extremity of the spleen, a portion of the anterior, and a portion of the posterior borders, can be circumscribed by percussion; hence, it is impossible to give an average measure of the normal dulness of the spleen, since the whole portion, that is about a third, lying above the border of the lung, cannot under normal circumstances be circumscribed by percussion. E. Seitz and Schuster have, therefore, recommended to judge of the size of the spleen only by the extent of the splenic dulness from above downward, and by the circumstance whether the anterior extremity of the spleen is thrust into the abdominal cavity more or less far, before or behind the axillary line, so that the splenic dulness forms a region limited on three sides—that is, above, in front, and below—and is open behind. Weil also judges of the size of the organ by the breadth of the dulness found in the axillary line (that is, according to length of the line d, h), as well as by the distance of the anterior extremity from the costo-articular line, or the arch of the ribs; but warns us especially to pay attention to the situation of the lower border of the left lung, lest it might be erroneously supposed that the upper and posterior border of the spleen had been reached.

The spleno-pulmonary boundary was placed by Avenbrugger at the seventh rib in the axillary line; by Strempel, at the seventh intercostal space; by Piorry, at the eighth; by Bamberger, at the ninth; by Schuster, at the eighth or ninth. Weil also found in most cases, in the diagonal or right-sided position, the spleno-pulmonary boundary, in the middle axillary line at the eighth intercostal space, or at the ninth rib; in many cases also at the eighth rib.

The distance of the lower border of the spleen from the upper in the middle axillary line, that is, the breadth of the splenic dulness, is usually, in health, 5 to 6 ctms. In rare cases it was found by Weil 7½ ctms.

The anterior border of the spleen—that is, the point of the splenic dulness lying nearest to the median line—lay in most of the cases examined by Weil exactly in the costo-articular line, or passed about one centimetre beyond it—that is, it was distant four or five centimetres from the arch of the ribs.

Leichtenstern has lately paid attention to the varying conditions of the thoracic circumference, since the distance between the vertebral column on the one side, the axillary and costo-articular line on the other, differs according to the circumference of the thorax, but the spleen does not become longer or shorter in the same ratio as the difference between the lines mentioned becomes more or less; therefore, the long diameter of the spleen must show in different cases a varying proportion to the amount of the distance between the vertebral column and the axillary line. And since the upper posterior end of the spleen, which is inaccessible to percussion, is found at a constant distance (2 to 4 ctms.) from the vertebral column, the distance between the anterior extremity of the spleen and the axillary and costo-articular line is subject to variations dependent upon the thoracic circumference. So the necessity arises of using none of the customary lines to limit the anterior end of the spleen, but of always founding an estimation of its size and length upon the absolute amount of the splenic dulness.

Notwithstanding this, according to Leichtenstern's very numerous examinations directed to this point, one or another of the usual lines, notwithstanding its dependence upon the thoracic circumference, is employed in most of the cases as a very useful starting-point in determining the size of the spleen, and he gives the following limits for the anterior end of the spleen.

This does not usually pass farther forward than the middle axillary line. When the periphery of the thorax is large, it lies somewhat behind; when smaller, in the axillary line; and only passes this when the thorax is very long and small, and at the farthest only to the costo-axillary line of Bamberger.

It cannot be denied that the determination of the size of the spleen belongs to the most difficult problems of percussion, and hence demands many cautions. For instance, in the percussion of the anterior border (margo crenatus), it may be mentioned that —especially in the rhomboidal form, which lies close to the wall of the thorax, with a larger surface accessible to percussion than the oval—this border grows gradually thin, as happens at the sharp edge of the liver. Under such circumstances only a moderately strong, or, when the thoracic wall is thin, even a weak percussion, can separate the region of relative dulness which corresponds to the thin edge of the spleen from the full tympanitic sound of the stomach and colon.

It should not ·be forgotten that in some cases—without the existence of emphysema or a pleuritic exudation on the left side—the normal dulness of the spleen cannot be found anywhere. This happened to Schuster only five times among eighty examinations. We cannot say in these cases whether we have to do with an abnormally situated, or diminished, or hemispherically formed spleen. A very flat, disc-shaped spleen, when the stomach and colon are resonant, may make the percussion difficult even unto impossibility (Leichtenstern).

Special difficulties in percussing the spleen arise from the various conditions of fulness of the neighboring organs. In the spleno-pulmonary angle mentioned above (o in the diagram) are situated the stomach and the colon—the first, when moderately distended, following with its great curvature the course of the eighth rib. Between the eighth and ninth ribs the colon lies against the thoracic wall, and runs along that part of the margo crenatus which is accessible to percussion.

Leichtenstern calls special attention to the fact that the omentum majus, which reaches to the left end of the transverse colon, to the splenic flexure, here and there covers the colon running along the margo crenatus in the spleno-pulmonary angle, and keeps it away from the thoracic wall (Braune and Luschka).

In this case one percusses, directly above the anterior border of the spleen, the colon covered by the omentum majus. Thus it is possible that we may get in the spleno-pulmonary angle, especially when the omentum is fat, a very dull, tympanitic sound, even when the stomach and colon contain air, which makes the percussion of the thin margo crenatus much more difficult. In the spleno-renal angle is found the descending colon (Braune and Luschka). Since, when the descending colon is strongly distended, even the anterior border of the spleen can be surrounded thereby, a condition is possible in which both the anterior and posterior border and the anterior extremity of the spleen are surrounded by the colon. When the stomach is largely distended, not only the whole spleno-pulmonary angle can be occupied by the stomach (Braune), but it may reach downward some distance, along the inner surface of the spleen.

This neighborhood of the spleen throws many difficulties in

the way of its percussion, since not only the colon, filled with fæces, but also the stomach, filled in its lower part with solid or fluid matter, may make percussion impossible, or its results faulty. Careful consideration of these circumstances justifies the advice of Piorry, always to make the percussion when the patient is fasting. The same thing is true in regard to the evacuation of the large intestine.

Slight changes in the volume of the spleen are often difficult to determine by percussion ; even when the spleen is completely normal, an enlargement may be counterfeited by other bodies, that give a dull sound, coming in immediate contact with it.

It not unfrequently happens, in consequence of the varying fulness of the colon and stomach, that we find a dulness of the spleen, which appears quite extensive on one day, reduced on the next to its normal size ; therefore, when its condition is doubtful, it is necessary to establish the diagnosis by repeated examinations.

On the other hand, a tumor of the spleen may be present, and its enlargement cannot be demonstrated. This happens if the diaphragm is placed high, and, in consequence, only a small part of the spleen lies against the ribs. Percussion of the splenic tumor may become absolutely impossible, from flatulent distention of the stomach and intestinal canal, as well as by dropsical effusions in the abdominal cavity. In a case of melano-leucæmia I was able to demonstrate the enlargement of the liver and spleen only after the considerable ascites had been reduced by puncture. In a case of well-marked splenic leucæmia in an old lady, I was unable, in the last stage of the disease, to determine by percussion the size of the enormously enlarged spleen, because an extensive ascites had been developed.

Less frequently enlargements of the liver or of the left kidney prevent the accurate percussion of the spleen ; still more rarely this happens by encapsulated peritoneal exudations in the neighborhood of the spleen ; here, however, palpation usually comes to the assistance of percussion, since the characteristic indentations of the spleen can generally be clearly felt. Diseases of the thoracic organs, like consolidation of the lungs, emphysema, collections of gas or fluid in the left pleura, occasionally embarrass the examination of the spleen; even then, if the right side is healthy, we may succeed in percussing the spleen. The position of the left lower border of the lung may be inferred from that of the right side. It is stated by many authors that the sound of the splenic dulness may be distinguished from that of a consolidation of the lung, or of a pleuritic exudation (Siebert). Even if a distinction can be made between the flat tone of a pleuritic exudation and the less dull sound of the spleen, yet in such cases the determination of the upper limit of the splenic dulness by percussion is always uncertain.

In general, we can suppose that the normal spleen, as well as small splenic tumors, on account of their less extent, give a less dull sound than the liver. On the other hand, if the splenic tumors attain a very considerable size, the percussion-sound over them is just as flat as over the liver. With these large splenic tumors the percussion, as a rule, is much easier than with smaller ones, the increase and decrease of size less difficult to determine. The method of percussion is precisely the same as that given above. It is very easy in this case to limit the circumference of the organ accurately on all sides; it is, of course, often possible to find the limits of large tumors more distinctly by palpation than by percussion.

Therapeutics of Splenic Diseases in General.

The therapeutics of splenic diseases establish the truth of the statement that the more obscure the insight into the physiology and pathology of an organ, the greater is the number of the remedies which are recommended for the cure, or, at least, the alleviation of its diseases; it would hardly be possible to mention by name all the drugs which, in earlier or later times, have been supposed to have an action on the spleen (Milzmittel—splenica). They belong chiefly to the vegetable kingdom, as diuretics, astringents, carminatives.

In favor of the splenic remedies praised by the ancients, like white mustard, watercress, and the spleenwort (Asplenium), referred to various kinds of plants, or the remedies used later, and then again forgotten, like Scolopendrium officinale,

Adiantum capillus, and Chrysosplenium, there is just as little proof as of the value of the splenic remedies of the homœopaths and Rademacher.

The older French physicians, Tournfort and Garidel, ascribed to the herb Geum urbanum, besides its febrifuge action, solvent powers in obstructions of the spleen. In further recommendation, Bouteille, Jr., describes the cure of a great ague-cake in a young woman who had suffered from it for a long time in consequence of a double tertian malarial fever, after she had been treated in vain with vegetable extracts of all kinds.

Rademacher assures us that he has proved vegetable charcoal to be curative in some undoubted cases of splenic diseases, but is unable to give any more accurate indications for these cases. In a man who suffered from a very tedious enlargement of the spleen, with secondary troublesome shortness of breath, and cough, other means failing, he tried the vegetable charcoal with brilliant effect, so that the patient was soon entirely freed from his disease. In other cases, however, the splenic asthma did not yield to the charcoal.

Among the splenic remedies furnished by the vegetable kingdom, St. Mary's thistle (Frauendistel), according to Rademacher, occupies a prominent place. Its beneficent action is celebrated in diseases of the spleen, which depend on sluggish circulation and enlargement of this organ, as well as upon disturbances of the circulation of the whole portal system. The efficacy of the seed of the St. Mary's thistle resides, according to Rademacher, not in the starchy portion, but in the envelopes.

Squill was praised by the older writers as a splenic remedy. This root was approved in painful obstructions of the spleen, and was said to act as a specific in splenic dropsy. In the latter affection also, acorns, in the form of a spirituous extract, continued for weeks, were said to be of special benefit (Rademacher) against chronic obstructions of the circulation and the enlargement of the spleen connected therewith. Belladonna root was recommended, as well as conium; which acts like the belladonna as a narcotic to the abdominal ganglia.

The number of remedies to which, according to my experience, an influence upon the spleen must be conceded, is a small one. If we ask for the causes, we must mention as among the most prominent, that, owing to its deep position, the spleen is less accessible to remedies than other organs, and that local means have so far been made useful only to a very slight extent.

Prophylactic Treatment.

Since abdominal obstructions, anomalies of menstruation, psychical influences, syphilis, intermittent, and other infectious diseases, are well known causes of splenic tumors, it is the first task of the practitioner to make use of prophylactic means against the so frequent occurrence of splenic tumors.

The connection of the spleen with the digestive organs is anatomically clear, and disturbances of the digestion react upon the spleen. We have been made aware by the works of Ludwig, Von Bezold, and their scholars, of the great capacity of the vascular territory of the abdomen in comparison with the total blood-mass; hence arises a special tendency to abdominal obstructions under various circumstances; hence, in a prophylactic point of view, exercise in the open air and gymnastic practice are to be recommended. Regular and careful expansion of the lungs contribute, as Ramadge has already remarked, indirectly to remove congestions of the stomach and intestinal canal, and their appendages, the liver, spleen, and pancreas. The value of deep inspirations as an important compensatory function in derangements of the circulation has been lately shown by Hermann.

Against the troubles occurring in advanced years, fulness of the chest, pressure in the abdomen, so-called abdominal plethora, derivative means are to be employed; laxative cures, especially long use of the Friedrichshall bitter-water, do good service in these cases. A carefully regulated diet is the most important point. I cannot say enough in favor of giving to such patients a definite bill of fare, which enjoins upon them to take only definite quantities of nourishment at prescribed times.

The influence of cold upon the stomach, as well as upon the abdomen generally, is often given as a cause of splenic troubles. The theory of taking cold has lately received a firmer basis from Hermann's physiological experiments on the danger of cold drinks when the body is heated. After the injection of a syringeful of ice-cold water into the stomach of a dog, Hermann observed the arterial pressure in the carotid, or femoral, almost doubled. This rise of the arterial pressure produces disturbances of the circulation in the interior organs, according to the point of least resistance; such disturbances take place in a similar manner by the action of cold upon extensive regions of the skin. I do not consider it impossible that tumors of the spleen may arise from the influence of cold upon the skin. I have observed a case of exceedingly well-marked splenic leucæmia which arose in consequence of a suppression of the menses from taking cold ; hence, the influence of cold deserves consideration among the prophylactic directions.

Disturbances of the sexual functions in the female sex have an unmistakable influence on the existence of splenic tumor, there is consequently a distinct call upon gynæcology to direct its attention to changes of the spleen in diseases of the female genital organs. If, in such cases, a tumor of the spleen can be detected at the same time with slight increase of the white blood-corpuscles, the possibility of a leucæmia in the formative stage may be suspected, and an energetic treatment of the splenic trouble should be begun.

The proof of the connection between syphilis and tumors of the spleen is of importance in the cure of the latter. In the specific treatment of syphilis a prophylactic measure is placed in our hands, by which we can effect the cure of an incipient tumor ; but for this we must demand that the patient should give himself up completely to a regular, methodical mercurial cure during complete abstinence from business for from four to six weeks ; diet, rest, warmth, a proper regulation of the secretions and excretions, must be held as the first conditions of treatment. Just here the welfare of the patient depends upon the correct management of the careful practitioner.

We should be especially observant of those measures which combat the diseases of the spleen arising from malaria ; these have been lately given with accuracy by Léon Colin.[1] Some of them are concerned with the soil, and are intended to prevent the development of the miasma itself, while others are supposed to limit the action of the miasm upon man.

As is well known in the various marshy districts of all parts of the world, better hygienic conditions are attained by extensive drainage ; however great may be the number of men sink-

[1] Traité des fièvres intermittentes, par L. Colin, méd. principal de l'armée, prof. à l'école imp. d'application de méd. milit. (Val-de-Grace). Paris, 1870. J. B Baillière et fils. 8. XVI. et 544 pp. 8 Francs. Beiträge zur Lehre von Malaria-krankheiten, nach neuern Untersuchungen von Dr. Oscar Berger in Breslau. Schmidt's Jahrbücher. 1871. 152. S. 29.

ing under these works, the prosperity and increasing health of succeeding generations will sufficiently outweigh the sacrifice. Large experience has shown that in general the simple drainage of the marsh is not sufficient, but the careful cultivation of the soil is demanded.

Among the physical conditions of the soil the development of malaria is particularly favored by the presence of an impermeable stratum of clay, preventing the soaking-in of the water, as well as a sandy condition of the superficial layers of the soil preventing vegetation. In many countries the extreme richness of the soil is looked upon as the cause of malaria. It may often be shown that when fever-epidemics occasionally arise in neighborhoods usually considered healthy, at the same time the soil exhibits an unusual sterility. It can easily be understood that regions which of themselves are very productive, but remain untouched by cultivation (Campagna Romana), are constantly unhealthy. In all countries it is universally recognized as a necessity that the population, in the interest of health, should be careful, after previous drainage of the soil, to maintain a sufficient vegetation. Hence, the advice is worthy of notice to plant in fever regions certain trees whose rapid growth is a sign of their great absorbing power; as, for example, trees of the family Eucalyptus, especially Eucalyptus globulus.

The growth of these trees is extremely rapid. In a short time they attain gigantic dimensions, and are said to possess unusual powers of destroying miasmatic influences in fever regions. The peculiar property is ascribed to them of absorbing ten times their weight of water from the soil and giving out antiseptic, camphorlike effluvia; if they are planted in a marshy soil, they are said to dry it up in a short time. The English were the first who made experiments with them at the Cape of Good Hope, and within two or three years they succeeded in entirely changing its climatic conditions of the unhealthy part of the colony. A few years later its cultivation was undertaken on a large scale in Algeria. At Pardock, a farm twenty miles from Algiers, situated on the Hamyze, and known for its infected air, were raised in the spring of 1867 about 13,000 plants of Eucalyptus globulus. In July of this year, at which time the fever had usually begun in former years, there was not a case, although the trees were only nine feet high. Since that time the place has maintained a complete immunity from disease.

In the neighborhood of Constantine the farm of Ben Marhillie was in bad repute; it was a marsh summer and winter. In five years the whole soil was made dry by 14,000 trees. The inhabitants and their children enjoyed excellent health.

In the factory Gue of Constantine, plantations of Eucalyptus globulus succeeded in changing twelve acres of swamp into a noble park; fevers entirely disappeared. In Cuba, malarial troubles are said to have disappeared from those districts where the cultivation of this tree has been introduced. A station-house at the end of a railroad viaduct, in the department of the Var, was so infected that officials could live there only for one year. After forty of these trees had been planted the place became completely healthy. Where this tree grows, it may be regarded as the surest and most beneficent destroyer of swamp-miasm.[1]

Colin considers himself, in consequence of his observations, justified in the statement that the farther south the climate from which an individual comes, the better can he resist the influence of malarial poisoning. While, for example, in the Antilles and regions of the Mexican coast, the Spaniards find themselves in good health, the English are much more subject to malarial diseases. According to Colin, it is well established that the greatest danger threatens those who first enter a foreign country infected with fever, while the later arrivals, in consequence of the prophylactic and hygienic regulations already in force, find themselves in relatively favorable conditions of acclimatization; of an habituation to the marsh-miasm we cannot speak, since a longer residence, on the contrary, increases the danger.

As a prophylactic measure for inhabitants of fever countries, protective arrangements, such as elevated sites and woods, are of great importance. Residence at elevated points is rightly looked upon as an important prophylactic measure. The level of protection varies according to the intensity of the poisonous influence. Sources of malaria in the neighborhood of a hill make its protective action vain. In fever countries, delay in the open field, especially at night, should be forbidden. The danger of the nocturnal emanations can be diminished by lighting great fires. Proper warm clothing, good nourishment, temperance, are under all circumstances to be expressly advised; for protection against the rays of the sun, a suitable covering for the head should be worn.

It is also important that a stranger should not travel to fever countries at the time of the yearly endemo-epidemic. In the febrile regions of the temperate zone, the first six months of the

---

[1] Med. Times and Gazette. 1873. No. 1218. 1st Nov. p. 502.

year are the least dangerous. Strangers can most safely visit Rome in the autumn, before the end of September. Earthworks and military expeditions should only be attempted in favorable times of the year.

Infected regions should be avoided during the time that the fever prevails. Residence at sea has been warmly recommended for a long time by observers in warm countries (Lind, Thévenot), so that floating hospitals on shipboard have been arranged for malarial patients. A radically prophylactic means is sending back the fever patient to his home. Colin has every year, in August and September, sent back hundreds of sick soldiers from Rome and Civita Vecchia to France. He was almost always able to learn of their subsequent recovery.

It is certainly very important to every physician and layman who lives in a malarial region, to have recourse at certain times to prophylactic drugs.

The last work of Prof. Dr. Ritter von Vivenot, Jr., lost to science by an early death, treats at length of the prophylactic use of quinine against malarial poisoning. He had set for himself the important task of inducing the Austrian government to act in restraining the spread of the disease in one of the largest and most notoriously malarial regions of Europe. This region stretches over the greater part of Hungary, the Banat, Sclavonia, and Croatia, and continues in a south-west direction along the coast of the Adriatic to Istria and Dalmatia. This tract is limited on the east by the mountains of Transylvania, and on the north by the Carpathian range, and includes the valleys of the Theiss, the Danube, the Drave, the Save, the Mür, and their tributaries.

The prophylactic power of quinia has long been a fixed fact for American physicians (Van Buren, G. B. Wood, and others). The valuable statistical reports on the health of the British navy, which contain a treasure of the most various experiences, collected from all parts of the globe, furnish a mine of important observations. The richest material for the English navy was furnished by the deadly climate of the West African station. The frightful amount of disease and death which the first Niger expedition, fitted out in the year 1843, for restraining the slave trade, experienced, was diminished during the later expeditions, when the prophylactic use of cinchona bark and its preparations was introduced. There were many cases in which only the few who did not use quinia fell sick with the fever, while all the others were spared.

Of the numerous facts which Vivenot has adduced in favor of the prophylactic action of quinia against malarial poisoning, this conclusion can be drawn without doubt: that the use of moderate doses of quinia, continued daily for a long time, is a measure which can materially reduce the susceptibility of the organism to the injurious consequences of the malarial poisoning. This proposition has the more importance from the fact that the continued use of preparations of quinia in suitable form is followed by no evil consequences (Dr. Newberry, Dr. H. de Saussure). Vivenot's statements certainly deserve general consideration. Trustworthy results may be obtained among the troops besieging the numerous fortresses situated in fever regions. Experiments should be made in febrile regions having a known time at which the epidemic commences, at least from two to three weeks before this time arrives, and should be continued from two to three weeks after the epidemic has abated.

During the whole time of the fever, according to Vivenot, a dose of three grains of sulphate of quinia is to be given daily to every man, and preferably dissolved in an ounce of wine, rum, or brandy. It may be supposed, under such circumstances, that the increased cost to the government of the quinine for prophylactic use might be looked upon as economy in comparison with the increased expenditure in cases of actual disease.

In this prophylactic treatment, matter of expense is of less consequence, since the cheaper succedanea of quinine may be very properly used for this purpose. According to my experience, the amorphous muriate of quinine (Zimmer) may be here recommended, as well as the quinoidin, which, in the form of quinoidin pills, obtained from Zimmer's quinine factory, costs very little. I shall again speak of its action. I will only mention in this place that the experiments[1] which were tried in the garrison hospital No. 2 in Vienna, to determine the therapeutic value of the preparations of quinoidin in intermittent, as well as my own observations, have shown that quinoidin possesses the action belonging to quinine as a febrifuge, and that preparations of quinoidin are borne by patients in general just as well as quinine.

The action of quinia as a febrifuge can be explained in different ways. Since the influence of this drug upon the germination, growth, and increase of the lowest

---

[1] Allgem. Militärärztliche Zeitung. Nr. 31. u. 32. 1871.

organisms, that is, upon septic and zymotic processes, was demonstrated by Binz, this property of quinia may be considered a consequence of an antizymotic action.

The French physicians attempted to solve the problem, in order to find a basis for the action of quinia in splenic troubles, by directing their attention chiefly to the contractile character of the tissue of the spleen. From experiments upon animals they assumed that quinia exerted an influence upon the tissue of that organ similar to that of the induction current on muscles. Kuechenmeister[1] undertook such experiments on rabbits, calves, and sheep, but arrived at no positive result. On the other hand, he saw in swine, which had been kept fasting, the exposed spleen plainly contract after large doses of quinia. Buchheim leaves it undecided whether a change in the spleen after the use of quinia, in healthy men and animals, can be proved or not. R. Schmidt expresses himself decidedly against the results obtained by Kuechenmeister.

I myself have undertaken a series of experiments and published them in my monograph of leucæmia; before and after the use of quinia, the size and condition of the exposed spleen in dogs was carefully examined. Since the sulphate of quinine is dissolved only in 800, but the hydrochlorate in 60 parts of water of the ordinary temperature, the hydrochlorate was chosen for all the experiments. The solution was injected under the skin, in the immediate neighborhood of the abdominal walls; the organ afterwards felt very solid and firm, and its surface exhibited no longer the normal polish, but a clearly granulated condition, changes from which a contraction of the contractile elements of the spleen may be suspected. After an increasing dose of the drug, I could determine a further increase of the resistance and hardness of the organ, as well as of the granulated condition of the surface, especially of the borders, and also a distinct diminution in size.

Splenic Drugs.

After Binz had succeeded, in the case of frogs, in which he had artificially excited a peritonitis and also an acute swelling of the spleen, in producing in almost all cases, by the injection of quinia, a contraction and diminution of this organ, I also examined the effect of quinia in a spleen pathologically enlarged by cutting the nerves; notwithstanding all the visible nerves were cut at the niches of the spleen, the contractile action of the quinia took place from contraction of the muscular elements.

Binz believes that the diminution in size of the morbidly enlarged spleen may be explained by supposing that the production of the colorless elements is paralyzed by quinia; thus

---

[1] Schmidt's Jahrbücher. Bd. LXX. S. 13.

the cessation of a principal cause of the swelling permits a proper activity of the contractile fibres and a diminution of the organ.

In the frogs which Binz arranged for the production of mesenteritis, an acute inflammation of the spleen was usually demonstrable, together with increase of colorless elements in the blood ; both were alike diminished by subcutaneous injections of quinine. This hypothesis of Binz is competent to explain the results which I have obtained in the treatment of leucæmic tumors by the exhibition of large doses of quinine. At any rate, these are an encouragement to make a trial of large doses of quinine in leucæmia more frequently than has been hitherto done. Here, as well as always in the treatment of splenic tumors, all the precautions in the use of quinine must be observed in order to have certainty of absorption.

In the so-called status gastricus I follow the old rule of preceding the quinia by emetics or cathartics ; neither should the drug be taken upon a full stomach. It may be assumed with great probability that the quinia which is not absorbed in the acid secretions of the stomach passes away in part with the fæces. Its salts are precipitated by alkalies ; in the small intestine they are probably reduced to a form which is absorbed with difficulty ; hence, it is important to prescribe the quinia in an acid solution, and to choose preparations which are easily soluble. According to Binz, the sulphate of quinine is soluble only in 800, the muriate in 60 parts of water of medium temperature. If a little more hydrochloric acid is added to the latter solution, in order to increase the solubility, we gain the additional advantage of an agent—normally present in the primæ viæ—the excellent effects of which are recognized in many disturbances of the digestion. The salt is best prescribed in the liquid form :

> ℞. Quiniæ muriatis..................... ʒ i.
> Acidi hydrochlorici............... f. ʒ ss.
> Aquæ destillatæ................... f. ℥ v.
> Mucilaginis acaciæ,
> Syrupi, ā̄ā......................... f. ʒ v.
> Tincturæ cinnamomi .... f. ʒ iiss.

M.—S. A tablespoonful at 6, 7, and 8 o' clock in the morning.

The cheaper sulphate of quinine may be advantageously prescribed in connection with hydrochloric acid. Many patients cannot bear the quinia mixture continuously, and another form must then be chosen. They become most easily accustomed to the pill form :

> ℞. Quiniæ muriatis................... Ə iv.
> Solve in
> Acidi hydrochlorici.............. guttis xv.
> Aquæ destillatæ quantum satis.
> Adde
> Althææ,
> Sacchari albi, āā, quantum satis,
> ut fiant pilulæ numero C.
> Consperge pulvere cinnamomi.
> S. Take from five to ten pills morning and evening.

It is better to drink a little hydrochloric acid afterwards, as well as when the quinine is given in the form of powder with wafers.

> ℞. Acidi hydrochlorici............... ℳ xlvi.
> Syrupi rubi idæi.................. f. ℥ iiss.
> M.—S. A teaspoonful in glass of water.

From the subcutaneous injection of the solution of quinine, against which I have formerly spoken, I have lately seen favorable results. It is desirable to inject as deeply as possible into the subcutaneous tissue, in order to avoid the formation of abscesses, which are otherwise liable to occur.   To illustrate the manner of its use and its practical value, I will mention the prominent points in the following case :

Wilhelmina K., forty-one years old, entered my clinic on the 16th October, 1873, for severe tertian intermittent, which had already lasted four weeks. After the condition of the fever had been accurately determined on the morning of the 17th October, a hydrochloric acid mixture was ordered in the evening, and twice a day a syringeful of a solution of hydrochlorate of quinine (twenty-five grains to the ounce) was injected.   On the 18th and 21st of October the attacks recurred with the same intensity. So far nearly four grains of hydrochlorate of quinine had been injected.   Since no decrease of the fever could be determined, the following solution was chosen :

> ℞. Quiniæ muriatis .... gr.xviii.
> Aquæ destillatæ............. f ℥ ij.
> Acidi hydrochlorici .... gtt. j.

After warming of the solution, morning and evening on the 22d of October, and on the morning of the 23d, immediately before the attack, two syringefuls were injected at each time. From this time the attacks completely ceased, and the patient felt perfectly well.

The punctures in the neighborhood of the spleen were somewhat painful. Indurations could be felt, but did not come to suppuration. On the 24th and 25th of October a syringeful was injected morning and evening. No further paroxysms of fever occurred, and, when the patient was discharged on the 3d of November, the splenic tumor was no longer to be felt.

In the form of subcutaneous injections, smaller doses seem necessary than when it is given by the mouth.

For economical reasons, I have frequently employed in diseases of the spleen the neutral sulphate of quinoidin (quinidia), the action of which has already been examined by experienced clinicians—Wunderlich and Hasse. I obtained in large quantities, from Zimmer's quinine factory at Frankfort-on-the-Main, pills prepared from pure sulphate of quinoidin, in the form of an extract. Instead of using an inert powder for their manufacture, precipitated cinchonia is employed, of which from twenty to twenty-five per cent. is required; thus, these pills contain exclusively cinchona alkaloids, in definite quantity (Kerner). Each of these pills weighs one and a half grains, and their action is nearly equivalent to that of a grain of sulphate of quinine. The experiments upon the action of these pills, which I once had made by my assistant physician in the medical polyclinic, Dr. Adam, gave the result that a larger quantity of sulphate of quinoidin (quinidia) than of sulphate of quinia was necessary for breaking up an intermittent; that the quinoidin acts more slowly, which may be partly due to the fact that large doses cannot be given at once without the occurrence of vomiting.

In order to make these durable, since they contain no other vehicle than pulverized, pure cinchonia, they must be made quite hard, and therefore always give some mechanical work to be done by the stomach. The physician is therefore compelled to extend the administration of large quantities of these pills over several hours. This drug is, therefore, not suited for cases where large doses of cinchona preparations are to be given at once.

Dr. Kerner has lately recommended the amorphous muriate

of quinine, prepared at Zimmer's factory in a chemically pure form—a light brown powder of the well-known quinine taste, which has the advantage over the sulphate that it is soluble in all proportions of water, and also easily absorbable. Kerner has determined in his numerous experiments that there is no combination of the cinchona alkaloids which, with an immense solubility, is so nearly equivalent in action to the ordinary quinia as the amorphous muriate (Zimmer). It is taken so rapidly into the circulation that intoxication therefrom is more to be dreaded than from ordinary quinine. It may also be used in powder in every form of administration. For supporting and increasing the action of quinine, Kerner recommends carbonic acid (soda-water) as a drink. Since the preparation is very hygroscopic, it must always be kept dry and well stoppered. A concentrated solution of known strength (1 : 3 or 1 : 5) may be prepared, which may be kept completely unchanged, and by dilution or concentration graduated for mixtures, enemata, pills, solutions for hypodermic injection.

In conjunction with Dr. Bickel, I have experimented upon the influence of amorphous muriate of quinine upon the spleen of dogs, just as was done with quinine in the experiments mentioned above. These experiments have shown that this agent is capable of contracting the normal, as well as the pathologically enlarged spleen, but, with equal doses, not to the same degree as the crystallized quinine.

For subcutaneous injections in man, I prefer, from my later experience, the amorphous muriate to the crystallized. Kerner recommends the concentration of 1 to 5; this I have often used. It produces, if injected carefully and deeply into the subcutaneous tissues, astonishingly little local irritation.

According to my experience, the action of the cinchona preparations in diseases of the spleen is made more effectual by applying at the same time cold water over this organ. It has been shown by Thomsa that the spleen contracts, not only upon electrical and chemical, but also upon thermic irritations. I have recently clearly shown by my experiments, published in the 57th Vol. of Virchow's Archives, that the immediate contact of cold water with the normal spleen produces a visible contraction of it ; according to the length of the application, the surface showed a granulated condition; the parenchyma a solid consistence, and a diminution of the organ followed. Probably the fibrous sheath, together with the processes given off into the interior of the true splenic tissue, in connection with the organic muscular fibres which are known to be abundantly developed in the dog, were contracted by contact with the cold water ; there seemed to be a difference if the cold were applied by means of ice-bags, or if at the same time the mechanical force of the cold douche came into play.

The action of cold water on the normal spleen was less distinct through the abdominal walls ; more with the cold douche, where the mechanical influence is to be taken into account, than when cold compresses or pieces of ice are laid over the spleen.

In acute as well as in chronic tumors of the spleen, I have seen favorable results from the application of cold to the splenic region, either in the form of douches or of ice-bags, since I could determine a diminution of the tumors immediately after.

I have been able to check paroxysms of intermittent by the cold douche, after the method of Fleury. By this method the patient receives for a long time a douche of from one and a half to two minutes, A. M. and P. M. The average duration of the bath upon spine, spleen, and liver was half a minute. The warmth of the water was 56.7° Fahr.

At the same time with the douche, a shower-bath was used, which allowed the water to fall from above upon the patient. On one patient this procedure was continued twice a day for forty-five days; the fever-paroxysms immediately ceased; but notwithstanding the continuance of the cold douche, a return of the fever, with increase of the tumor, took place. When no febrile attack returned within ten days, the patient was discharged at his own request, but the tumor remained. The patient had become tired of the trouble of so long continued treatment, and only by great persuasion was brought to continue the cure. I did not dare to use in intermittent a greater degree of cold or force of stream, because I feared the same ill effects of which I shall speak farther on in connection with the typhus spleen.

According to my previous experience, I think I cannot be wrong in supposing that the patients with intermittent, so far treated by me with cold douche, after Fleury's method, would have got well much sooner by the administration of large doses of quinine. I have not been able to convince myself that, either in recent or old cases of intermittent fever, the cold douche has the advantage over quinine, as is constantly stated by some enthusiasts. On the other hand, I by no means ignore the favorable influence of cold upon tumors of the spleen. Besides the contractile influence produced through the skin upon the elements of the spleen, the vigorous irritation of the cold douche upon the spleen itself is to be considered, which increases its action. Besides this it stimulates to deeper inspirations. By the sinking of the diaphragm there is produced a pressure on the spleen, and thereby a mechanical diminution.

I have used the numerous cases of typhus recurrens which have occurred of late years in my clinic to determine the influence of cold water upon the typhus spleen. In hardly any case have I neglected to determine accurately the limits of the spleen before and after the bath. This is not so easy in typhus abdominalis, on account of the meteorism. As a rule, I was able to demonstrate to my students in cases of typhus recurrens a distinct diminution of the splenic tumor after the use of cold water. I must, however, give a warning against the application of the cold douche over the spleen in typhus. It seems to exercise too abrupt an influence over the typhus spleen. Once I observed after it severe peritonitis; another time intense fluxionary hyperæmia of the brain. The baths—of from 90.5° to 54.5° F.—which, according to individual peculiarities, are given in my clinic in the various forms of typhus, fulfil the object of producing a lowering of the temperature and also a diminution of the splenic tumor; but I often use a combination of cold water and quinia in typhus.

It appears to me as if, according to the greater or less diminution of volume of the spleen after the use of cold water and quinine in typhus, the individual case has taken more or less rapidly a favorable or unfavorable course, so that I have often made use of this symptom in prognosis. In the severe cases of typhus, with unfavorable result, I have been able to find only a slight diminution of the splenic tumor after cold water and quinine, probably because the contractile elements are almost completely paralyzed by the great accumulation of the typhus poison in the spleen.

In chronic tumors of the spleen, with or without a leucæmic condition of the blood, I have shown the contractile action of the cold douche, as well as of cold in general, but have clearly convinced myself that this influence is materially increased if large doses of quinine are used at the same time.

According to my previous experience, a combined application of cold water upon the spleen, either in the form of cold baths, or ice-bags, or cold douche, with the simultaneous exhibition of quinine, possesses an advantage in the treatment of acute and chronic tumors of the spleen over the use of either of these means alone.

Since the removal of chronic tumors of the spleen is brought about only by the continued use of cinchona preparations, it is impossible, in many cases, on account of the high price, to give pure quinia for a long time. It is therefore advisable to try the much cheaper amorphous muriate of quinia (Zimmer), together with the application of cold to the spleen.

Besides the cinchona preparations, the internal administration of arsenic has been often tried against diseases of the spleen. Its febrifuge action has been long known (Paracelsus).

Since 1786 this drug attained its reputation through Fowler in England, and afterwards upon the continent, in Germany, through Harless, Heine, and von Schoenlein. The views of its action are various. Although quinia cannot be completely replaced by arsenic, yet most authorities are agreed that the two drugs supplement each other. There are cases of intermittent fever which are not cured by quinia, but yield to arsenic, especially persistent malarial troubles with irregular attacks. The cure often takes place rapidly if quinia is given after the arsenic (Morgandie): At particular times and in certain neighborhoods arsenic is the usual cure, while quinia does little or no good (Koehler[1]).

I was encouraged, by the results which have been obtained in chronic affections of the skin by arsenic given subcutaneously, when it had been given internally without manifest benefit, to try the injection of Fowler's arsenical solution in tumors of the spleen.

Since then I have used this plan of treatment with benefit.[2]

---

[1] Handbuch der speciellen Therapie. I. S. 212. Tübingen, 1867.

[2] I have often been told by patients of this neighborhood, that they had gotten rid of the most obstinate intermittent after the use of pepper used as a domestic remedy. My friend *Altdorfer* in Gingst, on Rügen, told me that he had permanently cured patients whose intense attacks of fever, sometimes of the quartan type. had yielded neither to quinine alone, or in combination with other remedies—nor to arsenic and phosphorus—by prescribing five times daily twenty drops of the tincture of pepper, still to be obtained in the pharmacies of this neighborhood. The curious magistral formula for this tincture is the following:

R. Piperis Hispanici................. ℥ i.
" Nigri,
" Albi,
" Longi.................... āā ℈ ij.
Liquoris potass. acetatis,*
" Ammon. vinosi........... āā f ℥ vj.
Macera. S. fever tincture.

Piperin has been often recommended by Italian and German physicians. I was thus induced to study its action on the normal spleen. By experiments similar to those described above, I determined, after the exhibition of large doses of piperin to a dog, a clearly granular condition and diminution in size of the spleen.

* Three parts contain one part of dry potassium acetate.—*German Ph.*

I have several times lately injected into the parenchyma of a spleen a dilute solution of arsenic by means of Pravaz' syringe, and with benefit.

Besides arsenic, iodine, bromine, mercury, and ammonia have been recommended against tumors of the spleen. I can give no observations of my own regarding them.

I have been assured by careful physicians, that they had observed a distinct diminution of spleen tumors after a long use of bromide of potassium. Many physicians like to prescribe iodide of iron and iodide of mercury.

The tincture of Eucalyptus globulus has lately been often mentioned as a splenic remedy, since it was so warmly recommended by Dr. F. Lorinzer, in Vienna, against intermittent fever.

Three ounces of fresh leaves bruised in a stone mortar, are covered with six ounces of alcohol, digested in a well-closed vessel for fourteen days at a moderate temperature, then strongly pressed, and filtered. The tincture thus obtained is of a dark greenish brown color, peculiar aromatic smell, and an aromatic, slightly bitter taste. This tincture is generally administered by giving two teaspoonfuls, mixed with some water, four hours, and again two hours before the expected attack. In rare cases, in which the fever returned after some days, three teaspoonfuls were given instead of two.

Lorinzer draws the conclusion from trials made by various physicians, which are collected in No. 27 of the Wiener medizinischen Wochenschrift, 1871, that the leaves of Eucalyptus globulus, or the tincture prepared from them, are a remedy of some value against intermittent.

This statement of Lorinzer has induced me to try the effect of the tincture prepared by Lamatsch, in Vienna. From one pound of leaves, half of them fresh and indigenous, and half exotic and dry, obtained from the tropics, a scant pound of tincture is obtained. My experiments, published in the Deutsches Archiv für klinische Medicin. Bd. X. S. 164, showed that the tincture of Eucalyptus globulus is able to contract the normal spleen in the same way as quinine.

This drug has been found to possess another resemblance to quinine. The ethereal oil of the leaves of Eucalyptus globulus—a clear, colorless oil, of agreeable smell, for which Cloëz has given the formula $C_{17}H_{26}O$, and which he names eucalyptol, was used by Binz in his experiments; it was found to be antizymotic. The body temperature fell after the administration of large doses, in healthy rabbits as well as in those suffering from an artificial fever produced by the injection of a glycerine extract of fresh pus. Equivalent controlled experiments being made for comparison, an equivalent result was obtained in healthy men after the internal administration of from sixty to eighty minims.

W. Mees [1] has lately reported similar results, obtained with the assistance of Huizinga and Rosenstein, as to the commercial ethereal oil of eucalyptus leaves. He found it even more antiseptic than muriate of quinia. It had more power in restraining the decomposition of glucose by yeast. He found that the colorless blood-corpuscles of the frog, at a temperature of from 77° to 95° F., were killed in a diluted solution of one-fifteenth per cent., after fifteen minutes; in a solution of one-tenth per cent., immediately. The oil of eucalyptus, injected into rabbits in a dose of thirty minims, manifestly reduced the temperature, both when they were free from fever, as well as when they were under the pyrogenic influence of putrid material or pus. In all the animals treated with the oil, the punctures of the canula healed immediately, while in the others they suppurated.

Mees treated thirty-five cases of intermittent of various types with tincture of eucalyptus (prepared with one part of leaves to eight parts of alcohol, at 77° F), giving in all up to five and three-quarter ounces (a teaspoonful several times daily). Thirty-one of these were walking cases; in thirteen patients, some of whom had used quinine without result, the cure was clearly determined; in twelve, who did not present themselves again, a cure is probable; ten cases are described as not cured, which probably remained exposed to malaria during the treatment.

Schlaeger [2] proved that the oil of eucalyptus has an action upon the spleen, by experiments upon dogs, in which he measured the spleen removed from the belly, replaced it, then injected the oil into the jugular vein, and a short time afterwards again measured the spleen. He found that after the injection of twenty minims of oil of eucalyptus, an evident contraction and firmer consistence of the spleen could be determined, a confirmation of the results obtained by me with the tincture of eucalyptus.

I have several times lately tried in my clinic, against intermittent fever, the "oleum eucalypti australe," obtained from Simon, in Berlin; the results are detailed in the dissertation of Dr. F. Petermann (Greifswald, 1874). The administration of large doses, even from sixty to eighty minims, in the non-febrile interval, were necessary to overcome obstinate attacks of fever. In

[1] Akademisch. Proefschrift. Groningen, 1873; Centralblatt. 1874. No. 15.
[2] Inaugural Dissertation. Göttingen, 1874.

some cases the action upon the febrile attack was less striking than upon the splenic tumor, just as Chvostek has observed of electricity.[1]

These experiments demand a further trial of the drug, and, if possible, of a better preparation. In the Deutsches Archiv I shall report in detail on this point.

Besides quinia, it has heretofore been usual to administer iron in chronic tumors of the spleen. It was supposed that iron directly made blood-corpuscles and healthy blood; and that, under the use of iron, the transformation of white blood-corpuscles into red was everywhere promoted. It was hoped that iron would prove a specific against anæmia splenica and against leucæmia—just as against the idiopathic chlorosis of the period of development. Unfortunately, we know too little of the chemistry of the human organism to specify under what circumstances and in what kind of splenic tumor the administration of iron brings about an increase of the red corpuscles. It is, however, advisable to make a trial of iron in chronic tumors of the spleen, although I cannot report cases in which a diminution of the splenic tumor after the use of iron was directly determined, yet I can state that I have often observed strengthening of the pulse, as well as an improved general appearance. Whether only small doses have attained the object and only a small part of large doses has been absorbed, I can give no exact statement, since I have been able to make no accurate experiments upon the elimination of iron through the intestine and kidneys in diseases of the spleen. I can only assert that large doses of iron are well borne in splenic leucæmia. The first condition for a favorable action of the iron is that the digestive organs shall not be disturbed thereby; therefore, I give easily soluble, mild preparations which are best borne by the stomach. I have derived special advantage from the lactate of iron, as well as from the reduced iron in combination with small doses of quinia and aromatic powder. Both preparations are well borne by almost all my patients, if I insist that they shall be taken at meal-times.

---

[1] According to *Defermon*, strychnia, morphia, and camphor diminish the spleen materially, and yet do not act as febrifuges. *Piorry* has asserted that sea-salt cures intermittent fever and diminishes the spleen. Schmidt's Jahrbücher. Bd. LXXVI. S. 25.

℞. Ferri lactatis,

Sacchari lactis................... āā ℨ ijss.

M.—S. With the noon and evening meal take from as much as will be held on the point of a large knife, to half a teaspoonful.

℞. Ferri redacti.................... gr. iss.

Quiniæ muriatis.................. gr. ss.

Pulv. aromatic;

Sacchari albi. .... āā gr. iij.

M. Fiant pulv. tal. No. xx.

S. One to be taken morning and evening in a wafer.

I am in general no friend to tinctures of iron ; they contain in commerce often much less iron, than they ought to, and the proportion of iron changes with time. When I have made use of them at all, I have selected the *tinctura ferri acetici ætherea*.[1] Of this I give fifteen drops, morning and evening, at meal-time, in a glass of red wine.

In the treatment of chronic tumors of the spleen it is advisable to vary the preparations of iron; without this precaution one should never say that the iron cannot be borne. Many preparations are sometimes badly borne because they have been used too long; then another preparation should be chosen, the diet and mode of life carefully regulated, and, if necessary, for a time the iron entirely omitted, in order to be able to begin anew.[2]

If one does not get satisfactory results from the use of pharmaceutical preparations of iron, he must send those patients

---

[1] Solution of acetate of iron nine parts; alcohol two parts; acetic ether one part. It contains six per cent. of iron.—German Ph.

[2] Drinking fresh ox blood sometimes revives the nutrition more rapidly than any other measure. The use of this simple remedy was anew recommended at Dresden, at the Congress of Physicians and Naturalists. It can, of course, only be used with such patients as live in the neighborhood of a butcher who kills at least two or three times a week. Like *Ferber* in Hamburg (Virchow's Archiv. Bd. LII. S. 103), I direct the blood to be drunk warm at the house of the butcher. Most persons soon conquer their disgust. They avoid the first repugnance by drinking out of an opaque vessel, or in the dark; some of my patients prefer to drink it mixed with a teaspoonful of brandy. As a rule, I have prescribed blood-drinking in anæmia splenica, at the same time with the internal use of iron. The transfusion of blood offers still greater advantages; in which operation, according to my past experience, I prefer the venous transfusion of defibrinated human blood. In order to attain a frequent transfer of blood without danger, I have quite lately made use of the subcutaneous injection of defibrinated blood by means of a large Pravaz' syringe, such as is used in veterinary medicine.

whose circumstances permit to one of the esteemed health resorts with iron springs. The activity of the stomach is rapidly regulated, the appetite becomes strong, the strength increases. A striking improvement in chronic splenic diseases is sometimes produced by iron baths. In such a cure it is very difficult to say whether the result is attained by the mountain air, the exercise, the baths, the changed nutrition, or the characteristic constituents of the iron baths ; special results may be expected in chronic tumors of the spleen from iron bog baths.

Local Treatment of Splenic Tumors.

Among the local measures which have been attempted against splenic tumors the total extirpation of the organ should be first mentioned, since in animals splenotomy, as has been shown by numerous experiments, has been very well borne ; the same operation upon man has been often discussed and performed. The most complete collection of cases of extirpation of the spleen in man are those of Kuechenmeister[1] and of Magdelain.[2] A distinction is to be made between partial and total extirpation. So far nine cases of partial extirpation are known which had a favorable result. They were called for by wounds of the left side, with protrusion of the spleen. It was removed in some of the cases without a previous ligature, in some after a ligature previously applied, and in some by ligature without the knife.

Clarke reports one case in which a butcher stabbed himself with a knife in the left side ; a portion of the omentum, some loops of intestine, and the spleen fell out ; probably the whole spleen and a portion of the omentum were removed ; the patient soon recovered. These cases have rather a surgical interest. Total extirpations of normal spleens, and even of splenic tumors which have protruded from a wound, experience has shown to be well borne. Kuechenmeister recommends for future cases torsion, ligature, and removal, with the knife, of the spleen situated outside the abdominal wound. Nothing can be said against such an operation, since all the total extirpations of the spleen which

---

[1] Die Wandernde Milz. Leipzig, 1865.   [2] L'Union. 146, 147. 1867.

had been performed after injury had a favorable result (Schumann[1]).

The prognosis is, however, different in splenotomy on account of internal diseases of the organ. Of the nine cases in which this operation was undertaken for splenic diseases six resulted fatally. It is to be mentioned here that death, in two of these cases (Koeberlé, Bryant), took place during or immediately after the operation; in three, some hours after it. After Bryant, in the case of a woman forty years old, with splenic leucæmia, had ligatured the pedicle, and cut it off without excessive bleeding, it appeared that, from a portion of the surface of the diaphragm which was connected with the spleen by adhesions, a severe capillary hemorrhage occurred which nothing could stop, and which, in a short time, cost the patient her life. Koeberlé also, who attempted the operation in a splenic leucæmia, lost his patient, a female, in consequence of abundant hemorrhage during the operation. These two cases, in which splenotomy was performed for splenic leucæmia, have given the most unfavorable results of all. In future, therefore, in cases where leucæmia is diagnosticated, extirpation of the spleen should not be ventured upon. In the first place it must be looked upon as exceedingly difficult of execution, on account of the hemorrhagic diathesis which usually complicates splenic leucæmia, and secondly, the operation promises no good result even if it succeeds, because the leucæmia is not limited to the spleen, but other glands and the osseous marrow are altered in the same way. If, besides, one remembers the case of Péan, who diagnosticated an advanced dropsy of the left ovary, but completely extirpated a unilocular cyst of the spleen; the great difficulties of diagnosis, which are always to be considered in operating for abdominal tumors; and further, that in Quittenbaum's and Kuechler's case, a commencing cirrhosis of the liver was found at the autopsy; and finally, if one bears in mind the possibility of excessive hemorrhage, there will appear but few indications for the extirpation of wandering as well as not wandering splenic tumors. Simon correctly says that it

---

[1] Die neueren Untersuchungen über die Exstirpation der Milz. Schmidt's Jaherbüchr. Bd. 144. S. 218. 1868.

woùld be a great mistake if extirpation of the spleen were recommended and introduced into surgery as equally valuable with
ovariotomy.

After this unfavorable experience it was natural to attempt a
local action upon tumors of the spleen in a less dangerous way.
The question first arose of producing a suppuration and cicatricial atrophy of the spleen by means of the needle operation recommended by Simon for echinococcus of the liver.

After the favorable results of subcutaneous injections of tincture of iodine in glandular tumors, especially in the thyroid
gland, one might think of extending the same treatment to
tumors of the spleen.

It was desirable, in the first place, to ascertain by experiments upon animals
whether the peritoneal covering of the spleen would permit such an interference; and,
since in the smaller animals, like rabbits and dogs, the position of the spleen cannot
be determined by percussion, I have, for the purpose of injecting tincture of iodine
into the spleen, withdrawn this organ from the abdomen by a wound in the linea
alba, and then with the hypodermic syringe injected larger or smaller quantities of
tincture of iodine into the substance of the spleen. The animals bore the operation
without intense peritonítis. One rabbit lived several weeks afterwards; another
died without evident cause on the ninth day. In a bird death followed on the day
of the injection, in consequence of bleeding from the puncture.

Up to the present time I have treated no tumors of the
spleen by injection of tincture of iodine.

I have often employed lately injections of dilute carbolic acid
into the thickened parenchyma of the lungs, for the local treatment of pulmonary diseases, especially putrid bronchitis. I have
treated a splenic tumor in the same way, and with such result
that I feel further experiment to be demanded.

Electricity has often been tried for tumors of the spleen.
Since Scudamore first called attention to the capability of the
continuous current in rapidly coagulating blood, Guerard, Ber-
tani, Milani, Baumgarten, Wertheimer, Steinlin, and Moritz
Meyer have succeeded in curing varicosities. After Althaus, in
London, had particularly recommended the electrolytic treatment of tumors, it seemed proper to try acupuncture in so vascular an organ as the spleen, especially when enlarged. Leyden[1]

---

[1] Virchow's Archiv. Bd. LII. S. 65.

thrust several needles, isolated to 'the points, through the skin, deep into a leucæmic spleen, connected them with the negative pole, while the positive was placed upon the abdomen. After every sitting, slight fever and slight, never alarming, peritoneal symptoms appeared. No permanent effect was obtained. Several times the spleen seemed afterwards to enlarge somewhat, but soon returned to its former dimensions. I have often attempted galvano-puncture in a non-leucæmic tumor of the spleen, with just as little result.

Chvostek[1] attempted to reduce the enlarged spleen through reflex action, by stimulation of the nerves, especially the vaso-motor and trophic fibres. He faradized the skin of the splenic region with two pencils and the secondary current of an induction apparatus. He found the influence of an electric current upon the febrile attacks less striking than its action upon the splenic tumor. Electricity, therefore, is little likely to compete with quinine in preventing the attacks of intermittent fever, and still less in curing the disease. Berger also failed in controlling the intensity or frequency of the febrile attacks, either by the application of electricity to the spleen or by the galvanization of the sympathetic.

Berger has reduced a leucæmic tumor of the spleen to considerably smaller dimensions by electric irritation of the skin of the splenic region. Continued pencilling of the skin, as well as the application of the constant current, could not bring back the spleen to its normal size, and the leucæmia remained unchanged.

In No. 10 of the Berliner klinische Wochenschrift for the year 1874, Moritz Meyer mentions a new procedure for reducing glandular growths by the electric current. He allows the most intense current which can be obtained from the sliding coils of Dubois to pass through for about a minute, interrupting them repeatedly by his interrupter.[2] The results are so striking as to call for the application of this method to splenic tumors.

Very lately Botkin[3] has spoken of the great therapeutic importance of electricity in splenic tumors. He considers the

---

[1] Wiener Medicinische Presse. XI. 34, 38, 41. 1870.
[2] *Ziemssen*, Elektricität in der Medicin. 1872. S. 221.
[3] Die Contractilität der Milz. Berlin. Aug. Hirschwald. 1874.

enlargement of the spleen to depend, to a certain extent, upon a diminution of its contractility, in consequence of which a retention of its contents takes place. Since the muscular fibres of the spleen can be excited to greater activity by the electric current, we think that one of the injurious consequences of the swelling of this organ may be diminished—that is, the increased stagnation of blood and the destruction of the red blood-corpuscles. From his previous experience, he thinks that these indications may be fulfilled by faradization of the spleen, not only in chronic, but also in the acute splenic tumors of typhoid, recurrent, and intermittent fevers.

SPECIAL PART.

Anomalies in the Structure and Position of the Spleen.

Giesker, Splenologie. I. Abth. Zürich, 1835.—*Heinrich*, Krankheiten der Milz. Leipzig, 1847.—*Fuehrer*, Archiv für physiol. Heilkunde. XV. — *Dr. Klob*, Zeitschrift der Ges. der Aerzte in Wien, 1859. 46.—*Rokitansky*, Lehrbuch der pathologischen Anatomie. Bd. III. S. 291. 1861.—*Foerster*, Pathologische Anatomie. Leipzig, 1863. S. 818.—*Dietl*, Wandermilz. Wiener med. Wochenschrift. 1854 u. 1856.—*Helm* und *Klob*, Wochenschrift der Ges. d. Aerzte in Wien. 1856. S. 37. — *Heusinger*, Hemmungsbildungen der Milz. Meckel's deutsches Archiv f. d. Physiologie. Bd. VI. S. 17.—*Otto*, Pathol. Anat. Bd. II. Abth, 1.—*Rokitansky*, Ueber die wandernde Milz. Wiener Zeitschr. N. F. III. 3. 1860.—*Dr. Rezek*, Wiener med. Wochenschrift. Nr. 27. 1856.—*Ullmann*, Ungarische Zeitschrift. VII. 35. 1856.

There is little practical interest in excess or deficiency of formation in the spleen. ·It has been often proved by experiment that the spleen is not absolutely necessary to the life of the animal, and that after its extirpation, as well as after an artificially produced atrophy, its functions are taken up by the other lymphatic organs.

Congenital absence of the spleen is observed in acephali and in rare cases, even in otherwise normal individuals. Heusinger has made an abundant collection of deficiencies of formation in the spleen. Atrophy of the spleen sometimes reaches such a degree that it looks like an original deficiency. I have several times mechanically produced a complete atrophy of the spleen in animals.

The opposite of this deficient formation occurs as duplicity of various degrees in double monsters, as well as in the form of accessory spleens (Lien succenturiatus, accessorius). These are seated in the gastro-splenic ligament, the omentum, or even in the head of the pancreas (Klob). They vary in size from a millet seed to a walnut, and in number from one to twenty or more. In the anatomical cabinet at Bonn are four accessory spleens which were found at the autopsy of a young man who died of phthisis. The largest number was observed by Otto, viz., 23—from the size of a pea to that of a small chestnut. Rosenmueller makes the remarkable observation, that among 400 bodies of persons of various ages and both sexes from North Germany there was only 1 accessory spleen of the size of a walnut; while among 40 bodies of Southern Europeans there were hardly 5 who were not furnished with an accessory spleen. I possess no statistics on this point.

The so-called accessory spleens appear to be sometimes new formations. After extirpation of the spleen in animals, some observers are said to have discovered newly-formed or accessory spleens. Among fifty extirpations I have only once had an opportunity to observe this. I found the great omentum completely strewn with dark, red nodules, from the size of a pea to that of a bean, which, both in their outward appearance and upon section, showed great similarity to the splenic tissue. The more minute examination of M. Roth[1] characterized them as pathological formations, as teleangiectatic-hemorrhagic lymphoma.

A transition to accessory spleens is made by indentations of the organ upon its anterior border, which may go so far as to cut off a portion by a horizontal fissure. A similar malformation, in the form of tuberosity and lobulation of the spleen, may result from the shrinking of inflammatory deposits. Everywhere the careful observer meets with the most various changes of form; not unfrequently a tongue-shaped, a roundish, a disk-shaped, an almost cylindrical, hemispherical, an obtusely triangular or quadrangular spleen (Rokitansky) may be met with.

The congenital anomalies of place consist in the position of the spleen outside of the abdominal cavity when the walls are ununited as well as in large umbilical herniæ, in the left thorax in defects of the diaphragm, or on the right side, when the position of the viscera is inverted.

---

[1] Compare *Mosler*, Leukæmie. S. 35.

In the year 1852, I.observed in the Wurzburg clinic a febrile affection, in which the liver, situated upon the left, had led to the assumption of a typhus tumor of the spleen. Since then, I have observed two other cases of inverted position of the viscera which could be recognized by the greater dulness of the liver in the left hypochondrium, and the smaller, splenic dulness in the right.

Very frequently, acquired changes in the position of the spleen are observed. Every physician who understands the percussion of the spleen, must have convinced himself that in enlargement of the left thorax, especially from pleuritic effusion, the spleen is thrust far downward into the abdominal cavity. On the other hand, it is forced upward by free or sacculated peritoneal effusion, by meteorism of the intestinal canal. In such cases the spleen is found in the immediate neighborhood of the vertebral column. The organ may be pushed in various directions by tumors, but it is usually difficult to find it on account of adhesions with the tumors. In penetrating wounds of the abdomen the spleen often falls outside of the abdominal walls, and has often been removed with good results. The position of the spleen in the left thorax in rupture or wounds of the diaphragm is much more rare, and also more dangerous.

A striking change of position occurs in almost every increase of volume of long duration; large spleens occupy at first the left lateral region of the abdomen, and almost a perpendicular direction, push up the diaphragm, and lie below in the hollow of the ilium. Upon further increase of volume, they turn from this direction, and push diagonally across the hypogastrium towards the right ilium. In such cases it very frequently occurs that the spleen is movable. This condition consists in an abnormal length of the splenic ligaments (ligamentum gastro-lienale and phrenico-lienale), so that the viscus is only loosely attached, the length of the ligament being either congenital or acquired by stretching during the growth of the tumor, and remaining after its reduction. The movable spleen is not to be confounded with the wandering spleen.

Wandering Spleen.

In the slighter degrees the spleen remains under the left arch of the ribs. By pressure and an appropriate position of the

body it may be pushed again backward and upward into its
proper place. In more advanced stages the spleen lies with its
hilus looking to the left and upward in the left iliac fossa, at the
entrance to the pelvis, even in the right half of the abdomen. It
can generally be pushed thence in all directions, even under the
right hypochondrium, or be turned upon its axis. It may thus
happen that the spleen is completely loosened from its attach-
ments, since the cord by which it hangs is atrophied by twisting.
As a consequence, shrivelling and atrophy may be observed.
Prof. Dietl, formerly in Cracow, has collected numerous observations upon wandering spleens, as well as upon movable kidneys. He mentions as remarkable its exclusive occurrence in
women. In the Wiener medicinischen Wochenschrift, No. 23,
1856, he communicates a case of great importance for the symptomatology and diagnosis of this condition.

A Jewess of about thirty years, the mother of several children, stated that she
had been pregnant more than a year, but, notwithstanding frequent pains, could
not be delivered. She was very anæmic, her legs almost paralyzed. Dietl found
the spleen three or four times enlarged, situated crosswise in the great pelvis, probably firmly held by adhesions; attempts at replacement were without result. He
ordered quinia and salt-baths, but heard nothing of the result of this treatment.

According to Dietl's view, adhesions with the neighboring
organs make the trouble worse. Such a spleen has no tendency
to return to its normal position, and an abdominal bandage will
not retain it there. Therapeutics can only reduce its volume.
This is of importance, since the symptoms from pressure are
thereby diminished.

Dr. Rezek observed a woman who thought she was pregnant.
The abdomen had in the median line the appearance of a hernia.
Upon palpation, a tumor could be felt through the normal abdominal walls, hard and smooth, not elastic, easily movable,
convex above; at the lower border, somewhat to the left, a fissure. The disease was at first considered abdominal pregnancy,
later, an ovarian tumor. Upon more careful examination, Rezek
found that the tumor was movable in all directions; could be
pushed into the right as well as the left hypochondrium, and
was not connected with the organs of the lesser pelvis. A wan-

dering spleen seemed all the more probable when he heard that the patient had suffered for five years from intermittent fever; had afterwards felt a hard growth in the splenic region, which, five months before, after falling down-stairs, had sunk into the abdomen. This mechanical origin distinguishes this case from many others.

The amount of trouble depends upon whether the gastro-splenic ligament is little or much elongated. In the first case, in the horizontal position of the body, the spleen, drawn by the stomach, may retreat towards its normal position. Not only its reposition, but its retention by an abdominal bandage is then much easier.

When the ligament is longer, the spleen continues to sink downward, and produces, by its pressure, disturbances of various kinds. Generally the continued dragging produces loosening of the pancreas, the splenic vein and artery form, with the remainder of the gastro-splenic ligament, a cord from which the spleen hangs with the hilus upward. As it sinks, the spleen turns several times around its horizontal axis (Rokitansky).

Corresponding to the amount of dragging, the splenic vessels are narrowed or obliterated. In the case of Quiquerez,[1] thrombosis of the splenic artery was dependent upon this twisting, and from this again the death of the organ. There is no doubt that the changes of the spleen, which consist sometimes in shrivelling, sometimes in pigmentary and fatty metamorphoses of the thickened parenchyma, depend upon atrophy of the vessels. In a case cited by Voigtel the spleen was found completely free in the abdominal cavity. After this withering of the spleen, the dislocation is often borne for a long time, and better than before.

Unfavorable consequences are mentioned by Rokitansky and Klob. In many cases death is produced by gangrene of the cul-de-sac of the stomach, which depended upon dragging of the stomach and injury to the calibre of the vessels. In one case compression of the duodenum was caused by a cord formed from the splenic vessels and the pancreas, in consequence of which considerable dilatation of the stomach had taken place.

---

[1] Oesterr. Zeitschr. für prakt. Heilkunde. IX. 52. 1863.

The diagnosis of the wandering spleen from other tumors of the abdomen is to be made from the characteristic form of the spleen, and the absence of splenic dulness in the normal place. In the case in my clinic the diagnosis was confirmed by feeling distinct indentations on the borders of the spleen.

The treatment is to be directed to diminishing the mobility of the spleen and the consequent dragging upon neighboring organs, as well as the pressure upon them. The first indication is to be met by accurately fitted, abdominal bandages of buckskin. For diminishing the tumor, the various drugs already mentioned are to be tried. The application of ice-bags in the horizontal position is to be specially recommended, as well as injections of Fowler's solution into the parenchyma. Kuechenmeister advises extirpation of the spleen, but the result is more than doubtful.

Inflammation and Hemorrhagic Infarction.

Heusinger und *Heinrich*, l. c.—*Voigtel*, Handbuch der pathologischen Anatomie. III. 153.—*Rokitansky*, Lehrb. III. 299.—*Cruveilhier*, Anat. path. Livr. 2. Pl. 5. Livr. 31. Pl. 4.—*Bamberger*, Virch. spec. Path. IV. 1. 657.—*Henoch*, Klinik der Unterleibskrht. II.—*Albers*, Atlas IV. Taf. 36.—*Cohnheim*, Untersuchungen über die embolischen Processe. Berlin, 1872.—*Jackson*, in Boston, On a Particular Derangement of the Structure of the Spleen, communicated (with some introductory remarks and comments) by Thomas Hodgkin, M.D. Transact. med. chirurg. Vol. XXIX. N. Ser. XI. 1846. Schmidt's Jahrb. Bd. LXIII. S. 41.— *A. Linas*, Gaz. hebd. II. 49. 1855. Schmidt's Jahrb. Bd. XC. S. 47.—*Dr. Mantell*, Dubl. Med. Press. July 26, 1865. Schmidt's Jahrb. Bd. CXXIX.— *Pleischel*, Oesterr. Zeitschr. für pr. Heilk. 1866.—*L'Hermite*, Mem. de l'acad. des scienc. 1753. p. 102.—*Zweifel*, Schmidt's Jahrb. Bd. LII. S. 172.— *W. Kernig*, Petersburg med. Zeitschr. XII. 177–215. Centralblatt. Berlin, 1867.— *Ponfick*, Virchow's Archiv. Bd. LX.

There is no point upon which the statements of writers have varied more widely than the frequency, symptoms, and course of inflammatory processes in the spleen. According to the frequent mention of splenitis in medical writings of Grecian antiquity this disease must have been far from rare. On the other hand, Fr. von Hildenbrand asserts that among numerous diseases of the spleen seen by him in Lombardy, he saw no case of a genuine inflammation of the substance of the spleen. Many modern physicians of great experience say the same thing. The question is therefore still to be answered.

It is not yet clear where we shall place the limits of inflammation of the spleen. At present it appears as if we ought to consider those changes which we now call acute tumors of the spleen—that is, those enlargements which arise in infectious diseases, as inflammatory conditions. Perhaps this view will be so readily received, will be supported by so many new proofs, that, even when diseases of the spleen shall be next thoroughly treated of, the large part of all these tumors will be considered among the inflammatory processes. The same thing is true of many chronic tumors; cases of splenic leucæmia have been observed, which owe their origin to inflammation of the spleen. I have seen this disease occur in a man who fell with the left hypochondrium upon the pommel of a saddle while mounting a horse. Practical ends, however, will for the present be best subserved by treating acute and chronic tumors of the spleen separate from its inflammation.

Etiology.

Inflammation of the spleen occurs very seldom spontaneously; in a great majority of cases it is metastatic. It then affects larger or smaller portions; only exceptionally the whole spleen, sometimes only the peripheral layer of substance to a greater extent.

Traumatic causes produce rupture more frequently than inflammation of the spleen. Violent bodily exercise is said to give rise to the latter, as in a case communicated by Berlyn, where an abscess of the spleen formed in a young soldier after a forced day's march, was opened and discharged a large quantity of pus and several pieces of the spleen, and was completely cured.

Idiopathic inflammation of the spleen is so rare that in every apparently spontaneous case, most careful inquiries should be made after some primary morbid condition. Bamberger observed one case of a splenic abscess as large as a hen's egg, which had

ruptured into the abdominal cavity, and for which **absolutely no**
further cause could be found.   No case of idiopathic **inflamma-**
tion of the spleen has so far occurred to me.   In former times,
before Virchow's pioneer works on the embolic morbid processes
were known, many apparently spontaneous cases of inflammation
of the spleen were published.

> For instance, *Linas,* so late as the year 1855, communicated a remarkable case
> of spontaneous splenitis in a man forty-six years old, who suffered for a long
> time with dyspeptic troubles, followed by pains in the left hypochondrium, ema-
> ciation and frequently repeated rigors.   The pains in the splenic region increased
> in violence and frequency ; percussion, which was very painful, showed consider-
> able enlargement of the spleen.   After apparent improvement, there followed left-
> sided paralysis of the extremities, right-sided of the face, and sudden death from
> œdema of the lungs.   The autopsy disclosed in the neighborhood of the right cor-
> pus striatum a collection of pus as large as a nut, in the posterior part of the
> spleen an abscess as large as an orange.   The aortic valves were insufficient.

Linas calls this case spontaneous splenitis—since he did not
at that time know the connection between diseases of the heart
and inflammation of the spleen, which has been so brilliantly
shown by Virchow.

Even in 1832 Hodgkin had noticed a circumscribed change in
the structure of the spleen, which he considered the consequence
of extravasation of blood from mechanical injury, but which
Rokitansky, when he was in England, explained as the result of
an altered condition of the blood from endocarditis.

A marked progress in the etiology of splenic diseases was made
in the year 1840, when Rokitansky, in a treatise on the combination and mutual exclusion of various morbid processes, called
attention to the frequent occurrence of endocarditis and secondary inflammation of the spleen and kidneys.   Among one hundred and sixty-five cases of endocarditis splenitis alone occurred
thirty-two times ; splenitis and nephritis together seventeen
times ; and nephritis alone, eleven times ; Rokitansky deserves
the credit of having very accurately portrayed the changes in the
spleen.   He gave as an explanation at that time, that the whole
process of splenic inflammation acted in the essential points
throughout like the inflammation of a vessel, especially a vein,
and that these secondary processes consisted essentially in stasis

of the blood mass, poisoned by resorption of an inflammatory product, and the reaction in the neighboring tissues consequent thereon.

In Virchow's classic works, which were published together in his collected essays, the close connection of the metastatic forms of inflammation of the spleen with diseases of the heart, was first demonstrated. Convincing proof was there given that primary inflammation of the walls can give rise in the heart as well as in the vessels to secondary coagulation of the blood, and that coarse and large bodies, pieces of obstructions, fragments of thrombi, and the walls of the vessels can be dislodged and again wedge themselves in. These wedged-in and obstructing bodies Virchow named plugs (Stopfen), emboli. After he had first followed out their history on the venous side of the vascular system, and had proved the occurrence of embolism of the pulmonary artery, he afterwards described its occurrence upon the arterial side, and therewith, embolism of various internal and external organs.

The anatomical arrangement, the form of the origin of an arterial lateral branch from a larger vessel contributes to the specially easy entry of plugs into some arterial branches;—metastatic deposits are hence observed with special frequency in the spleen and kidneys. As is well known, the calibre of the splenic artery is larger in comparison to the size of the blood-glands supplied by it than in any other organ of the human body, the thyroid gland perhaps excepted. These are the physiological reasons why the metastatic form of inflammation of the spleen is by far the most frequent.[1] It occurs not only in endocarditis of the left side, but with all valvular diseases of the heart, with the formation of clots in the left ventricle, and with changes of the aorta accompanied by thrombotic deposits, and is in these cases produced by emboli in the larger or smaller arteries of the

---

[1] The statistics of endocarditis have received an important contribution from the inaugural dissertation of Sperling, based upon 300 autopsies at the Berlin Pathological Institute. As to the seat of the emboli it appeared that, contrary to the usual idea, the kidneys rather than the spleen were most frequently affected. Embolic lesions were proved 58 times in the kidneys, only 39 times in the spleen, 15 in the brain, 5 times each in the liver and intestines, 4 times in the skin.

spleen. Also in pyæmic, puerperal, and allied processes, in typhus and Bright's disease, such emboli are generally concerned, although the proof is in most cases more difficult to furnish.

Splenitis is often caused secondarily by the spread of inflammatory and ulcerative processes from the neighborhood, in circumscribed peritoneal exudations, ulcers of the stomach, toxic gastritis, etc. In these cases inflammation is generally limited to the capsule of the spleen. A part of the errors of former times in the definition of inflammation of the spleen must hence be connected with the fact that diseases of the splenic substance could at that time be less accurately separated from those of its serous covering, as well as from the diseases of neighboring organs. The pain, as the most striking symptom, sufficed for the diagnosis of an inflammation of the spleen.

As remains of perisplenitis, we frequently observe the so-called tendinous spots on the surface of the spleen. The parenchyma of the spleen may be completely unaffected. In other cases the latter may be made to participate by gradual shrinking and contraction on the surface. An atrophic condition of the spleen is thus produced.

The condition is different in the cases of perisplenitis which arise from inflammation of the splenic substance. Since this generally occurs in the outer portion of the organ, the transition from the affection of the substance to that of the capsule takes place so much the easier. In leucæmic splenic tumors, beginning with inflammatory symptoms, I found the spleen firmly adherent to the neighboring parts. In recurrent fever, exudations, and adhesions of the serous covering with the neighboring organs occur in the later attacks, and with ordinarily small spleens. Peripheral inflammations of the parenchyma have involved not only the capsule of the spleen, but frequently also the adherent neighboring organs, diaphragm, lungs, pericardium, colon, etc. In one case (Kuettner) it had even given rise to gangrenous pneumonia of the lower lobe of the left lung, and to a perforation of the adherent colon. A portion of the decomposed splenitic parenchyma lay in the ulcerated and partially destroyed colon, so that the remainder might have passed during life in the bloody stools.

Pathological Anatomy.

In cases where the inflammation takes the form of diffuse infiltration of the whole parenchyma, the spleen appears considerably enlarged. Upon section the parenchyma runs together as a discolored pultaceous mass of pus, blood, and decomposing splenic elements.

The inflammatory foci (hemorrhagic infarctions), from one to three or more in number, are formed chiefly in the periphery of the spleen. By the gradual spreading or running together of several circumscribed foci, the affection sometimes becomes so extensive that finally the greatest part of the organ is involved in the morbid process. The form of the single infarction is usually wedge-shaped, corresponding to the branching of the arteries; the broad end looks outward towards the capsule, while the point of the wedge is directed inward. Their size varies from that of a pea to that of a dove's or hen's egg.

According to Billroth, the inflammatory foci are found as frequently in the interior of the organ as on the surface; they are usually sharply defined from their surroundings; they are at first dark blue, or brownish red in color, tough, as if hepatized; but later, they become lighter, especially in the middle, while on the periphery they become dark red. Over the inflamed spot, the peritoneal coating of the spleen frequently shows vascular injection, or it is covered to a greater or less extent by fibrinous exudation. The organ at first appears congested and swollen, according to the size and number of the foci, and sometimes remains to a later period enlarged, or returns to its normal dimensions.

Next to the classic works of Virchow, Cohnheim's excellent investigations upon the embolic process have served to explain the special conditions upon which the occurrence of a hemorrhagic infarction is usually dependent, since, after the entry of the branches of a splenic artery into the hilus of the organ, no further arterial anastomoses are formed, as can be clearly shown by injections. The formation of hemorrhagic infarctions in the spleen is especially favored by the exclusive presence of terminal

arteries (Endarterien). A further necessary condition for com-
pleting the stagnation, the want of valves in the veins of the
obstructed region, is completely fulfilled in the spleen, since we
have not here a completely closed capillary system, as in the
rest of the body, but W. Mueller's wall-less system of blood-
paths intermediate between arteries and veins. These are the
reasons, as Cohnheim correctly states, why the spleen is an
organ in which plugging the arteries almost invariably produces
a genuine hemorrhagic infarction. This is, according to Cohnheim, not the result of coarse rupture of the vessels, but of a
hemorrhage *per diapedesin*. The migrating red blood-corpuscles
are so numerous only because their emigration is made easier by
alteration of the vascular walls. The stationary layer of blood,
under strong pressure, and surrounded by very thin walls, gives
off at an earlier period serum into the tissues. Thus is formed,
in the region of the embolism, a sero-hemorrhagic infiltration.

According to the special circumstances, we observe further
secondary results in the hemorrhagic infarction. Under favorable conditions, the affected part gradually shrinks to a fibrous
callus, which draws the capsule with it. At other times the
infarction, while retaining its form, is changed into a yellow
mass looking like tubercle, at a later period sometimes becoming
calcified. Suppuration of the spleen is, according to the numerous observations in question, no rare appearance. It occurs as a
result of the primary traumatic, as well as secondary inflammation. It has already been demonstrated by Virchow's first work
upon Embolism, that embolic abscesses are produced by the
specific nature of the plug itself.

One abscess may arise alone, or several at the same time,
which, later, run together. All observations have been made on
splenic abscesses already complete. These abscesses, small at
the beginning, but gradually extending peripherally, increase in
circumference. Having arrived at a certain size, they sometimes
remain for a long time unchanged, while a fibrous capsule is
formed around them, and the parenchyma shrinks. In many of
these cases the pus at a later period becomes caseous, then calcified, and the abscess completely dries up.

Usually, however, the pus is not encapsulated, but constantly increases. Enormous masses of pus are often formed within the distended capsule. In a case of l'Hermite, already mentioned by many authors, the abscess is said to have contained about 30 lbs. of pus. Pleischel describes a splenic abscess in a patient sixteen years old, which reached extraordinary dimensions. The growth stretched downward to the iliac bone; on the right, to the umbilicus; was painful on pressure, and everywhere fluctuating. A puncture discharged 33 oz. of pus. The data were verified at the autopsy.

If the pus reaches the capsule, inflammation of the peritoneal coating takes place, which extends in the neighborhood, and leads to adhesions with the neighboring organs. Not unfrequently sloughing follows, when the contents of the abscess are either discharged free into the abdominal cavity, soon causing fatal peritonitis, or form sacculated abscesses by adhesions and false membranes, in which the remains of the destroyed spleen are often hard to find. The walls of the abscess are formed partly by the spleen, partly by neighboring organs—the fundus of the stomach, the transverse colon, the diaphragm, and the anterior abdominal wall. If suppuration of the adherent abdominal wall takes place, the pus is discharged through a fistulous opening.

Zweifel gives the history of a splenic abscess discharging outward through the abdominal walls, which got well. He says that he found pieces of the spleen in the pus, and thereby confirmed his diagnosis. In other instances the diaphragm is perforated, and the pus is discharged into the thoracic cavity. Nasse, in Bonn, has seen recovery after expectoration of the pus. Dr. Mantell mentions a fatal result from a splenic abscess which opened into the left lung. In the case of Newnham a fistulous passage was formed through the lung, so that the pus was discharged through the skin below the collar-bone. Perforation of the stomach and of the colon, with evacuation of the pus through them, have also been observed. In his Pathologia Indica, Dr. Webb mentions a case of recovery from a splenic abscess which opened into the intestinal canal. He recognized the nature of the trouble by the spleen diminishing rapidly in circumference in one night, while before the beginning of the purulent evacuations

it had been quite large. Suppuration of the spleen very rarely
affects the kidneys, and the pus is said then to have been evacuated through the urinary passages.

In the older writers gangrene of the spleen is frequently
mentioned. These observations seem to refer to simple softening
of this organ. Gangrene of the spleen is only rarely observed as
a metastatic deposit in septicæmic affections of internal or external organs.

A very instructive case of this kind was observed in my clinic in the year 1866,
in a girl of twenty-five years, as a consequence of gangrene of the lungs and of the
diaphragm. During a double croupous pneumonia a thrombosis was formed in the
veins of the right thigh ; this had been the source of an embolism of the left lung,
which produced gangrene. This extended to the diaphragm, the spleen, and partially to the neighboring muscles. In consequence of this, an acute peritonitis
arose, to which the patient finally succumbed. The spleen was mostly changed
into a dirty, dark-green, offensive, decomposing mass. In the neighborhood of the
hilus there was found a zone, perhaps half an inch thick, which still possessed a
normal splenic parenchyma, but also had already taken a blackish brown color.
This case has been carefully described in Virchow's Archiv, Bd. XL., S. 580, by
H. Hertz, at that time prosector of the pathological institute in this place.

Finally, we have to mention here another peculiar form of
circumscribed splenic inflammation which sometimes occurs in
typhus and recurrent fever, but has not been mentioned in
typhoid. In the latter disease C. E. E. Hoffmann has found in
181 bodies the wedge-shaped infarction 9 times. It led either to
contraction and adhesion with the neighboring organs by adhesive peritonitis, or to softening with general peritonitis. In
typhus fever Bamberger observed a peculiar change of the
spleen, which appeared to him as an inflammation of the Malpighian corpuscles. In the swollen organ the Malpighian vesicles
appeared uniformly hypertrophied to more than the size of a
pin's head, and discharged, when punctured, a little drop of
puriform-looking fluid, which consisted of numerous cellular
forms and nuclei—a condition which has been already described
by Rokitansky[1] and Hodgkin.[2] In typhus Griesinger found
the same change, and it has since been frequently confirmed.

---

[1] III., page 284.   [2] Sammlung auserl. Abh. Bd. XL. S. 613.

Very lately Ponfick[1] has thoroughly described the circumscribed morbid changes which occur in the spleen from recurrent fever. He has separated those of the arterial and of the venous tract.

The venous foci of disease — the so-called infarctions — on account of their much greater frequency, their considerable size, as well as the frequent evil consequences connected with them, have always specially interested the observer. Ponfick found them in the epidemic upon which he founded his description in almost forty per cent. of all the cases. They found sharply circumscribed, most variously shaped deposits of very different sizes. The larger and largest, which may include two-thirds of the whole spleen, are generally situated immediately underneath the capsule, and are more or less clearly wedge-shaped, while the smaller, roundish, or irregularly polygonal, lie scattered more in the depth of the organ. Their color is at first a dark, variously speckled, blackish red. This gradually fades into a grayish red, grayish yellow, and finally whitish yellow, and, consequent upon this change, the originally slightly granular, prominent surface of the section assumes more and more that smooth, homogeneous appearance, which, in connection with the yellow color, characterizes the typical caseous condition of the older deposits.

In the outer appearance of these deposits, a close correspondence exists with the appearance of the embolic infarctions of the spleen, but the stoppage of the arteries leading to them is wanting. The absence of this condition, as well as of any valvular disease which could cause it, is, according to Ponfick, a distinction from the processes arising from embolism, and, consequently, pathognomonic for their recurrent character.

The smaller foci may be healed quite rapidly, by progressive resorption of the disorganized tissue—some of them leaving behind a thick scar, colored yellowish brown by a deposit of pigment. If, on the other hand, they are larger, a zone of reactive inflammation is soon formed, which first provokes a capsulation of the portion destined to destruction, and then, by destructive

---

[1] Virchow's Archiv. Bd. LX.

suppuration, a loosening and progressive softening of the seques-
trium, up to its complete fluidification. The more this is dissolved into a mass—always becoming more fluid, and finally
completely puriform,—so much the nearer is the danger that the
corresponding peritoneal coating will be sympathetically infected, and, by simple conduction, a fibrino-purulent peritonitis
will be developed. Sometimes this becomes rapidly diffuse ; at
other times it remains limited to the spleen and the neighboring
parts, but can easily attack the pleura of the left side, and thus
give rise to new complications.

The danger of peritonitis becomes greater and more immediate
if that portion of the capsule closing the cavity of the abscess is
involved as a whole in the decay ; for then a most active peritoneal exudation must follow close upon the perforation of the
sack, and any discharge of its puriform contents into the cavity
of the abdomen. Even in the more favorable case of a purulent
effusion remaining capsulated, new complications threaten in the
gradual suppuration of the diaphragm, with final perforation.

According to Ponfick's view an embolic origin of this peculiar
splenic affection is not to be thought of in the ordinary sense—
that is, from migrating portions of valves or thrombi.

In no single case has an endocarditis or any other source for
the displacement of emboli been proved. Ponfick found the
splenic artery and its larger branches completely permeable into
the deposit. On the other hand, there were often found, in the
splenic veins leading from the deposit, thrombotic, obstructive
masses of not very recent origin. Although it can, of course, be
assumed that these were developed secondarily, originating in
the capillary thrombi, yet the other possibility should not be overlooked, that a venous thrombosis may have occurred primarily,
and that such an event may have caused the hemorrhagic infarction of the region of tissue lying behind and belonging to it.
Since Cohnheim has directly examined the infarctions under the
microscope, and followed out the individual phases of this complicated phenomenon, both independently and in their causal
connection with each other, we are, as has been already mentioned
above, clearly informed as to the mechanical basis of such a common final effect. The suggestion which Ponfick first made free

use of—that the hemorrhage which causes the infarction arises from the intrusion of Obermeier's fibrillæ into the splenic pulp, and thus, although in another sense, has its origin in embolism—has so far found no support in facts.

The much rarer, arterial circumscribed diseases of the spleen were found in five per cent. of all the cases; in recurrent fever they are always found within the follicular tissue, sometimes in such abundance that the dark background appears sprinkled with them; at other times they are limited to a comparatively small section of the organ, which corresponds to the distribution of some particular artery. Unlike the foci of the venous terri-tory, they occur in the form of small, dull white or more yellow-ish spots and stripes, which include sometimes only a part, some-times the whole extent of the section of the affected follicle. As Ponfick has very clearly shown, even in the latter case, their size only exceptionally exceeds that of a pin's head; but soon the color becomes more and more yellowish, the tissue looser, like pus, and in the centre can be seen a little, irregularly bordered cavity. Whether the pulp directly meets the inflammatory tis-sue, or whether a layer of gray follicular tissue still remains between them, the neighborhood is always free from secondary inflammatory appearances.

The microscopic examination of these diseased spots seated in the Malpighian corpuscles taught Ponfick that, in all the places thus altered, an increased accumulation of the same small lym-phoid elements is found as is normally present in the follicular tissue. The opaque, dirty white or whitish yellow color is ex-plained by the irritation of these cells; and the cavity in the centre by their complete separation, occurring in the further progress of degeneration. In the later stages, beside these small cells, much larger forms show themselves, which are distinguished by their richness in large and small fat-granules. These are situated partly in the true follicular tissue, partly in the adven-titia of the artery. Ponfick is so far of the opinion that we have here to do with inflammatory softening.

Symptoms and Diagnosis.

For the most part the symptoms of inflammation of the spleen are so obscure that a positive diagnosis can hardly be made. Mistakes arising from other morbid processes certainly form the basis of the symptomatology of the older pathology. For the sake of completeness I will begin with a sketch of the disease as it was formerly drawn.

After previous chills and sometimes rigor, as in most inflammations, a feeling of heaviness, fulness, and pain shows itself in the left side, which reaches upward to the left shoulder, and is increased by all pressure and cough; sometimes the patient is affected with thirst, nausea, dry cough, and other febrile symptoms; hæmatemesis, fainting, or pain on breathing are sometimes observed, but are, however, seldom connected with the simple form of this disease. In many cases the disease reaches a crisis by a bleeding from the nose or the stomach, by a copious sediment in the urine, by the return of piles or the menses, and sometimes by a profuse lochial flow. In very severe cases of splenitis, such as rapidly produce the complete destruction of the splenic tissue, persistent vomiting—often accompanied by the evacuation from the stomach and bowels of a grumous, coagulated blood—is a characteristic appearance.

According to Marcus, the symptoms vary as one or another part of the spleen is specially affected; if the lower and anterior part is particularly inflamed, the hardness and swelling can sometimes be felt on the left side, beneath the short ribs. The pains shoot downward towards the back and kidneys. If the upper part of the spleen is more inflamed, where the stomach, the diaphragm, or even the heart itself sympathize, we find oppression, anxiety, cough, nausea, vomiting, sighing, and fainting.

We must, unfortunately, confess that the medical progress of late decades has completely wiped out this picture of the disease, but, on the other hand, has substituted no other characteristic symptoms of inflammation of the spleen. The shrewdest and most scientific physicians must confess that they have found at autopsies extensive inflammatory processes, and even large abscesses of the spleen, where in life not a single symptom has attracted attention thereto. Where suspicion of inflammation of the spleen is aroused, an attempt should be made to obtain proof of it by finding the following changes:

I. Pain in the splenic region.

I have already mentioned, in the general part of this treatise, that actual pain only occurs in diseases of the spleen when the serous envelope is changed; even in the ordinary wedge-shaped inflammation, or in abscesses, it may remain absent so long as secondary peritonitis does not occur. Strong pressure or percussion in the splenic region usually excites pain in such cases, before any complaint is made of spontaneous pain. Radiation of the pain towards the left shoulder and half of the thorax is very rare.

II. Evident enlargement of the spleen cannot be considered a constant symptom of its inflammation; it is dependent on the number and size of the inflammatory foci. The increase of volume produced by simple inflammation is seldom more than double the normal size (Bamberger). If a portion of the enlarged spleen can be felt, it appears harder and more resistant, without reaching the high degree of resistance observed in chronic tumors. When the splenic tissue is already changed, the demonstration of an added inflammation is generally much easier than when the organ is completely normal. I observed in one patient with splenic leucæmia, frequently repeated febrile attacks, which depended on inflammatory processes in the spleen, for after each febrile attack a distinct increase of the size of the spleen could be shown. This opinion was afterwards shown to be correct by the autopsy.

III. Febrile symptoms belong only exceptionally, as in the case mentioned above, to splenitis alone, and then assume the character of an inflammatory fever. They are usually entirely or partly dependent on the original disease, the endocarditis, or other pyæmia, and have little value for diagnosis. If the inflammation of the spleen has gone on to suppuration, then, as a rule, the characteristic rigors make their appearance, and the fever assumes the so-called hectic character; the patients usually emaciate rapidly; severe sweats, œdema, slight icterus, and diarrhœa make their appearance. Kernig describes, as favoring the

probable diagnosis of splenic abscess, after previous recurrent
fever, a remittent fever, progressing with moderate temperature,
and marked morning remissions, with persistent splenic dulness.
Among 400 cases of recurrent fever he has seen 5 splenic abscesses;
Zorn, among 600 cases, only 1.

Only very rarely can the splenic abscess be recognized as a
fluctuating tumor felt externally. Its diagnosis is problematic,
even when pyæmic appearances are present, since the same·
symptoms can be produced by purulent inflammation of other
organs which are inaccessible to physical examination. They
can only be referred to the spleen when severe pains in the
splenic region, together with gradually increasing splenic dulness,
can be clearly determined. The difficulty of diagnosis is so very
great, because the symptoms of splenic abscess are so little characteristic and constant. It should be mentioned that splenic
abscesses have existed for a long time, during several years,
without any symptoms. All at once their course may be modified by the signs of perforation. If the abscess breaks into the
abdominal cavity, death follows either immediately or with the
phenomena of a very acute peritonitis.

Rupture into the stomach, with the discharge of bloody pus,
by vomiting and stool, has been comparatively often observed.

Cozé found at an autopsy the spleen firmly connected with the stomach, forming a sac with walls six lines thick, filled with purulent fluid and lumps of blood,
in connection with the cavity of the stomach by means of quite a large opening at
the place of adhesion. Rupture into the colon has been seen by Jacquinelle and
Grottanelli, both cases terminating fatally. Heusinger saw, in two cases, the discharge take place through the kidneys. Grottanelli observed the case of a man
who had an enlargement of the spleen remaining after several attacks of intermittent fever, and suffered from hectic fever, night sweats, and petechiæ. In a quarrel,
the patient received a blow in the left side, the growth rapidly began to disappear, while a thick, stinking mass was discharged with the urine with great pain.
The urine consisted chiefly of a dark gray, partly blackish mass, and was so thick
that it seemed like the intestinal discharges of little children. This evacuation
lasted three weeks. The patient recovered, and seven years after was perfectly well.

If the pus discharged from the splenic abscess is capsulated
in the neighborhood of the spleen, the same extremely obscure
appearances arise as are observed in similar sacculated purulent

exudations in general. Febrile symptoms of varying character, sometimes rigors like intermittent, circumscribed pain, varying in intensity, rapid emaciation, loss of strength, impairment of digestion, cachectic appearance, œdematous swelling, point to a deep-seated lesion, the exact position of which can only be shown with certainty when the sac is large enough and so situated as to be accessible to physical examination.

This glance at the symptoms of splenic inflammation has given us the assurance that a certain diagnosis can be made only when, after traumatic causes or in consequence of pyæmia, and especially when endocarditis is present, local and general symptoms arise which can be referred to the spleen. In every case of endocarditis the attention should be directed to this organ from the beginning, even when local symptoms do not point to it. This demand is the more peremptory if sudden swelling of the spleen, dull pain, or tenderness on pressure, arise in the splenic region. The diagnosis increases in probability if metastatic inflammations of other organs are developed at the same time. This is most frequently the case, for reasons given above, in the kidneys; hence, albuminuria and hæmaturia are, under such circumstances, very valuable signs for forming a diagnosis of splenitis.

Prognosis.

The fact that we so often find at autopsies, cicatricial depressions, as the remains of splenic inflammation, shows that they may run a favorable course; most cases are betrayed during life by no symptom which endangers life or health. If suppuration occurs, which may happen in cases arising from pyæmia, or under unfavorable circumstances in any case, or if the process ends with the formation of putrid matter, the prognosis is highly unfavorable. It has been repeatedly mentioned that perforation with general peritonitis always causes death; and also, that the non-perforating splenic abscess, as well as the sacculated abscess produced by perforation, or the opening into neighboring organs, although life may continue for some time, finally lead to death by various consequences and complications.

Healing and disappearance of a splenic abscess, its opening outward or inward, with favorable result, belong to the exceptions.

Therapeutics.

The older physicians called for very energetic treatment in acute splenitis. General bleeding should be employed so long as the inflammatory pain was severe, provided that the health of the patient permitted. At the same time mild laxatives should be administered to diminish the inflammatory activity. A copious application of leeches, followed by blisters, were suitable to complete the treatment.

At the beginning of every recognized splenic inflammation I think that we should chiefly recommend the continuous application of ice-bags to the splenic region, and the evacuation of the intestinal canal by saline cathartics. With severe stabbing pains local bleedings may be employed. In long-continued dull pain, blisters or painting with iodine may be used. Some of the splenic remedies mentioned above may be used with caution.

The cure of the original disease, the endocarditis or pyæmia and their symptoms, is the principal object of treatment.

Acute Tumors of the Spleen.

Rokitansky, Lehrbuch. 1861. III. S. 292.—*Bamberger*, Krankheiten des chylopoët. Systems. 1864. S. 613.—*Griesinger*, Infectionskrankheiten. 1864.—*J. C. Lehmann*, Ueber d. Verhalten d. parenchym. Entzündungen zu den acuten Krankheiten. Bibliothek for. Laeger. Jan. 1868. Schmidt's Jahrb. 1868. 193.—*Oertel*, On Diphtheria. Volume I. of this Cyclopædia, 619.—*Birch-Hirschfeld*, Der acute Milztumor. Archiv für physiol. Heilkunde. Bd. XIII. 1872. S. 389.—*N. Friedreich*, Der acute Milztumor und seine Beziehungen zu den acuten Infectionskrankheiten. Volkmann's Vorträge. Nr. 75.—*Trojanowsky*, Centralblatt für die med. Wissenschaft. Nr. 53. 1871. S. 842.—*Dr. A. Weil*, Ueber das Vorkommen des Milztumors bei frischer Syphilis. Deutsches Archiv für klin. Medicin. XIII. 3.—*Ponfick*, Ueber die Schicksale körniger Farbstoffe im Organismus. Virchow's Archiv. XLVIII. — *C. E. Hoffmann*, Untersuchungen über die path. anat. Veränderungen der Organe im Typhus abdom. Leipzig, 1869.—*Buhl*, Zeitschrift für Biologie. 1871. VI. 129.— *Waldeyer*, Virchow's Archiv. LII. S. 54.—*E. Wagner*, Ein Fall von tödtlicher

Pilzkrankheit. Festschrift. Leipzig, 1872. — *W. O. Leube* und *W. Mueller,* Drei Fälle von Mycosis intest. etc. Deutsches Archiv für klin. Medicin. XII. Bd.—*Billroth,* Virchow's Archiv. XXIII. S. 460.—*Ponfick,* Virchow's Archiv. LVI. S. 532.—*Dr. Carl Wenzel,* Die Marschfieber in ihren ursächl. Beziehungen während des Hafenbaues im Jahde-Gebiete von 1858-1869. Prager Viretel-jahrschrift. CVIII. S. 1. 1870. — *Ponfick,* Anatomische Studien über den Typhus recurrens. Virchow's Archiv. LX. Bd.—*Mosler,* Ueber die Wirkung des kalten Wassers auf die Milz. Virchow's Archiv. LVII. Bd.—*Virchow,* Die Fortschritte der Kriegsheilkunde bes. im Gebiete der Infectionskrankheiten. Berlin, 1874. A. Hirschwald.—*Botkin,* Die Contractilität der Milz u. die Beziehung der Infectionsprocesse zu Milz, Leber, etc. Berlin, 1874. A. Hirschwald.

Frequency. Anatomical Appearances. Mode of Origin.

With classic precision Rokitansky thus sketches the anatomical character of acute splenic tumors : "Moderate enlargement (three or four fold) ; a swollen appearance and feeling with tense, thin capsule ; sometimes a fluctuating feeling ; loose, mushy consistence of the pulp while the trabeculæ can easily be torn ; dark red color of the pulp and hyperæmia ; often the Malpighian corpuscles are especially swollen, when they coalesce with the red splenic pulp without definite boundary."

Notwithstanding several valuable works, our knowledge of the more minute changes of the acutely enlarged spleen is still incomplete. There is nowhere any sufficient statistical material for the comparative size and weight of the spleen in acute diseases.[1] What pathological anatomy has lately done for the knowledge of certain kinds of tumors will be mentioned under the proper heads.

Acute splenic tumors arise in the course of acute diseases,

---

[1] *Birch-Hirschfeld* has very lately enriched the statistics of splenic tumors on this point by a valuable contribution (compare Tageblatt der Breslauer Naturforscher-Vers. 1874. S. 100). For determining the normal weight of the spleen, the average weight from sixty cases of accident and suicide, of the average age of thirty-seven years, was found to be 150 grms. (0.26 per cent. of the body-weight). The variations in weight observed in splenic tumors are stated in the adjoining table. According to them, the weight of the spleen was most increased in amyloid degeneration (348.0) : in the pyæmic form of puerperal fever (331) ; metastatic pyæmia (302) ; typhoid (296) ; congestive tumor, in cirrhosis of the liver (296) ; variola hemorrhagica (291) ; croupous pneumonia (217).

especially infectious diseases. Since Virchow, with the glance of genius, recognized parenchymatous inflammation as such, in which the process calls forth no exudation between the elements of the tissue, but runs its course within them—the cells, taking up a greater amount of nutriment, increasing in size, and becoming hypertrophied; the acute splenic tumors are also to be looked upon as parenchymatous inflammations. In many acute diseases, other organs besides the spleen show similar parenchymatous changes. A special disposition to affect particular organs exists with certain morbid processes.

Among the infectious diseases, the recent intermittent fever tumor holds the first place. Next are the various forms of typhus, in which parenchymatous alterations of the spleen, the liver, the heart, and the kidneys, are found. The spleen and kidneys are especially exposed to attack; they are affected sooner than the liver—the heart last of all. In puerperal fever, the parenchymatous changes are observed as frequently, if not more frequently, than in typhus. The previous pregnancy seems to be not without influence; these affections often reach a high degree, so that far advanced fatty degeneration is found. In the liver, the process takes the form of acute atrophy with jaundice. The spleen shows on an average a greater enlargement than in typhus. In puerperal fever it is much oftener soft than hard; generally entirely diffluent. The follicles for the most part appear unusually large and distinct.

The parenchymatous changes occurring during pregnancy appear to be the consequences of the greatly changed composition of the blood, rather than of the anomalies of the abdominal circulation caused by this condition.

Puerperal fever and pyæmia are nearly related, and hence we almost always find in traumatic pyæmia the parenchymatous changes, especially of the spleen.

In malignant, or typhoid jaundice (icterus gravis), the spleen, according to Lebert, was enlarged two or three fold, and softened in a third of all the cases collected by him. Frerichs also mentions, as a rule, a considerable swelling. The spleen is usually much enlarged, but, with the access of considerable gastric or intestinal hemorrhage, rapidly diminishes again.

	Number of Cases.	Average Age.	Average Weight of Body, Kilo.	Weight of Spleen, Grammes.	Percentage of Weight of Body.	Dimensions of Spleen, Centimetres.	Weight of Liver.	Percentage of Weight of Body.
I. In otherwise healthy persons, accidents and suicides (chiefly males)	60	37	59	150	0.26	13:8:3	1625	2.7
II. In the bodies of patients where the disease could be supposed to have no influence upon the spleen. a. Males..............	62	40	50.6	140	0.27	12.0:7.5	1534	3.0
b. Females..............	53	43	43.0	137	0.31	....	1488	3.4
III. In the bodies of patients over sixty..........	89	70.6	42.0	99	0.23	10:6	1131	2.6
IV. Congestive tumors in cirrhosis of liver	20	47	62.0	296	0.47	....	1355	2.1
V. Amyloid degeneration of spleen.............	41	37	48.4	348	0.7	15:9:4½	1718	3.8
VI. Typhoid..............	46	27	47.0	296	0.63	15:9:3	1702	3.6
VII. Variola. a. Ordinary form..........	20	30	43.0	177	0.41	.....	1669	3.3
b. V. hæmorrhagica..........	16	24	50.0	291	0.58	.....	1690	3.3
VIII. Croupous pneumonia..............	28	45	51.0	217	0.42	14:8	1896	3.7
IX. a. Pulmonary tuberculosis, where there was no ulcerative destruction, or where the cavities had become encapsuled..............	194	39	40.9	142	0.34	12:7	1432	3.5
b. Recent ulcerative (non-capsulated softening).	148	35	44.0	230	0.5	14:8	1634	3.7
X. Metastatic pyæmia..............	71	33	51.0	302	0.6	15:9	1908	3.7
XI. Phlegmonous, gangrenous, diphtheritic affections of wounds without metastases..........	36	43	48.0	174	0.35	13:7	1716	3.5
XII. Puerperal peritonitis (without metastases)	55	24	51.6	174	0.33	....	1707	3.3
XIII. Pyæmic form of puerperal fever..............	33	25	53.0	331	0.61	....	2066	3.8

In regard to diphtheria, observations are still much at vari-
ance. Oertel found the spleen in some cases enlarged, the capsule tense and covered with extravasations of blood, the parenchyma dark, cherry red, soft, and easily torn. The Malpighian
bodies are indistinct, or in other cases enlarged. Nuclear hyperplasia has been repeatedly demonstrated in the spleen by Buhl.
On the other hand, Oertel found, in cases of which the diphtheria
ran its course with a high degree of blood-poisoning, the spleen
only slightly enlarged, and its parenchyma of normal texture
and color.

Among the acute exanthemata, small-pox deserves especial
mention; like Friedreich, I have clinically determined, in a series
of cases, evident tumors of the spleen in the ordinary as well as
in the hemorrhagic form of variola.

E. Wagner has demonstrated lymphatic new formations in the liver and spleen
in variola. The splenic tissue was of normal consistence, brownish red, anæmic,
containing very numerous grayish spots, as large as a millet-seed, which were shown
by microscopic examination to be lymphatic new formations, situated especially on
the sheaths of the middle-sized and small arteries, as well as on some of the Malpighian corpuscles in connection with them.[1]

Trojanowsky has demonstrated the presence of considerable
enlargement of the spleen in scarlet fever and measles; he says,
however, that he has only found it in cases where a second eruption followed a short time after a primary incomplete outbreak
of the exanthem. In Greifswald scarlet fever and measles are
observed almost every winter; in a large number of cases I, like
Friedreich, have been able to convince myself that clinically
demonstrable tumors of the spleen may be found in most cases
of these exanthemata, which run a regular course from the beginning. In epidemic cerebro-spinal meningitis I have found
tumors of the spleen, as well as parenchymatous changes of
other organs. In acute miliary tuberculosis the occurrence of
the splenic tumor is almost constant, so that its absence cannot
be made of much value for the diagnosis of typhoid, as was formerly sometimes attempted. The same thing may be said of
many other acute diseases, like coryza, erysipelas, pneumonia

---

[1] Arch. der Heilkde. V. S. 90. Schmidt's Jahrb. 126. S. 159.

(Friedreich). Weil has lately succeeded in proving that the spleen is affected in many cases of syphilis, even during the existence of the primary induration, before the development of the first eruption. As a proof of their causal connection, he mentions the important fact that the enlargement of the spleen diminished during an antisyphilitic treatment.

We are not at present in a position to explain fully the mode of origin of these parenchymatous changes, and especially of the splenic tumor; there can be no doubt that the cause must be sought in the blood. When one remembers how rapidly the parenchymatous changes in various organs are developed during acute diseases, a sort of hint is thereby given of the nature of the cause.

According to Liebermeister, the increased temperature is put forward as a peculiarity common to acute diseases; certainly, the abnormally warm blood, when brought in contact with the tissues, must cause many changes in them. Many facts indicate, however, that the excessive rise of temperature is not the only cause upon which the anatomical changes depend. Our knowledge of these processes has been advanced by the study of acute poisoning, as by phosphorus and arsenic, and of the action of the biliary salts; just as in poisoning by these agents, we must, in infectious diseases and other acute processes, look upon poisonous material contained in the blood as the cause of the changes of the parenchymatous organs. All acute diseases in which such poisonous materials are met with in large proportion are probably to be looked upon as infectious diseases. As regards the precise way in which the anatomical changes in the elements take place, whether the poisonous material acts upon them as an irritant, or influences their nutrition in some other manner, no definite opinion can be given at present. We are not justified in giving up the older view according to which these anatomical changes are considered acute irritative processes.

Why the spleen should be so prominently involved in infectious diseases may be explained from its anatomical arrangement. The size of the splenic artery, as well as its distribution, favors the invasion of infectious materials; and besides, these are probably detained longer than in other organs, by the pecu-

liar conditions of the circulation in the spleen, as we may conclude from Ponfick's admirable inquiries on the behavior of
granular coloring matters in the organism.

Birch-Hirschfeld has attempted the solution of the problem
by experiments on the infection of rabbits with putrid blood, in
which he had demonstrated the presence of micrococci.

On the introduction into the blood of considerable quantities of fluid containing
micrococci, these minute organisms were first taken up by the white corpuscles in
considerable numbers. After the lapse of a certain time, the duration of which probably depended upon the quantity injected, an increase of the free cocci, steadily
progressive until death, was observed. The spleen retained in its pulp-cells a portion of the micrococci, and when their number was considerable, a distinct swelling
of the organ appeared. When putrid fluids were injected into serous cavities,
Birch-Hirschfeld observed a local inflammation, from which the animal sometimes
died before micrococci were taken into the blood in large numbers. In these cases
no swelling of the spleen took place. This experiment explains why we do not find
tumors of the spleen in all cases in man where an infection of the system is assumed.

According to the results of these experiments, the examination of tumors of the spleen in acute infectious diseases from this
point of view is a matter for further and more accurate investigation than has yet been made. Birch-Hirschfeld has already
brought forward a series of pathologico-anatomical cases, and
given special prominence to those in which an undoubted mycosis within the body was observed; he draws, hence, the conclusion that in infectious diseases the micrococci accumulate in the
spleen, and are, in part, taken up and retained by the protoplasm
of the pulp-cells.

The cases of intestinal mycosis thus far observed have all disclosed advanced alterations of the spleen.

In the well-known case of Buhl, who demonstrated in the stomach and small
intestine a permeation of numerous portions of the mucous membrane by groups of
zoogloea, in the submucous tissue numerous fine-jointed and branched threads of
fungus, and the same in the corresponding varicose lymphatics, all the blood in
the body showed abundant isolated particles, and all the organs, including the enlarged spleen, were impregnated with isolated granules. Waldeyer published two
more cases of intestinal mycosis, with considerable enlargement of the spleen. In
the splenic vessels he found an enormous quantity of very small zoogloea elements.
In the case of E. Wagner the spleen exhibited the ordinary characteristics of intense
hyperæmia, and numerous small hemorrhages; fungi were not found in it. Wilhelm

Mueller found in a case of intestinal mycosis, "the splenic pulp very rich in many nucleated cells; in the protoplasm of the pulp-cells, at the bruised-looking places, very numerous fine points, like those of the intestinal pustules; in the fluid found between the cells, besides colored and colorless blood-cells, numerous fine points, together with scanty, small bacteria, 0.004-0.006 mm. long. A portion of the venous epithelium was also impregnated with fine, punctiform bacteria."

Wilhelm Mueller made use of his observations to answer—by experiments on the infection of animals—the inquiry previously raised by Waldeyer and Bollinger as to the relation of intestinal mycosis to charbon or the anthrax of animals (Milzbrand). In these infected animals also he found the spleen swollen, congested, and somewhat fragile; the pulp-cells large, in part thickly pervaded by punctiform bacteria. In the blood of the splenic vein, besides free punctiform bacteria, a few bacterial rods. From his inoculation experiments, Wilhelm Mueller believes that there is now no sufficient ground for separating intestinal mycosis from the other forms of charbon.

As is known, Pollender and Brauell discovered small corpuscles in cases of charbon so long ago as 1855, which were made more generally known by Davaine under the name of bacteridia. This last named distinguished observer also stated that these bodies were found in special abundance in the spleen.

The view of Davaine is supported by Tiegel. Tiegel inoculated subcutaneously a rabbit with the splenic pulp of a slaughtered cow; the animal dying in twenty-four hours, bacteridia were found in the blood and in the splenic pulp. Grimm also asserts that the spleen is the headquarters of the bacteria in charbon. He found there such a mass of these organisms of the most various sizes that it was difficult for him to study the histological elements of the organ. "One might often almost be led to think that the spleen consisted only of trabeculæ, bacteria, and their germs, if in some cases parts of the spleen had not remained comparatively normal." He found the bacteria chiefly in the spleen when the animal examined had suffered long from the disease.

For the traumatic diseases, especially pyæmia and septicæmia, the near relation to putrid infection has been often insisted upon already, and an important rôle in the development of these diseases has been assigned to the little organisms sometimes called micrococci, sometimes bacteria, sometimes monads, by von Recklinghausen, Klebs, Hueter, and Waldeyer. In an address upon the progress of military surgery, especially in the department of infectious diseases, delivered at Berlin on the 2d of August, 1874, on the anniversary of the foundation of the medical school for military surgeons, Virchow discusses this question thoroughly.

In an enlarged spleen of pyæmia, examined a short time after death, Birch-Hirschfeld found enlargement of the pulp-cells, and micrococci within them. The same observer also, during an epidemic of puerperal fever, which is known to have the greatest similarity to those surgical diseases, was able to confirm the former observations of Waldeyer. In three cases, which he was fortunate enough to be able to examine from one-half an hour to two hours after death, he found in the blood free micrococci, both isolated, in the chain form, and in little masses; besides these, increased white blood-cells, which also contained them. The spleen in all three cases was considerably enlarged, its tissue moderately soft, containing hemorrhages, alternating with paler spots. In all three cases there was swelling of the pulp-cells, which also contained micrococci, and upon tearing up portions of the spleen, the fluid added, which had been previously examined, also contained them in large quantities. Since Birch-Hirschfeld was not able to establish the last conditions in all the cases which he examined, he thinks he has a right to assume that, in patients who died with splenic tumor, the infectious material was early introduced into the mass of the blood; while in others the infection advanced more in the lymphatic circulation, and the blood was reached only at a later period.

In only one case of hemorrhagic small-pox Birch-Hirschfeld examined the spleen fresh enough to attach much importance to the result. It differed from the condition of the septicæmic tumor only by the circumstance that, besides the single, punctiform elements, a considerable number of rod-like, jointed elements was present in the spleen.

In typhoid the splenic enlargement is an almost constant symptom, but a special demonstration of its anatomical condition is wanting. Billroth found the venous sinuses of the typhoid spleen only moderately distended, the capillaries and arteries not dilated. In the veins large cells (the largest of from 0.04 to 0.05 mm. in diameter), containing from two to six granules, occurred in much larger number than in the normal spleen; the venous epithelium was not visibly altered, the Malpighian corpuscles were compressed and poor in cells. Circumscribed foci of newly formed cells could not be demonstrated in the pulp tissue ; whether the cells of the pulp in general were enlarged is not stated ; while Billroth remarked in the pyæmic splenic tumor a slight enlargement of all the cellular elements.

C. E. E. Hoffmann[1] has carefully measured the spleen in typhoid 181 times. He refers the increase of the cellular splenic elements to a proliferation of the original lymph-cells.

Accurate observations on the splenic tumor in typhus exanthematicus are up to the present time wanting.

In recurrent fever the condition of the spleen has been more thoroughly studied. This has a special interest of its own since Obermeier discovered peculiar formations, endowed with independent movement, within the circulation of living patients with recurrent fever. As is known, this observer has also proved that the presence of these formations in the circulation, on the one side, and the beginning, as well as the duration of the attack, on the other, constantly coincide, and thus very probably stand in the relation of cause and effect. We thus have given us, not only a contribution to a mechanical theory of the fever, but a possibility of explaining the origin of the splenic tumor.

The St. Petersburg epidemics had already called out a series of works which, in part, treated very thoroughly of the pathological appearances of recurrent fever (Herrmann and Kuettner, Zorn), and also gave special attention to the changes of the spleen (Kernig).

Very recently our knowledge of the splenic tumor occurring in recurrent fever has been essentially advanced by Ponfick's anatomical studies. They proved that the splenic affection forms a constant condition, besides which we have certain changes of the osseous marrow and of the blood, also of the liver and kidneys, and finally of the muscles, especially of the heart.

According to Ponfick, the diffused disease of the spleen is never wanting in recurrent fever. It betrays itself by considerable enlargement, which is always greatest during an attack, and sometimes reaches a degree which is never heard of except

---

[1] Untersuchungen über die pathol.-anat. Veränderungen der Organe beim Abdominaltyphus. Leipzig, 1869.

in leucæmia. The increase of size affects the organ in all directions; the weight is considerably increased, the capsule dense
and shining, the tissue softer than normal, but not diffluent; the
pulp dark, bluish red, swelling out strongly on section; the
follicles moderately enlarged, often effaced—their color chiefly
gray, sometimes pure white or more yellowish; in the later
stages they again stand out more sharply, as the shrinking of
the pulp advances. Even four weeks after the last attack a distinctly recognizable enlargement of the organ is always present.
The type of the simple recurrent tumor corresponds, according
to Ponfick, so completely in every respect to that of typhoid,
that he doubts whether it would be possible to distinguish two
such spleens from each other. This swelling of the pulp depends, as is usual in acute splenic tumors, upon two factors:
first, the great engorgement of the vessel, and, secondly, a very
copious increase of the cellular elements, among which large
forms, containing many granules, occur in special abundance,
which stand in immediate local relation to the cavernous veins.

Starting from his results obtained by experiment upon the
transit of fine particles suspended in the blood into the cells
of the pulp-tissue, Ponfick took great pains, in his anatomical
studies on recurrent, to find again in the pulp-cells of the spleen
the thread-like bodies discovered by Obermeier. For this purpose he chose chiefly such cases as died during the attack.
Although Ponfick never succeeded, either at this or any other
stage of the disease, in demonstrating their presence in the parenchyma of the spleen, yet he cannot give up the belief that they
are actually hidden in the pulp-cells. Ponfick thinks that no
one need be astonished at the previous negative result of his
labors who has once perceived with his own eyes the deceptive
minuteness of these threads, since the difficulty of bringing these
delicate structures to view is not unfrequently great enough
even in the blood-plasma. Since the much coarser granules of
the cell conceal and overshadow them, Ponfick fears that their
demonstration in the pulp-cells will not generally be reached, so
long as no characteristic reagent has been found.

A material progress in the knowledge of acute splénic tumors
was made when Ponfick demonstrated other abnormal elements

in the pulp-cells. He first found therein red blood-corpuscles, which, according to the stage of the disease, were fresh or in the various stages of regressive metamorphosis. Besides these pulp-cells, containing partly blood-corpuscles, partly pigment, which are, indeed, found in smaller numbers in the whole series of acute diseases, especially the infectious, he found others similarly formed, of a peculiar character ; they were distinguished by containing a greater or less number of fat-granules and globules, usually of considerable size, and reminded one exactly of granulation-cells. These forms are found, although by no means in so distinct development and in such numbers, in other infectious diseases of the most various character; hence, Ponfick did not consider their mere presence, but their abundant accumulation, as something peculiar to recurrent fever.

Precisely the same granular cells can also be constantly found in the splenic and portal veins, and their quantity usually stands in a definite proportion to a general enlargement of the spleen and to the richness of the pulp in the same elements. The fatty nature of the granules of each granulation-cell is clearly shown by chemical tests, since they disappear if ether is allowed to act for some time upon fine fragments hardened in alcohol. These same large granulation-cells Ponfick has demonstrated in specimens of blood which were taken during life from any vein of the greater circulation. In well-marked cases they were found in every specimen, sometimes in great numbers. The presence of these large cells in the blood—a proof of its contamination with formed organic matter—is considered by Ponfick, like the presence of Obermeier's filaments, as a phenomenon pathognomonic of recurrent fever.

Besides the general enlargement, and the anomalies of the pulp connected therewith, as well as the consequent affection of the portal, as compared with the general circulation, recurrent fever not unfrequently gives rise to circumscribed diseases of the spleen which may be considered pathognomonic. We may distinguish foci of the arterial and of the venous tracts, which have been already minutely described in another place.

Ponfick has rendered a further service in the study of acute splenic tumors by carefully studying the changes of the osseous marrow occurring in connection with them. In twenty-one bodies of patients dead of recurrent fever, examined for this purpose, he found more or less clearly marked, constant, generally microscopic changes of the whole structure of the marrow, but in six, that is in about 30 per cent. of the bodies, gross anatomical anomalies in the form of discrete foci, some of them of considerable size.

The first, which generally affected diffusely the whole mass, could be studied in their most extreme development in the spongy bones, sternum, ribs, and vertebra. In these places they were not visible to the naked eye, but were so in the marrow of the long bones, especially in the diaphyses. In advanced degrees of the affection of the marrow they are sharply marked off, even to their finer ramifications, as chalk-white lines, resembling the delicate filaments and cords which cross the cavities in softened spots of the brain. Just as in the latter region, so in the present case, the characteristic color depends upon a multitude of large granular cells and free fat granules embedded in the adventitia, which surround the vessel itself like an opaque sheath; besides this, just as in the spleen, the muscular fibres of the middle coat, especially of the small arteries, are the seat of a thick accumulation of fat granules, which continues as far as the capillary wall. The tissue in the immediate neighborhood of the vessels is not spared; we find here also, between the large fat cells, single granulation globules, and here and there small masses of fatty granulation.

The limited affections in the medullary tissue are not, like those in the spleen, to be referred to hemorrhagic infarctions; their whole appearance is against such a theory, especially their color and their position in the deep portion of the medullary cavity, and in particular the absence of every trace of the constituents of the blood within the altered tissue. Ponfick considers it a peculiar kind of softening which, in this place, must lead to destruction of the tissue the earlier that it occurs in a purely adipose structure. The circumscribed lesions of the marrow, discovered by Ponfick in recurrent fever, are of great importance from an etiological point of view in explaining the origin of the various affections of the bones after infectious and acute diseases.

Ponfick, in the fifty-sixth volume of Virchow's Archiv, has communicated numerous observations on the sympathetic morbid alterations of the marrow in internal diseases generally, but especially in typhoid, intermittent, pneumonia, pleurisy, pericarditis, peritonitis, meningitis, and pyæmic fevers. It follows that in these severe constitutional or acute inflammatory diseases, all the organs to which we usually ascribe the most intimate connections with the formation and destruction of the blood are actively concerned.

Intermittent fever ought to be more particularly mentioned here as a disease which has a long recognized relation to the spleen. The most frequent of all the tumors of the spleen is found in this disease; it is observed at every age, equally in both sexes, and is sometimes congenital. This last fact is very important in regard to the mode of origin of splenic tumors. They are induced in this case by transmission of the malarial poison from the maternal blood to the embryo; in such children, attacks of intermittent fevers have been observed.

Many hypotheses have been brought forward as to the mode of origin of splenic tumors in intermittent fever. Piorry, as is well known, considered the spleen the primary seat of the disease. When the view put forth by Salisbury (Amer. Journal of Med. Sci., Jan., 1866), that intermittent fever was caused by a fungus, received currency, Piorry's theory appeared justified in a certain point of view. If the spleen retained the fever-causing organisms, it was easy to suppose that the typical febrile attacks were caused by a periodical emigration of the spores; an attack of fever would then take place as soon as the development of the fungi exceeded the capacity of the spleen. The greater enlargement of the spleen, which can be determined before the beginning of the attack, and especially in the cold stage, favors such a view. It could then also be explained why persons who come from a malarial district into a region free from fever may be attacked with intermittent after months of apparent good health. Such persons must carry in their body the material which gives rise to intermittent. It needs no proof to show that its prolonged latency can be more easily explained by its deposit in a tissue than by its continued circulation in the blood (Birch-Hirschfield). Unfortunately these speculations upon intermittent fever belong as yet solely in the realm of hypothesis; neither anatomical inquiry nor experiment have given us any positive starting-point. A long series of clinical observations, however, make such a mode of origin of the splenic tumors occurring in intermittent very probable, and the importance of the subject requires that some of them should be given more minutely.

We have obtained, through Dr. Carl Wenzel, a very valuable contribution for the genesis of malarial diseases and their accompanying tumors.

The conditions for obtaining statistics were very favorable during the period of twelve years which elapsed from the commencement of the construction of the harbor in the Province of Jahde in 1858, to its completion in 1869; the demonstration that the temperature was the most important factor in producing malaria was of special importance. The highest point of the fever curve fell almost without exception in that month in which the highest point of the yearly temperature was reached.   Cold put a check to the epidemics in their intensity and extent.   In the summers, distinguished by a uniformly high temperature, in which the malaria was particularly widespread, the severe malarial affections—the pernicious and remittent forms—were especially seen.   The various modifications of the affections could be referred to a varying intensity in the cause of the disease.   The quicker types of fever were relatively more frequent with increasing heat of the weather than in the cool seasons, while, corresponding to the diminished malarial intensity, the slower types of the tertians and quartans occurred specially in the colder months.

All the facts given by Wenzel, which I cannot fully detail here, force us to the supposition that a low—that is, vegetable organism, is the cause of malaria.   Prof. Thomas, of Leipzig, in his excellent essay on intermittent fever, has brought forward a great number of arguments for the probability of such an assumption; first is the fact that the morbid principle, as a rule, stands in special relation to swampy soil.   The fever has been seen to become frequent in certain localities where it was before unknown, near newly-produced marshes, while it completely disappeared when the marsh was redeemed, and returned again when stagnation of the water again took place.   Damp places are generally a home for malaria, hence intermittent fever abounds in the neighborhood of rivers, on overflowed land, on clay and alluvial soil.   In the marshy regions, specially fitted for the production of malaria, we find not only moisture, but also a large amount of organic and particularly vegetable substances; the more their decomposition is favored by outward circumstances, the more widely spread and intense is the malaria.   The gases arising from the decomposition of vegetable substances may be of various kinds.   They are carbonic acid, carburetted hydrogen, ammonia, sulphuretted and phosphuretted hydrogen.   Circumstances under which these gases arise in other places are not of such a kind that their production is regularly followed by that of intermittent fever, since it is presumably not the gases alone which are active, but it must be looked upon as probable that the lower organisms contained in the marshes have an influence. Numerous late mycological studies have shown that these organisms specially thrive under conditions which we know to favor the production of malaria.   Organic life flourishes only under certain conditions of warmth and moisture; its development is checked by too great dryness or too great cold. Intermittent fevers then begin in our latitude with the starting vegetation, sometimes even in February, but sometimes not until March. As the months go on the heat increases, they entice from nature more and more abundant organisms, and intermittent fevers soon reach their height. But the surface of the earth is dried by the July sun ; notwithstanding the favorable conditions of the earth, moisture becomes less in the soil. Whenever showers in September and October supply the dampness, and evaporation takes place more slowly, if the temperature of the soil is high enough a new period of development may begin. With the oncoming of the winter's cold the new vital thread of vegetation becomes inactive. In the tropics the fevers are developed just at a time when the conditions favorable for the germs lying in the soil begin to be developed, not at the time of the inundation, but in the early part of the dry, or just at the beginning of the wet season, in which the most favorable conditions of warmth and moisture are found. Just according to the degrees of dryness or of flood they will prevail for a longer or shorter time in the various years. In hot springs and summers, which follow wet years, malarial diseases are most frequently observed, since the vigorous germinating processes aroused at such times by the abundant moisture of the soil, is, up to a certain point, only increased by the subsequent heat.

For the same reason malarial diseases are increased after inundations, to recur oftener in years with floods than in years without them. The greater moisture which remains after them must encourage a freer development of the fever germs. We see then, that only by the coöperation of air, moisture and warmth, the soil plays its important rôle in the production of malaria, by becoming the breeding place of innumerable lower organisms of a specific character.

The hypothesis of a miasma animatum (Henle) cannot therefore at this time be considered inadmissible, merely because the specific lower organisms have not been found in the blood or in the spleen in intermittent fever. Perhaps they are not present therein in very large quantities. Perhaps it is the lower organisms, in connection with the specific products of decomposition formed by them, which impress upon the fevers their **peculiar** character. The disease seems to depend upon a chemical change, which has affected every part and every cell of the body. The successive affection of the glands, intended for the formation of blood and lymph, is very striking. The reception of the mala-- rial germs by the blood-corpuscles in the lungs seems to be the first effect which the infection produces ; then the infected blood-corpuscles are deposited in the blood-forming glands and pro-duce an enlargement of them.

It is generally admitted that the spleen shows the most con-stant changes in malarial processes, but whether its affection is the first and most important event of the whole intermittent process is not certainly determined. The changes appear to consist at first of simple congestions, especially great fulness of the venous vascular territory. I have had as yet no opportunity to see a recent intermittent tumor in the dead body. Griesinger found it after a few attacks, generally very soft, sometimes diffluent, of a dark gray to violet black color. Wedge-shaped inflam-mations of the spleen sometimes occur in such cases without any ground for assuming their metastatic origin. According to Wedl, a diffuse exudation occurs in the parenchyma, is usually followed by hemorrhages from the small vessels, and makes-itself manifest at a later period by reddish brown pigment, which is deposited free in the parenchyma. According to this, the acute splenic tumor of malaria is to be looked upon as a diffuse paren-chymatous inflammation.

As I have mentioned above, the conditions found in acute infectious diseases, and in the ordinary forms of poisoning, dis-play in many points of view a striking coincidence, so that we are compelled to refer the alterations of parenchymatous organs in acute infectious diseases to the irritating action of poisonous substances circulating in the blood. Unfortunately, pathologi-cal chemistry has so far failed to furnish the proof that chemical alterations of a specific character take place in infectious dis-eases. We must, however, assume them, since it is not probable that the course and the symptoms of acute infectious diseases depend simply on the presence of little organisms in the blood, as corpuscular particles, either from their physical action, or, perhaps, from the mechanical irritation which they produce in the parenchyma of the organ. According to my view, it is the lower organisms, in connection with the specific products of decomposition formed by them, which impress upon the fevers their peculiar character. For many reasons certain fluid materials, secreted by the lower organisms during the time of their life in the blood, may be looked upon as the essential injury.

The acute enlargements of the spleen, arising from simple fluxionary hyperæmia in derangements of menstruation, are entirely different from the tumors occurring in the acute infectious diseases. In the general portion of this work I have set forth this mode of origin of splenic tumors. Fluxionary hyperæmia may also arise from injuries, inflammations, and new formations. The enlargement then usually takes place by way of hemorrhagic infarction.

Symptoms and Diagnosis.

The phenomena of acute splenic tumors are generally so little prominent, that they are completely concealed by the symptoms of the primary disease. Complaints of trouble caused thereby are seldom loud; sometimes a dull pain is perceived in the splenic region, which is increased by pressure, especially in recurrent fever. Deep breathing is often rendered difficult, and causes increase of the pain. If intense pains arise in the course of typhus or intermittent, this may depend upon the capsule of the spleen having been rendered thick and resistant by former attacks; or upon the fact that inflammatory processes, which may also occur in the course of those diseases, have taken place in the spleen or its capsules.

Since the importance of splenic tumors in the diagnosis of infectious diseases, and especially for their early recognition, sometimes even in the stage of incubation, is very great, all the means described in the diagnostic portion of this work for the discovery of enlargement of the spleen gain a special value. Only rarely can an acute splenic tumor be discovered by inspection; on the other hand, one can frequently succeed in finding it by palpation, especially if the apex projects below the ribs.

When meteorism is present, the demonstration may become difficult or impossible, even by percussion. In typhoid the splenic dulness is to be sought farther back towards the vertebral column.

I have often heard peculiar murmurs in the recent tumors of intermittent fever, and once in recurrent fever. It is easy to suppose, considering the great vascularity of the spleen, that from pathological alterations, such as tumors originating very acutely, murmurs might arise in the splenic vessels. I have often auscultated the normal spleen in man, and have never perceived a special murmur in that region. Since it is possible that murmurs existing in the spleen should not be transmitted outward through the abdominal wall, I have not neglected, in my numerous experiments, to auscultate the exposed surface of the spleen in animals by means of a stethoscope. I learned, however, nothing special thereby. I further auscultated the spleen in congested tumors, which had been caused by compression of the splenic veins, and also after its vessels had been tied, or after the nerves had been cut. In all these cases I perceived nothing specially abnormal. I have further auscultated a series of chronic splenic tumors, very pronounced leucæmic spleens, without finding special murmurs. That friction sounds can occur in such cases is a well-known fact, which I have often confirmed.

I heard for the first time, in June, 1871, a peculiar humming murmur in a patient with intermittent fever, during the cold stage. I have since succeeded, in almost every case of the kind, in demonstrating to my students murmurs during the cold stage. These murmurs were heard, not only in the splenic region, but upward and downward in the abdominal region; they became less in the febrile stage, and vanished completely during the apyrexia. Griesinger has also frequently heard over the spleen, in attacks of intermittent fever, especially at the beginning of the febrile stage, a continuous hum, or an intermittent, more blowing murmur, like the so-called placental or uterine murmur of pregnant women, and believes that it comes from one of the great vessels, especially the venous trunks of the abdomen, but hardly from the spleen. According to my view, it owes its origin to the contraction of the splenic artery, as well as other arteries, during the cold stage of intermittent. On a dog's spleen, outside of the abdomen, I have heard precisely the same sound after the administration of large doses of quinia.

A consideration of the history of the case, the perceptible increase of the splenic growth on repeated examination ; the greater sensitiveness to pressure—are generally sufficient to prevent acute tumors of the spleen from being confounded with longer existing chronic enlargement.

Acute tumors of the spleen end, if the primary disease is not fatal, in gradual return to their normal conditions of size and consistence. Not unfrequently the enlargement becomes chronic, especially after intermittent fever exists in this condition for years, and causes chronic splenic cachexia.

In rare cases, acute tumors of the spleen lead to a fatal result by a rupture of the distended organ. This disastrous event has been observed in attacks of intermittent fever as well as in typhus. Even at birth, hemorrhages of the splenic veins may take place by pressure on the congenital tumor. Rupture of the spleen will be more minutely treated in another place.

Therapeutics.

Separate treatment is seldom demanded for acute tumors of the spleen. The means used to combat the fundamental disease, usually contribute to the removal of the tumor ; this is specially true of the treatment of typhus and intermittent. My numerous experiments have shown that quinia and cold water, besides their antipyretic action, have an influence in contracting the spleen, so that the application of cold water to the spleen, combined with the administration of quinia, is especially recommended in the treatment of acute and chronic splenic tumors.

I must, however, give warning against the application of the cold douche to the splenic region in typhus. It seems to have too sudden an action upon the typhus spleen. The baths from 26° to 10° R., as they are given in my clinic in typhus, according to the particular case, fulfil the double object of reducing the temperature and diminishing the size of the spleen. According to the greater or less decrease in volume in the spleen after the action of cold water and quinine in typhus, each case appears more or less rapidly to take on a favorable or unfavorable action.

If, after the fever has run its course, the tumor, as frequently happens, still remains, its transition into the state of chronic enlargement is to be dreaded. All the remedies useful in diseases of the spleen, and mentioned in the general portion of this work may then be tried in succession. According to M. Meier and Botkin, faradization of the spleen deserves special consideration.

Numerous observations have convinced me that treatment, energetically continued, often attains the desired end. The enlargement of the spleen is removed, the chronic cachexia avoided.

Chronic Tumors of the Spleen.

We place in this category pure hypertrophy, amyloid degeneration, the syphilitic spleen, tuberculosis, cancer, and echinococcus of the spleen.

I do not think it necessary to retain the division into primary and secondary tumors of the spleen. Among the primary are generally reckoned the leucæmic tumors, as well as the cases of pure hypertrophy, very similar to them morphologically, but without the condition of the blood occurring in leucæmia (pseudo-leucæmia). Neither of them, however, is exclusively of spontaneous origin, but often arises secondarily, after disease of the lymphatic glands, or usually in consequence of acute or chronic infectious diseases, such as the syphilitic spleen, amyloid degeneration, tuberculosis and cancer.

Hypertrophy of the Spleen (Pseudo-leucæmia).

Hypertrophy or hyperplasia of the spleen is diffuse or circumscribed; the latter has been carefully described by Friedreich in Virchow's Archiv, Bd. XXIII., 1865, as multiple, nodular hyperplasia of the spleen and liver.

The spleen was enlarged, its capsule thickened and opaque; embedded in the soft brownish red pulp, innumerable little points of granulations from the minutest size, to that of a pea, which were clear, grayish red, firm and projected above the surface. The splenic tumors proved to be granular and nodular hyperplasias of splenic pulp. They consisted of small delicate elements, identical with the cells of the splenic parenchyma, which were filled with large nuclei, often in process of division, and sometimes single fat-granules or fat-molecules. In the nuclei were usually to be found two or three vesicular nucleoli—some of the cells were very large, resembling the liver cells, in their dull yellowish-gray appearance, their sharp angular contours, and large nuclei. Here also were to be found transitions from the smallest to the largest cells. The nodules were grouped to form larger tumors, and were not seldom surrounded by a collateral circle of vessels; growths precisely similar were found in the liver.

According to Friedreich, the occurrence of innumerable hyperplastic nodules in the spleen is very rare, since only Rokitansky and Griesinger have found single encapsuled tumors, the structure of which agreed almost exactly with that of the spleen. These tumors appeared to have developed in a latent manner without known cause.

The diffuse hypertrophy of the spleen consists either in excessive multiplication of the splenic cells or in increase of the trabecular tissue (reticulum). The organ retains its usual form; the capsule is usually somewhat thickened, opaque, its consistence sometimes normal, sometimes more dense; upon section the organ sometimes retains its normal appearance; sometimes appears more brown or grayish red; the greater the degree of hypertrophy, the less usually is its fulness of blood. In the hypertrophy produced by obstacles to the circulation, a greater degree of hyperæmia is found—the color is blue or dark red; upon section the surface is full of blood, and the venous sinuses appear dilated. The hypertrophy is then connected with a copious deposit of pigment in the form of brown or black granules, which are generally enclosed in cells.

Pure hypertrophy occurs especially after long-continued intermittent, or even simply from the action of marsh miasma, without actual febrile attacks having occurred. It is found also after obstructions in the circulation; in uncompensated mitral insufficiency, a not inconsiderable enlargement of the spleen usually occurs, while in insufficiency of the aortic valves the size of the spleen is nearly normal (Birch-Hirschfeld). In interstitial hepatitis, Frerichs saw in thirty-six cases enlargement of the spleen eighteen times, Birch-Hirschfeld in twenty cases fourteen times. I have seen congestive tumors of the spleen in more than half of my cases, frequently even in the early stages. I have occasionally seen something similar in chronic disease of the stomach. I can easily understand this, since during vivisections I have seen the spleen swell very rapidly to a considerable degree, after slight pressure on the splenic vein.

In the cases mentioned the degree of hypertrophy is usually moderate. It is most developed in those cases which stand nearest to the leucæmic tumors in their appearances, and are only separated from them by the absence of the characteristic condition of the blood, and have therefore given occasion for establishing a pseudo-leucæmia. English, French, and German authors have described this form of disease under various names : Hodgkin's[1] disease (Wilks), Anæmia lymphatica (Wilks[2]), Cachexie sans leucémie (Bonfils[3]), Adénie (Trousseau), Pseudo-leucæmia (Cohnheim, Wunderlich), Anæmia splenica (Griesinger), Malignant lymphosarcoma (Langhans).

Hodgkin first pointed out the simultaneous occurrence of certain changes of the spleen, and all, or nearly all, the lymphatic glands. In the year 1856 Wilks directed attention to the same condition.

After him, Bonfils described a clear and accurately observed case of " Hypertrophie ganglionaire générale, cachexie sans leucémie," with a report of an autopsy. He gave a clear sketch of the disease in question. In the year 1859 he was followed by Pavy,[4] with a further description of anæmia lymphatica. After him, Cossy[5] published three further cases of " Hypertrophie simple plus ou moins généralisée des ganglions lymphatiques sans leucémie." In a work which appeared in 1865 Cornil[6] gave a collection of the previously observed cases, with the addition of

---

[1] On Some Morbid Appearances of the Absorbent Glands and Spleen. Med. Chir. Trans. XVII. 68. 1832.

[2] Guy's Hospital Reports. 3d Series. Vol. II. 1856.

[3] Receuil d. travaux de la Soc. méd. d'observ. I. 157. 1857–1858.

[4] The Lancet. Aug. 1859. p. 213.

[5] Echo Médicale. t. V. Neuchâtel. 1858.

[6] Arch. génér. des Méd. Août, 1865.

two new ones, observed and examined post-mortem by Dr. Hé-rard and Leudet, which is of great interest, particularly in regard to the pathological anatomy of pseudo-leucæmia. In the same year Trousseau, who had at his command four additional cases, undertook, on the slender basis of twelve observations, to clear up accurately and thoroughly the nature of the new disease, to which he gave the name of Adenia, and devoted to it a special chapter in his Clinique Medicale.

The knowledge of pseudo-leucæmia has been very materially advanced by the cases published in Germany. After Cohnheim[1] and Gressel[2] had published single cases, Wunderlich,[3] while add-ing three further observations, gave the first thorough discussion of pseudo-leucæmia in German journalism. Since then seven new cases from Niemeyer's clinic, of which two underwent post-mortem examinations, were reported by Mueller.[4] Quite lately a very interesting case of pseudo-leucæmia, which had a striking similarity to leucæmia, has been communicated by Ollivier and Ranvier.[5] I[6] have myself published a highly typical case, and three other cases from my clinic were communicated by Dr. Hommelsheim in his dissertation.

The pathological anatomy of this highly important affection, which ought to interest physicians much more generally than heretofore, has been most excellently treated by Langhans in the fifty-fourth volume of Virchow's Arch., p. 509; he has there drawn the distinction that the malignant, metastatic lymphosarcoma (maligne metastasirende Lymphosarkom, Pseudoleukæmie) occurs in two forms, a soft and a hard. The first of these is distin-guished from leucæmia only by the condition of the blood ; but the second also by the very hard, sometimes almost cartilaginous, consistence of the lymph-glands and follicles.

In other respects the organs are found as in leucæmia, so that the description of their anatomical condition may be omitted in this place.

---

[1] Virch. Arch. 1865. XXIII.
[2] Berl. klin. Wochenschrift. 1866. No. 20.
[3] Arch. der Heilkunde. 1866. 6.
[4] Berl. klin. Wochenschrift. 1867. Nos. 42, 43, 44.
[5] Gaz. méd. 1868. No. 27.
[6] Pathol. u. Therapie der Leucæmia. S. 188.

Etiology.

The male sex is affected by pseudo-leucæmia in the much larger proportion. The cases of this affection are pretty uniformly distributed among the various classes and occupations; the ages vary from one to sixty-nine years; most cases occur in the middle period of life; the beginning of the disease is usually obscure; the persons affected have usually had no special sickness, and have been in fact always healthy, many of them even of a strikingly blooming and powerful appearance. In some cases Trousseau mentions inflammatory affections in the neighborhood of the lymphatic glands first attacked, otorrhœa, dacryocystitis, coryza chronica. In one patient clearly marked scrofulous affections had previously existed, one suffered from syphilis, two made habitual use of alcohol.

Symptomatology.

The phenomena involve not only the spleen, but also the lymphatic glands. The morbid relationship of each to the other is as various in pseudo-leucæmia as we shall see it in leucæmia. Trousseau observed in all his cases enlargement (primary) of the lymphatic glands; in eight of his twelve cases they were alone affected, *without* simultaneous hypertrophy of the spleen. The inverse was true of the patients of Niemeyer; three cases, of which two after a long duration of the disease were examined post-mortem, ran their course without hypertrophy of the lymphatic glands.

But in those patients of Niemeyer's, in which the spleen as well as the glands were diseased, the enlargement of the spleen was in excess compared to the degree and extent of the glandular hypertrophy.

In pseudo-leucæmia, as in leucæmia, a splenic and lymphatic form can be separated. The most frequent condition is a combination of both. According to Neumann, in pseudo-leucæmia the disease of the bony marrow is wanting, but Wood has lately found in it the same changes as in leucæmia.

The disease is developed in the same way as in leucæmia. After one or several lymphatic glands have increased in size, new glands gradually and constantly become affected, and the disease is generalized by slowly progressive development. Sometimes a larger number of glands is involved from the beginning, and the hypertrophy advances rapidly to a high degree. Marked hypertrophy of the spleen seems never to have been developed in so short a time as has been many times observed in the lymphatic glands. Pains of a severe character are not continuously present, either in the spleen or in the lymphatic glands, but an unpleasant feeling of pressure and fulness in the left hypochondrium has been often noticed. In a number of cases the commencement of the swelling was accompanied by febrile symptoms.

Besides the palpable changes of the spleen and lymphatic glands, a grave disturbance of the general condition, a peculiar cachexia splenica et lymphatica shows itself as a constant symptom. Usually the general weakness is very prominent; gradually increases to complete physical incapacity, and the functions in general decrease in intensity or cease; death has frequently taken place by exhaustion after the disease has lasted from four to twenty months, without any special local symptoms having been observed, with the exception of slight dropsical swellings and not very marked emaciation. The duration of the disease, up to the development of a well-marked cachexia, was in most cases so various that a systematic division into stages cannot well be made.

The cachexia can be present during the development of the hypertrophic enlargement, or even precede it. Most patients suffer from difficulty of respiration; the shortness of breath probably depending in part on the changed condition of the blood, but sometimes on a compression of the trachea and the bronchi by the swollen lymphatic glands of the neck and thorax. Nervous dyspnœa has been observed from pressure on the vagus; symptoms of obstruction are frequently developed in the form of œdema of the lower extremities and abdomen; in consequence of their defective nutrition, the vessels show great inclination to rupture. Among eighteen cases, petechiæ occurred four

times; once frequent and abundant bleeding, and once each
bleeding from the gums, and circumscribed hemorrhages in the
intestinal walls. One patient died from œdema of the brain,
probably from a cerebral hemorrhage. One patient observed by
me showed for a long time symptoms of melæna. The digestive
organs, as a rule, were not materially disturbed, and the same is
true of the renal function.

Prognosis.

Trousseau believes that the patients, if they are not carried
off before by local troubles, inevitably perish from exhaustion in
from eighteen to twenty-four months. The cases communicated
by Mueller, as well as those observed by me, showed a less rapid
progress of the disease. Wunderlich reports one case, which
was, to be sure, in the early stages of development, which ended
with complete recovery and return of the glands to their normal
condition. I have also observed a distinct improvement in
splenic pseudo-leucæmia.

In most cases death took place with the appearances of general exhaustion, without previous local symptoms; twice in consequence of compression of the air-passages by swollen lymphatic
glands. Death, in the other fatal cases, seems to have been produced by intercurrent diseases. Prognosis, in pseudo-leucæmia,
is to be considered, in general, unfavorable.

Therapeutics.

The measures mentioned on a previous page are to be put
in force from the very beginning of the disease. In one case of
pseudo-leucæmia lienalis I have produced considerable diminution of the splenic tumor by large doses of quinia. The preparations of iron are to be recommended as a subsequent treatment. The iron bog baths deserve especial confidence.

Lardaceous Spleen.—Amyloid Degeneration of the Spleen.

Rokitansky, Lehrbuch. III. Bd. 3. Aufl. S. 305. 1861.—*Virchow*, Archiv für pathologische Anatomie. Bd. VI. u. VIII.—*Meckel*, Annalen des Charité-Krankenhauses. 1853.—*Friedreich*, Archiv für pathol. Anatomie. Bd. XIII.—*Pagenstecher*, Ueber die amyloid. Degeneration. 1858.—*Traube*, Medizin. Centralztg. 14. Aug. 1858. Deutsche Klinik. 1859.—*Kekulé*, Ueber die chemische Constitution der Amyloid-Substanz. Verhandlung des naturhistor. medic. Vereins zu Heidelberg. 1858. S. 144.—*C. Schmidt*, Ueber die chemische Constitution des thierischen Amyloid. Annal. der Chem. und Pharm. LX. S. 250. 1859.—*E. Wagner*, Beiträge zur Speckkrankheit. Archiv der Heilkunde. 1861.—*Grainger-Stewart*, "On the Waxy or Amyloid Form of Bright's Disease." Edinburg Med. Journal. 1864.—*Kuehne* und *Rudneff*, Ueber die chemische Natur des Amyloid. Virchow's Archiv. Bd. XXXIII. Heft 1.—*E. Kyber*, Studien über die amyloid. Degeneration. Inaug.-Dissert. Dorpat, 1872. 154. S. 77.—*Cohnheim*, Virchow's Archiv. Bd. LV. S. 271. 1871.—*A. Fehr*, Ueber die Amyloid-Degeneration. Bern, 1867.—*Steiner* und *Neureuter*, Prager Vierteljahrschrift. 91. S. 115. 1866.—*Grainger-Stewart*, Brit. Rev. XLI. p. 201. Jan. 1868.

Anatomical and Chemical Characters.

Statements may be found in the older literature (Bonetus, Malpighi[1]) which favor the supposition that this alteration in the organs had not entirely escaped the observation of the early inquirers. But it was reserved for the present century to attain scientific data for understanding them. The progress of inquiry in this direction is closely connected with the names of Rokitansky and Virchow. While the former, under the idea of lardaceous degeneration, brought together the most of the conditions appertaining thereto, the latter, by the discovery of the characteristic reaction, gained a firm basis for the investigation. A certain confusion still exists in the nomenclature. The designation amyloid degeneration should, for the present, be retained, although the investigations of Kekulé and Carl Schmidt have proved that the substance obtained from lardaceous spleens is, in its chemical behavior, not a non-nitrogenous hydrocarbon, akin to cellulose, but a nitrogenous albuminate. The analyses of Kuehne and

---

[1] The historical material has been carefully collected by *Frerichs*, Klinik der Leberkrankheit. II. S. 165.

Rudneff have further shown that this substance, obtained as pure as possible, dried at 120°, gave, after incineration, 0.79 per cent. of ash, and contained 15.53 per cent. nitrogen, 1.3 sulphur. In its further behavior, also, the same authors found this sub-stance characterized as an albuminoid body.

According to Rokitansky, the characters of amyloid degeneration are as follows : enlargement of the spleen, with rounding off of its borders ; smooth, tense capsule ; tough, doughy consistence ; homogeneous surface on section, interrupted only by the trabeculæ ; with a lustre like bacon ; and translucent nodules, with a color varying from dark to light red.

In the beginning of the disease the degeneration sometimes occurs in the form of a granulation like swollen sago, projecting upon section—the so-called sago-spleen (Virchow). It often undoubtedly depends upon a degeneration originally affecting the Malpighian vessels. In the progress of the disease, this granulation disappears, and is changed into the homogeneous affection above described (Rokitansky).

"In the diffuse degeneration, the true lardaceous or waxy spleen, the organ often appears materially enlarged;[1] feels unusually hard and firm ; the color is, for the most part, dark brownish red, but sometimes paler, even of a light brownish yellow. The surface is anæmic, with a strong waxy or lardaceous lustre—smooth, may be easily cut with a knife, but not scraped down, as in the normal spleen, to a bloody mush. Microscopic examination shows the trabeculæ of the true splenic tissue thickened and uniformly permeated by a homogeneous, shining, bacony mass, in which the cells themselves are lost. The bacony mass is most largely deposited around the cavity of the venous sinuses, and forms around them thick, shining rings. Lardaceous degeneration can also be noticed in the middle coat of the larger and smaller arteries ; the Malpighian bodies generally also show degeneration.

"In the degeneration occurring in the form of small local deposits—the so-called sago-spleen—the size of the spleen is also, for the most part, enlarged, the consistence increased. In the reddish brown parenchyma may be seen a large number of gray, soft granules, from the size of a millet- to that of a hemp-seed, projecting upon the surface like boiled sago granules. The larger they are, the nearer they

[1] Birch-Hirschfeld found in 41 cases of amyloid degeneration of the spleen, with an average age of 41 years, and weight of 48.4 kilogrammes, the average weight of the spleen = 348.0 grammes (0.7 per cent. of the body-weight). The dimensions = 15 : 9 :: 4½ ctms. He found the normal weight equal 150 gr. (0.26), and the dimensions, 13 : 8 : 3 ctms.

are to each other, so that they are sometimes separated only by small isthmuses. On the cut surface of a hardened sago-spleen may be seen, besides these roundish bodies, long, cylindrical, and branched deposits of degeneration, in the middle of which the transverse or longitudinal section of an artery may be perceived. Microscopic examination shows that in this form the degeneration is limited especially to the immediate neighborhood of the arteries and the Malpighian bodies.

"In the most marked degree of the degeneration, the deposits are so large that they almost touch; in other cases each deposit is still surrounded with a zone of normal tissue. In the middle of the degenerated focus no more normal tissue is to be seen, but only a multitude of shining flakes and lumps, thickly crowded together, and among them twisted and winding bodies, which represent degenerated small arteries. In the periphery of the deposits the degeneration of the splenic tissue is to be seen in the same form as when it is diffuse—only in a much higher degree. In the Malpighian bodies the lardaceous degeneration appears to affect partly the colorless cells, partly the vascular network, while the reticulum and its nuclei seem to resist the longest. In the splenic tissue the cells and the reticulum, even to the nuclei, pass into degeneration. Virchow saw also the trabeculæ thickened" (Foerster [1]).

It is generally known that the terminal branches of the blood-vessels are the favorite seat of the degeneration.

Kyber was the first to show that the principal trunks and the large branches of the arteries and veins were also frequently affected. The aorta and pulmonary artery degenerate most decidedly and earliest in the portions situated nearest the heart. In their outward appearance they are not perceptibly changed. Solution of iodine on the yellow ground color of the inner coat brings out reddish points. Sulphuric acid there produces a thick, blackish punctuation on a yellow ground. Of the branches, those arising from a branch of the aorta first become amyloid. Beyond the axillary artery and the common carotid, the degeneration never occurs; below, it can still be found in the common iliac arteries—never in the femoral and popliteal. Thus, a considerable part of the vascular system remains free, until the degeneration again begins in the smaller branches.

In the smaller arteries the muscular coat is the special seat of degeneration. In many places, especially in the spleen, the intima is almost as often the seat of the disease; the capillaries are often affected; on the other hand, a direct continuation of the degeneration to the veins is rare.

[1] Handbuch der speciellen pathol. Anatomie.

For the slighter degrees of degeneration the gross examination often leaves us at fault. The reaction, stated by Virchow, alone gives a sure criterion.

E. Kyber has lately called attention to a series of circumstances which are important for the success of the reaction. In the macroscopic examination one must not, as is usual, be content with the iodine reaction ; after the section to be examined has been washed, it is treated with a solution of iodine 0.6, iodide of potassium 1.2 to 120.0 water, until it becomes of a clear yellow ground color, on which the amyloid portions stand out red or reddish brown. The addition of dilute sulphuric acid (1 : 10-20 aq.) then gives to the latter a dark violet color, while the non-amyloid portions remain light yellow.

In applying the amyloid reaction under the microscope, the employment of concentrated reagents is particularly to be avoided. Kyber recommends the aqueous solution of iodine. The section to be examined is thoroughly treated with it by being shaken to and fro. In the slighter degrees of the degeneration the iodine solution must be renewed from four to six times. The color of the amyloid substance ranges from reddish yellow to violet. The object thus treated with iodine is then covered with the thin glass, the fiftieth part of a drop of concentrated sulphuric acid is placed upon the object-glass, diluted with a drop of distilled water, and is then led up to the edge of the covering glass. Since in this method of procedure the reaction takes place very slowly on slightly degenerated organs, repeated examination is necessary ; hence, in order to preserve the preparation from drying, the addition of glycerine for preservation in a moist atmosphere is to be recommended. Like nitric and chlorhydric acids, chloride of zinc and chloride of barium, according to Kyber, concentrated tartaric acid also is capable of replacing the sulphuric acid.

As to the nature of the amyloid degeneration, Fehr favors the theory of a purely local degeneration of the small vessels. The only support of this view is the fact that the demonstration of amyloid substance in the blood is wanting. The facts which speak in favor of infiltration ; viz., the origin from elements, histologically so different from each other, the commencement at those points at which secretion goes on—the capillaries and small arteries,—the progress from the inner to the middle coat of the arteries, remain unnoticed. Kyber also favors the view that the amyloid substance is a product arising in loco by metamorphosis of the tissues, so that a general swelling of the constituents of the tissue takes place instead of a deposition of granular masses, as in other metamorphoses. According to Kyber, the amyloid organs, contrary to what is seen in other metamorphoses, show an increase of size; from which he draws the conclusion that in amyloid degeneration some substance comes to the tissues from the blood or the nutritive fluid, this view being supported, in his opinion, by the fact that the degeneration in question occurs only where the passages for the blood are more or less open. By this concession Kyber's opposition to the view of those who speak of an amyloid infiltration, like Frerichs, Billroth, Rindfleisch, and others, is materially weakened. Although we have as yet vainly sought in the blood of persons whose organs have undergone the amyloid degeneration to the most marked degree, for any albuminous body of similar reaction, we must, on the ground of the arguments brought forward by the authors mentioned, still retain the view of amyloid degeneration sustained by Virchow. How can we otherwise explain the perfectly uniform nature of its occurrence in such different histological points, and the progress of the degeneration in the various organs?

Etiology.

The knowledge of the causative influences has a special interest in the diagnosis of this form of chronic tumors of the spleen. Age and sex have some influence; middle life is especially disposed thereto. These conditions are in close connection with the diseases to which amyloid degeneration owes its origin. To these causative pathological processes belong, first of all, the diseases of the bones, connected with tedious suppuration; caries, necrosis in the articular extremities of the vertebral column; affections of the bones of traumatic origin may have the same effect.

As to the time within which amyloid degeneration begins, we owe some recent interesting facts to Cohnheim.

At the autopsy of a soldier, wounded on the 16th of Aug., 1870, by a shot in the thigh, who died on the 28th Jan., 1871, a sanious cavity was found in the affected limb, which communicated with the hip- and knee-joints; the spleen had undergone amyloid degeneration. An amyloid spleen was also found at the autopsy of a soldier who had received a complicated fracture of the right leg, from being run over on the 18th of August, 1870, and died on the 21st of December, 1870.

Since neither the histories nor the autopsies disclosed facts which could refer the degeneration to any other cause than to the suppuration occurring in consequence of the wound, it appears that in these cases a degeneration took place in the course of some months, a length of time which, compared with the usual idea of the chronic development of amyloid degeneration, appears very short.

Dickinson endeavored to show that the amyloid infiltration depended upon impregnation with fibrine deprived of alkali, and that tuberculosis and other cachexiæ were not to be looked upon as causal influences, but that a close relation existed only between suppuration and amyloid degeneration, which was to be referred to the loss of the blood in albumen and alkalies produced by the suppuration.

A series of observations by myself, as well as others, has taught me that the amyloid degeneration not unfrequently accompanies many other constitutional affections, in which one can unqualifiedly assume as a basis a discrasic condition of the blood. In the collection of 152 cases, given by Fehr, among the causative pathological processes, constitutional syphilis (34) stands at the head. Next come chronic affections of the lungs. According to my experience in Greifswald, chronic bronchitis and bronchiectasis are followed by amyloid degeneration just as frequently as phthisis and tuberculosis of the lungs.

In the dissertation of Dr. Taesler is given the history of a patient in my clinic, twenty-nine years old, who, in the course of twelve years, had recovered fourteen times from croupous pneumonia, and died from another attack of this disease in March, 1865. At the autopsy there were found, besides the pneumonic infiltration of the lungs, a very remarkable amyloid spleen, as well as amyloid degeneration of the liver and of the vessels of the intestinal mucous membrane. None of the thus far recognized primary diseases, except the frequently recurring pneumonia, could be discovered as a causative influence for this amyloid degeneration.

Among the causes are still to be mentioned scrofulosis, intermittent, alcoholism, atonic ulcers of the feet. There are many forms of chronic inflammations which are connected with the deposit of amyloid substance. Among them belong, besides the chronic inflammation of the lungs, mentioned above, chronic nephritis and peritonitis, as well as cirrhosis of the liver.

In consequence of chronic intestinal catarrh in children, the spleen is usually somewhat enlarged, somewhat hard or tough like muscle, more rarely flabby; the color pale brownish violet, sometimes dark red, brown and marble; the pulp scanty; the stroma predominant. The so-called sago spleen is observed with unusual frequency. This degeneration may be the reason why, after almost complete disappearance of the symptom of chronic intestinal catarrh, in many non-rhachitic children, a general anæmia, which cannot be removed, remains behind, so that the children continue to atrophy, and finally die with secondary hydrocephalus (Steiner).

Symptoms.

Since the amyloid degeneration usually extends to several organs which are important in the preparation of the blood and in nutrition—spleen, liver, lymphatic glands, mucous membrane of the stomach and intestinal canal, a pale cachectic appearance in patients with well-marked amyloid spleen is scarcely ever wanting. Symptoms of anæmia and hydræmia are the more clearly marked, since the primary disease is generally of a severely debilitating character. The type of the disease varies according to the variety of the primary affection, and according to the direction and extent of the amyloid degeneration.

The physical signs of chronic tumors of the spleen have been already stated several times. With the amyloid spleen enormous enlargement may often be determined. In a boy of thirteen years, in my clinic, I observed, some years ago, a tumor of the spleen, arising from hereditary syphilis, which filled almost the whole abdominal cavity, had a firm consistence, perfectly smooth surface, and rounded edges.

Abnormal sensations exist in the region of the spleen only so far as the feeling of fulness is disagreeable to the patient. More acute pains occur rarely in consequence of perisplenitis. A more frequent accompaniment of amyloid degeneration of the spleen is an enlargement of the liver of the same kind, which often reaches considerable size. The two tumors usually touch.

After the etiology, the simultaneous enlargement of the

spleen and liver, together with the condition of the urine, is of special importance in the diagnosis.

In 129 cases, collected by Fehr, the liver, spleen, and kidneys were degenerated in 63 ; spleen and kidneys in 29 ; liver and kidneys in 8 : the kidneys in 25 ; the spleen in 3 ; the liver in 1.

The functions of the stomach and intestinal canal are disturbed in several ways; the appetite is lost, and vomiting takes place. Without special cause, loose discharges of pale color and mucous consistency also occur, and last for weeks. The autopsy then shows amyloid degeneration in the walls of the smaller arterial vessels, in the mucous membrane of the stomach and intestines. The intestinal villi may be made to stand out very clearly by Virchow's reaction. Considerable losses of substance may frequently be found in the mucous membrane.

Grainger Stewart describes among the symptoms the inclination to hemorrhage present in many cases of amyloid degeneration, in consequence of the fragility of the vessels. He found repeatedly extravasations in the spleen, as well as hemorrhage of the stomach and intestines. In a syphilitic girl, twenty-six years old, where the autopsy showed extensive amyloid degeneration, death took place with violent hematemesis and profuse intestinal hemorrhage.

Prognosis.

Prognosis is usually unfavorable, especially if the process has lasted long and extended far. Once begun, the degenerative process of the spleen usually continues till death. Recovery takes place seldom, and when the degeneration is far advanced it is questionable whether the degenerative tissues ever become again capable of discharging their functions. It has been determined that more recent infiltrations may, under certain circumstances, retrograde. Especially surgical procedures upon suppurating surfaces have sometimes had an astonishing result in the resolution of amyloid tumors.

Therapeutics.

The treatment of the amyloid spleen is not essentially different from that of the other tumors of this organ. It is highly important that special attention should be given to the cause.

Syphilitic Tumors of the Spleen.

Virchow, Ueber die Natur der interstitiellen syphilitischen Affectionen. Virchow's Archiv. XV.—*E. Wagner*, Das Syphilom der Milz. Archiv der Heilkunde. IV. S. 430.—*Biermer*, Schweizerische Zeitschrift der Heilkunde. I. 1862.—*Pleischl* and *Klob*, Beitrag zur Pathologie der interstitiellen Syphilis. Wiener mediz. Wochenschrift. 1860. Nr. 8, 9, 10.—*Frerichs*, Klinik der Leberkrankheiten. II. Bd.—*Weil*, Ueber das Vorkommen des Milztumors bei frischer Syphilis. Deutsches Archiv für klinische Medicin. XIII. 3.—*Mosler*, Syphilis und Leukämie. Berl. klin. Wochenschrift. 1864. S. 15.—*Hecker*, Syphilis congenita. Monatsschrift für Geburtskunde. XXXIII. 1869.—*S. Gee*, Brit. Med. Journal. 1867. p. 435.—*Eisenschitz*, Wien. mediz. Wochenschrift. 1873. 49.

Syphilitic affections of the spleen are of the most various kinds. They are more frequently the object of anatomical inquiry than of clinical observation. They occur, besides the forms of amyloid degeneration just mentioned, in which the syphilitic cachexia is often well marked, in the nodular and diffuse forms. The syphilitic nodules, generally called gummata, which are on the whole rare, have been accurately described by E. Wagner. The spleen is usually enlarged. The number of the tumors designated by this observer as syphilomas is various, and generally inversely proportioned to their size. They are always sharply circumscribed, generally round or roundish, seldom irregular, sometimes very small, most frequently one-half to one line, rarely one to one and a half inches, in diameter. Recent syphilomas are grayish red, homogeneous, generally containing considerable blood. The older forms, much more frequently observed, are gray or grayish yellow, homogeneous, somewhat dry, tough, almost cheesy. The surrounding splenic tissue is somewhat compressed, the remainder usually somewhat harder.

In the diffuse syphilitic disease Virchow has distinguished

two forms of hyperplastic tumor of the spleen ; one soft and
flabby, the other indurated.   The latter may be referred to interstitial inflammation of the spleen ; the soft form, on the other
hand, arises from the increase of the cellular contents, especially
of the pulp, and hence probably corresponds to a slighter degree
of irritation.

Some of the changes described may be diagnosticated during
life, or at least suspected with more or less probability.   Cases
have been observed in which splenic tumors have been found
together with syphilitic hepatitis.   In two patients in my clinic
syphilis of the liver was so clearly pronounced, that the splenic
tumor also could be confidently stated as of specific origin.
Sometimes the splenic tumor is more likely to confuse the diagnosis of syphilis, that is, when ascites, existing at the same time,
leads one to think first of the ordinary cirrhosis of the liver.
Oppolzer, Frerichs, and Lancereaux consider the splenic tumor
as a usual accompaniment of syphilis of the liver.   Aside from
the cases in which the splenic tumor can be demonstrated, together with syphilitic hepatitis, sometimes an enlargement of the
spleen, occurring in the course of constitutional syphilis, may be
correctly designated as amyloid spleen, or as simple hyperplasia
of the organ, according to the presence or absence of amyloid
degeneration of the liver, the kidneys, and the intestines.   My
observation of syphilis and lieno-lymphatic leucæmia, to which
I shall again refer when considering the latter disease, is very
remarkable.

The diseases of the spleen which usually accompany hereditary syphilis have been often described.   They are subject to
the same anatomical classification as the analogous affections in
acquired syphilis, and may also be considered clinically from a
similar point of view.

In seventeen children who were born with syphilis, living and active, except in
one case dead and decomposed, Hecker found the spleen in five cases diseased,
considerably enlarged, of a waxy lustre, without localized affections. The skin
was diseased in seventeen cases, the lungs in fourteen, the thymus in eight, the
supra-renal capsules in eight, the liver in seven, the brain in four, the peritoneum
in three, the pancreas in one.

S. Gee has also found enlargement of the spleen in about one-fourth of all the cases of hereditary syphilis. He considers the degree of enlargement as a measure of the syphilitic cachexia. Very lately Eisenschitz has attached special weight to the enlargement of the spleen as a symptom of latent hereditary syphilis. According to this author, this condition may very frequently be demonstrated even before the first eruption has taken place, and also exists during the latent stage between the different eruptions. For discovering the enlargement of the spleen in suckling children Eisenschitz specially recommends palpation, since the syphilitic tumor is a chronic one, and on account of its greater weight usually takes a low position.

Hereditary syphilis leads much earlier than acquired to disease of the internal organs, which then attains a considerable degree. Except in leucæmia, I have never seen so far advanced a splenic tumor as in the thirteen-year-old boy mentioned above, in whom hereditary syphilis was known to be present.

The splenic tumor of acquired syphilis is generally observed at a period far distant from the infection, at which other symptoms of the syphilitic cachexia are generally present at the same time. In opposition to all previous observations, so far as known, Weil was able to determine the presence of a considerable enlargement of the spleen, even during the existence of the primary induration. He considers the enlargement of the spleen as produced by an irritation of its tissue by substances circulating in the blood of syphilitic patients, so that I have already treated of the splenic tumors occurring in recent syphilis among the acute tumors. It will be the task of pathological anatomy to fix positively the nature of this recent splenic tumor.

In a practical point of view, Weil considers the knowledge of the early occurrence of syphilitic tumors of the spleen not without importance for the discrimination of lesions upon the genital organs; for the sake of the early diagnosis of syphilis, such a splenic tumor might be of value for prognosis and therapeutics. Before the spleen has attained its normal size, no syphilitic patient can be considered cured. Recent tumors of the spleen are possibly still susceptible of recovery, while in the chronic, therapeutics has done little.

Tuberculosis of the Spleen.

Andral, Anat. Pathol. II. 92.—*Barthez* and *Rilliet*, Mal. des enf. III. 467.—*Roki-tansky*, Lehrbuch. III. S. 304.—*Heinrich*, l. c. p. 394.—*Foerster*, Pathol. Ana-tom. S. 826.

The tubercles occur in the form of numerous granulations—translucent, sometimes whitish and opaque, small, very often scarcely as large as a poppy-seed—with which, in some cases, especially of acute tuberculosis, the spleen is very thickly sprinkled, but which may also appear very isolated. The spleen is swollen, and when the granulations are numerous is denser than normal. Billroth found the seat and starting-point of the miliary tubercles in the true splenic tissue—very seldom in the Malpighian corpuscles.

In chronic tuberculosis they form gray, or very often yellow, cheesy, roundish nodules, from the size of a millet-seed to that of a pea—an alteration which is frequently met with in scrofulous persons, and even named scrofulous spleen. The number of nodules varies from some single scattered ones to a complete crowding of the splenic parenchyma.

Both forms are the expression of a general affection arrived at a high degree of development. They never occur independently of tuberculosis in other organs. As a rule, they kill by the advanced development of the general affection, or by the disease of other organs, before they can reach the stage of metamorphosis ; hence, we seldom observe in the spleen a transition of tubercle into softening, or the formation of cavities.

The diagnosis is very difficult, and generally impossible. The deposit of miliary tubercles in the spleen during acute tuberculosis may be suspected when this organ is painful upon pressure and considerably enlarged. We have, however, mentioned above that in acute tuberculosis acute enlargement of the spleen may take place without a deposition of tubercles in its tissue.

Since chronic tubercle, as a rule, betrays itself by no symptoms whatever, the diagnosis is still more difficult. The size of the spleen is increased only when very numerous masses of tubercle are deposited. As to any efficient therapeutics, nothing can be said.

Carcinoma of the Spleen.

Andral, Clin. méd. T. IV. 1131. p. 441.—*Bright*, Guy's Hosp. Rep. Vol. 3. p. 401. 1836.—*Cruveilhier*, Anat. path. liv. XX.—*Walshe*, On Cancer. p. 312.—*Guensburg*, Path. Gewebslehre. Med. Zeitschrift f. klin. Medicin. IV. 5. 1853.— *Baccelli*, Presse méd. 7. 1858 (Primitiv carcinom).—*Rokitansky*, Lehrbuch. III. 303.—*Foerster*, Handbuch. S. 827.—*Dr. Th. Eiselt*, Prag. Vierteljahrschrift. XIX. 4. 1862. S. 26.

Cancer of the spleen is rare ; it occurs most frequently as a secondary growth with cancer of the liver and of the abdominal lymphatic glands, in the form of scattered or numerous encephaloid nodules, from the size of a pea to that of a hazel-nut—or of single ones, as large as a walnut or the fist.

In pigmentary cancer the spleen is usually only affected at the last, and then grows so rapidly that its size may be doubled in a few days. The pigment nodules are generally very pale, so that they are like medullary cancer. In fifty cases they were present thirteen times (Eiselt).

In some cases cancer of the spleen appears as a diffuse inflammation, propagated from the fundus of the stomach. It is very seldom a primary growth. Guensburg and Baccelli describe such cases. I have myself observed a primary carcinoma of the spleen in my clinic, in a workman forty-five years old. He was at first treated for troubles arising from a very extensive dilatation of the bronchi ; besides this, there existed, without any special cause having been found therefor, a far advanced, very dense tumor of the spleen, on the surface of which, during life, no prominences could be discovered. As the autopsy afterwards showed, icterus and ascites had supervened in consequence of secondary enlargement of the mesenteric glands, especially of the transverse fissure of the liver ; also, rapid failure of the powers of life followed. From increase of the jaundice, death occurred, with cholæmic, comatose symptoms.

The spleen was found to be considerably enlarged in all its dimensions, and showed upon its surface clearly marked, light yellow spots, of the size of a thaler, the nodules being firmer than the substance of the spleen. Upon section, they had a diameter of two or two and one-half inches ; were round, often projecting irregularly into the parenchyma, and of a light yellowish red. In the liver only a few small, scattered nodules were found.

The diagnosis is possible only when the cancer has been demonstrated in other organs, and the uneven and knobby surface of the enlarged spleen can be felt, while the irregular and unusual contours of the organ are found by percussion.

The prognosis is very unfavorable, and the therapeutics purely symptomatic.

Echinococcus of the Spleen.

Heinrich, Krankheiten der Milz. S. 376.—*Davaine*, Traité des entozoaires. p. 486. *Dr. M. Wolff*, Berl. klin. Wochenschrift. VII. 5. 6. 1870.—*Dr. C. Uterhart*, Berl. klin. Wochenschrift. VII. 4. 5. 1869.—*Dr. Wilde*, Deutsch. Archiv für klin. Medicin. VIII. 1. S. 116. 1870.—*Dr. Schroetter*, Wiener medizin. Jahrbüch. XXVI. 2. 3. S. 216. 1870.—*Lebert* u. *Berger*, Berl. klin. Wochenschrift. VIII. 3. 4. 1871.

The echinococcus sac is not frequently observed in the spleen. Among the older writers great obscurity and confusion reign as to the various forms assembled under the names, hydatids, acephalo-cysts. We must separate the formation of serous cysts not inhabited by living beings, which arise from local causes, from the formation of the cysticerci. Heinrich has made a collection of the earlier literature upon the occurrence of cysticerci in the spleen. Most of the cases were accidental discoveries, made upon post-mortem examination; they have no great practical interest.

Echinococcus of the spleen is observed, either alone or together with a similar formation in other organs—partly in the form of isolated cysts, partly in the form of large mother-cysts, with numerous daughter-vesicles, so that the parenchyma of the spleen is almost completely destroyed.

Dr. Saeller describes, in November, 1826, an abscess of the liver opening through the lungs, with seventy-four hydatids in the spleen, in the same individual. In the place of the spleen was found a round, tense body, and, when this was lifted out, upon its lower posterior surface was found the whole spleen shrunken together. The tense, elastic growth was seated at the hilus of the spleen, and weighed 3 lbs.

and 2 oz. The sac contained seventy-four larger and smaller hydatids, of from half an inch to an inch in diameter.

The causes of the occurrence of echinococci in man have been cleared up by more recent investigations. It is now known why this disease is more frequently observed in many countries. According to the statement of H. Krabbe, in his "Recherches helminthologiques en Danemark et en Islande," among 70,000 inhabitants of Iceland, at least 1,500 carry around with them an echinococcus tumor. According to other reports, one-seventh of the entire population suffers from echinococci. This enormous frequency of hydatid growths is referred to the very great number of dogs, and the intimate relations with them on the part of the inhabitants, who often shelter in their huts, during the winter, nine or ten dogs. G. Simon has called attention to the frequent occurrence of echinococci in Mecklenburg; there, however, dogs are no more frequently kept in the house than in South Germany, where echinococcus growths of recognizable dimensions are seldom observed; it is probable that in Mecklenburg a greater percentage of dogs are affected with echinococcus tapeworms, as has been shown to be the case with the dogs of Iceland in comparison with those in Copenhagen (Wolff). In Greifswald I have very frequently found this tænia, upon examining dogs, in so great numbers that the surface of the intestinal mucous membrane was almost completely covered with them, while in Giessen this state of things did not exist. Here I have seen echinococcus tumors of the liver four times in ten years, but during the same time in Giessen not at all. Even here, however, I have not yet observed their presence in the spleen. Why this organ is so seldom attacked, I am unable to explain.

The symptoms of echinococcus in the spleen are exceedingly variable. They are often to be recognized only from the trouble caused by their bulk; at other times by an inflammation of the sac. The subjective painful symptoms are very variable; often very severe pains are felt long before the patient has remarked the swelling; then disappear for years, to break out anew with increased intensity. In another series of cases, and, indeed, in the larger number, severe pain is wanting. The only feeling present is that of fulness and weight at the place where the growth has developed, which increases with the increasing tension ; gastric symptoms often occur, which depend upon mechanical compression of the stomach and the intestines. These are : want of appetite, nausea, constipation, sometimes persistent vomiting of portions of the food, or even bloody masses. To these are sometimes added, as signs of the commencing inflammation of the sac : chills, succeeded by fever,[1] sweating, delirium, and emaciation.

In all cases which were diagnosticated during life one tumor was present, of the existence of which the patients usually became aware accidentally, and, as a rule, long after the first symptoms had shown themselves. The tumor is usually visible to a greater or less extent as a single prominence, but sometimes with several conical projections. Its boundaries may be accurately made out by palpation and percussion.

In the case described so clearly and thoroughly by Wolff the examination showed a large abdominal tumor, which had distended the left posterior half of the thorax, had pushed out the last intercostal space upon the left side, and appeared as a palpable projection, immediately below the edge of the ribs, inward from the line of the nipple. The tumor, as limited by percussion dulness, began in the left anterior axillary line, at the upper border of the sixth rib, went obliquely downward nine centimetres to the right epigastrium, where it was distinctly separated from the liver by the clear, tympanitic sound of the fundus of the stomach, which had been pushed forward, then bent to the left and downward, beyond the umbilicus, where its lower limit was three fingers' breadth distant from the anterior spine of the ilium, and two inches from the vertebral column at the level of the eleventh dorsal vertebra. The greatest length of the tumor was forty-seven, the greatest breadth, twenty-five centimetres. At the place where it arched forward decided fluctuation was found over an extent of several inches, but no hydatid thrill. Upon a full inspiration the tumor was thrust far downward.

Upon *palpation*, as a rule, fluctuation may usually be determined, at least in one spot, which, however, does not always correspond to the most prominent part of the tumor. In other portions the tumor has an elastic and often quite resistant character. Hydatid trembling, upon which special weight has often

---

[1] *Cruveilhier* mentions a patient who suffered for eighteen months from a tertian intermittent, returning at intervals, and in whom acephalo-cysts were found in the liver and spleen after death ; he assumes that the febrile symptoms made their appearance as the thrusting out or inflammation of the cysts began.

been laid among the symptoms, is seldom perceived. Finsen, whose observations were based upon 255 cases of various echinococcus tumors, has never observed this symptom. Wolff makes the same statement as to seven cases observed in Rostock. Frerichs also found it wanting in half the echinococcus tumors examined by him. He found it clearly only in those cases where the echinococcus sac enclosed a large number of vesicles, and was not too tensely stretched; where only one cyst was present Frerichs was never able to detect the hydatid thrill. As in other splenic tumors, a peritoneal friction sound is often observed in these cases in the left hypochondrium. For the differential diagnosis of this kind of splenic tumors, important data are found in the continuance of the disease for years; the slow growth of the tumor; in most cases the comparatively slight disturbance of the general health; the favorable conditions of nutrition; and the enduring ability of the patient to labor, notwithstanding the immense tumor. The exploratory puncture affords greater certainty. Wolff remarks that every one who has made a diagnosis of echinococcus experiences a certain feeling of uncertainty if, after puncture, he finds in the evacuated fluid neither scolices, nor hooks, nor pieces of membrane, which justify him in his diagnosis, and if, besides, the fluid contains albumen instead of being free from it, as is expected. The absence of scolices and hooks is not so very rare an occurrence. In twelve cases of echinococcus at the Rostock clinic they were found only twice. According to Wolff, their absence points either to an incomplete development of the echinococcus or to sterile hooks, or to destruction of the scolices or hooks which had been present at an earlier period. In the cases without scolices and hooks, the evacuated fluid was often purulent or albuminous; it appears that the scolices are destroyed by altered or purulent fluid in the cysts. The albumen contained in the echinococcus fluid may be referred to the albuminous serum of the pus, and consequently to suppurating connective tissue, even when only few or no pus-corpuscles can be demonstrated.

As to the *prognosis* and *therapeutics* of echinococci of the spleen, the same may be said as of those of the liver. The double puncture recommended by G. Simon has been twice per-

formed in Rostock : once with a favorable result (Hueter) ; once
with an unfavorable termination from copious hemorrhages of
about 600 grms. from an eroded vessel of the spleen (Koenig).
Dr. Wilde has also obtained a favorable result from the same
operation. On the other hand, Dr. Schroetter, in Vienna, reports
a case of echinococcus of the spleen, in which he obtained a very
favorable result from simple puncture followed by the injection
of iodine.   Lebert and Berger mention the favorable effect of exploratory puncture in echinococcus colonies.

Rupture of the Spleen and its Vessels.

Heinrich, Milzkrankheiten: S. 402.—*Bamberger*, L. c. p. 621.—*Dieffenbach*, Med.
    Zeitung des Vereins für Heilkunde in Preussen. 1833. Nr. 4.—*Herrick*, London
    Med. Gaz. 1845. April.—*Buss*, Med. Times and Gaz. Nr. 7. 1868.—*Simpson*,
    Edlnb. Med. Journ. Sept. 1866.—*Aufrecht*, Virchow's Archiv. XXXVII. 3.
    1866.—*Cohnheim*, Virchow's Archiv. XXXVII. 3. 1866.

Anatomical and physiological peculiarities combine to render
the parenchyma of the spleen more disposed to rupture than
that of other glandular organs.   Its decided richness in blood
during every digestion should be remembered, as well as the very
marked increase in size when it receives the masses of blood
driven from other parts of the body.   It might be supposed that
it would more frequently burst if it had not a fibrous capsule
which appears to be capable of a certain amount of stretching.
A diseased condition and an increase in size of the organ are generally found as a further disposing cause.   The number of cases
in which a perfectly healthy spleen has been ruptured or injured
is small.[1] In regions where intermittent fever is endemic—as in
the East Indies—swelling and softening of the spleen are said to
occur to such a degree that rupture takes place from the slightest exertion, from vomiting, from blows upon the left side, or
even without any external occasion ; thus Playfair reports that
he saw in the East Indies, during two and a half years, twenty
cases of rupture of the spleen, and that in Bengal every third

---

[1] *Dieffenbach*, Med. Zeitung des Vereins für Heilkunde in Preussen. 1833. No. 4.

person has a fever-spleen, which is inclined to softening and rupture. Stadkowsky, in Volhynia, in the course of ten years, had an opportunity to make seven examinations of persons who had died in consequence of injuries to the spleen—the death, in all cases, resulting from hemorrhage. This question is important in the consideration of medico-legal cases.

Herrick [1] states that after a blow of the fist in the left hypochondrium, and a consequent fight, the death of one of the men took place within twenty-five minutes. The examination made twenty-four hours afterwards showed no trace of external violence. On opening the abdominal cavity, it was found to contain two to three quarts of dark, partly coagulated blood. The spleen was some five times as large as usual, and so soft that a slight pressure of the finger was sufficient to crush it, and on its posterior surface was found a fissure, some five inches long, extending deep into its substance. The assailant was indicted for manslaughter, but acquitted, because the spleen was already much diseased. In the case related by Salluce, the prisoner was condemned to death. The spleen of normal character was in two places ruptured in consequence of a violent blow in the lumbar region received in a fight, the man immediately falling dead.

The immediate cause consists, when coming from without, in some sudden mechanical violence. Aside from penetrating, punctured, and gunshot wounds, it may be a concussion of the splenic region or of the whole body, as in violent blows and shocks, a fall, or leap of considerable height. Injuries in the splenic region, may, as Portal remarks, cause a rupture without leaving any visible signs externally. In pathological conditions, the rupture may be either spontaneous or occur from some external cause. The spontaneous ruptures are almost always a consequence of acute swelling rapidly reaching an extreme degree. Rokitansky saw a rupture of the spleen suddenly swollen above its maximum, most frequently in typhus and the cold stage of intermittents.

Buss observed hemorrhage of the spleen in consequence of the hemorrhagic diathesis (hæmophilia) in a man twenty years old, who had had from his early youth great losses of blood succeeding every injury ; and after an abundant bleeding from extraction of a tooth and lasting several days, suddenly experienced, without any outward injury, severe pains in the left iliac region, where a tumor was to be felt ; moderate fever, vomiting, consti-

---

[1] London Medical Gazette. 1845. April.

pation were present. On the sixth day after the beginning of the pains, death took place. At the autopsy a quantity of coagulated blood was found in the abdominal cavity. The spleen, enlarged to twice its normal size, soft, and dark red, lay upon the left internal iliac muscle, and showed only a deep tear in the inner surface, the rest of the organ being anæmic.

Rupture of the spleen was observed in three cases in women, by Simpson, in connection with pregnancy and childbirth. Aufrecht reports a case of miliary tuberculosis of the abdominal organs; scrofulosis of the mesenteric glands, with death from rupture of the spleen in a man forty-two years old, addicted to drink, who occasionally suffered from diarrhœa and dropsy of the lower extremities, but no further symptoms, in whom collapse and death occurred after abundant watery evacuations. The spleen exhibited upon its lower surface a rent two and a half lines long and four inches wide, filled with clots; the portions of the spleen surrounding were thickly sprinkled with whitish miliary granulations, others being more thinly scattered in the remainder of its tissue.

The form of the rupture is either straight, angular, or round. The spleen is torn either in one or in several places, and the separation may extend throughout the whole parenchyma. In Thomson's case the spleen was divided into several pieces. A considerable amount of blood, partly coagulated and partly fluid, is found in the abdominal cavity.

Many cases which have been described as spontaneous rupture of the spleen seem to have been occasioned simply by softening and suppuration of hemorrhagic infarctions. In others, there is a rupture of the splenic artery or vein, with or without dilatation. Cohnheim has lately described a very interesting rupture of varices of the spleen.

A man twenty-seven years old was treated for several months for indefinite symptoms referred to a syphilitic lesion of the brain; for the last three days he had complained of a stitch in the left side. A short time after eating, he fell with a cry of distress, and died in a few moments. The autopsy showed almost a litre of bloody fluid in the peritoneal cavity, and a large quantity of soft, firmly coagulated blood, especially in the left hypochondrium. The spleen was six inches long, five wide, and two thick. The surface was rendered uneven by numerous, roundish, dark blue, soft elevations, in the middle of one of which was a slit three-quarters of an inch long, opening easily, and filled with clot. In the interior were irregular, rounded cavities, from the size of a pea to that of a goose's egg, communicating freely with each other, filled with coagulated blood and thrombi, both recent and old. In a side cavity of the largest of these dilatations was the slit found on the outside. The wall of the cavities was smooth, of a reddish white color, resembling that of the veins; only in certain places the smooth wall could not be continuously followed, and the clots were immediately surrounded by the torn splenic pulp. The parenchyma was tolerably tough, grayish red, with large and numerous follicles. The splenic artery and vein were empty, and, up to their entry into the hilus, normal. Upon one side of a branch of the artery in the hilus was situated an aneurism as large as a pea, which had no connection with the cavities in the interior. The connection of these cavities, on the other hand, with the branches of the splenic vein, could be very clearly made out. Similar, but smaller and more oval, varicose cavities connected with the branches of the portal vein were found through a small space in the right lobe of the liver, close beneath its convex surface. The other organs, which were normal, furnished no basis for an explanation of the dilatation of the veins. Under the microscope, the walls of these showed clearly the structure of normal veins; an epithelium could not be demonstrated.

As to the origin of such varices, my discovery of dilatation of the splenic veins in animals, after cutting the nerves in the hilus, possesses some interest.

Rupture of the splenic artery sometimes happens when this vessel is diseased, or has a tendency to the formation of aneurisms. Parker[1] observed in a man whose health, with the exception of occasional dyspeptic symptoms and pains in the back, had been usually pretty good, sudden death a few hours after a hemorrhagic discharge from the bowels. The post-mortem disclosed as the source of the bleeding an aneurism arising from a branch of the splenic artery, forming a tumor of the size of a small orange, which projected into the stomach and had ruptured therein. Pfeuffer also observed a hemorrhage from the splenic artery communicating with the stomach. I have observed the same thing in ulcers of the stomach.

The symptoms of rupture of the spleen are in general those of the rupture of an internal organ. The patients experience a severe pain, which is most intense in the region of the spleen, but not unfrequently extends over a large part of the abdomen.

---

[1] Edinburgh Journal. 1844. July. p. 132.

Many patients describe their feelings as if something burst inside. The splenic region is exceedingly sensitive to pressure. In a very short time the symptoms of hemorrhage appear, such as paleness, small pulse, cold extremities, fainting, distention of the abdomen, and usually rapid death. According to Vigla, peritonitis is never observed, even when life is prolonged several days after the rupture.

When the previous disease of the spleen is known, or a severe injury in the splenic region has taken place, the diagnosis, according to Bamberger, can be made with great probability from the combination of symptoms mentioned. Rupture of the spleen may be distinguished from ruptures and perforations of the stomach and intestinal canal by the extravasation of air into the abdominal cavity, which can always be demonstrated by the physical signs in the last mentioned accident, and the rapidly following general peritonitis. The peritonitis is never wanting in rupture of the liver, the biliary passages, the kidneys or their pelves, the ureters, or the bladder, and, in addition, symptoms of an affection of the organs mentioned are present, while the seat of the most intense pain does not correspond to the position of the spleen.

Death is the usual result of rupture of the spleen, generally within twenty-four hours. No authentic case of recovery is yet known, although not beyond the limits of possibility. Among seventeen cases which Vigla has collected, death occurred four times suddenly, three times after some hours, and three times before the end of the first day. The longest duration was in one case—six days.

The *therapeutics* must be directed towards checking the bleeding, and combating the symptoms of collapse resulting from hemorrhage with secondary action upon the nervous system; the application of ice-bags in the left hypochondrium is the most important measure. At the same time, several litres of ice-water are to be poured into the colon by means of the intestinal tube and a funnel while the patient lies upon his back, in order to exercise pressure from below upon the spleen. In accordance with previous experience in other hemorrhages, a subcutaneous injection of a solution of extract of ergot might be combined therewith. If the pain is severe, opium in large doses, as recommended by Vigla, is suitable: for internal exhibition, the pill form is to be chosen ; in other cases, the subcutaneous injection of morphia. If the collapse increases, stimulants are to be used internally, such as wine, ether, musk, and camphor, the latter also as a subcutaneous injection in the form of camphorated oil (1 to 5).

The question has been raised whether splenotomy is indicated in rupture of the spleen, especially in malarial districts. A natural recovery from ruptured tumors of the spleen has so far not been observed. The operation, however, on account of the uncertainty of the diagnosis, is usually out of the question.

Leucæmia.

Nasse, Untersuchungen über Physiologie und Pathologie. Bonn, 1835.—*Virchow*, Weisses Blut. Froriep's Notizen. 1845. Nov. N. 780.—The same, Weisses Blut und Milztumoren. Medic. Zeitung. 1846· Nr. 34–36.—*Bennett*, Edinb. Journ. October, 1846.—The same, Edinb. Monthly Journ. 1851. Vol. XII. p. 326.— The same, Leucocythæmia, or White Cell-Blood in Relation to the Physiology and Pathology of the Lymphatic Glandular System. Edinb., 1852.—*Julius Vogel*, Ein Fall von Leukämie mit Vergrösserung von Milz und Leber. Virchow's Archiv. III. S. 570.—*Virchow*, Zur pathologischen Physiologie des Blutes. Die Bedeutung der Milz- und Lymphdrüsenkrankheiten für die Blutmischung (Leukämie). Virchow's Archiv. I. 567. V. S. 58.—Würzburger Verhandlungen. II. S. 325.—*Uhle*, Ein Fall von linealer Leukämie. Virchow's Archiv. 1853. V. S. 376.—*Griesinger*, Zur Leukämie und Pyämie. Virchow's Archiv. V. S. 391.—*de Pury*, Virchow's Archiv. VIII. S. 289.—*Heschl*, Virchow's Archiv. VIII. S. 353.—*Schreiber*, De Leukaemia. Regiom. 1854.—*E. Vidal*, De la leucocythémie splénique, ou de l'hypertrophie de la rate avec altération du sang, consistant dans une augmentation considérable du nombre des globules incolores du sang. Gaz. hebdom. III. 7, 10, 12, 14, 15. 1856.—*B. Schnepf*, Des globules incolores du sang, de leur valeur physiologique et pathologique (Leucocythämie) du sang blanc (Leucaemie). Gaz. méd. de Paris. 14, 15, 16, 20, 21, 22. 1856.—Handbuch der speciellen Pathologie und Therapie von Rudolph Virchow. Störungen der Blutmischung von *J. Vogel*, I. Bd. S. 392.—*R. Walther*, Ueber Leukämie. Schmidt's Jahrbücher. 1858. Vol. 97. S. 203–227.—*Friedreich*, Ein neuer Fall von. Leukämie. Virchow's Archiv. XII. S. 37. 1857.—*Boettcher*, Virchow's Archiv. 1858. XIV. S. 483.—*v. Recklinghausen*, Virchow's Archiv. XXX. S. 375.—*Scherer*, Verhdlgn. d. Würzb. physikal.-medic. Gesellsch. II. 325. 1852 ; VII. 225. 1857.—*Folwarczny*, Allg.

Wiener med. Zeitung. N. 29–31. 1858.—*Mosler* and *Koerner*, **Virchow's** Archiv. XXV. S. 142.—*Salkowsky*, Virchow's Archiv. Bd. L. S. 174.—*Martin Ehrlich*, Ueber Leukämie. Inauguralabhandlung. Dorpat, 1862.—*Mosler*, Klinische Studien über Leukämie. Berl. klin. Wochenschrift. 1864. 2, 3, 12, 13, 14. 1867. 10, 11, 12.—*E. Neumann*, **Wagner's Archiv der Heilkunde. Bd.** XI. —*Waldeyer*, Diffuse Hyperplasie des Knockenmarkes: Leukämie. Virchow's Archiv. LII. Nr. 305.—*Kottmann*, Die Symptome Der Leukämie. Bern, 1871. —*Mosler*, Die Pathologie und Therapie der Leukämie. Klinisch bearbeitet. Berlin, 1872. A. Hirschwald.

Historical Sketch.

It was in the year 1845 that Virchow correctly explained and interpreted without prejudice a case of leucæmia, since he looked upon the corpuscles occurring in leucæmic blood and characterizing the disease as white blood-corpuscles, and not, like Bennett, Bouchut, and, much earlier, Velpeau, as pus-corpuscles. That the blood, from its whitish color, might become similar to pus, mucus, chyle, or milk, was known long before Virchow. There was no neglect in forming numerous theories, such as purulent absorption (Ribes), inflammation of the blood (Piorry), purulent fermentation of the blood (Engel); in fact, these theories had taken deep root in pathology, notwithstanding Nasse's discovery, in the year 1835, that colorless, white corpuscles were present in normal blood, besides the red ones; full ten years passed by during which the theory of pus in the blood was firmly held. By a singular coincidence of events it happened that just at the time when Virchow, by his works, "White Blood" and "White Blood and Tumors of the Spleen," assigned the correct meaning to the white corpuscles in the blood, Bennett, by a simultaneous observation, thought that he had placed the keystone to the pus theory by explaining the condition as a suppuration of the blood; hence, many physicians incorrectly look upon the discovery of leucæmia as having been made simultaneously by Virchow and Bennett. The fact is, that while Virchow and Bennett each, almost simultaneously (1845), observed a case of leucæmia, the latter considered his a suppuration of the blood (pyæmia), and only six years later, after Virchow had explained his immediately as white blood (leucæmia), accepted the doctrine of Virchow. There can be no more dispute at the present day that the discovery of leucæmia belongs to Virchow alone. Through the services of Virchow alone we are at present in the condition to judge correctly of the older observations on "white blood," "purulent blood," "blood of a peculiar appearance," which occurred in what Walter calls the "ante-leucæmic" period, and make them useful, as Virchow himself has done, in enlarging the catalogue of cases. Here belong the cases of Bichat, Velpeau, Oppolzer and Liehmann, Rokitansky, Wintrich, Caventou, Harless, Andral, and Bricheteau.

The doctrine of leucæmia received important support from Julius Vogel, at that time professor in Giessen, who, in 1849, made for the first time the diagnosis of leucæmia in a patient of his clinic. Afterwards, Bennett also gathered a series of cases, which were first collected in the Monthly Journal of Med. Science, 1851, and afterwards in a special work. It has already been properly shown that with the *new name*, lèucocythæmia, which he bestowed upon the disease, he gained no claim to the priority of the discovery. Bennett did good service, however, in spreading the knowledge of this disease in England and collecting twenty-one new observations, partly his own, and partly from Robertson, Chambers, Quain, Walshe, Hislop, Douglas, Gairdner, Wallace, Drumont. He also added four cases of hypertrophy of the spleen without the development of leucæmia, described several examinations of the blood, and gave a valuable analysis of the anatomical and symptomatic conditions.

In the year 1853, in a longer article, Virchow communicated a series of new cases, and indicated the necessity of separating two different forms of leucæmia. In consequence of Virchow's works, numerous cases of leucæmia were published by German physicians, as Uhie, Griesinger, Heschl, Schreiber. The last-mentioned author has shown that the follicles of the intestine also, especially the Peyer's patches, may show the same changes in leucæmia which we meet with most distinctly in the external lymphatic glands.

In the year 1856 two very complete treatises upon this subject appeared, one by E. Vidal, the other by B. Schnepf. The former treated especially the clinical side of the subject, the

latter the pathological. In the same year the knowledge of leu
cæmia was essentially advanced in Germany. Virchow's collected contributions to scientific medicine, which were published
in the year 1856, contained a new essay on leucæmia, in which
the author gave a general sketch of the disease, and demonstrated the connection of the diseases of the individual organs
with the leucæmic dyscrasia.

The peculiar lesions in the digestive tract, as well as in the
pleura, the liver and kidneys, were more carefully studied by
Friedreich, Boettcher, and Von Recklinghausen. The chemical
side of the question was not neglected. After the condition of
the normal constituents of the blood had been determined from
the analysis of leucæmic blood, by Julius Vogel, Robertson,
Parkes, Becquerel, Laveran, and Robin, Scherer, from the examination of a case of leucæmia observed by Bamberger and Virchow, furnished the chemical proof of the near relation in which
leucæmia stands to changes in the activity of the spleen, since he
found in leucæmic blood several soluble constituents of the splenic pulp, viz., hypoxanthin, uric acid, lactic acid, leucin, and
formic acid. These statements were confirmed by the investigations of Folwarczny, Koerner, and myself. Salkowsky has lately
undertaken chemical investigation in the same direction

Special attention was given to the etiology, symptomatology
and therapeutics of this disease in the observations communicated by me to the Berliner klinische Wochenschrift. The
subject has recently received a most thorough elaboration from
Virchow, in his Lectures on Morbid Growths, II. Bd. Berlin,
1864 and 1865. In the twenty-first lecture on lymphatic growths
the leucæmic lymphomas are thoroughly treated.

Quite lately an important contribution to the pathological
anatomy of leucæmia has been made by E. Neumann. After he
had been led, in consequence of his investigations upon the function of the osseous marrow in the formation of the blood, to
consider its connection with leucæmia, a necropsy of a case of
this kind made by him on the 3d of July, 1869, convinced him of
the existence of a myelogenous form of this disease. Very important confirmation of this discovery of Neumann has already
been made by Waldeyer. In a case since observed by me I found

considerable pain in the sternum, produced by the myelogenous degeneration of the bone. All the previous observations upon leucæmia are carefully detailed in the monograph upon this disease published by me in 1872.

Nature of Leucæmia.

There is hardly a disease which furnishes so many points of interest, both to the physiologist and the pathologist, as leucæmia. The name chosen by Virchow, rightfully belongs to it. The number of the colorless cells is so much increased that the blood has a whitish color. The fact of the highest importance in the genesis of this alteration is that, according to all previous observations, the phenomena begin with the hyperplasia of a lymphatic organ.

According to Virchow, the progress of the leucæmic disease is as follows: "First, a lymphatic organ becomes hyperplastic, then from this organ certain changes affect the blood, and indeed changes in a two-fold direction; partly purely chemical, since certain substances which usually occur in this organ as parenchymatous juices, are found in greater quantity in the blood; partly morphological, since cellular elements pass into the blood; then comes, in the third place, the heteroplastic affection of other organs, or, so to speak, a kind of metastasis."

According to this, we have in leucæmia a very complete picture of the gradual generalization of an originally local process, the separate stages of which we know more accurately than of any other kind of generalization (Virchow).

Kottmann, on the other hand, defines leucæmia as a disease in which we have primarily to do with a hyperplasia of the white blood-cells, which increase takes place in the blood itself, and is followed by metastases of these cells in nearly all the organs, but especially in those which, like the glands and the osseous marrow, stand in the most intimate connection with the blood. This view is supported, according to Kottmann, by various observations in which a considerable increase of the white cells existed without change in the blood-forming organs (glands, osseous marrow, lymph-spaces), and by the cases of pseudo-leucæmia, where these organs have become considerably hyperplastic without leading to increase of the white corpuscles. Hence Kottmann concludes that leucæmia and pseudo-leucæmia, notwithstanding their remarkable resemblance, are far removed from each other; and that

the designation of tho latter leads only to error, and ought to be given up. Leucæmia, according to Kottmann, is a neoplasm in the fluid tissues of the blood, which,
like other new formations in the solid organs, is connected with numerical increase
of some parts and atrophy of others (tho red blood-corpuscles). It has clinically a
great resemblance to carcinoma, since it, like this, increases rapidly and secondarily
infects the most various organs, most frequently the spleen and the lymphatic
glands, then the liver, the kidneys and the osseous marrow, and more rarely the
lungs, the submucous tissue of the intestines and of the pharynx. Other diseases,
like intermittent, tuberculosis, carcinoma, and syphilis, stand, according to Kottmann, in no genetic connection with it. Leucæmia is rather a disease sui generis,
and not simply a symptomatic condition; for which reason Kottmann considers the
usual separation of splenic, lymphatic, and myelogenic forms as not well founded,
but prefers rather a division into large cell, small cell, or mixed leucæmia. Even
this separation he considers to be due only to a more or less rapid progress of the
disease.

Clinical observation has often confirmed Virchow's view of
the progress of development. After a stage of prodroma or
gradual development of the leucæmic process in the lymphatic
organs, a stage of complete leucæmic cachexia, with secondary
disease of other organs, can be clearly made out.

According to the origin of the leucæmia in the spleen, or the
lymphatic glands, and the gradual change of the blood arising
from them, Virchow has separated two forms—the splenic and
lymphatic; of which the first introduces into the blood elements
resembling the constituents of the splenic pulp; the second,
bodies like the parenchymatous nuclei of the lymphatic glands.
In the lymphatic form—lymphæmia (Virchow)—may be found, in
large numbers, colorless elements, which are in the average
smaller than the ordinary colorless blood-corpuscles, most of
them, however, having larger, more simple, and more strongly
granulated nuclei. In the splenic form (splenæmia, Virchow),
the cells usually resemble the ordinary colorless blood-corpuscles; most of them are larger, and show, upon the addition of
acetic acid, multiple or divided, smoother, or more rarely, single,
round, and somewhat granular nuclei (Virchow).

The cases in which the distinction between these two forms is
clearly marked are rare. More frequent than the purely splenic
and purely lymphatic cases are the mixed forms, in which the
spleen and lymphatic glands both become hyperplastic. Virchow

has lately embraced all the lymphatic growths occurring in leucæmia, under the title of Leucæmic Lymphoma. Those which form the starting-point of the leucæmic dyscrasia are to be considered primary lymphomas.

According to previous observations, there can no longer be any doubt that the changes in the bony marrow described by Neumann also play a part in the pathogenesis of leucæmia. To Virchow's splenic and lymphatic leucæmia, Neumann's myelogenous form must be added, which will obviously be rarer as an unmixed form than as a complication of the others.

It is all the more probable that all three forms of leucæmia may occur together in òne and the same individual, because, after extirpation of the spleen, a change in the marrow has been observed, where lymphatic glands and marrow seem to take up together the function of the spleen.

It is probably the colorless blood-corpuscles or lymph-corpuscles which determine the spread of the leucæmic process from the organs first affected. According to Virchow, it may easily be assumed that some contagious material is transported by the colorless elements as carriers of the dyscrasia and as conditions of the metastasis, and an inoculation follows at some place which determines there a development analogous to the primary lesion. According to my own experience, this appears probable.

Unfortunately, attempts made by Bollinger [1] and myself to inoculate healthy animals with leucæmia, partly by transfusion and partly by injection with Pravaz' syringe, have so far given only negative results; they ought, however, to be continued, since the occurrence of leucæmia has recently been determined in dogs, swine, and horses (Bollinger, Fuerstenberg, Leisering).

The origin of secondary leucæmic tumors has been lately explained in another way, that is, by extravasation of white blood-corpuscles. Many of the appearances in leucæmia may be explained in this way, and our knowledge of the disease has been advanced by the proof of the diapedesis of the white blood-corpuscles; but, according to my experience, all the secondary lymphomas in leucæmia cannot be explained by this process. For the others, we must retain Virchow's explanation, that the

---

[1] Virchow's Archiv. Bd. LIX. p. 341.

elements of the metastatic lymphomas are developed in loco from the connective tissue, so that we have to deal, not with deposits, but with new formations.[1]

Etiology.

Since we have recognized the spleen, the lymphatic glands, and the bony marrow, as the starting-points of leucæmia, we must direct our attention to those disposing causes which are able to produce primary diseases of these organs.

It appears from previous observations, that no age, neither sex, and no social position is free from leucæmia. It occurs as well in the male as in the female sex; from the tenderest childhood to old age; in nearly all ranks of society, from the poorest day-laborer to the richest proprietor. Notwithstanding this universality, a greater disposition of the male sex cannot be denied. In ninety-one cases collected by Ehrlich, there were sixty males and thirty-one females. Among the sixteen cases observed by me, there were four females, that is, one-quarter. Derangements of the generative functions in the female sex have no inconsiderable influence on the occurrence of this disease. Actual leucæmia was noticed a short time after delivery in the observations of Bennett, Vidal, Virchow, and Leudet. I observed an exceedingly well-marked case after several miscarriages and difficult labors; another in consequence of a suppression of the menses from cold. Among the twenty-one cases of leucæmia in women which have come under my notice, there are in all sixteen in which disorders in the activity of the generative organs have occurred.

As to the *age*, statistical observations have shown that in the male sex the disposition to leucæmia gradually increases from childhood until it reaches its highest point, between the ages of thirty and forty, and from the fiftieth year again declines. In the female sex, the greatest number are found in the ages from forty to fifty. After many irregularities in the sexual life of the

---

[1] This view has been lately confirmed by the observations and examinations which are recorded in the dissertation of *Reimond Granier* (Die lymphat. Neubild. d. Leber. Inaugur. Dissertation. Berlin, 1868), as well as by Dr. *Gustav Wolfhuegel* ("Zur Kenntniss leukämischer Neubildungen." Würzb. Inaug.-Abhandl. Carlsruhe, 1871).

woman have gone before, the fully developed disease is often observed for the first time at the climacteric period.

The youngest ages at which leucæmia has been observed were eight and ten weeks; the oldest, sixty-eight and sixty-nine years. On account of the connections with scrofulosis and rachitis, mixed forms occur in children more frequently than in adults, in which we observe at the same time hyperplasia of the spleen and lymphatic glands. I have seen a case of splenic leucæmia in a boy, sixteen months old, as a consequence of chronic intestinal catarrh.

Chronic intestinal catarrhs lead to hyperplasia of the solitary glands and Peyer's patches, from which leucæmic infections of other lymphatic and non-lymphatic organs may then arise.

Behier [1] describes a new form of leucæmia under the name of "leucémie intestinale," where the spleen and lymphatic glands were normal, but genuine lymphomas were present in the Peyer's patches and in the solitary follicles of the small intestine, which were supposed to have given rise to a continuous increase of the white blood-corpuscles.

In a statistical review of 124 cases, there are only eight or ten in which it can be distinctly shown that they followed intermittent, which shows the infrequency of their occurrence. These cases have, however, shown that there are certain forms of irregular, obstinate, long-continued intermittent fever, which, among other consequences, may also give rise to leucæmia.

The same thing is true of syphilis, which may also be mentioned among the causes of leucæmia. In a case treated by Bamberger, the influence which previous depressing mental impressions exercised upon the course of the disease was unmistakable, and the patient himself, a well-to-do merchant, believed that the cause of his disease was to be sought in domestic troubles. In a case observed by me in 1867, in Schwalbach, no other cause could be found than excessive bodily and mental exertions and continued excitement. The influence of the nervous system on the production of leucæmia has become more probable since the experiments on the innervation of the spleen and its relation

---

[1] L'Union. 99, 100. Aug. 1869.

to leucocythæmia, published by Prince Tarchanoff in the Eighth
Volume of Pflueger's Archiv für Physiologie.

In many cases, notwithstanding the most careful examination, no direct cause can be found for this most mysterious
affection. The attempt has been made to discover whether any
constitutional peculiarities furnish a predisposition to leucæmia,
but the results are negative. In several cases a robust build, and
once, remarkable obesity, are mentioned, as well as, on the other
side, a delicate frame and tardy development.

The largest proportion of cases have come from the lower and
working classes. In eighty cases in which the social position and
occupation of the patients are mentioned, only eight are from the
higher and well-to-do classes, the others belong to the working
class. No trade or occupation seems to have any special disposition to this disease. From the causes so far known, it may
be assumed that persons who are most exposed to the weather, to
want, grief and care, and other unfavorable conditions, acquire a
certain disposition to leucæmia.

Finally, I must mention one special cause—traumatic injury.
In the cases communicated by Velpeau and Wallace, a blow upon
the splenic region is mentioned. In a case mentioned by me, the
leucæmia began by bruising the spleen against the pommel of a
saddle in mounting a horse. In a case observed by Virchow,
fracture of the thigh is mentioned as a cause. I have seen leucæmia in a boy ten years old, for which the cause assigned was
over-exertion in pushing a wheelbarrow. Myelogenous leucæmia
seems to be specially often developed from injury to the bones.

As to the immediate cause of leucæmia, notwithstanding all
the hypotheses which have been set up, we can give no sufficient
explanation. From some of the predisposing causes just mentioned, one or several of the lymphatic organs is first affected
with hyperplasia, and thus changes in the blood are brought
about, partly of a chemical, partly of a morphological character.

According to the view of W. Müller, that the spleen has no
other function than to be the brooding-place of the white blood-
corpuscles, and to keep up a continual supply of them to the
blood, the increased introduction of white blood-corpuscles in
the leucæmic hyperplasia of the spleen could be easily explained.

We should certainly have no doubt as to the mode of origin of leucæmia, if the same pathological changes of the spleen and lymphatic glands—exactly this hyperplasia—did not occur without any increased supply of white corpuscles in the blood having been observed. Hence, in the leucæmic hyperplasia, some specific distinction must exist—some sort of specific irritative condition—by which the exportation of white corpuscles into the blood is favored. One may well doubt whether it is specific nervous activity, or chemical influences acting upon the splenic tissue, which make this distinction.

Pathological Anatomy.

The splenic tumor of leucæmia always shows a considerable increase in size, often of four-fold the normal measurement, and ten or fifteen times the normal weight. It generally retains the normal form with its indentations, and develops itself proportionally in all its dimensions. In other cases the enlargement takes place more in one direction. Not unfrequently the capsule shows thickenings and opacities, whitish patches, or even papillary new formations.

The consistence of the leucæmic spleen is increased, scarcely ever diminished. Upon section, the parenchyma is bluish red, often homogeneous, dry, with a dull lustre, and frequently somewhat granular. Whitish granules are either scattered throughout the whole spleen, or arranged in rows. Sometimes the fibrous trabeculæ are scarcely visible, at others very prominent. Occasionally the parenchyma is covered with yellowish masses of fibrine and exudation. The Malpighian corpuscles are often distinctly marked from the red pulp by their whitish appearance, the latter being present in comparative abundance, but not very compact. The microscopic examination shows everywhere the normal elements, only in very close combination, so that the intermediate substance of the pulp-cells appears to be richer and firmer (Virchow). Towards the outer surface are occasionally found more or less extensive regions of tougher consistence, in which Virchow demonstrated all the characteristics of older and newer hemorrhagic infarctions.

From these appearances the conclusion may be drawn that
this enlargement, usually so marked, of the organ results from
the congestion with new formations taking place in it. The
number of the cellular elements increases more and more; the
cells themselves reach a considerable size and greater development, while the vessels and the stroma also increase. In the
course of time two stages may be distinguished: a softer stage,
more rich in cellular elements, and a harder, more indurated.

In the lymph-glands the leucæmic process declares itself also
by a hyperplasia of their constituent parts, and first, of the cells;
later, an increased formation of connective tissue may be added.
The process seems, just as in the spleen, to begin with a greater
flow of blood and an increased vascularization, under the influence of which the multiplication of glandular elements takes
place.

The single lymphomas often attain the size of a goose-egg or
a man's fist. They are found very often in the hilus of the
spleen and liver. Sometimes all the lymphatic glands in the
body are involved in the process. Externally they are distinguished by a usually soft, unelastic, smooth, sometimes almost
fluctuating feeling; they have a rather smooth, often somewhat
shining surface, with a whitish, yellowish, or gray look. Upon
section one may distinguish much enlarged, properly glandular
cortex, and the cavernous connective tissue of the hilus also
somewhat more voluminous. The surface, upon section, is gray
or reddish white; the expressed juice sticky, milky, with single
nuclei and nucleated cells. The mass is most like the pulpy infiltration in typhus.

Besides the lymph-glands already mentioned, there are others
which may take part in the leucæmic process. The thymus has
been found still remaining, much enlarged, partly in a condition
of fatty degeneration, and in the juice the same elements as in
that of the lymphatic glands. In the case of Dr. Cnyrim the
enlargement of the thymus gland was so huge that it covered
the whole heart. In another case the thyroid gland was enlarged, nodular, and tough. The follicles of the tongue and the
tonsils are also sometimes much enlarged, whitish, pulpy upon
section. Even upon the posterior surface of the epiglottis many

pulpy nodules, up to the size of a pea, have been found which projected above the surface of the mucous membrane. Similar nodules have been observed on the mucous membrane of the larynx and the trachea in great numbers. Still more often than at the entrance of the digestive tract, leucæmic changes of the glands occur in the mucous membrane of the ileum, and even of the stomach and duodenum. The observations of Schreiber first proved that the intestinal follicles—especially those of Peyer—may show the same change in leucæmia which we observe in its most striking form in the external lymph-glands.

The pathological anatomy of leucæmia has received an important contribution in the discovery of the changes in the bony marrow, by E. Neumann. Both in the central cavity of the long bones and in the cancellated structure of the ribs, the sternum, and the vertebræ, the marrow has the same greenish yellow, purulent color, and just the same consistence as thick mucous pus in a purulent osteo-myelitis involving the whole skeleton. Upon microscopic examination it may be seen that cellular elements of the same nature as those occurring in leucæmic blood form the principal constituents. There may also be found, just as in the blood, but in greater number, cells distinguished by a sharply-marked, vesicle-like, clear nucleus, with a nucleolus. Transitional forms between colored and colorless cells were found by Neumann no more frequently than in the normal red marrow. The complete absence of the normal, richly developed vascular net-work, which usually serves as the frame-work in the meshes of which the cell-masses are imbedded, was a very striking circumstance; the only vessels which could be found were arterial branches. The larger among them showed a wall infiltrated with lymph-corpuscles. In the smaller, the walls seemed to be formed of loosely connected, long, small spindle-cells, which could also be frequently seen isolated in the preparation, and much reminded one of the well-known spindle-cells of the splenic pulp. The contents of these vessels which remained consisted of blood, in which the red cells predominated. Outside the vessels the number of the latter was exceedingly small, compared to that of the colorless elements.

The pathological changes which the marrow exhibits favor

the theory of a continued and abundant importation of lymph-corpuscles into the blood from the marrow. Neumann explains their passage into the blood, by saying that the pathological alteration of the marrow facilitates the intercourse between it and the blood, so that the blood-corpuscles, before they have attained maturity in the bones, as under normal circumstances, get into the general circulation in a state of incomplete develop-ment. The same observer also believes that an abnormal transit of the chemical constituents of the marrow into the blood may be considered probable.

We owe to Waldeyer a valuable confirmation of Neumann's discovery of the relation between disease of the marrow and the leucæmic condition of the blood. It depends, as it appears, on an affection of the bones of a peculiar form, hitherto undescribed, which Waldeyer has considered a simple hyperplasia of the mar-row; since, according to Neumann's investigations, the marrow is to be placed in the same category with the lymphatic glands and the spleen.   Waldeyer believes that hyperplasias of the marrow also, which are associated with enlarged conditions of the spleen developing in the same way, ought to be more strictly separated from the inflammatory conditions, which end in indu-ration or suppuration.

At the Leipzig meeting of naturalists, I made a report upon a primary splenic leucæmia, upon which had supervened a secon-dary affection of the marrow, resembling purulent osteo-myelitis. A specially interesting point in this case was great pain over the sternum without previous injury. When this bone was sawed through at the autopsy, the marrow appeared dirty gray; the spongy substance showed several irregular cavities as large as peas, and one place as large as an almond, like an abscess in the lower part.   The external layer above the cavities was every-where intact; the medullary tissue of a lumbar vertebra, of the femur, and of other bones was degenerated in the same way in the form of the same hyperplasia. The medullary vessels in places were filled full with white blood-corpuscles. There were also numerous giant-cells, but none of Neumann's transition-forms from the white to the red corpuscles. The spleen was in a condition of leucæmic degeneration, very hard, with numerous inflammatory foci; the lymph-glands were everywhere normal.

. Neumann's suggestion that the affection of the spleen and lymphatic glands in leucæmia has only an accidental importance, while the disease of the marrow is the only constant appearance, is not in harmony with previous clinical experience. In a case of leucæmia reported by Ponfick, the change in the marrow was not so marked in comparison with the decided enlargement of the lymphatic glands and the spleen, that the former could be considered the primary, and the latter the accidental affection.

The further spread of leucæmia in non-lymphatic organs happens partly in consequence of an infiltration of those organs, produced by the emigration of colorless cells. More frequently actual leucæmic heteroplastic tumors are observed.

The liver is extremely often diseased; in ninety-two cases collected by Ehrlich, fifty-four times. It weighs from four to five, or even from eight to fourteen pounds—generally only in consequence of hyperplastic increase of the cells; but when the disease has lasted longer, in the form of lymphatic new formations, which occur as an infiltration, or, more rarely, in the form of grayish white, soft nodules, like miliary tubercles. The follicular form is often connected with the trabecular infiltration described by Virchow, starting from the portal connective tissue.

According to Rindfleisch, the leucæmic new formation of lymphadenoid tissue in the liver is to be considered as an infiltration produced by the emigration of white corpuscles—since it everywhere closely follows the course of the vessels. The leucæmic cells force their way through the lobule from the outside inward, and press the liver-cells away from the vessels, so that these are atrophied and destroyed, leaving behind them only masses of pigment-granules.

In a case of leucæmia with jaundice, observed by me, the liver presented the appearances of cirrhosis, whence it may be assumed that the change took place by a proliferation originating in the elements of connective tissue.

The kidneys are in most cases normal; sometimes there is found in them an infiltration of the parenchyma with lymphatic

elements, beginning at the surface and running parallel to the
uriniferous tubes, in grayish white lines and streaks, or pulpy
nodules, often with a central hemorrhage, and formed by the
deposition of lymph-cells in the circumference of the glomeruli,
which, like the tubes, are choked by the growing new formation
(Virchow, Friedreich, Boettcher). Here also the origin of the
nodules from the interstitial connective tissue, especially the
stroma, in the neighborhood of the Malpighian tufts, can be followed by the microscope.

In a case reported by Vogel, the kidneys were normal, but the
supra-renal capsules were changed into a grayish yellow, cheesy
mass, which showed under the microscope numerous drops and
granules, and between these, here and there, rust-colored remains
of extravasations of blood.

Among the changes in other organs are still to be mentioned
colorless or pale yellow clots in the vessels of the meninges (according to Ehrlich, five times in 100 cases), emboli of white corpuscles in the meningeal arteries (Bastian), serous and sanguineo-
serous effusions in the subarachnoid space and ventricles of the
brain (according to Ehrlich, nine times in 100 cases), more rarely
effusions of blood into the substance of the brain and sclerosis of
the fibres of the optic nerve (Von Recklinghausen), retinitis leu-
cæmica (Roth and Reinecke), frequently serous exudations in the
pleuræ, pulpy patches on the pleuræ, consisting of colorless
blood-corpuscles (Friedreich), which originate in pre-existing connective-tissue corpuscles of the pleuræ, frequently œdema, more
rarely hypostatic congestion in the lungs, sometimes leucæmic
lymphomas on the mucous membrane of the air-passages, which,
according to Virchow, are to be distinguished from tubercles
only by having no tendency to fatty or cheesy degeneration. In
one of Boettcher's cases caverns were formed—that is, ulcerating
bronchiectatic cavities, which arose from the breaking through
of the lymphoid collections of cells into the branches of the
bronchi.

At the heart may be found, besides its dislocation by the enlarged abdominal organs and the exuberant lymph-glands in the
thoracic cavity, not unfrequently pericardial effusions and peri-
and endo-cardial ecchymoses, with occasionally lymphoid nod-

ules along the vessels under the pericardium (Wolffhuegel). In the usually dilated cavities often a completely coagulated, sometimes puriform blood ; while in other regions of the vessels the blood contains more red elements. A diapedesis of white blood-corpuscles has been demonstrated by Roth in the retinal vessels, and made probable by A. Boettcher in the leucæmic ulcerations of the ascending colon.

In the digestive organs a leucæmic inflammation of the mouth and pharynx has been observed by me as a characteristic change. Friedreich found numerous leucæmic tumors as large as a cent or a dollar in the mucous membrane of the stomach, without being able to show a genetic connection with the pre-existing follicles of the mucous membrane ; he also found in the small intestine that the closed follicles were partly atrophied and the development of the colorless elements had taken place in the connective-tissue bodies of the intestinal mucous membrane. These pulpy swellings of the intestinal mucous membrane, especially of the ileum, frequently ulcerate, form ulcers with raised borders, and can then hardly be separated from the pulpy typhus infiltration.

Character of the Leucæmic Blood.

The changes of the blood in leucæmia are so characteristic that they form the most prominent mark of the disease; the lighter color is more and more marked as the process advances. It is produced by an increased supply of colorless elements to the blood. Max Schulze has accurately described various kinds. Virchow discovered its varying condition in splenic and lymphatic leucæmia. Klebs, Erb, Von Recklinghausen, Boettcher, Eberth, Neumann, have referred to the occurrence of transition stages between colored and colorless cells ; the latter refers them to the osseous marrow. The same observer has also found in leucæmic blood a formation of peculiar, colorless, shining, elongated, octahedral crystals.

The increase of the white corpuscles occurs in very different degrees, the relation of the white to the red corpuscles being usually defined by numbers. In this way it has been attempted to separate leucæmia from those conditions of slight and transitory increase of the white cells known as leucocytosis; these occur in the course of pregnancy, in typhus, in febrile diseases, and many others where irritation of the lymphatic glands exists.

Since only a gradual distinction exists between leucæmia and leucocytosis, the diagnosis of a commencing leucæmia, from an examination of the blood, is often difficult. Whether Magnus Huss is entirely right in assuming the existence of a leucæmia only when the proportion of the colorless to the colored blood-corpuscles equals 1 : 20, is not yet quite certain. For the diagnosis of leucæmia is demanded the proof of a continued and progressive increase, finally reaching a considerable amount, of the white corpuscles in the blood, corresponding to the increasing enlargement of the lymphatic organs affected. This dyscrasia, as so far observed, is continuous, leading in its regular progress to the death of the patient. The proportion of colorless corpuscles finally reached is very great. Virchow estimated their proportion to the red as 2 : 3; Julius Vogel, in another, at 1 : 3 to 1 : 2; Schreiber, in a third, at 2 : 3. I have several times observed these proportions in my patients.

The red blood-corpuscles are not only relatively, but absolutely, considerably diminished, as is shown by Welcker's blood-color scale and method of estimation by settling. The specific gravity of the blood seldom reaches the physiological minimum of healthy blood; the water and fibrine are increased, the iron considerably diminished. According to the examinations of Scherer, Folwarczny, Koerner, leucæmic blood contains glutin, formic, lactic, and acetic acids, leucin, tyrosin, uric acid, hypoxanthin; of these lactic and formic acids and hypoxanthin are the only substances constantly found. Besides these, Salkowsky found an organic acid containing phosphorus—probably glycerin-phosphoric acid. Although an acid reaction of the leucæmic blood has been hitherto assumed, I have lately found the reaction of leucæmic blood just drawn from the vein not acid, but alkaline.[1]

---

[1] Zeitschrift f. Biolog. VIII. 1. S. 147. 1872.

Symptomatology.

Leucæmia is usually developed with such various symptoms that a symptomatology suited to every case cannot be given. On pathological-anatomical grounds, we distinguish a splenic, a lymphatic, and a myelogenous form. It would be most reasonable to consider each of these forms separately in the symptomatology. Of the cases so far observed, the splenic form furnishes the majority; the purely lymphatic cases, without a tumor of the spleen, are so few that Schnepf believed that this form should be entirely ignored. The occurrence of the myelogenous form alone has not yet been clearly determined. Most frequently these forms have been observed together, and we may distinguish a splenico-lymphatic leucæmia, when the hyperplasia has begun in the spleen and set up secondary leucæmic processes in the leucæmic glands; and a lymphatico-splenic form, when the primary process took place in the lymphatic glands. But we are still not quite clear as to the relation of the myelogenous form to those just named. In a case observed by me the spleen appeared primarily, the marrow secondarily, and the lymphatic glands not at all affected.

From the place of the first appearance of the leucæmia arises a difference in the symptoms in the early stages; later, the appearances are more accordant.

A strict division of leucæmia into different periods has been already attempted. Walther, however, is perfectly right in looking upon Vidal's arrangement as too artificial, since it does not suit most cases. As a rule, only two stages are to be recognized in the course of all the forms of this strange disease : first, a stage of prodromes, and of the development of the leucæmic process in the organs primarily affected, and in the blood; and next, a stage of the extension of the leucæmia to other organs— the condition of developed leucæmic cachexia.

The prodromal and developmental stage appears in various forms. The beginning is usually latent — may be merely suspected—when a leucæmia of the spleen or the lymphatic glands is developed without previous disturbance of the health. It is

otherwise when the disease begins as a consequence of intermittent or syphilis, or when it arises from disordered function of
the sexual organs in the female, or after violent mental excitement.

For the first time, in the year 1865, I was successful in carefully following the
development of a leucæmia—that is, in being able to observe how, with the growth
of the splenic tumor, the number of the white corpuscles gradually increased.

The subjective symptoms—weakness, prostration, dislike for
work, a feeling of heaviness, dull pains in the splenic region or
throughout the abdomen, headache, dizziness, ringing in the
ears, palpitation—show, in the beginning, striking alternations
of improvement and aggravation. After a longer or shorter
duration of these symptoms, there are developed objective signs
of disturbance of the general health—emaciation, paleness, intumescence of the skin, dyspeptic symptoms, difficulty in breathing. The signs of enlargement of the lymphatic glands, on
account of their superficial position, are much earlier remarked
by patients than tumors of the spleen. The glandular tumors
occur at the most various points.

If the leucæmia is a sequel of other diseases, the transition is
an immediate one.

The duration of the stage of development may vary from
three weeks to eight years—from one to two years being about
the average. In children, the course is usually more rapid, and
hence we observe in them almost exclusively the second stage,
that of the fully developed leucæmic dyscrasia, in which the
process has already extended to many organs.

In the second stage occurs an increase of all the symptoms, or
the development of entirely new appearances, under the influence
of which the patients either gradually waste away, or are destroyed in a short time by losses of the nutritive fluids occurring
in paroxysms or continuously.

Besides weakness and exhaustion, the patients complain
chiefly of shortness of breath, which arises in part from the capacity of the lungs being diminished by the glandular and splenic
enlargement, but chiefly from the diminished respiratory power
of the blood. According to Pettenkofer and Voit, there is, to be

sure,. no essential difference in the metamorphosis taking place in the body of a normal and leucæmic man with the same nourishment. The person affected with leucæmia may be able, with the same nourishment, while at rest, to fix as much oxygen as a healthy person, but is nevertheless powerless and capable of no exertion, because the blood-corpuscles in him are capable of doing no more than they are already doing during rest.

Complaints of headache, dizziness, oppression of the head, are less frequent than of dyspnœa. To these are added hypochondriacal mental conditions, melancholy, psychical disturbances; these are often only consequences of the diminution of the red corpuscles, but are sometimes produced by the hinderance offered to the return of the blood by glandular tumors. More frequently still, they are to be explained by the resistance to the circulation of the adhesive blood in the finer vessels of the brain, and the capillary embolisms produced thereby. Just so various causes give rise to the visual disturbances of leucæmia which have been minutely investigated with the opthalmoscope by Liebreich, Becker, Leber, Saemisch, and others. Roth assumes, on the basis of the observations so far made known, that two series of changes in the retina may occur, partly separate, and partly combined—a simple irritative, in which, of course, a disturbance of the circulation plays an essential part, and another arising from the specific and peculiar products of leucæmia.

The most noticeable symptoms on the part of the skin are, besides the paleness, an inclination to profuse sweating, to various eruptions, and to dropsy. The respiratory organs, notwithstanding the great dyspnœa, only rarely exhibit striking changes, occasionally pleuritic effusions, and, in the case of Boettcher, specific miliary nodules. In the heart, one may sometimes observe anæmic murmurs with the systole. The temperature, the pulse, and the respiration show a slight increase only in the evening, and nothing else remarkable.

Among the most striking symptoms of splenic leucæmia, which are frequent in the second stage, are to be reckoned hemorrhages; sometimes, before the occurrence of splenic or glandular tumors, a hemorrhagic diathesis has been observed (Huss, Jacqot, Mohr, and Mueller). These hemorrhages are caused not only by the obstruction to the circulation in the capillaries caused by the collecting of white corpuscles, but also by the weakness and friability of the vessels, arising from deficient nutrition.

As to the abdominal organs, in most cases a very considerable distention of the belly is noticeable, and may often be perceived through the clothes. When the walls are lax, the shape of the splenic tumor stretching from the left hypochondrium into the anterior region of the abdomen may be seen and felt. Percussion, however, gives more accurate results; generally the liver also is enlarged, though seldom giving rise to prominent symptoms. Jaundice is mentioned only four times among the earlier cases. I have observed in my clinic a very interesting case of icterus and leucæmia; when the icterus had lasted some time, a decrease of the white corpuscles took place—that is, a diminution of the leucæmia.

Sometimes the enlarged mesenteric glands may be felt through the walls as hard nodules which can be moved from side to side. Ascites supervenes later. The glands in the groin are, as a rule, enlarged, and in many other parts of the body enlarged lymphatic glands make their appearance. From the glands under the jaw the specific changes are sometimes transmitted to the glands of the mouth and throat. An exceedingly well-marked case of leucæmic pharyngitis and stomatitis was described by me in Virchow's Archives. The pharyngeal and tonsillar lymphomas appear as large, pulpy tumors, of tough structure and shining appearance. They give rise to difficulty in swallowing, and are apt to set up inflammation. The leucæmic stomatitis does not appear until after the pharyngitis. It may be supposed to be only the consequence of the change in the secretions of the mouth arising from the lymphatic leucæmia. In its symptoms it shows the greatest similarity to scorbutic stomatitis. In general, the disturbances of the digestive tract are not so constant as those of the respiratory organs. The tongue is only seldom coated, the appetite in most cases normal, more rarely diminished, often increased to perfect voracity. The thirst also is usually normal. Troubles in swallowing frequently occur as symptoms of pressure from the enlarged glands. The intestinal evacuations are frequently interfered with. At first, constipation alternates with diarrhœa, while later the diarrhœa predominates, becomes copious and frequent, sometimes bloody, and accompanied by tenesmus.

The urinary excretion is in most cases normal in quantity, in many cases even increased, but towards the end always diminished; more rarely oliguria exists during the whole course of the disease. In external appearance, also, it is not strikingly different from the normal. When first passed, the urine is generally clear, of a yellowish red, or somewhat darker color, of somewhat acid reaction, and considerable specific gravity (1020 to 1027). After cooling, it usually becomes turbid, deposits a clay-colored sediment of urate of soda and ammonia (sedimentum lateritium); frequently large, rhombic tables of pure uric acid, partly colored and partly uncolored, may be found therein. Virchow first stated that in leucæmia the secretion of uric acid was increased. Later, H. Ranke found the same thing, and drew thence the conclusion that uric acid was formed, in part at least, in the spleen, in the juice of which Scherer has demonstrated uric acid as a normal constituent. More minute statements on this point may be found in the general symptomatology.

Of the other derivatives of the spleen, hypoxanthin has been found in the urine by almost all observers in splenic, but not in lymphatic leucæmia. As to lactic, formic, and oxalic acids, which Scherer has found in the spleen, the urinary analyses of Koerner, Jakubasch, Salkowsky, have given different results. Further examinations must determine whether the presence, or at least the presence in increased quantity, of these bodies in the urine during leucæmia is to be considered a consequence of in-complete oxidation or of increased action of the spleen.

Complications.

Complications occur in all the forms and stages of leucæmia; among them are to be found some which may be considered consequences of the disease, and others which seem to have no special connection with it. Ehrlich has considered this relation in his excellent dissertation, in which 100 cases of leucæmia are collected. In the first class of complications are to be reckoned those occurring in the cachectic stage, or as symptoms preceding the fatal termination, such as serous, or sanguineo-serous exudations in the pleuritic cavity (17 times); in the pericardium (15 times); cranial cavity (11 times); peritoneal cavity (21 times); œdema of the lungs (15 times); hypostatic congestion of the lungs (8 times); pulmonary catarrh (11 times); then the frequent pleuritic and peritoneal inflammations and adhesions; and finally, inflammations of the skin, muscles, lymphatic glands and vessels (15 times); and the cerebral apoplexies probably occurring from the influence of the hemorrhagic diathesis.

As complications which seem to have no demonstrable causal connection with leucæmia, are found tuberculosis of the lungs, the liver, the kidneys, and the intestinal canal (12 times); Bright's disease and amyloid degeneration of the kidneys (7 times); jaundice (11 times); fatty liver (12 times); cirrhosis of the liver (once); and among the acute diseases, pneumonia (12 times), usually appearing late in the disease, and hastening death.

Diagnosis.

The difficulties of diagnosis may be inferred from the fact that leucæmia has only been known for some thirty years; all the auxiliaries of physical examination must be employed for this purpose, notwithstanding which the recognition of the disease in its early periods is still surrounded with difficulties. One is often in doubt whether he has to do with chlorosis, symptomatic leucocytosis, or commencing leucæmia.

The first stage of this disease is often completely latent. Practitioners who are not familiar with physical exploration as a means of diagnosis are often obliged to assume the existence of an essential anæmia, in cases where a more practised physician, from the demonstration of a splenic tumor and a coincident increase of the white corpuscles, already thinks of the possibility of a commencing leucæmia.

Hence, many cases of leucæmia are at first diagnosticated and treated as chlorosis; the long duration of the affection and the inefficacy of treatment lead to the suspicion of some other disease; the attention is often directed to the actual disease by frequent nose-bleed, by distention of the abdomen in consequence of a splenic tumor, or by enlargement of the lymphatic glands. All the points of distinction of splenic tumors mentioned in the general part of this treatise may be made useful in the diagnosis. Splenic tumors occurring in females have several times been mistaken for ovarian tumors, in consequence of which at least one splenotomy has taken place.

They have also been mistaken for tumors connected with the kidneys; in the latter cases the analysis of the urine generally gives accurate information. For establishing the diagnosis, the relation of the intestine to the tumor, especially after pouring large quantities of fluid into the intestine, may be made useful.

When one has, with all the necessary caution, convinced himself of the existence of a splenic tumor, there is no specific character to be found, either by the clinical or the anatomical examination, which permits it to be recognized with certainty as leucæmic. Many other tumors give exactly the same physical signs. It is only rarely that a mistake can take place between leucæmia and tuberculosis, cancer, or echinococcus of the spleen. Tuberculosis and cancer almost never occur, except combined with the same affections in other organs, especially the abdominal. In acute tuberculosis one may suspect with probability the deposition of miliary tubercles in the spleen, when it is considerably enlarged and painful on pressure; but it must not be forgotten that, in acute tuberculosis, an acute enlargement of the spleen occurs without deposition of tubercles in its tissue, although this condition is much more rare. The diagnosis of chronic tubercles is generally quite impossible, since it betrays itself by no local symptoms. Cancer of the spleen can only be recognized when it has already been demonstrated in other organs; when inequalities and nodules can be made out upon the enlarged spleen by palpation, or irregular outlines, unlike the usual splenic dulness, can be determined by percussion. An echinococcus sac of the spleen can, under some circumstances, be diagnosticated by its physical peculiarities.

Among the older writers, inflammation of the spleen is so frequently mentioned, that one might suppose that confusion would exist between the leucæmic tumor and inflammation of the spleen. Primary inflammation of the spleen is rare. Secondarily it occurs more frequently from the effects of inflammatory ulcerative processes from its vicinity, as in sacculated peritoneal exudations, gastric ulcers, toxic gastritis. Under these circumstances it could hardly be mistaken for leucæmia. We meet most frequently with the metastatic form of splenitis. Endocarditis, valvular disease, the formation of coagula in the left heart, give rise to it ; the symptoms are usually completely latent. The organ is enlarged in proportion to the number and size of the inflammatory foci ; it only exceptionally reaches a considerable degree, except in the cases where the embolism has taken place in an already enlarged organ. Such large tumors are seldom seen in these cases as occur in leucæmia ; mistakes can occur only in the early stages of leucæmia, since the examination of the blood can settle the question. A splenic tumor of this kind is more sensitive to strong pressure and percussion than a leucæmic one ; a spontaneous pain over the spleen, increased by the movements of respiration, occurs only when the inflammation has gone on to suppuration. Patients generally emaciate rapidly. Chills occur with severe sweats, œdema, diarrhœa, and very rarely a fluctuating tumor to be felt externally. Abscesses of the spleen, however, may last for years without such striking symptoms, and may then possibly be mistaken for commencing leucæmia, especially if typhoid or a childbirth have preceded.

Pure hypertrophy of the spleen, the physical appearances of which completely coincide with those of the leucæmic tumor, often remains behind after the diseases mentioned, as well as after intermittent, and there is frequently some doubt whether a leucæmia may be developed therefrom. Splenic enlargements arising from syphilis may also have a special interest in the way of differential diagnosis ; the special point to be noticed is whether the splenic tumor is increasing. The change in the blood may often be discovered for the first time when the tumor has attained a certain size. There is as yet no possibility of distinguishing a leucæmic tumor from any other by chemical analysis ; therefore the diagnosis of a commencing leucæmia, since other kinds of splenic tumors may occur with a transient increase of the white corpuscles, presents many considerable difficulties. Unfortunately, there is no symptom which can be referred with certainty to leucæmia. The numerous cases which I have observed and reported have sufficiently proved this for me.

Even in far advanced cases the same macroscopic and microscopic changes of the spleen and lymphatic glands may be present; the same group of symptoms and the same course of the disease may be observed, and yet the examination of the blood gives a negative result; the relative proportion of the colorless and colored blood-cells is and remains normal, on account of which this condition of things has given the occasion for establishing the disease called pseudo-leucæmia.

Since the certain diagnosis of leucæmia can only be made by an accurate examination of the blood, the knowledge of this disease would be materially advanced if the microscope were used in practice even more than now, and if a microscopic examination of the blood were made more frequently by physicians. Every day adds to our conviction that among the local and general symptoms of leucæmia there is not a single one which can make the diagnosis absolutely certain; thus, without a microscopic examination, mistakes of two kinds are possible; either, from the various and anomalous symptoms of leucæmia, some other affection may be suspected; or, from phenomena completely coinciding with the symptoms of leucæmia, the existence of this disease may be falsely assumed.

It is regarded by many physicians as a difficult task to determine an increase of the white corpuscles in the blood; any one who is at all skilled in the use of the microscope may undertake such an examination. I generally choose the little finger of the left hand for a somewhat deep prick with the needle, and use the issuing drops of blood by collecting them singly on an object-glass; the blood is best mixed with a one per cent. solution of common salt, then covered with the thin glass, and examined with a power of 300. I have also used the undiluted blood for microscopic examination, spreading it with much care upon the object-glass. The blood to be examined should not be pressed out of the prick, nor be taken a short time after a meal, since in both cases too many colorless corpuscles or chyle come out, and make the result of the examination doubtful.

Advanced leucæmia is easily diagnosticated by the micro-scope. The blood has the same appearance as pus. The color-less blood-corpuscles are so numerous that the colored ones are often in great part concealed by them ; only the origin can sep-arate blood and pus from each other. It is difficult for most physicians to recognize the various forms of colorless corpuscles and pick out with certainty those which come from the spleen as distinguished from the corpuscles of the lymphatic glands, which are smaller, and have a completely developed nucleus. Hence, the diagnosis of splenic and lymphatic leucæmia can be better made from the macroscopic appearances, according to the extent in which spleen and lymphatic glands participate in the leucæmic process ; for the diagnosis of the myelogenous form Neumann suggests the occurrence of forms intermediate between the red and white corpuscles ; I, as well as W. Eales,[1] was una-ble to find these. Pain in the sternum, as well as in other bones, may be of importance in the diagnosis.

The greatest difficulty is in interpreting correctly a slight increase of the colorless blood-corpuscles ; only a continued observation can determine whether such a case is to be consid-ered commencing leucæmia or transitory leucocytosis. Enumer-ations of the blood-corpuscles have only a relative value, and are considered useless by many physicians. Welcker has suggested an approximate estimation of the proportion of the colored and colorless blood-corpuscles by observing their settling in small graduated vessels.

Course of the Disease, and Prognosis.

The course of leucæmia is almost always lingering and con-tinuous ; sometimes an intermittent accelerated progress is ob-served. First the patients complain of dulness, heaviness of movement, shortness of breath, pressure and fulness in the abdomen, while the healthy complexion is likewise lost. Physi-

[1] Inaugural Dissertation. Leipzig, 1870.

cal examination gives considerable enlargement of the spleen, and, more rarely, of the lymphatic glands. The swelling of the spleen has been developed either without pain and fever, so that the time of its first appearance cannot be determined, or it has appeared in separate attacks, during which the region of the spleen was painful and the patient had fever. In the lymphatic form, the enlargements of the lymphatic glands in the neck, in the axilla, and in the groins, which are developed either slowly or in successive attacks, direct attention to the trouble at a much earlier period. If a drop of fresh blood is now brought under the microscope, the difficulty may often be recognized from the increased number of white corpuscles; during the further growth of the splenic or lymphatic tumors, their number considerably increases. Inflammatory irritation of the capsule, or hemorrhagic infarctions when they are associated with the hypertrophy, produce occasional pains in the region of the spleen, and febrile symptoms.

To these symptoms are frequently added those of a hemorrhagic diathesis; the patients have repeated hemorrhages, which take place especially from the nose; more rarely, from the intestinal canal, the lungs, into the tissue of the skin, or in many cases into the brain, by which complication the result is much accelerated. The patients either die suddenly with symptoms of apoplexy, or are so debilitated by repeated and abundant losses of blood, that they soon die with the symptoms of exhaustion and anæmia. If no hemorrhagic diathesis is developed, the disease, with few exceptions, takes a tedious course, and may last for years; in such cases, the enlargements of the spleen and lymphatic glands reach a very high degree; the patients emaciate greatly; their pale, cachectic appearance becomes very striking; the dyspnœa increases and becomes extremely distressing; in the urine sediments of urates and pure uric acid are observed; in many cases bronchial catarrh is developed, with violent cough and mucous expectoration—sometimes intestinal catarrh appears and leads to obstinate diarrhœa; dropsical symptoms often appear towards the end, and death follows, if there are no complications, from gradual exhaustion, being often preceded by symptoms of disturbed cerebral functions, delirium, or sopor.

I have stated above that, in the course of all the forms of leucæmia, only two stages, as a rule, are to be recognized : first, a stage including the prodroma—that is, of development of the leucæmic process in the organs primarily affected, and in the blood ; then a stage of extension to other organs, that is, of fully developed leucæmic cachexia. The course of these stages may be different, as the disease begins with the splenic or lymphatic form, or as its development is accompanied, or not, with febrile symptoms.

The prodromal stage of the splenic form has an average duration of one or two years.

The shortest duration was about three weeks (Shearer) ; the longest, nearly eight years (Velpeau) ; in most of the cases observed by me it was not possible to determine with accuracy the length of the developing stage.

The duration of the second stage of splenic leucæmia is as various as the first.

Among my observations the longest time was eighteen months. The leucæmic cachexia usually has a much shorter course, from about three weeks to six months. The presence or absence of febrile symptoms and hemorrhages has much influence upon the duration ; cases which run their course without fever exhibit fewer violent symptoms than when the disease assumes a febrile character, the disease is then more protracted ; the patients die, greatly wasted away, in consequence of the frequent and exhausting hemorrhages and intestinal evacuations, accompanied by excessive dyspnœa, œdema, and ascites.

The lymphatic leucæmia pursues a course similar to that pursued by the splenic ; the same exacerbations and remissions occur ; fever and hemorrhage may be present or absent. As a rule, the tumor of the spleen is associated with enlargement of the lymphatic glands ; hence, the lymphatic form displays the same objective and subjective symptoms as the splenic, though the dissemination of the glandular enlargements is greater, both on the surface of the body and in the interior cavities. Hence, the result is not different from that already described, according to the presence or absence of fever.

There are too few observations on the duration and course of the myelogenous form to permit an exact distinction from the others.

It is sufficiently shown by the preceding statements, that the course and duration of leucæmia cannot be brought within definite limits, and may vary in duration from one month to four or eight years; most cases end fatally within from one to three years, so that the average may be assumed as being twenty-two or twenty-three months. In children the course is usually more rapid.

Prognosis, according to the observations which have been so far made, may be looked upon as unfavorable as soon as the disease has reached the second stage, that of the leucæmic cachexia; all cases in which this stage has been clearly marked have ended fatally. Leucæmia, however, is not in the least to be regarded as an incurable disease. Recoveries in the first stage have been clearly established. These cases will increase, and we shall become more successful and more certain in the treatment of them when proper attention shall be given by physicians to the etiology of leucæmia, and the miscroscopic examination of the blood shall be more frequently employed for diagnostic purposes.

Therapeutics.

The therapeutics of leucæmia have never been very thoroughly treated, since it was not supposed that any method of treatment could be recommended with a prospect of a favorable result. Julius Vogel has already suggested that, in the earlier stage of this disease, certain remedies might produce better results than in the latter. By my observations the etiology of leucæmia has been advanced, a number of new causes have been discovered, and I believe that I have thus rendered essential service in the therapeutics of this disease. Since then, we are not only in a position to recognize the earlier stages of leucæmia, but we can direct our attention to the causal indications, as it has been clearly shown that abdominal obstructions, anomalies of menstruation, psychical influences, syphilis, intermittent, intestinal catarrh, may all be causes of leucæmia; prophylactic rules may be derived therefrom, which are to be well considered, and have been carefully laid down on page 406.

Since the influence of large doses of quinia upon the spleen has been directly proved, they ought to be employed, not only

for the leucæmic tumors of the spleen connected with intermittent, but for others.   I call to mind in this connection the
expression of Binz, that we ought not to suppose that quinia is
of no especial advantage until we have been to the limits of possibility ; if no clear results are seen, too small doses of the remedy or incomplete absorption are to be suspected.

Many physicians still have considerable dread of large doses
of quinia, although permanent injury has very seldom been observed from them.   That quinine can be of material advantage
in splenic leucæmia, when it is given in large doses, is shown by
the following cure obtained from it by me :

Heinrich D., a boy of ten years, from Heyger, in Nassau, was treated by me with
large doses of quinine, in October, 1862, for a clearly demonstrated leucæmia, with
a considerable splenic tumor and an increase of the white blood-corpuscles, in the
approximate proportion of 1 : 20.   The sulphate of quinine was given from the 7th to
the 11th of October in the following mixture :

> ℞. Quiniæ sulph........................ ʒ ss.
> Ac. sulph. dil..................... ℳxx.
> Syr. cinnamomi.................... ʒ ij.

M.—D. Sig. Teaspoonful dose.

In the days mentioned the mixture was taken three times (in all, one and a half
drachms of quinine); in the first two days fifteen grains each, in the last three
twenty grains each.

On the 12th of October the quinine was omitted for two days, since the symptoms of intoxication had reached a marked degree; during these two days the
patient recovered from its effects.   The spleen had become smaller within five days.
From the 12th to the 19th October the patient again received ten grains a day, and
the tumor had then become four-tenths of an inch smaller.   A diminution of the
white corpuscles could not be clearly demonstrated.   Then from the 20th to the
31st of October the boy got six grains of quinine a day, besides iron and nourishing diet.   Although the patient had taken within three weeks more than two hundred grains of quinia, no symptoms of a threatening character had appeared.   On
the other hand, the marked improvement of the leucæmia, which went on to complete recovery, dated from this time, and afterwards no enlargement of the spleen
nor increase of the white corpuscles could be discovered.   Some time ago I received
intelligence that no traces of the former trouble had returned, so that the cure may
be looked upon as complete.

Ehrlich reports in his excellent dissertation a second case of
leucæmia, also in the commencing stage, cured by the persistent
use of iron and quinine.

The action of quinia in splenic tumors is materially assisted by the application at the same time of cold upon the region of the spleen, as I have mentioned at page 416. After this procedure I have observed a striking diminution of a large leucæmic tumor.

Instead of the crystallized quinia, the amorphous hydrochlorate (Zimmer) is to be recommended for long-continued treatment. All the drugs employed instead of quinia, on account of their low price, have been rendered almost superfluous by the introduction of the amorphous quinia. The internal and subcutaneous methods of administration, or its use as an enema, dissolved in carbonic acid water, as recommended by Kerner, are to be tried in turn. If it is desirable to suspend the use of the quinia preparations, oil of eucalyptus or piperine is in place. I have lately ordered both of these drugs in the following prescription:

> ℞. Olei eucalypti.................. gtt. 100
> Piperinæ,
> Ceræ albæ................... āā ℨ i.
> Althææ .... ℥ ij.
> M.—Div. pil. no. 100. Consp. pulv. cort. cass. cin.
> S. Three to five to be taken three times a day.

The preparations of arsenic ought not to be left untried.

According to the method described by me in the Deutsches Archiv für klin. Med. Bd. XV. Heft 2, the parenchymatous injection of Fowler's solution into the leucæmic, splenic and glandular tumors is to be tried, since the contractile elements seem to be excited to stronger contraction in this way than after the internal use of splenic remedies.

Botkin, on grounds mentioned upon page 427, has recently set forth the great therapeutic importance of electricity in leucæmic tumors of the spleen.

As soon as he applied the induced current upon the neighborhood of the spleen, he saw this organ grow smaller in all its dimensions; with the diminution, its consistence became tougher, its surface irregular. After each electrization, the number of white corpuscles in the blood increased, while the general condition, the appearance, and complexion of the patient decidedly improved. Simultaneously with the diminution of the splenic tumor, under the action of the induction current, the liver clearly increased in size. The latter diminished again as soon as the

spleen began to increase, after the cessation of the electric current. " Although
the continued faradization always produced a decrease in the volume of the spleen,
as well as of the lymphatic glands, yet it clearly lost, little by little, in activity,
for the most striking and beautiful results were always obtained in the first
sittings."

Dr. Elias,[1] of Breslau, who treated a leucæmic spleen by faradization, in twelve
sittings, exactly according to the recommendation of Botkin, could easily convince
himself that the considerable change in form of the abdomen and the apparent
diminution of the spleen depended only upon a strong contraction of the abdominal muscles, which pressed up the still movable splenic tumor against the yielding diaphragm. He made the same experiment in a typhus patient, whose enlarged
spleen could be felt almost three fingers' breadth below the edge of the ribs. Here
also the organ disappeared upon faradization, with strong contraction of the abdominal muscles, but, upon removal of the electrode, immediately resumed its former
position, as determined by percussion. Elias draws from his observation the conclusion that the induction current has not the slightest action, and that the apparent
diminution of the splenic tumor depends, in fact, only upon its being pushed
upward; so that he cannot recognize in this process any progress in the therapeutics
of leucæmia.

Among local remedies, splenotomy has been attempted. The
two cases in which extirpation of the spleen has been undertaken on account of leucæmia gave the most unfortunate results
of all, and hereafter, when leucæmia is diagnosticated, splenotomy ought not to be ventured upon.

When it was believed that iron made blood-corpuscles and
healthy blood, and that, under the use of iron, the change of
white to red corpuscles was everywhere facilitated, it was hoped
that iron would be a specific against leucæmia; but I have
never been so fortunate as to see in fully developed leucæmia
any decrease of the white blood-corpuscles or diminution of the
splenic tumor, after the use of iron; yet I do not omit in any
case the prescription of this remedy, since a stronger pulse and
better appearance are generally observed after it.

The transfusion of defibrinated human blood promises more
than mere palliation. The experiment should be made whether
a complete cure cannot be obtained from a frequently repeated
transfusion. The consequences described in my monograph
justify this hope.

---

[1] Deutsche Klinik. 1873. No. 5.

To remove the distressing symptoms which occur in the course of leucæmia, many other remedies may be of value ; but, since the treatment of leucæmia differs as little in this respect as in the dietetic rules, which point chiefly to nourishing food, from the therapeutics of other chronic diseases, I have not given special attention to the particulars of the symptomatic and palliative treatment.

Melanæmia.

Literature.

Reil, Memor. clinic. med. pract. fasc. III. 54.—*Heusinger*, Untersuchungen über anomale Kohlen- und Pigmentbildung im menschlichen Körper. Eisenach, 1823. *Lancisi*, De noxiis paludum effluviis.—*Stoll*, Ratio medendi. Tom. I. p. 196.— *Bailly*, Traité anat. pathol. des fièvres intermittentes. Paris, 1825. p. 181.— *Billard*, Archives génér. 1825.—*Popken*, Historia epidem. malignae Jeverae observ. Bremae, 1827.—*Fricke*, Bericht über seine Reise nach Holland im Jahre 1826.—*Rich. Bright*, Reports of medic. Cases. London, 1831.—*Haspel*, Maladies de l'Algérie. I. 335. II. 318.—*Stewardson*, The Americ. Journ. Med. Sc. April, 1841. 42.—*Dr. H. Meckel* in Halle, Ueber schwarzes Pigment in der Milz und im Blute eines Geisteskranken. Zeitschrift für Psychiatrie von Damerow. IV. 2. 1847. Schmidt's Jahrb. LVII. S. 282.—*Dr. Meckel*, Körniger Farbstoff in der Milz und im Blute bei Wechselfieber. Schmidt's Jahrb. Bd. LXXI. S. 176. —*Virchow*, Die path. Pigmente. S. Archiv, Bd. I. II.—*Heschl*, Zeitschrift der Gesellschaft der Aerzte in Wien. 1850.—*J. Planer*, Ueber das Vorkommen von Pigment im Blute. Ebendas. 1854.—*Frerichs*, Die Melanämie u. ihr Einfluss auf die Leber u. ardere Organe. Günsb. Zeitschrift. VI. 5. 1855. Klinik der Leberkrankheiten. 1858. II. S. 326.—*F. Grohe*, Virchow's Archiv. XX.—*v. Basch*, Wiener med. Jahrb. II. 1873.—*Arnstein*, Ueber Melanämie u. Melanose. Tageblatt der 45. Versammlung deutscher Naturforscher in Leipzig. 1872. S. 219. Virchow's Archiv. Bd. LXI. S. 500.—*Valleix-Lorain*, Guide de Médecin practicien. 1866. III. 316.—*L. Colin*, Traité des Fièvres intermitt. Paris, 1870.

Historical Sketch.

Galen supposed the so-called black bile, which was an important element of the earliest humoral pathological theory, to accumulate as a side product of cell-formation in the spleen, and, starting from here, to produce stoppages of the vessels, engorgements of the intestines, and severe nervous disturbances. This view held its ground, with some modifications, until towards the end of the last century (Van Helmont, Sylvius). Reil first noticed the contradictions between the theory of black bile and the experiences of physiology. Heusinger referred it to the abnormal formation of pigment. The more accurate observations on melanæmia belong to the most recent period, and have been collected by Frerichs, to whose classic description I am much indebted in the following statement. It appears from this, that Lancisi found the liver of a person, dead from intermittent fever, colored blackish. Stoll describes the dark pigmentation of the brain and the liver of a woman who died after several febrile attacks. The observations which Bailly gives in his pathological anatomy of intermittent fever are more abundant. Billard described, at the same time, the same change in the brain of three patients dying with acute cerebral disturbance. Similar experiences are recorded in Montfaucon's Hist. Medic. des Marais, 306, 322. During the epidemic of fever which prevailed, in 1826, on the coast of the North Sea, black pigmentation of the spleen, the liver, and the brain was several times observed. Richard Bright gives a masterly representation of a brain the cortex of which was of a dark slate color. Physicians who have observed intermittent and remittent fevers in hot climates have repeatedly described a blackish coloration of the spleen and liver (Annesley, Harpel, Stewardson, and others).

For the first time, in 1837, Meckel recognized that the dark coloration of the organs depends upon an accumulation of pigment in the blood. Two years later Virchow found numerous pigment-cells in the blood and in the enlarged spleen of a man who had become dropsical after long-continued intermittent fever. The scientific basis of melanæmia was established by these two authors. Heschl and Planer published further interesting observations. Frerichs deserves the credit of having presented a clear picture of the disease. Very lately Colin and Arnstein have published valuable investigations on this affection.

Etiology.

In melanæmia a granular pigment is found in the blood. It is either free or enclosed in cells, also imbedded in little hyaline coagula; it probably originates only in consequence of previous intermittent fever; it often circulates for a long time without doing any harm, until, by suddenly sticking in some capillary province, especially in the brain, it gives rise to local symptoms. Its color is black, more rarely yellow or brown. It has been found in the largest quantities in the portal vein.

It generally appears in the form of small, roundish granules; often several granules are united by a translucent hyaline substance, which disappears in acids and alkalies. They form masses of a roundish, oval, or sometimes entirely irregular form. Somewhat more rarely, besides the granular masses, true pigment-cells have been observed; some of these resemble in form and size the colorless blood-corpuscles, while others consist of larger, spindle-shaped or rounded cells, with a round nucleus and sharp outlines, like the forms which are usually found in the spleen besides the free granules; in the interior of these cells lie the black granules in greater or less number. Planer could not convince himself of the existence of such pigment-cells, which Virchow carefully described. Frerichs seldom failed to find them in the blood of the portal vein. Meckel and Planer figure pigment-flakes, up to the size of 0.05''', which showed the most various forms, and sometimes had so sharp a border upon one side that they looked as if they had been broken off. Frerichs found them sometimes cylindrical, with straight parallel boundaries on two sides, while the ends were irregularly broken off. They called to mind the cavity of some small vessel, of which they seemed to be moulds.

· In the fully developed forms of melanæmia, pigment is found wherever the blood goes. Planer found the pigment quite equally distributed in the blood of the heart and large vessels. He could not convince himself of any special collection of them in the blood of the splenic or portal vein; the largest quantity he always found in the spleen, so that this appeared dark brown, chocolate color, or almost black, even in cases where very little pigment could be found in the liver and in the blood. The various stages of the change of the red coloring matter of the blood into melanotic material are represented by the color of the organ, varying from yellowish red to black. The gradually progressive metamorphosis may be recognized not only in the color, but also in the behavior towards reagents. The resistance which the black substances offer to acids and caustic alkalies varies very much. The more recent products are rendered paler and lose their color more or less rapidly; the older ones, on the other hand, withstand their influence for a long time.

Besides the pigment, there may be found in the blood hyaline coagula, which are free from coloring matter. There is nothing unusual to be remarked in the blood-corpuscles; the number of the white ones appears occasionally increased (Meckel), though this is not constant.

The appearance in the blood of large quantities of pigment points to an extensive destruction of red blood-corpuscles. It is assumed as well established by most observers that this process takes place in the spleen—that the spleen is the place of formation of the melanotic material. Frerichs believes that this function cannot be exclusively claimed for the spleen, since the change of the red coloring matter of the blood into black pigment may take place anywhere in the vascular system and even outside of it. Arnstein and Colin absolutely deny the special function of the spleen in the production of melanæmia.

Many circumstances favor the view that pigment is formed in the spleen, thence reaches the portal vein, is partly arrested in the capillaries of the liver, and partly passes through it and reaches the greater circulation. Even in the normal condition, cellular structures occur in the spleen of men and animals, which contain blood-corpuscles or pigment-molecules. In melanæmia the accumulation of pigment is nowhere so constant as in the spleen. This fact has been determined by all observers. Next to the spleen comes the liver, then in succession the other organs: lungs, brain, kidneys. According to Frerichs, the cases are not rare in which the spleen alone is rich in pigment. Cases have also been seen where only the spleen and the liver contained a considerable quantity of dark coloring matter—while the other organs retained the normal color. Frerichs, on the other hand, never observed accumulation of pigment in the blood of the heart, in the capillaries of the brain or of the kidneys, without the participation of the spleen and liver. The form also in which the black coloring matter is found in the blood, points to its origin in the spleen, since the same elements which occur in the splenic pulp, colorless blood-corpuscles, with simple or divided nuclei and spindle-shaped cells, are, besides the fragments of coagula, carriers of the pigment. Frerichs, who assigns to the spleen in melanæmia this function of sending out the pigment-material, believes that he could clearly prove only in one case that formation of the black pigment is not exclusively connected with the splenic parenchyma, but can also take place in the liver.

Colin has arrived at other conclusions from his observations. If pernicious fever were connected with the transit of splenic pigment to the brain or other organs, distinct proof of this pigment ought to be found more frequently in the circulation, which he could not establish. According to his view, Frerichs had been observing very complicated circumstances, in which he was not dealing with purely malarial affections. Colin considers the pigment in the spleen as the product of an extreme destruction of red corpuscles, caused by violent congestion of the blood in this organ. He assumes the same for the other organs — liver, spleen, and kidneys. The elements of the blood suffer dissolution and decomposition just as in other infectious diseases, typhus and dysentery, where the intestinal glands are often found filled with pigment. This decomposition is more rapid in malarial fevers than in other infectious diseases. According to Colin, the deposits of pigment have no connection with each other, but are simply the results of a local change of the red blood-corpuscles. He simply admits that the metamorphosis of coloring matter of the blood into melanotic material takes place more rapidly in the spleen than elsewhere.

Arnstein, who has observed, after intermittent fever, amyloid spleens which contained a little pigment, while at the same time the liver and the bony marrow showed considerable quantities, believes that in melanæmia the pigment is formed within the circulation by the destruction of the red corpuscles, and is very rapidly taken up by the white corpuscles. According to his view it remains only for a time in the capillaries and veins of the spleen, liver, and marrow, and is finally, enclosed in the white corpuscles, carried into the tissues. In favor of this view, Arnstein brings forward the correspondence in the distribution of the pigment with that which is observed from the artificial introduction of granular coloring matter into the vascular system.

According to Arnstein,[1] the process goes on in some such way as the following: During a febrile attack, red corpuscles are decomposed and destroyed within the vessels. The pigment formed in this way is very rapidly—that is, after some hours, taken up by the white blood-corpuscles. These then accumulate in the capillaries and veins of those organs in which the current of the blood is less rapid. In the liver the rapidity of the current is considerably diminished, because the blood of the portal artery, which has already passed through one capillary system, is again distributed over a large territory. In the spleen and in the bone marrow the capillaries pass into very wide veins, a circumstance which must act in diminishing the rapidity of the blood-current. From the blood-vessels of the spleen and the marrow the pigment-bearing blood-corpuscles pass into the tissues of these organs, while the capillaries of the liver retain the pigment a longer time. At the next febrile attack the same process is repeated, and the patient again becomes for a short time melanæmic. Melanæmia, according to Arnstein, is a transitory condition which is replaced by another—that is, melanosis of the spleen, the liver, and the marrow; so that it is not astonishing that one so frequently finds, post-mortem, melanosis, and so seldom melanæmia. The distribution of the pigment in the separate organs is a different one, in those cases where death occurs soon after the febrile attack, from that found in chronic cases. In the acute cases the capillaries of all the organs contain more or less pigment; in the chronic cases, only the spleen, the liver, and the marrow. Hence, Arnstein distinguishes an acute and chronic melanosis, or, more correctly, an acute and chronic stage of melanosis. In this way may be explained the varying and partly contradictory conditions described by the different authors, while, according to the views heretofore prevalent on the origin of melanæmia, this could not be easily done.

The milder forms of intermittent fever seem to give rise to the formation of pigment in the spleen, either not at all, or in a very slight degree. For the production of melanæmia the severer and more obstinate forms of intermittent are necessary, since its occurrence is connected chiefly with the pernicious forms of this disease; it may be supposed that in these cases, in consequence

---

[1] Virchow's Archiv. Bd. LXI. S. 500.

of a thorough infection of the organism with swamp-miasm, a certain chemical influence is followed by extensive necrosis of the red corpuscles and the formation of pigment (Griesinger). It is not difficult to imagine that the minute structure of the splenic pulp predisposes to the formation of pigment therein; even in the normal condition, the blood, passing from the narrow capillaries into the intermediate blood-passages, flows more slowly, and not unfrequently stagnates in some places, so that collections of blood-corpuscles take place, which gradually change to pigment. These stagnations soften in the intense congestions which take place in intermittent fever, and then lead to the formation of pigment on a large scale. Probably the acid condition of the splenic juice is not without influence upon the metamorphosis of the red coloring matter of the blood. In pernicious intermittents the composition of this juice may perhaps be changed in some striking manner. It is perhaps for some such reason that in many other congestions of the spleen, as in typhus, pyæmia, or simple intermittent, the pigment is wanting, or is present only to a slight extent.

Pathological Anatomy.

As already mentioned, the form and color of the pigment in the blood corresponds with that found in the spleen. This organ has always undergone some morbid change in melanæmia, as it has in general after old intermittent fever. It is considerably enlarged, of varying consistence, tough, and brawny, if the attacks have ceased for some time, but softer if they are still recent; the color is always dark grayish brown to blackish brown. When the intermittent attacks have for some time ceased, black pigment is found, in recent cases more yellow. According to Arnstein, the pigment is accumulated chiefly around the veins, so that they appear surrounded by black borders. The arteries are also accompanied by streaks of pigment, and if much pigment is present, the whole splenic pulp appears pervaded with it. It is connected with lymphoid cells and with the large splenic cells, which frequently contain blood-corpuscles. The Malpighian corpuscles, as well as the lymphatic sheaths of the arteries, generally remain free from pigment. Here and there a pigmented cell is to be found; it is also to be found within the arteries and veins (Arnstein).

Similar changes take place in the lymphatic glands, especially in the neighborhood of the liver and spleen. They are considerably enlarged, composed of a pulpy, white, easily-crushed mass, like encephaloid, of a clear white color, or yellowish brown, blackish brown, or bluish black. The granular pigment, of a color varying from yellow to black, is often found enclosed in the cells.

According to Arnstein, the marrow also contains considerable quantities of pigment; it is partly contained in the vessels and partly in the tissue itself, connected with lymphoid cells, and with larger cellular structures analogous to those of the spleen.

The liver shows a steel-gray or black, not unfrequently chocolate color, upon the dark background of which may be seen brown insulated figures. The accumulations of pigment are either uniformly distributed, or crowded thickly together in particular regions. Sometimes the brownish colored lobules appear surrounded with black borders, on account of the distention of the inter-lobular veins with colored particles. Oftener the pigment is more uniformly distributed, since it crowds in from the circumference of the lobule to the commencement of the hepatic veins at its centre, and spreads thence into the vena cava (Frerichs). Arnstein also frequently found in the periphery of the acini much pigment accumulated. In such cases the branches of the portal vein and of the hepatic artery, between the acini, contain much pigment. Not unfrequently he found pigment also in the central vein. As has been indicated above, Arnstein's investigations are distinguished by his finding the granular, frequently agglomerated pigment, everywhere contained in the white blood-corpuscles, and, in addition, pigmented cells in the tissue itself, in the immediate neighborhood of the vessels. The liver-cells themselves, according to the statements of both Frerichs and Arnstein, contain no black pigment. According to Frerichs, they are of normal appearance, or filled, and often completely infiltrated, with brown biliary coloring matter; rarely, and only when the disease is of long duration, do they contain colloid or amyloid material. The size of the whole organ appears, in the cases running a rapid course. either normal or enlarged ; the glands enlarged by congestion, here and there containing many extravasations of blood, and softened. Later, the size diminishes, and frequently a true atrophy follows, unless amyloid infiltration is developed.

In the kidneys the pigment appears in large quantity, in the Malpighian capsules and in the capillaries of the cortical substance; much less in those of the pyramids. Planer saw in the kidneys the smaller vessels filled with old clots and small hemorrhages.

In the vessels of the lungs the quantity of pigment is exceedingly variable, being often considerable, without the usual deposit of black pigment in the lungs themselves. In other cases only a very small quantity was to be found.

Next to the spleen and liver, the brain receives the largest amount of pigment ; the cortical substance takes the color of chocolate and graphite, while the white substance remains unchanged. Only when the color was very intense, a gray appearance could also be perceived in it, the fine vessels being visible as brown lines. Under such circumstances the microscopic examination shows the capillaries filled with black corpuscles and scales, which are sometimes uniformly distributed, and sometimes crowded together in masses. Meckel saw, in the body of a person dead of comatose intermittent, innumerable punctiform extravasations of blood, like flea-bites, distributed through the whole substance of the cerebrum and cerebellum. At the same time an extraordinary quantity of black pigment was found in the blood-vessels, by the blocking up of which, and the thereby increased blood-pressure, the walls of the smallest capillaries were probably ruptured. Planer observed several cases like that described by Meckel, where capillary apoplexies were produced by a stoppage of the pigment ; larger hemorrhages did not occur.

In the vessels of the other organs and tissues the pigment is not accumulated to any remarkable extent, although in many cases a marked coloration of the skin, the cellular tissue, and the mucous membrane is perceptible.

Symptoms.

Many cases of melanæmia exist without disturbance of the functions of the organs overloaded with pigment; in these cases the anomaly is discovered upon post-mortem examination. This happened in a third of the cases observed by Planer. We should not, however, on this account entirely underestimate the importance of the obstruction of certain capillary districts by pigments. Under favoring circumstances capillary embolisms, congestions, rupture of vessels, inflammations, softenings, may be observed as consequences. This process may be developed in a single organ, or in several at the same time; hence, melanæmia makes its appearance under various forms of disease, according to the predominance of symptoms on the part of the brain, the kidneys, or of the intestinal mucous membrane and the liver; or by simultaneous occurrence develops a complicated affection, which presents a different type according to its origin during or immediately after attacks of pernicious intermittent, or after a longer interval; hence, it is impossible to give a clear picture of the disease which shall suit all cases.

In fact, there is only one symptom which is common to all the observations: this is the splenic tumor, demonstrable to physical examination, which, in connection with the special anamnesis—the previous occurrence of intermittent fever—has a real diagnostic value. As a rule, it is accompanied by marked splenic cachexia, which is chiefly produced by the destruction of considerable quantities of blood-corpuscles.

Since the amount of pigment formed is proportional to the loss of blood-corpuscles, the signs of anæmia, either acute or chronic, are clearly marked in well-developed cases of melanæmia.

The attention of the physician is chiefly arrested by such cases as begin with severe cerebral symptoms; they resemble, in many cases, typhoid or inflammatory diseases of the brain, though they may be of various kinds. Sometimes the disturbances of the cerebral function appear in intermissions, and diminish with the febrile paroxysm, but more frequently they extend over the time of the intermission, and are continuous.

According to Frerichs, whom I have followed in this sketch, the cerebral disturbance expresses itself in various forms: in the lighter cases, as headache and dizziness; in the more severe, as delirium, but generally as coma. Not unfrequently motor disturbances, convulsions, or paralyses were present; dull headache, with attacks of giddiness, formed the most constant symptom; delirium was less frequent, sometimes quiet, as is generally seen in typhoid, but sometimes active, with great excitement and restlessness, so that the patients had to be restrained. The excitement gradually passed into stupor and deep coma, which was the most usual form of cerebral disturbance. The slighter degrees of stupor, from which the patient could be aroused by loud calling, and gave rational answers, generally increased after a short time to deep sopor. Occasionally this condition abated at the time of the intermission, to return during the paroxysm. Convulsions and paralyses were much more rare than the disturbances of consciousness; the former always appeared as light twitchings of single muscles of the trunk and of the extremities; sometimes as rolling or slinging movements of the extremities and head; sometimes as epileptiform convulsions, which lasted five or ten minutes, and returned at longer or shorter intervals. The paralyses, which were only exceptionally present, affected sometimes the muscles concerned in articulation or in swallowing, and sometimes the extremities. They were developed suddenly or gradually. In fifty-one cases of melanæmia observed by Frerichs in the Silesian intermittent endemic of 1858, severe brain-symptoms occurred twenty-eight times, either simultaneously with the febrile paroxysm—abating with the febrile symptoms during the intermission—or, more frequently, continuous. It is not difficult to bring them, as Planer did, into causal connection with a flooding of the brain with pigment; Frerichs, however, adduces against the assumption of such a causal connection the following facts: that, in many cases, in which the coloration of the brain is well marked, no considerable disturbance of the circulation can be demonstrated; further, that, notwithstanding the decided coloration of the brain, frequently no cerebral symptoms occur; and, finally, that severe brain-symptoms were observed without any pigmentation of the brain. Among twenty-

eight cases of cephalic intermittent which Frerichs observed, a
dark coloration of the brain was wanting in six. Another important argument against the dependence of these brain-symptoms on pigmentary obstruction of the cerebral vessels appears
in the typical sequence of these phenomena, as well as in their
partially successful treatment with quinine.

In the present condition of our knowledge, nothing certain
can be stated as to the causal connection of melanæmia and the
disturbance of the cerebral functions. It is very possible that in
the malignant forms of intermittent a specific decomposition of
the blood takes place, which, besides an accumulation of pigment
in the cerebral vessels, is followed by cerebral disturbances not
dependent upon the former lesion.

Irregularities in the action of the kidneys were observed in
another series of cases; in some of them albuminuria, or even
hæmaturia, being present, while in others the secretions were
suppressed.

Von Basch has recently reported the case of a physician in the Banat, thirty-two
years old, who, after long continued irregular attacks of intermittent fever, suffered
from a peculiar burning in the urethra, especially in the fossa navicularis, of a well-
marked intermittent type. Upon a microscopic examination of the urine, when
recently passed, he found, besides numerous crystals of uric acid, pale scales, of
which some had the form and size of cells, though most of them were much larger,
and presented the irregular forms of fragments; these were less solid and filled with
dark brown, finely granular pigment. He found in the blood also, the same hyaline
pigment-bearing scales and cell-like structures. Probably the scales of pigment
found in the urine had left the circulation within the kidneys.

In this case, which was, however, not completed by an autopsy, the typical, vesical and urethral neuralgia might have
been in some way connected with pigmentary obstruction. In
general, however, the assumption of the dependence—at least, the
constant dependence—of functional disturbance of the kidneys,
upon an obstruction of the renal arteries, is open to the same
objections which were made to the dependence of cerebral disturbances upon an obstruction of the cerebral vessels; that is,
that we often observe other disturbances of nutrition after intermittent.

Frerichs also observed in melanæmia exhausting intestinal

hemorrhages, profuse diarrhœas, acute serous effusions into the peritoneal sac, and congestions of the serous coat of the intestines; it is certainly highly probable that the melanæmic liver, when a large number of its capillaries are obstructed, leads to considerable disturbance in the portal vein and its branches. But, according to the preceding observation, some doubt must exist on this point also, for, although the liver in all cases observed by Frerichs showed, next to the spleen, the largest amount of pigment, the appearances which seemed to point to an interrupted circulation in the roots of the portal artery were by no means constant, and far from being so frequent as the cerebral symptoms. To this it should be added that the intestinal hemorrhages which Frerichs observed in these cases were clearly intermittent, and, while they resisted the remedies applied directly against the bleeding, yielded to large doses of quinine. Should we not rather in these cases think of some chemical changes in the blood, as in the hemorrhagic diathesis which accompanies leucæmia, as well as splenic cachexia in general. At any rate, it is difficult to believe in an intermittent obstruction of the vessels.

Only a few appearances remain to be mentioned, of which we know with certainty that they belong to actual melanæmia, and are not the immediate consequence of malarial infection. Here belongs the dark color of the skin, which is produced by the abundance of pigment in the vessels of the cutis. The complexion, in the slighter degrees, is ashy gray; in the more severe forms, yellowish brown. When such a color is found in a person who has suffered recently or remotely from obstinate and severe intermittent fever, and if it further appears that this fever occurred during a malignant epidemic and presented the appearances of a "febris comitata," a very strong suspicion of melanæmia is likely to be aroused and lead to a microscopic examination of the blood.

Diagnosis. Course. Prognosis.

The diagnosis of melanæmia can only be made with certainty by a direct examination of the blood. A drop of blood is obtained in the way already mentioned, carefully avoiding impu-

rities, and examined by the microscope. I have myself made
these examinations in a very large number of suspicious cases,
without ever having discovered a decided case of melanæmia, for
which reason, to my great regret, I can base this description on
no observations of my own. I have always felt called upon to
make such examinations upon the occurrence of severe brain-
symptoms with simultaneous albuminuria or hæmaturia, in persons who presented the gray complexion, and in enlargement of
the spleen, which could be looked upon as the remains of previous attacks of intermittent fever.

The *course* of melanæmia is various ; there are cases which
kill in a few hours or days, while others last for months. The
cephalic forms are almost always acute, the others are just as
often chronic. Among fifty-one cases which Frerichs observed,
twenty-four were acute and twenty-seven chronic.

Prognosis is always doubtful. The remission of the fever
does not justify a favorable prognosis, because not unfrequently
sudden and unexpected relapses occur which may be immediately fatal. In addition, cachexia and hydræmia impend as
consequences of the changes usually undergone by the spleen
and liver.

Therapeutics.

The prophylactic and causal indications are answered by the
rules laid down in the general therapeutic portion of this work.
The method of administration of quinine, which was there thoroughly discussed, deserves the preference before other remedies.
In all severe cases of intermittent fevers its action is so far unsur-
passed. The remedies used to replace it are only to be considered
when there is no necessity for rapid and energetic action.

After the removal of the fever, the second task remains of
removing the remaining local disturbances in the spleen, the
liver, and the brain. We are not in a condition to fulfil the *indicatio morbi*, since we possess no direct means of removing the
pigments from the blood. We should, however, use all energy
and diligence to remove, or at least to diminish the enlargement
of the spleen by a systematic application of the remedies already
described.

I have very recently had an opportunity to observe a case of melanæmia which affords some interest in a therapeutic point of view, so that I will here add a preliminary sketch of it: A ship's carpenter, thirty-six years old, who had acquired an intermittent fever in September, 1874, at Wilmington, N. C., was received in December into my clinic. The very severe attacks recurred irregularly, at intervals of from two to eight days. After long use of oleum eucalypti, with piperin, they became less frequent and less severe.

During the severest attacks the microscopic examination of the blood showed larger and smaller dark pigment-scales, the number of which was less during the apyrexia. They were still found in the blood of this patient by myself and my colleague on the 20th of February, after the febrile attacks had ceased for some time. They were free in the blood, not enclosed in white blood-corpuscles.

I have applied electricity to the clearly perceptible splenic tumor, in the manner recommended by Botkin, and made a microscopic examination of the blood both before and afterwards, but no increase of the pigment in the blood nor diminution of the tumor could be perceived as a result of its electrization. In another place I shall report more minutely this very interesting case, which is still under my treatment.

For the symptomatic indication many remedies are suitable, which are to be chosen according to time and circumstance. Not the least important is the persistent use of iron preparations, ferruginous waters, bog-baths, since the wholesale destruction of red corpuscles leads to an extreme anæmic and hydræmic condition of the blood.

ISEASES OF THE PANCREAS.

FRIEDREICH.

DISEASES OF THE PANCREAS.

I. General.

Alberti, De morbis mesenterii et ejus quod παγκρεας appellatur. Dissert. Wittenberg, 1578.—*Heurnius*, De morbis mesenterii et pancreatis. Ludg. Batav. 1599. *Schenckius a Graefenberg*, Observ. medic. tom. unus. Frankofurt, 1600. Observ. 291. p. 742.—*Boë Sylvius*, Praxeos medicae idea nova. Ludg. Batav. 1667-74. Tom. III.—*De Graaf*, Tractat. anat. med. de succi pancreatis natura et usu. Lugd. Batav. 1664.—*Bonetus*, Polyalthes sive Thesaurus medico-practicus. Tom. II. Genevae, 1691. p. 666.—*Chr. Barth. Holdefreund*, De pancreatis morbis. Dissert. Hal. 1713.[1]—*Brunner*, Experimenta nova circa pancreas. Amstelodam, 1682. Edit. nova. Lugd. Batav. 1722.—*Buechner*, De damnis ex male affecto pancreate in sanitatem reduntantibus. Hal. 1759.—*Barfoth*, De morbis pancreatis affect. Dissert. Lund. 1779.—*Lieutaud*, Histor. anat. med. edit. Schlegel. Vol. I. Longosalissae, 1786. p. 296.—*Th. Cawley*, Lond. Med. Journ. 1788. Sammlung auserlesener Abhandlungen. 13. Bd. Leipzig, 1789. S. 112.—*Conradi*, Handbuch der patholog. Anatomie. Hannover, 1796. S. 219.—*J. R. Rahn*, Scirrhosi pancreatis diagnosis observationibus anat. pathol. illustr. Götting. 1796.—*J. B. Siebold*, Dissert. inaug. med. sistens historiam systematis salivalis physiologice et pathologice observati. Jenae, 1797.—*Voigtel*, Handbuch der pathol. Anat. 1. Bd. Halle, 1804. S. 543.—*G. Hoffmann*, De pancreate ejusque morbis, etc. Altdorf, 1807.—*Chr. Fr. Harles*, Ueber die Krankheiten des Pankreas, mit besonderer Berücksichtigung der Phthisis pancreatica. Nürnberg, 1812. —*Fleischmann*, Leichenöffnungen. Erlangen, 1815.—*Schmackpfeffer*, Observ. de quibusdam pancreatis morbis. Dissert. Hal. 1817.—*Pemberton*, Abhandlung über verschiedene Krankheiten des Unterleibes. Uebers. von *Gerhard von dem Busch*. Bremen, 1817. S. 71.—*C. Vogel*, De pancreatis nosologia generali. Hal. 1819.—*Baillie-Soemmering*, Anatomie des krankhaften Baues von einigen der wichtigsten Theile im menschlichen Körper. Aus dem Engl. Berlin, 1820. S.

---

[1] This oftquoted dissertation is by all authors wrongly attributed to *Fr. Hoffmann*. The mistake is possibly due to the fact that Hoffmann's name, as Dean and President, is printed in large letters, while the name of the author typographically remains in the background.

158. Anhang. S.·106.—*Eyting*, Pancreatitis chronica. Hufeland's Journal. 54.
Bd. 4. Stück. 1822. S. 3.—*Abercrombie*, Edinb. Med. and Surg. Journ. LXXIX.
1824. p. 243. Sammlung auserlesener Abhandlungen. 8. Bd. Leipzig, 1824.
S. 660.—*Annesley*, Researches into the Causes and Treatment of the more Prevalent Diseases of India. Vol. II. 1828. Sammlung auserlesener Abhdlgen. 12.
Bd. 2. Stück. Leipzig, 1829. S. 210.—*Gendrin*, Anat. Beschreibung der Entzündung und ihrer Folgen. Deutsch von *Radius*. 2. Thl. Leipzig, 1829. S.
191, 213, u. 233.—*Bardenhewer*, Dissert. de insania cum morbis pancreatis
conjuncta. Bonn, 1829.—*Urban*, Hufeland's Journal der prakt. Heilkde. 1830.
Nov. S. 87.—*Bécourt*, Recherches sur le pancréas, ses fonctions et ses altérations
organiques. Thèse. Strasbourg, 1830.—*Dawidoff*, De morbis pancreatis observ.
quaedam. Dissert. Dorpat, 1833.—*R. Bright*, Cases and Observations Con-
nected with Disease of the Pancreas and Duodenum. Med. Chir. Transact. Vol.
XVIII. London, 1833. p. 1.—*Lloyd*, Case of Jaundice with Discharge of Fatty
Matter from the Bowels. Ibid. p. 57.—*Elliotson*, On the Discharge of Fatty
Matter from the Alimentary Canal. Ibid. p. 67.—*Hohnbaum*, Zur Diagnose der
Krankheiten der Bauchspeicheldrüse. Casper's Wochenschrift. Nr. 16, 17. 1834.
—*Eberle*, Physiologie der Verdauung. Würzburg, 1834.—*Bigsby*, Observ. on
Diseases of the Pancreas. Edinb. Med. Journ. No. 124. 1835.—*Pollack*, De
pancreate ejusque inflammatione. Diss. Prag, 1835.—*Medicus*, Nonnulla de
morbis pancreatis. Diss. Berol. 1835.—*Mondière*, Recherches pour servir à
l'histoire pathol. du pancréas. Arch. génér. de méd. Mai. 1836. p. 36; Juillet.
p. 265.—*Perle*, De pancreate ejusque morbis. Diss. Berol. 1837.—*Lappe*, De
morbis pancreatis quaedam. Diss. Berol. 1838.—*Hesse*, De morbis pancreatis.
Diss. Berol. 1838.—*Buerger*, Was ist in den neueren Zeiten für die Diagnose
der Krankheiten des Pankreas geschehen? Hufeland's Journal. 89. Bd. 2. St.
1839. S. 104.—*Landsberg*, Einige Bemerkungen über die Krankheiten des un-
teren Magenmundes und der Bauchspeicheldrüse. Ebendas. 91. Bd. 1840. S.
15.—*Bressler*, Die Krankheiten des Unterleibes. 2. Bd. Berlin, 1841. S. 251.—
Jos. Engel, Ueber Krankheiten des Pankreas und seines Ausführungsganges.
Oesterreich. med. Jahrbücher. 23. Bd. 1840. S. 411 ; 24. Bd. 1841. S. 193.—
Claessen, Die Krankheiten der Bauchspeicheldrüse. Cöln, 1842 (Hauptschrift).
—*Jos. Frank*, Praxeos medicae universae praecepta. P. III. Vol. II. (De morbis
systematis hepatici et pancreatis.) Lips. 1843.—*Schlesier*, Zur Lehre vom Scirrh.
der Bauchspeicheldrüse. Med. Zeitung des Vereins für Heilkde. in Preussen.
Nr. 10, 11. 1843.—*Abercrombie*, Pathol. u. prakt. Untersuch. über die Krankh.
des Magens, u. s. w. Uebersetzt von *G. v. d. Busch*. Bremen, 1843. S. 501.—
Battersby, Two Cases of Scirrhus of the Pancreas. Dubl. Journ. of Med. Sc.
Vol. XXV. 1844. p. 219.—*Melion*, Beitrag zur Erkenntniss und Behandlung
der Bauchspeicheldrüsenkrankheiten. Oesterreich. med. Wochenschrift. Nr. 17.
1844.—*Aran*, Observation d'abscès tuberculeux du pancréas. Arch. génér. de
méd. Sept. 1846. p. 61.—*Canstatt*, Spez. Pathol. und Therapie. 2. Aufl. 4. Bd.
2. Abth. Erlangen, 1845. S. 735.—*Gould*, Anat. Museum of the Boston Soc.
Boston, 1847, p. 147.—*Fearnside*, Illustrations of Pancreatic Disease. London

Med. Gaz. 1850.—*Lussanna*, Bulletino delle science med. Bologna. Aug. Sett. 1851. p. 182.—*Moyse*, Étude historique et critique sur les fonctions et les maladies du pancréas. Thèse. Paris, 1852.—*Eisenmann*, Zur Pathologie des Pancreas. Prager Vierteljahrschrift. 40. Bd. 1853. S. 73.—*Reeves*, Ueber Vorkommen von Fett in den Excrementen. Monthly Journ. March, 1854.—*Herbst*, Ztschr. f. ration. Med. N. F. III. Bd. 1853. S. 389.—*Handfield Jones*, Observations Respecting Degeneration of the Pancreas. Med. Chir. Transact. XXXVIII. 1855. p. 195.—*Cl. Bernard*, Mémoire sur le pancréas. Paris, 1856.—*Fauconneau-Dufrèsne*, Précis des maladies du foie et du pancréas. Paris, 1856.—*M. Schiff*, Ueber die Rolle des pancreatischen Saftes und der Galle bei Aufnahme der Fette. Moleschott's Untersuchungen zur Naturlehre. 2. Bd. 1857. S. 345.—*Gross*, Elements of Patholog. Anatomy. Philadelphia, 1857. p. 626.—*Corvisart*, Collection des mémoirs sur une fonction méconnue du pancréas, etc. Paris, 1857-1863.—*Klob*, Zur pathol. Anat. des Pancreas. Oesterreich. Zeitschr. für prakt. Heilkunde. VI. 33. 1860.—*G. Harley*, On Jaundice, its Treatment and Pathology. London, 1863. p. 82.—*Danilewsky*, Ueber spezifisch wirkende Körper des natürlichen und künstlichen pankreatischen Saftes. Virch. Arch. 25. Bd. 1862. S. 279.—*Foerster*, Handbuch der speziellen pathol. Anat. 2. Aufl. Leipzig, 1863. S. 213.—*Fles*, Ein Fall von Diabetes mellitus mit Atrophie der Leber und des Pankreas. Archiv für die holländ. Beiträge zur Natur- und Heilkunde. 3. Bd. Utrecht, 1864. S. 187.—*Hartsen*, Noch Ewas über Diabetes mellitus. Ebendas. S. 319.—*Griscom*, Transact. of the American Med. Association. Vol. XIV. Philadelph. 1864.—*Maurice Besson*, De quelques faits pathologiques pour servir à l'étude du pancréas. Thèse. Paris, 1864.—*O. Wyss*, Zur Aetiologie des Stauungsicterus. Virch. Archiv. 36. Bd. 1866. S. 455.—*Ancelet*, Études sur les maladies du pancréas. Paris, 1866.—*Maigre*, Des phénomènes cliniques de la digestion à propos d'une obsérvation de tumeurs du pancréas. Thèse. Paris, 1866.—*Oppolzer*, Ueber Krankheiten des Pancreas. Wiener medic. Wochenschrift. Nr. 1, 2. 1867.—*Kuehne*, Ueber Verdauung der Eiweissstoffe durch den Pancreassaft. Virchow's Arch. 39. Bd. 1867. p. 130.—*Klebs*, Handbuch der pathol. Anat. Berlin, 1870. p. 529.—*Bernstein*, Zur Physiologie der Bauchspeichelabsonderung. Arbeiten des physiol. Instituts zu Leipzig. IV. p. 1–36. 1870.—Sitzungsberichte der sächsischen Akad. der Wissenschaften zu Leipzig, 1869. p. 96.—*Silver*, Trans. Pathol. Soc. Lond. XXIV. 1873.

Historical Sketch.

We find but few and vague references to the pancreas and its diseases among the writings of the older physicians. It was only towards the close of the sixteenth century that Alberti (1578) and Heurnius (1599) endeavored to describe the diseases of the pancreas in a more comprehensive manner—an attempt, however, which naturally 'was not followed by any permanent results, seeing that all useful and reliable clinical and anatomo-physiological knowledge of the subject was quite wanting, and further, that the most indefinite notions as to the nature and physiological function of the organ still prevailed. At one time the pancreas was regarded as a structure evidently for the protection of the neighboring vessels, at other times as the seat of the most varied diseases, such as ague, hypochondriasis, melancholia, etc. (Fernelius). But later (1642), when Wirsung had discovered the excretory duct, the pancreas had to be looked on as a special organ, and this must be considered as the first step to a definite and successful investigation of its physiological and pathological importance. But notwithstanding this, the oddest views as to the nature of the organ and its relation to disease continued to prevail for a long time, and it was especially the so generally accepted theories of Le Boë Sylvius and his school, which at all events thus far stood in the way of further progress, by teaching that the cause of digestion lay in an intestinal fermentation (effervescentia intestinalis) brought about by mixture of the acid pancreatic fluid with the alkaline bile, and that the origin of most diseases was due to an interference with this process.

It is the medical literature of the eighteenth century which supplies the earliest reliable facts on the pathology of the pancreas. Among the authors of this period, who furnished important clinical contributions may especially be mentioned Holdefreund (1713), Buechner (1759), Barfoth (1779), Rahn, 1796, and J. B. Siebold (1797), while to Morgagni, Lieutaud, and Conradi we are indebted for an exhaustive retrospect of all the facts then known relative to the pathological anatomy of this subject. Among the authors of the beginning and first half of the present century, who have advanced the pathology of this organ, the following are the most prominent: G. Hoffmann (1807), Harles (1812), Schmackpfeffer (1817), Bécourt (1830), R. Bright (1833), Mondière (1836), Jos. Frank (1843), but it was especially Claessen, through his well-known monograph on the diseases of the pancreas, in which he reviewed and criticised the earlier recorded cases with marvellous ability and learning. Among later works may be mentioned those of Fauconneau-Dufrèsne, on concretions in the pancreas (1851), and of Ancelet (1866) on diseases of the pancreas, but with especial reference to cancerous induration.

It is, however, only quite recently that any really reliable facts on the clinical pathology of the diseases of the pancreas have been obtained; and this through a number of carefully observed single cases, and also through the labors of numerous investigators in pathological anatomy (Cruveilhier, Rokitansky, Virchow, Klebs) and in physiology (Bernard, Schiff, Corvisart, Danilewsky, Kuehne, Senator, and Bernstein). The great rarity of diseases of this organ considerably hinders a more rapid development of the knowledge of their clinical bearings and pathological characters, so that, as compared with other organs of the body in these respects, we are necessarily behindhand.

Preliminary Remarks, Anatomical and Physiological.

Seeing the intimate anatomical relation in which the pancreas stands with some of the most important organs of the abdomen, it may be well to begin with a short exposition of the topographical anatomy.[1] The large number of possible symptoms of pancreas disease depends, no doubt, on this intimate relation of the pancreas with neighboring organs, and both the knowledge and a proper appreciation of the symptoms will be best facilitated if the more intimate of these relations be here plainly laid down; nor will an epitome of some important points in the physiology of the gland be entirely without interest to the pathologist.

The pancreas is a long, narrow, acinous gland, which lies crossways behind the stomach and left lobe of the liver. It can be exposed in its entire length by cutting through the gastro-colic omentum, parallel with the lower border of the stomach, and by drawing the stomach upward, and the transverse colon downward.

---

[1] Compare *Henle*, Handbook of Systematic Anatomy. 2 vols. Brunswick, 1862. p. 218. *Luschka*, The Human Abdominal Organs. Carlsruhe, 1873. p. 30. *Ruedinger*, Topograph. Surgical Anatomy. 1st and 2d parts. Stuttgart, 1873. p. 136.

The pancreas will now be seen at the bottom of the sac of the omentum (Bursa omentalis), covered by peritoneum (ascending layer of the transverse meso-colon). The middle portion of the gland (the body) lessens towards the tail, which reaches as far as the hilus of the spleen, with which, as also with the kidney and suprarenal capsule, it is connected by loose areolar tissue ; towards its right extremity (the head) the gland increases in size, especially in an upward and in a downward direction, so that the entire organ has, in some measure, the appearance of a hammer (Henle). The ascending portion of the head lies in the concavity of the duodenum, and is connected with the ascending and descending portions by means of dense areolar tissue. The descending portion, the so-called pancreas parvum, inclines backward and outward, and sometimes even forms an almost complete ring around the duodenum.

The length of the pancreas in adults averages 23 ctms., its breadth 4.5, and its thickness 2.8 ctms. Its weight varies from 90 to 120 grms. The remarkably granular appearance of its surface on section is due to the unusually loose areolar tissue which surrounds its acini.

The arteries of the pancreas are derived from the pancreatico-duodenal branch of the hepatic, from the splenic, and from the superior mesenteric. They penetrate between the lobules, and surround the ultimate vesicles with a capillary net-work, from which veins arise, which empty themselves into the vena portæ and the splenic vein. The lymphatics join those of the spleen, and terminate in the upper lumbar glands. The nerves are derived from the hepatic, splenic, and superior mesenteric branches of the solar plexus. It is probable, also, that branches of the right vagus reach it.

The posterior surface of the pancreas lies on a level with the first lumbar vertebra, on the pars lumbalis (pillars) of the diaphragm. Its anterior surface is covered with peritoneum (the posterior layer of the lesser omentum). Behind the pancreas, and connected with it by areolar tissue, are found the vena cava, the abdominal aorta, and the commencement of the vena portæ. With its lower border it covers the commencement of the superior mesenteric artery and the termination of its accompanying vein, and across its upper border is the cœliac axis, so that the pancreas runs between the cœliac axis and the origin of the superior mesenteric artery. A shallow groove along its upper border serves for the splenic artery and vein, the former running in a very tortuous course from right to left. The anatomical relation of the pancreas to the solar plexus and its ganglia is of considerable importance in the estimation of certain pathological phenomena, as these nerves, lying on the pillars of the diaphragm, in front of the aorta, are covered by it. Not less important is a knowledge of the topographical relation of the pancreas to the ductus choledochus, on which point we are indebted to Wyss for exact details. As a rule (fifteen times in twenty-two), the bile-duct descends near the head of the pancreas, towards the duodenum; not rarely it goes through the head, but in such a way as sometimes to be only partially, sometimes entirely surrounded by gland substance. It is obvious, therefore, that the bile-duct, when it simply passes over the pancreas, would be pushed aside by any enlargement of this gland, unless the enlargement were very considerable, in which case the duct might then be compressed and interfered with; whereas, in the cases in which the bile-duct passes through gland-substance, a comparatively small enlargement of the pancreas would suffice to close the duct entirely, and so cause jaundice. The principal excretory duct, called the canal of Wirsung, is about as large as a goose-quill; it is lined with columnar epithelium. It commences by the union of five branches at the tail-end, and runs from left to right through the entire length of the gland, nearer the posterior than the anterior surface. The comparatively small branches of the individual lobes unite at acute angles with the principal duct. In the head the duct curves slightly downward, and, as a rule, opens with the bile-duct (though it sometimes opens separately) into the duodenum. Before the main duct opens into the duodenum, it is generally joined by a large, curved branch from the upper part of the head, which, however, sometimes opens independently into the duodenum (D. pancreat-recurrens, Bernard; canalis pancreaticus azygos, Verneuil; ductus pancreaticus accessorius). In other cases this accessory duct joins with the ductus choledochus in a common opening, while the main duct opens separately. It also happens that both ducts, about equal in size, may run through the pancreas, and only be connected by a single small branch; and even this branch may be absent, so that the secretion is conveyed by two entirely separate ducts, each one opening independently into the intestine, as is the rule in dogs.

Many controversies as to the minute structure still require settling. It is not yet decided whether the alveoli are surrounded by a membrana propria, or not, or whether the secreting cells possess a special investment; nor how the cells behave during the various phases of functional activity; nor whether a system of fine capillary tubes (without walls) is to be found between the alveoli, which carries the secretion into the central duct of the acinus (Saviotti, Gianuzzi, Langerhans, Ewald), or whether such a net-work is artificial (Latschenberger). The statement by Boll, that from the interior of the membrana propria, which lines the alveoli, there is given off a reticulum, consisting of branched cells, which spreads out between the epithelial cells, and supports them in its meshes, requires further confirmation. Pflueger's idea, that the secreting cells are in direct communication with nerve-twigs, has been freely disputed. However desirable for the progress of pathological anatomy that these points concerning the minute histological structure of the pancreas should be settled, they are questions of less moment to us, from a clinical point of view, than the topographical relations of the entire organ, to which we have already alluded.

Concerning the physiology of this, the abdominal salivary gland, it is certain that it plays a most important part in the digestion of all kinds of organic food. We now know that the pancreatic secretion assists both in the transformation of starch into dextrine and sugar, and in the digestion of albumens and of fat, and Danilewsky has shown that each one of these three functions is brought about by a special ferment which is contained in the pancreatic juice.

The power of the pancreatic juice, as proved by Eberle,[1] of quickly converting starch into sugar exceeds that of the salivary

---

[1] Physiologie der Verdauung. Würzburg, 1834. p. 245.

glands, nor is its action further down the intestine in any way interfered with by the admixture, either of bile or of gastric juice. It was discovered by Prospero Sonsino[1] and Korowin,[2] and recently confirmed by Zweifel,[3] that the pancreatic juice possesses absolutely no sugar-forming power over starch during infancy; and that this power is not acquired until after the earlier months of life; and that it is not perfectly developed until towards the close of the first year, a fact not devoid of pathological interest.

The second function of the pancreatic juice, viz., to emulsify neutral fat, and so facilitate its absorption by the lymph-glands of the intestine, did not escape Eberle's[4] notice. Herbst (1853), however, showed by experiment that even after ligature of the pancreatic duct, neutral fat still found its way into the lymph-vessels in not inconsiderable quantities, thus proving that the pancreas, although the most important, was not the only means of promoting fat absorption as taught by Cl. Bernard. Bile also possesses the power of emulsifying fat and aiding in its absorption. Lenz, Bidder, and Schmidt have proved by experiment that during the absence of bile from the intestine the amount of fat absorbed is less in quantity, and Steiner[5] has lately shown that the intestinal juices also emulsify fat and make it absorbable. The peristaltic action of the intestine must be considered as an important factor in the production of a permanent emulsion and of its absorption.

Now, although the larger quantity of fat taken in with our nourishment is absorbed in a highly divided but yet otherwise unaltered condition, as was first shown by Cl. Bernard,[6] a smaller portion of it is converted by the pancreatic juice into fatty acids and glycerine, and this would seem to be a special function of the pancreas, and one peculiar to it. This process is not interfered

---

[1] Imparz. di Firenze. 16. Agosto. 1872.

[2] Centralblatt für die medic. Wissenschaften. Nr. 17. 1873. S. 261.

[3] Untersuchungen über den Verdauungsapparat der Neugeborenen. Berlin, 1874. S. 37.

[4] Loc. cit., p. 251.

[5] Archiv f. Anat., Physiol. und wissenschftl. Med. 1874. p. 286.

[6] Mémoire sur le pancréas. Paris, 1856.

with by mixture with the gastric juice, since, even in presence of abundance of gastric juice, a considerable quantity of free fatty acids has been found after eating fat, both in the large and small intestines, as well as in the fæces (Hoppe). The fatty acids, however, for the most part, recombine in the intestine and form with the alkaline salts of the bile, and also of the pancreas itself, and of the intestinal juices, soapy compounds, which, by their presence, materially assist the emulsifying action of the pancreatic juice (Bruecke). What further rôle these soaps play in the blood, after absorption by the radicles of the vena portæ and lacteals, is not yet settled. They may either be directly oxidized in the blood or the fatty acids may again be set free, and by combination with glycerine be converted into fat, either to be burnt off in this form, or to be stored up in the tissues for future use.

In virtue of its third function—that of digesting albuminous compounds,—as was believed by Purkinje and Pappenheim, proved beyond all doubt by Corvisart (1857), and since confirmed by Meissner, Kuehne, Senator, and others, the pancreas must be looked upon as an accessory organ to the stomach thus far, that the peptonizing of such parts of the albuminous bodies as has not been completed by the gastric juice devolves on it. The co-operation of free acid is not necessary; on the contrary, the peptonizing pancreatic ferment seems to lose its digestive power in the presence of any large amount of acids. The gastric juice has no disturbing effect, because all its free acid is at once neutralized and the pepsin precipitated by the bile. By the continued action of the pancreatic secretion the peptones are again broken up, chiefly into leucin and tyrosin; these are at last voided as fæcal matters (Kuehne), which are the ultimate products of the prolonged action of the pancreatic juice.

When fresh pancreatic juice is clear and colorless, it contains fifteen to twenty per cent. of solid constituents, and when exposed to the air, deposits a jelly-like clot; it is strongly alkaline in its reaction; its chief constituent is albumen; besides this, there is potassium albuminate (Kalialbuminat), and certain quantities of those three peculiar organic ferments—sugar-producing, peptonizing, and fat-destroying—of which, however, only the first two have been definitely isolated.[1] It also contains considerable quantities of leucin (Virchow, Scherer, Frerichs, Staedeler), which, since it is found abundantly in the fresh secretion, would seem to be formed by the action of the peptonizing ferment on the protoplasma of the secreting cells. We must, at all events, admit that the leucin found in the intestine is only partly the result of the decomposition of the protein bodies taken in as food.

As to some other amides which are found in pancreatic juice, such as tyrosin, guanin, xanthin, etc., it is doubtful whether they exist in the fresh secretion, and are not rather the result of decomposition. Lastly, the pancreatic juice contains a small quantity of saponaceous compounds, and some inorganic materials, chloride of sodium, carbonates and phosphates of the alkalies and alkaline earths.

The formation and secretion of pancreatic juice is not continuous, but commences shortly after the reception of food into the stomach (Bidder and Schmidt, Bernard, Frerichs, Bernstein). Schiff describes a period of rest, and one of activity. During the period of rest, such as is found in fasting animals, the gland is pale, flabby, and shiny, its secretion very scant; its cells are transparent, and its veins contain dark blood. In the stage of activity it is opaque, turgescent, and if digestion be going on, is secreting; then it is reddened, and its juice flows in rapid drops, or even in a small stream if an artificial opening be made for it. It is only the active pancreas that contains and secretes the real ferments, according to Schiff and Corvisart, though Kuehne believes that the gland, even when inactive, exerts a powerfully digestive action in alkaline solutions on albuminoid bodies. Schiff believes that this charging (Ladung) of the gland is brought about by the absorption of peptones from the stomach, a circumstance that would satisfactorily explain its taking place during and towards the end of stomach digestion. Even more

---

[1] According to the most recent researches of *Heidenhain*, the peptonizing ferment does not exist as such preformed and perfect in the living gland, but is formed during secretion from a substance contained in the secretory gland-cells, which *Heidenhain* calls "Zymogen."—Berliner klin. Wochenschrift. No. 15. 1875. p. 198.

than peptones, the pancreas seems able to take up dextrine,
but only when it has passed through and from the stomach.

According to Bernstein's observations, the secretion of the
pancreas becomes considerable during the first hour of digestion,
attains its maximum during the second or third hour, and decreases again, until from the fifth to the ninth hour, when it
again increases; about fifteen hours after taking in food, it
gradually sinks to *nil*. The two separate secretory flows, the
one shortly after a meal, the other after the lapse of a few hours,
correspond to the entry of the food, firstly, into the stomach,
and later on, into the intestine. The increased blood-flow during
the activity of the gland must be explained as due to the stimulus of the ingesta on the sensory nerves of the mucous membrane of the stomach and of the intestine, acting by reflex action
not only on the secreting nerves of the gland itself, but also by
causing at the same time a dilatation of its afferent arteries.

A remarkable fact was observed by Weinmann and Bernard,
and more recently also by Bernstein, namely, that the pancreas
secretion is arrested by the act of vomiting, also during the
nausea which precedes. The last named investigator succeeded,
after section of the vagus and irritation of its central end, in
entirely arresting the secretion; an arrest which continued for a
long time after the irritation had been discontinued. Irritation
of the peripheral end of the cut vagus produced no effect. The
simple section of one vagus or of both was also without result.
On the contrary, section of the nerves accompanying the arteries
produced a free and continuous secretion of normal juice, with
redness and even œdema of the gland, and, under these circumstances, no inhibitory action could be produced on the secretion
by stimulating the vagus. It would seem, then, from these experiments that the arrest of secretion during vomiting, as also
from irritation of the vagus, is due to reflex action of the spinal
cord and sympathetic nerve. But, as before mentioned, it is
certain that irritation of the mucous membrane of the stomach
by food brings about, and increases, the pancreatic secretion,
and so it would appear as though this organ were under the
influence of two sets of nerves from the vagus, one of which
inhibits, while the other excites the secreting power (Bernstein).

General Pathology and Symptomatology.

In passing from the consideration of such points in anatomy and physiology as were most important to the pathologist, to the general symptomatology of diseases of the pancreas, it must be remarked, in spite of the very important and manifold part which the pancreas takes in the digestion of all kinds of food, that in only very rare cases shall we be able, from an analysis of the functional disturbances, to diagnose pancreas disease. The obvious reason for this is, that the pancreas does not possess singly and solely any one special function, but rather shares them with many others of the digestive organs. Thus, it shares its saccharifying power with the saliva, perhaps also with the secretion from Brunner's glands, its peptonizing properties with the gastric juice and succus entericus, and its power of emulsifying neutral fats with the bile; while its power of breaking up fat into fatty acids and glycerine is the only one which, as far as our knowledge of to-day goes, can be said to be peculiar to the pancreas.

It seems no longer doubtful that, in disease of the pancreas, its deranged or even entirely suppressed function can be undertaken and compensated for by the other digestive fluids, provided these be sufficient in quality and quantity ; and indeed, the observation of those cases in which the pancreas has been found to have been the only organ, or chiefly affected, has disclosed no appreciable disturbance in the functions which are assigned to the pancreas. On the other hand, morbid disturbance of these peculiar functions ought not to be considered as an absolute proof of disease of the pancreas, seeing how often similar disturbances have been observed in diseases of the stomach, duodenum, liver, etc., when no complication of the pancreas has *post-mortem* been found. In the majority of cases of pancreas disease, it happens that other and neighboring organs, either the stomach, duodenum, liver, gall-duct, or peritoneum, are in some way or other implicated, so that we get a complexity of symptoms which point to one of these organs rather than to the pancreas. The intimate relation of the pancreatic nerves and vessels with those of other organs in the upper belly produces a most complicated and ever-changing picture of disease, out of which specific symptoms the less readily show themselves and can be isolated, seeing that the pancreas does not possess any special function the disturbance of which would produce not pathogno-monic, but even appreciable symptoms. Then, if we consider the depth at which this organ lies and the difficulty of any examina-tion from without, we shall understand the difficulties and some of the hinderances which stand in the way of a knowledge of pan-creas diseases.

But the great rarity of this disease must be looked on as the greatest obstacle in our way. Primary and uncomplicated dis-ease, from the observation of which our knowledge would be best furthered, is unusually rare ; there is scarcely any other organ in the body so little liable to idiopathic disease. No doubt quite different views were held on this subject by the older physi-cians. After Wirsung had discovered its secretory duct, and Le Boë Sylvius had founded his theory of intestinal fermenta-tion, medical men for a long time believed that the pancreas was frequently diseased, and became affected in almost all chronic complaints ; they were even inclined to regard it as the source of the most diverse symptoms. Even in 1713, Holdefreund believed that the pancreas was more often the seat of cancerous indura-tion than any other organ in the body, and this leads to the suggestion that the gland, on account of its compact, granular appearance, has often been considered indurated, while it was really normal. In presence of such views, it behooves us to use the greatest care before utilizing any data furnished by older writers bearing on the pathology of diseases of the pancreas. Later physicians have come to an opposite opinion as to the relative frequency of these diseases, and Baillie assures us that during many years of active practice he had only seen one single case in which pancreas disease was verified by *post-mortem* ex-amination.

All these facts explain why our knowledge of the pathology of the pancreas is so scant and so far behind that of all the other internal organs. How little we have to rely upon for our diag-nosis will be seen from the following description.

One symptom of disease of the pancreas which has been chiefly, and, I believe, was first urged by Pemberton, is emaciation of the whole body, beginning early and proceeding to an unusual degree. The recorded cases of primary, uncomplicated, non-cancerous affection of the pancreas are by no means rare in which there had been great emaciation; and this is easily intelligible in the absence of the fat-absorbing, peptonizing power so largely attributed to the pancreas. We must not, however, allow ourselves on this account to attribute too much importance to this symptom, since the same degree of emaciation not unfrequently accompanies various organic diseases of others of the digestive organs, where the pancreas is quite intact, such as the stomach, duodenum, liver, etc., and we must not forget, further, that disease of the pancreas may be complicated with organic changes, such as obstruction of the pylorus, or duodenum, or gall-duct, which of itself would be sufficient to account even for a high degree of general marasmus. There is, however, a chief point which materially affects the importance of this symptom, namely, that there is a series of well-authenticated cases of affection of the pancreas and closure of its duct, in which not only has there been an entire absence of emaciation, but in which even a certain amount of corpulence has been preserved. Abercrombie and Claessen had already drawn attention to these cases when Schiff collected and published a series of similar instances. Again, in very corpulent subjects, the pancreas is occasionally found in such a state of complete fatty degeneration that scarcely any of its real gland-tissue remains, and consequently there must be an entire absence of all secretion. No doubt, in these and similar cases, it is the bile which, in the absence of the pancreatic juice, is able to sufficiently emulsify and render fit for absorption the fat; and so it would seem that the greatest emaciation is found in those cases in which, together with disease of the pancreas, the function of the liver or a flow of bile is interfered with; or where the disease mechanically interferes with the general nutrition, either by compressing the pylorus or the duodenum; or, lastly, where the disease itself is such that in any other place or organ a high degree of marasmus would result (cancer, for instance).

In proof of this assertion, that an absence of the pancreatic fluid does not alone suffice to cause marked emaciation, we might refer to results obtained experimentally, in which the pancreas of dogs has been extirpated or caused to atrophy by the injection of different materials into its ducts. Brunner[1] is generally regarded as the first who noticed that young dogs recovered and might so thrive after extirpation of the pancreas, that nothing unusual could be noticed about them ; and Colin[2] and Bérard are both said to have performed similar experiments with a like result. But these experiments are not convincing, because only a portion, not the entire gland, was removed, and because more recent experiments by Bernard and Schiff, in which the entire gland was removed, have been resultless, owing to rapid death of the animals from acute peritonitis.[3] Schiff only succeeded in saving birds (ravens and pigeons) for any length of time after complete extirpation of the pancreas ; digestion did not seem in any way disturbed, and after death the intestinal epithelium was found charged with fat-globules.

Of more importance are the experiments of Bernard[4] and Schiff, who sought to injure the secreting function of the gland by injecting different substances into its ducts. But although some of the animals lived a considerable time afterwards, no especial emaciation was observable. Bernard, who injected fat, found that a portion of the fat taken as food was passed in the fæces. Schiff used paraffine for injection ; this solidified, and the gland gradually but completely atrophied. Dogs which had been so treated took their food again after a few days, their appetite kept good, and they rapidly gained flesh, and neither their power of digesting in general, nor that of digesting fat in especial, was in any way altered; neither was there any change observed in their fæces.

---

[1] Experimenta nova circa pancreas. Amstelod. 1682. p. 10.

[2] Compare *Besson*. De quelques faits pathologiques pour servir à l'étude du pancreas. Thèse. Paris, 1864. p. 6.

[3] Only one case of partial extirpation of the human pancreas is known to me. It is reported by *Kleberg* as occurring in a man æt. 60, from whom the head of the pancreas, protruding through a wound in the abdominal wall, was removed. . Recovery followed uninterruptedly. (Archiv für klin. Chirurgie. IX. Bd. 1868. p. 523.)

[4] Mémoire sur le pancréas. Paris, 1856. p. 99.

A second symptom which, from a diagnostic point of view, must be considered as important, has been mentioned by Rahn, J. Frank, Fourcroy, Wichmann, and many others, viz., a flow of saliva-like fluid from the mouth, either as eructations or by frequent spitting. This was at one time considered as a hyperse-cretion from the salivary glands—the expression of an especial sympathy[1] between these glands and the pancreas; at another time this fluid was considered as an access of pancreatic fluid (Portal, Wedekind, Harles, Schmackpfeffer), and on that account it was thought justifiable to speak of a " Salivatio s. Sia-lorrhœa pancreatica." But we must be careful in considering such an increased salivary secretion as due to disease of the pancreas, for as yet there are no recorded cases of primary uncomplicated pancreas disease in which this symptom was definitely present.

The observations are few and have no good foundation, on which it was tried to base the theory that a consensual, sympathetic or vicarious relationship existed between the pancreas and the salivary glands. On the contrary, we have in the literature of this subject definite data to show that there has been no ptyalism; and many observers, including Annesley and others, have even quoted cases in which an unusually dry condition of the mouth and throat has been observed. An increased secretion of saliva, as is well known, is often present in some chronic diseases of the stomach where there is no implication of the pancreas (chronic gastric catarrh, cancer); and it has been shown by Frerichs[2] that in these cases the watery vomiting (vomitus matutinus aquosus, Wasserkolk) which occurs in the early morning is due to the large quantities of saliva which have been secreted and swallowed during the night. And if we just consider for a moment how often disease of the pancreas is complicated with disease of the stomach, we shall be the more inclined to look upon this flow of saliva as a strong argument in favor of such

[1] *Regnerus de Graaf*, a pupil of Sylvius, also refers to a sympathetic relationship between the pancreas and the salivary glands (Opera omnia. Lugd. Batav. 1678. p. 282. De succo pancreat. Cap. I.)

[2] Art. "Verdauung" in *R. Wagner's* Handwörterbuch der Physiologie. III. B. 1. Abthlg. 1846. S. 791.

complication, and under these circumstances, therefore, the symptom loses all its diagnostic value, as concerns the pancreas.

Besides which, we have as yet no sufficient grounds to assert even the existence of a pancreatic salivation; we certainly possess no knowledge of any diseases in which this hypersecretion occurs, even if it occur at all.   But, if we allow the existence of such a thing, it will then be impossible to deny that any unusually large secretion into the duodenum may be brought up as eructations or by vomiting; still, at present we have no positive proofs, and should guard ourselves from accepting such fluids as pancreatic juice, unless a very careful examination of the same reveal the presence of abundance of leucin.   Neither must we forget the fact already alluded to (p. 562), that the secreting function of the pancreas is almost at a standstill, not only during the act of vomiting, but also during the stage of nausea which precedes it.   The same doubts must be expressed as to the existence, as a symptom of disease of the pancreas, of a thin, viscid and constant diarrhœa, spoken of as "Diarrhœa pancreatica," "Fluxus cœliacus," "Fluxus pancreaticus," the assumption of which is unproved and hypothetical.   As we have said before, the possibility of hypersecretion of the pancreas (salivatio abdominalis) is by no means proved; and to say, as did earlier physicians, like Wedekind, that a fluxus cœliacus is the result of a slight temporary inflammation of the pancreas with increased flow of pancreatic juice, is altogether arbitrary, as was the doctrine of Portal, that most kinds of diarrhœa are due to this same cause.   Only one single case has been brought forward which would support the idea of a "fluxus pancreaticus" in the sense of the earlier pathologists, viz., a report by Levier "On the Presence of Large Quantities of Leucin in the Fæces during a Cholera Epidemic in Bern in 1863 and 1864."[1]   The leucin was found in the discharges, partly in the well-known form of concentrically sheathed globules, and partly as small crystalline rods and plates (scales), some single, some in the form of wheels, and others aggregated into clusters.   It is, however, by no means

---

[1] Schweizerische Zeitschrift für Heilkunde. 3. Bd. Bern, 1864. S. 140.   This remarkable cholera-epidemic followed immediately upon one of measles, and was accompanied with cases of epidemic parotitis with secondary orchitis.

certain that this was hypersecretion of the pancreas, accompanying as it did a severe epidemic form of intestinal catarrh, though
it will no doubt serve to draw the attention of pathologists to
this very interesting question.

The presence of fat in the stools, however, is a symptom of
much greater diagnostic importance. Kuntzmann[1] (1820), so far
as I am acquainted with the literature of the subject, seems to
have been the first to draw attention to the relation between this
symptom and induration of the pancreas, and described the passing, at different times, of large quantities of fat with the stools,
in a man who died of jaundice and dropsy, with induration of
the pancreas and obliteration of the canal of Wirsung.[2] But it
was not until after Bright had published (1833) his seven cases
of pancreas disease, in which this symptom had been present
three times, that the attention of pathologists was especially directed to it, and then, from various quarters, confirmatory observations came in. First to be mentioned are the cases of Lloyd
and Elliotson (1833) ; also the case, reported by Gould (1847), of
a man, æt. forty, with calculi and cysts in the pancreas, and
stools highly charged with fat; then came the case published by
Lussanna (1851). Reeves collected sixteen fatal cases where there
had been fat in the stools ; of these, in eleven cases there was
disease of the pancreas or of its duct (fatty induration ; cancer ;
induration of the head of the gland, with obliteration of its excretory duct ; cysts in the head of the gland, with obliteration of
the duct of Wirsung and of the bile-duct ; concretions in the
pancreatic duct ; cancer of the liver, causing obstruction of the
pancreatic duct); in five cases only was the pancreas healthy.
Griscom collected twenty-four cases of fatty stools, of which fourteen died, and in eight cases disease of the pancreas was proved
by post-mortem examination ; in fourteen cases no examination
was made. Moyse also, who ventures to attribute an almost pathognomonic importance to this symptom, collected a number of
cases, in support of Bernard's doctrine that the pancreas is really

[1] Hufeland's Journal. 1820.

[2] It is true that two cases with fatty stools are recorded by *Tulpius* (Observ. anat
Amstelodam. 1652. Lib. III. Cap. XVIII. and XIX. pp. 216 and 218), but as there
was no autopsy it is doubtful whether the pancreas was really affected.

the only fat-digesting organ in the body. In the cases of total atrophy of the pancreas in diabetic patients, recorded by Fles (1864) and by Silver (1873), fatty stools were present.[1] It is obvious, from the list of cases given above, which makes no pretence at being complete, that a remarkable coincidence exists between disease of the pancreas and the presence of fat in the stools, and we may here again refer to the confirmatory experiments of Bernard, who found considerable quantities of fat in the excrement of dogs, whose pancreas-function had been suppressed by the injection of various substances into its ducts.

The appearance and the amount of fat so passed has been variously described by different authors. At one time it has appeared in small lumps, pale yellow or whitish in color, and varying from a pea to a nut in size, soluble in ether, and easily melted and burned if thrown into the fire. At another time, when the fæces had cooled, it had formed a thick cake around the edges of the containing vessel, or more or less completely smeared the surface of the masses of fæces, or even swam in a fluid oleaginous condition on the surface of the liquid fæces. In many of the cases it was stated that the fat appeared, with scarcely any fæcal admixture, to have flowed from the rectum like oil (stearrhœa). I have myself observed one case in which the stools consisted entirely of fat—partly amorphous, tallow-like lumps, and partly crystalline. We had here undoubtedly to deal with a case of plugging of the ductus choledochus for several days, with biliary concretions, and where the mouth of the pancreatic duct had also been occluded.

A man, æt. 60, very corpulent, and a great beer-drinker, was taken ill five days before his admission—August 8, 1874—with paroxysmal and increasing pains in the region of the liver, faintness, and constant hiccough. On admission, he was found to have marked jaundice, pain on pressure over the somewhat enlarged liver region. In spite of his fatness, the greatly distended gall-bladder could be felt through the abdominal wall. Urine contained bile and albumen. Spleen normal. A stool passed on the day of his admission consisted of a whitish gray, thick, slimy material, without any fæcal admixture or odor. The microscope showed it to consist of a large number of irregularly shaped, amorphous, tallow-

---

[1] In reference to all the authors here quoted, consult the list given at the commencement of this essay.

like lumps, with enormous masses of needle-crystals aggregated into sheaves and tufts; other constituents were altogether absent, except here and there a single crystal of triple phosphate. A more minute examination showed it to be fat. The addition of ether reduced the masses and crystals to oil-globules. Acetic acid produced a similar result, as did also hydrochloric and sulphuric acids; and under the microscope it could be seen how these masses and crystals break up into oil-globules under their action. (It seemed as though, by the action of these acids, the neutral fats were broken up into fatty acids and glycerine.) In potash solution these crystals became converted into an amorphous, saponaceous material. It ought to be stated that this patient, both just before and subsequently to his admission, took considerable quantities of milk. During the night of the 10th of August—up to which time he had had frequent stools of the above-described character—the pain in the liver ceased, and from this time he passed, several times daily, highly bilious, watery evacuations, from which all traces of fat quickly disappeared. The jaundice gradually passed off, and in the course of a few days the patient was quite convalescent. (For the purpose of comparison, I dissolved some margaric acid in warm glycerine. On its cooling, a tallow-like substance separated, which, on the addition of ether and of the above-mentioned acids, underwent the same microscopic changes as did the masses composing these stools.)

In estimating the value of fatty stools as diagnostic of disease of the pancreas, we must carefully remember that healthy human fæces contain a certain amount of fat after the ingestion of a rich, fat diet, as also after the use of castor or cod-liver oils, for it appears that the secretions of the liver and pancreas, although normal in quantity and quality, do not always suffice to render digestible any unusual amount of fat, so that these fatty stools can only be looked upon as a pathological condition, provided that they occur without there having been any unusual or large ingestion of fat. From the very important part which the pancreatic juice plays in the digestion and absorption of fat, these well authenticated cases are easily intelligible, in which primary and uncomplicated diseases of the pancreas were followed by fatty evacuations, either because the pancreatic juice was no longer normal in its composition, or because its flow into the intestine was interfered with. But large and frequent fatty evacuations are especially found in such cases of pancreas disease as are complicated with hepatic disease, in which therefore, in addition to the want of pancreatic secretion, there is obstructive jaundice, the result of a simultaneous interference with the flow of bile, and consequently a deficiency in the intestine of the two fluids so essentially necessary for the proper absorption of the fats.

And although numerous cases are on record, in which, in spite of disease of the pancreas, no fatty stools occurred, it is no ground to detract from its pathognomonic value, partly because in the disease the formation and secretion of the fluid may be only partially interfered with, or because a less quantity in conjunction with bile may be sufficient to bring about the absorption of the ingested fat, provided it be not taken in too great quantity. It seems possible that the bile alone, under certain circumstances, may suffice to emulsify and absorb considerable quantities of fat, and Hartsen failed to detect any unusual amount of fat in the evacuation of two diabetic patients, who had daily taken from eight to ten spoonfuls of cod-liver oil, though at the post-mortem examination the atrophied pancreas had scarcely left any traces behind.

Another circumstance, however, which cannot be passed over in silence, is that cases are known of disease confined to the liver and its ducts, where the pancreas was quite healthy and yet fatty stools occurred, although no large quantity of fat had been indulged in. Bright has brought forward such cases, and among the eighteen cases collected by Reeves there were six in which this condition was said to exist. However much, therefore, such observations may lessen the diagnostic value of fatty stools as a means of diagnosis of disease of the pancreas, it will nevertheless be allowed, seeing the frequent coincidence of the one with the other, that the presence of such evacuations speaks strongly in favor of this disease, especially if other symptoms be present, and if at the same time it be possible to exclude with some certainty coincident disease of the liver.

It is obvious that the amount of fat excreted will be in direct proportion to the amount which is taken in. But by a comparison of the recorded cases we every now and then hit on cases in which the amount of fat excreted in the stools is out of all proportion to that which is ingested. If the possibility of such a condition of things could really be proved by careful observation, provided it were not the result of a mistake on the part of the observer, nor of wilful misrepresentation on the part of the patient, we should be obliged to look about for another source than the food from which the evacuated fat could be obtained.

Considering, then, the rapid and extreme emaciation which not unfrequently accompanies pancreas disease, ought we not to think of the possibility of large quantities of fluid fat from the adipose tissues of the body passing directly into the blood, and hence through the vessels of the intestinal mucous membrane being set free. In connection with this, we might refer to some hitherto unnoticed cases of pancreas disease, in which, either with or without fatty stools, fat was passed along with the urine. In Tulpius[1] there is the report of a case in which there were not only fatty stools, but also fat in the urine; but here, as in a recorded case of Elliotson (loc. cit. p. 80), owing to the want of a post-mortem examination, there is the uncertainty as to whether pancreas disease was really present. Clark[2] reports the case of a woman who, for a length of time, passed with the urine a greasy substance, which on cooling floated about like masses of butter; later on there was also a large quantity of this fat in the stools. The post-mortem revealed medullary cancer of the pancreas and nutmeg liver, with a remarkable absence of bile from the gall-bladder; the remaining organs were healthy. Bowditch[3] relates the clinical history of a man who for months had suffered from abdominal troubles. The urine showed floating on its surface numbers of oil-globules; it is not said whether fatty stools were also present. At the autopsy, cancer of the liver and of the greater part of the pancreas was found. The possible occurrence of lipuria in diseases of the pancreas, as here shown, is well worthy of further investigation.[4]

Fles (loc. cit.) has drawn attention to the presence of large quantities of undigested striped muscular fibres in the faecal discharges as a symptom of disease of the pancreas. In this case, which the author had carefully observed, the patient, who was

---

[1] Observ. med. Amstelodam. 1652. Lib. III. Cap. XIX. p. 218.

[2] The Lancet. August, 1851. Schmidt's Jahrb. 72. Bd. p. 304.

[3] Americ. Journ. Jan. 1852. Schmidt's Jahrb. 74 Bd. p. 307.

[4] In a woman, who had died of marasmus senilis, I once found the renal glomeruli with their afferent arteries filled with fluid fat, as though it had been injected. Unfortunately, I am not in a position to say whether lipuria had been observed during life.

diabetic, was in the habit of eating a great deal of bacon and fat meat, and passed such quantities of fat with the stools that it could be scraped off the fæces by ounces. The fæces also contained very large quantities of unaltered striped muscular fibres. They soon disappeared, as did also the fat, after the patient added a calf's pancreas daily to this same kind of food. The experiment was made several times with a similar result. At the necropsy the pancreas was found so atrophied that little else than connective tissue remained, and no traces whatever of its duct could be discovered. It would seem from this case, though at present an isolated one, that, in the absence of the pancreatic juice and of its peptonizing properties, such muscular fibres as escape the action of the gastric juice may circulate through the intestine in large quantities and pass away with the fæces. However, this condition is worthy of consideration, and it may perhaps lead to the establishment of new points for diagnosis.

A fact of great importance is the by no means rare combination of pancreas disease and diabetes mellitus. The oldest of these cases is probably the one described by Cowley (1788) ; it occurred in a man aged thirty-four, who had been much addicted to drink, and was very fat and diabetic. At the autopsy his pancreas, on section, was found studded with small calculi, white in color, and with a mulberry-like surface ; they were firmly embedded in the substance of the gland. Later on, Dr. R. Bright recorded the history of a young clerk aged nineteen, who suffered from well-marked diabetes mellitus, with jaundice and fatty stools ; he died of marasmus. At the autopsy, the pancreas with several of the adjacent lymph-glands was found converted into a hard, lumpy, knotty mass, firmly adherent to the duodenum ; the gut orifice of the ductus choledochus was closed, and the gall-ducts were dilated with retained bile. Elliotson (l. c.) found the pancreatic duct, as high up as its larger branches, filled with white calculi, in a diabetic patient aged forty-five, who had passed fatty stools. Frerichs,[1] in nine cases of diabetes, noted atrophy, or fatty degeneration of the pancreas, five times, and specially refers to the case of a diabetic man aged fifty, in whom jaundice

---

[1] Klinik der Leberkrankheiten. 1. Bd. 1858. p. 153.

and hemorrhage from the bowels occurred, death resulting from marasmus ; at the autopsy, carcinoma of the head of the pancreas with closure of the common duct and of the duct of Wirsung, with dilatation above the seat of closure. We must also add the cases mentioned in the bibliography of this subject (Fles, Hartsen, Silver), in which such complete atrophy of the pancreas was found, that scarcely any remains of gland-substance could be distinguished.[1] Recklinghausen[2] describes two remarkable instances of diabetes, one in connection with a large cystic dilatation of the pancreatic duct, the other with dilatation of the gland-ducts, owing to concretions within them and erosion of the glandular parenchyma. Munk[3] once saw in a diabetic patient atrophy of the pancreas with atrophy of the solar plexus, and considerable swelling of the spleen. Seegen[4] collected thirty cases of diabetes mellitus from the records of the Vienna General Hospital, and in thirteen of the cases found more or less well-marked simple or fatty atrophy of the pancreas, and in one case its duct was filled as high as its smaller branches with a multitude of small white cylindrical or prickly calculi about the size of hemp-seeds, and sometimes 10''' in length. I myself have recently seen in a diabetic woman, who died in my wards, a most marked example of fatty degeneration of the pancreas, as follows:

The patient, a wet-nurse, æt. 47, who had suffered from diabetes mellitus for the past five years, had been treated at various times as an out-patient. Urine, specific gravity 1037-39, containing plenty of sugar, but no albumen. Lungs, liver, and spleen, normal. Her only complaint was of constant thirst, with a feeling of great weariness. Glycerine treatment had availed nothing. Under the use of opium and carbonate of soda she had felt herself comparatively well, and the conditions of strength and general health were maintained. On the 10th April, 1857, the patient was admitted into the wards. On the previous night she had been seized, suddenly

[1] A case recorded by *Langdon-Down* (Union med. No. 60, 1869 ; Centralblatt für die med. Wissenschaften. Nr. 38. 1869. p. 608), of a man fifty-two years of age, suffering from mellituria, fatty stools, and great emaciation, but who completely recovered from his disease, can scarcely be quoted as one of disease of the pancreas, because there was no autopsy to confirm the diagnosis.

[2] Virchow's Archiv. 30. Bd. 1864. p. 360.

[3] Tageblatt der 43. Versammlung deutscher Aerzte und Naturforscher in Innsbruck. 1869. p. 112.

[4] Der Diabetes Mellitus. 2d. Edition. Berlin, 1875. pp. 134 and 138.

and without any known cause, with urgent dyspnœa, headache, and pain in the region of the spleen. She died the day after admission, the above given symptoms continuing so that she was unable to answer any questions. At the time of admission there was subnormal temperature, 35.4° C. (96.8° F.) ; pulse, 100 per min. The autopsy showed some œdema of lung and of the aryteno-epiglottic ligaments. Heart, liver and kidneys normal. The follicles of the intestinal mucous membrane were a little swollen. Calvaria was thickened ; the pia mater also thickened and opaque. Brain and medulla oblongata natural. The pancreas alone was altered ; it was contracted in all its dimensions, of a very soft consistence and flabby, yellow in appearance, and almost entirely converted into large-celled fat-tissue, in which here and there could be detected small, grayish white points, which proved to be the remains of gland structure, the acini of which were undergoing fatty degeneration.

It is scarcely probable that in all these cases the combination of diabetes and pancreas disease was an accidental one, though at present it would be difficult to determine the precise connection between them. Popper[1] would explain it as a disturbance of that function of the pancreas through which fat is broken up into the fatty acids and glycerine ; and he believes, as little or no fatty acids can get into the liver, where, in combination with the glycogen, they go to form the biliary acids, that this glycogen becomes converted into sugar, and being in excess, that it then appears in the urine. Popper, in support of this view, shows that diabetes is common in corpulent individuals, and seeing that the ingestion of hydrocarbons and fats generally are such important factors in the production of corpulence, he believes that the fat-reducing function of the pancreas, being constantly and excessively called into action, becomes weakened, and, as above explained, this gives rise to diabetes. Against this theory must be borne in mind the fact that combinations of diabetes and pancreas disease by no means always or even often occur in corpulent persons ; besides which, total degeneration of the pancreas, or complete obliteration of its excretory duct through disease, ought to be more frequently observed in diabetes than is actually the case. Again, the experiments of Munk and Klebs tell against this view ; also the case, already quoted, of Klebs, in which the daily administration of a calf's pancreas arrested the

---

[1] Oesterreich. Zeitschrift f. prakt. Heilk. No. 11. 1868.

fatty stools and restored the power of digesting fat, while the diabetes continued unrestrained.

It will be more generally conceded that we must look to the nervous system for an explanation of the connection between diabetes and diseases of the pancreas, and especially to the solar and cœliac plexuses, which appear to play such an important rôle in the production of diabetes. Of great importance in this direction are the joint experiments on dogs, of Munk (loc. cit.) and Klebs, in which, even after partial extirpation of the solar plexus sometimes permanent, sometimes only temporary diabetes was set up, while extirpation of the pancreas or ligature of its duct invariably gave negative results, as far as diabetes was concerned. Neither could diabetes be produced by section of the hepatic or splanchnic nerves. From the above experiments we are justified in assuming the occasional supervention of diabetes in previously existing pancreas affections to be the result of secondary implication of the solar ganglion and plexus ; and Munk's case, just quoted, in which, together with diabetes and pancreas disease, there was found atrophy of the solar ganglion, has a most important bearing on this point. Owing to the intimate and close anatomical relation between the pancreas and the above-named nerve-structures, one must allow that diseases of the former will probably give rise to secondary changes in the latter, either by the direct pressure (as in cancer and the formation of calculi) of the enlarged pancreas on the solar ganglion, causing atrophy, or from extension of the inflammatory or other trophic changes in the pancreatic plexus along those nerves which connect it either with the solar or the cœliac plexuses. In a second class of cases, in which, to already existing symptoms of diabetes, later on have been superadded those of disease of the pancreas (e. g., fatty stools), and in which the autopsy only reveals either simple or fatty atrophy of the pancreas, as, for instance, in Fles' case, we must regard both affections—the diabetes as well as the pancreas disease—as the common result of primary disease of the solar plexus and its large ganglia, the atrophy being brought about in much the same way that it occurs in the submaxillary gland after division of its vaso-motor nerves (Bernard). And, indeed, in Munk's case there were very obvious signs of vaso-motor paralysis in the inordinately dilated branches of the hepatic, splenic, and gastric arteries; and in this, as in other cases of pancreas atrophy, there was considerable enlargement of the spleen.

In my opinion, therefore, we shall have to interpret the combination of pancreatic affections and diabetes in different ways. We must distinguish those cases of already existing disease, such as cancer, chronic inflammatory induration and formation of calculi, which, in their progress, give rise secondarily to mellituria, from cases of primary diabetes followed by trophic changes in the gland, such as simple atrophy or fatty degeneration.

It must be the object of clinical investigation, by a careful examination of individual cases, to determine as accurately as may be the chronological order of the various symptoms; we may then hope, from a larger and more comprehensive record of cases, taken hand in hand with the results of anatomical, pathological, and experimental research, to arrive at more definite conclusions on this as yet very obscure subject.

It will not be out of place here just to glance at the possible connection of diseases of the pancreas with bronze-skin (Addison's disease), and probably similar conditions to those described by Addison in supra-renal disease may exist. Indeed, Aran[1] has described the case of a woman, aged twenty-five years, who for a long time suffered from faintings, bilious vomiting, and epigastric pain, and who at last died of marasmus. The formerly white skin of the patient had gradually assumed a mulatto color, which was due to deposit of pigment in the rete Malpighii. The liver was enlarged, spleen normal, and the urine free from albumen. The autopsy showed cheesy infiltration of the pancreas, with formation of (detritus) cavities, swelling, and partial calcification of the cœliac and spleno-pancreatic glands. Aran is doubtful whether he should regard the bronze skin as accidental or in connection with pancreas disease. In a case of cancer of the pancreas, recorded by Jenni,[2] mention is made of

---

[1] Archiv. général de méd Sept., 1846.
[2] Schweizer Zeitschrift. 2. Bd. 1850; Schmidt's Jahrbücher. 69. Bd. p. 38.

the existence of ashen gray color of skin. Unfortunately, in neither of these cases is the condition of the supra-renal capsules noted, so that the participation of these glands in the disease cannot be excluded. However, we must all allow that diseases of the pancreas, if they lead to secondary changes in the great sympathetic ganglia of the abdomen and in the solar plexus, may possibly give rise to skin-pigmentation without directly affecting the supra-renal capsules, and we must further remember that the most recent experimenters on Addison's disease ascribe, and on good grounds, a greater share in the production of bronze-skin to the great abdominal sympathetic nerves than to the pathological changes which are found in the supra-renal capsules.[1] Here, too, is another point to which the attention of pathologists may be directed in future cases.

Another very frequent symptom in various pancreas affections is chronic jaundice, with all its usual sequelæ. It is sometimes due to the presence of complications which bring about changes in the liver, but more frequently to the mechanical compression of the ductus choledochus by the enlarged head of the pancreas, and must be thus classed as simple stenotic jaundice. We have already (p. 557) pointed out the intimate topographical relations which exist between the ductus choledochus and the head of the pancreas; hence may easily be understood the predisposition to jaundice, which exists in those forms of pancreas disease which lead to enlargement of the gland, and especially in their later stages. In some rare cases, therefore, the supervention of jaundice might assist in the diagnosis, but more frequently would tend rather to put us off our guard, and, by complicating the case, would render the diagnosis more difficult and more uncertain.

The same may be said regarding possible stenosis and closure of important neighboring blood-vessels in consequence of the pressure of the pancreas, or of thrombosis. Several cases are recorded in our literature, in which, owing to pressure on the vena portæ, ascites, hematemesis, blood in the stools, etc., occurred, and so we find symptoms more suggestive of cirrhosis of the liver. In

---

[1] Compare *Virchow*, Die krankhaften Geschwülste. 2. Bd. 1864. p. 701.

some cases there was obliteration of the superior mesenteric artery and vein, or of the splenic vein ; compression of the abdominal aorta has even been observed [1] in a case of enlarged pancreas. In Portal's book [2] may be found a case in which the aorta was found to be aneurismally dilated with excentric hypertrophy of the left ventricle of the heart, above the place on which it was pressed towards the spine by an enlarged pancreas. The exceedingly frequent occurrence of œdema of the lower extremities, which comes on sooner or later in the course of pancreas disease, in the large majority of cases must be due to pressure on the inferior cava. In a few cases there has been pressure on the right ureter and consecutive hydronephrosis.

Among the subjective symptoms of these diseases must first be mentioned pain in the epigastrium ; but we must nevertheless remember that, in a great variety of diseases of the abdominal organs—stomach, liver, lymphatics, aorta, spine, etc., etc.—this symptom may be present ; and it will be allowed, therefore, that it is only with great reserve that we can attribute any real diagnostic value to it. It not infrequently happens, even in extensive disease, that pain is entirely absent, or that the patient simply complains of a peculiar feeling of weight or pressure at the epigastrium, with or without a sense of præcordial oppression and discomfort. At times it is only on deep pressure that a dull feeling of some unusual oppression is produced. Again, certain peculiarities, which by some authors are considered as diagnostic—for instance, their deeply seated nature between pit of stomach and navel, their shooting character either upward or downward, and so on—are decidedly unreliable, as also their varying intensity and quality in different positions of the body. Sometimes the pain would come on or get worse when the patient was on his back or left side ; at other times the sitting posture could not be borne, while other patients were comfortable only when in this position, turning to the right side at once increasing the pain. In some cases inclining forward, or stooping, was painful ; in others, on the contrary, it was impossible to assume the erect

---

[1] Comp. *Claessen*, Die Krankheiten der Bauchspeicheldrüse. Köln, 1842. p. 114.
[2] Observations sur la nature et le traitement de l'apoplexie. Paris, 1811. p. 390.

position without pain. The pain is sometimes of a stretching, dragging character, as though caused by a weight attached to the stomach, and patients, on rising into the erect posture, experience a feeling as though something heavy were sinking into the abdomen, or, when turning over upon the side, as though some heavy body were moving about.

No one will doubt that such abnormal sensations may be produced by a diseased pancreas, if an enlargement and increase of weight take place. No one, however, would be able to distinguish these from similar sensations which may undoubtedly be caused by chronic induration of the neighboring organs—stomach, epigastric lymphatic glands, or omentum. This uncertainty increases when we consider that diseases of the pancreas occur alone more rarely than in combination with simultaneous changes in other organs of the epigastric region, and especially when we consider that they are all covered by the same peritoneum, and that this is almost always implicated. It is, therefore, only in such cases—where other symptoms, among which fatty stools and mellituria are to be especially mentioned, and in which affections of the neighboring glands can be excluded with tolerable certainty—that we should be justified in diagnosing disease of the pancreas by the presence of pain and other subjective signs, as already given, in the epigastrium ; the absence of these signs, however, would not justify us in excluding pancreas disease.

The paroxysmal pains, with a feeling of intense anxiety, indescribable restlessness and oppression, a tendency to faintings and collapse, all point so clearly to a neuralgic character that we are bound to regard them as attacks of cœliac neuralgia, and caused by pressure of the enlarged and degenerated pancreas on the solar plexus. Such like attacks of pain, under certain circumstances, must be allowed to have greater weight than the subjective symptoms already described, or the irritative pain caused by chronic peritonitis.

The epigastric pains, increased by slight pressure, present in acute pancreatitis with fever, are no doubt due to the inflammation of the peritoneal covering of the pancreas, and naturally have no further diagnostic indication. The sensations of indescribable anxiety and oppression which accompany the pain, together with the disposition to collapse—so acute as sometimes to cause death—suggest an inflammatory participation (Neuritis propagata?) of the solar plexus and its large ganglia. That the presence of concretions in the duct of Wirsung, tightly griped at the place of arrest, may give rise to paroxysms of pain analogous to bile colic, can scarcely be doubted, though there are no definite facts in support of this view.

No elaborate proofs are required to show that the various dyspeptic difficulties (loss of appetite, coated tongue, pyrosis, flatulence, faintness, and vomiting), so often found in pancreas diseases, must be attributed to secondary changes in the duodenum (catarrh, stenosis, etc.), and that we should not be justified, in presence of such and similar symptoms alone, in concluding that we had to deal with pancreas disease. Especially with regard to vomiting it must be remembered that enlargements of the head of the pancreas, either from chronic inflammation, cancer, or the formation of cysts, frequently cause stenosis of the duodenum, less frequently of the pylorus, and that the most obstinate forms of vomiting are thus produced. In a case recorded by Petit[1] the cancerous mass in the head of the pancreas pressed the stomach so forcibly against the anterior abdominal wall as to give rise to symptoms of internal strangulation. It happens, too, not infrequently, that primary malignant neoplasms of the pancreas spread by contiguity to the stomach or duodenum, giving rise to stenosis, or, in the later ulcerative stages, to hæmatemesis and blood in the stools. But, even without ulceration, pancreas disease with enlargement may give rise to hæmatemesis from pressure on the vena portæ or to blood in the stools from pressure on the superior or inferior mesenteric vein, of which there are many examples in our medical literature. In Battersby's cases primary carcinoma of the pancreas, which had invaded the colon, caused symptoms of obstruction in this gut. Whether we are to expect constipation or diarrhœa will, as a rule, depend more on the nature of the secondary changes in the mucous membrane than on the immediate results of the pancreas disease.

---

[1] Compare *Ancelet*, loc. cit. page 130.

We have already touched on the most important points as to the diagnostic value of the vomiting up of quantities of saliva-like fluid (page 569), and also as to the semiotic signification of certain anomalies in the stools (page 571).

Lastly, we must allude to the opinion held by the older physicians since Fernelius, who regarded the pancreas as the seat of hypochondria and melancholia, and still to be found expressed in Harles' works (1812), that probably chronic disease of the pancreas existed in those individuals who were the subjects of melancholy madness. Such an opinion scarcely requires contradiction, and the predisposition to melancholy and suicide mentioned in some cases of pancreas disease [1] may also occasionally occur in chronic diseases of other abdominal organs.

Of the physical methods of examination, palpation alone furnishes anything like reliable evidence on which to base a diagnosis of pancreas disease. But even these results are negative, or, at best, must be accepted with great care and hesitation. The deep position of the pancreas, its being covered by the stomach and liver, renders it difficult of access, even when the stomach and intestines are completely empty and the abdominal walls quite relaxed, and even when this organ is considerably enlarged palpation with a positive and satisfactory result only succeeds in a small minority of cases. As regards the head of the pancreas, which is most frequently the seat and starting-point, do these remarks especially apply. Any considerable swelling of the head of the pancreas often displaces the left lobe of the liver forward, and may so give rise to diagnostic errors.

Palpation of the pancreas will be best accomplished when the stomach is empty, and after the administration of either purgatives or clysters so as to clear out the colon, and the usual precautions adopted in examination of the abdomen must be carefully carried out. Occasionally palpation leads to positive results, when performed with both hands by lateral pressure on the hypochondriac regions, or in the knee-elbow position. At times it may be desirable to administer chloroform in order to relax abdominal tension (rigidity). In one of these positions, then, the

---

[1] Compare *Claessen*, loc cit. p. 118.

altered pancreas may be discovered lying crosswise in the epigastric region as a slightly movable swelling, or as a round, firm, or
fluctuating tumor, either smooth or nodular on its surface, and
which, owing to the underlying aorta, may receive a pseudo-
pulsatile movement. Complications with diseases of the stomach,
of the liver, epigastric glands, or with ascites, may interfere with
the examination and lead to all sorts of diagnostic errors.

Percussion gives rise to distant dulness only over very large
tumors, but palpation in such cases will very probably have
afforded some definite result. Piorry's opinion that, in the knee-
elbow position, the pancreas may be clearly mapped out by percussion (percussion lombaire) in the lumbar region, belongs to
some of the many peculiarities and exaggerations which characterize this author.

Auscultation is only useful as a means to differentiate a
tumor of the pancreas and an aneurism of the abdominal aorta,
or of the cœliac axis. But we must clearly remember that a blowing murmur may be produced by the pressure of a tumor on the
aorta.

From what has been said, it is evident that no single one of
the possible symptoms of pancreas disease can be said to possess
any pathognomonic importance, and that even some or several
of them may be present and then not lead to a certain diagnosis.
Sometimes the disease may remain absolutely latent, while many
of the enumerated symptoms may be caused by disease of the
stomach or of the liver, the pancreas being quite healthy. At
other times, in consequence of the pressure of the hardened and
enlarged pancreas on the neighboring organs (blood-vessels, bile-
duct, intestine, solar plexus, etc.), there results such a complicated and ever-changing symptomatology that the most experienced clinician gets quite astray. Among the symptoms which
furnish the most reliable " points d'appui " we must especially
mention fatty stools, mellituria, darting pains in the epigastrium
(cœliac neuralgia), together with a palpable tumor. Sometimes, by
the method of exclusion, disease of the stomach or of the liver

may be shut out with tolerable certainty, and the diagnosis of pancreas disease thus indirectly aided. But even with the greatest care, and in spite of a combination of the most favorable conditions, errors cannot always be avoided.

Etiology.

Very little is known as to the cause of these diseases. Men seem to be more frequently affected than women; in Claessen's table of 322 cases, there were 193 males and 129 females. Old and advancing age seem decidedly to predispose. But yet cases are met with during early life; childhood even affords no immunity, and many examples of pancreas disease have been found in new-born infants, and even in the fœtus. Rokitansky[1] once found induration of the pancreas in a new-born child; Cruveilhier[2] in a fœtus; Schoeller describes a cartilaginous induration of the pancreas in a female child, nineteen days old, who had died of phlebitis hepatica. In another section I shall myself describe what was very probably syphilitic degeneration of the pancreas taken from a seven months fœtus, which was born dead.[3] It is at present uncertain whether heredity play any part in the production of pancreas disease; some of the cases observed by Claessen, though rather doubtful, incline rather to this view. Pregnancy is believed by some authors to predispose to this disease. As occasional causes, excesses in eating and drinking, more especially alcoholic drinks, great smoking or chewing of tobacco, the abuse of purgative medicines, excessive or long mercurial treatment, too long a use of the cinchona bark, sup-

---

[1] Handbuch der pathol. Anat. Vienna. 1840. 3d. vol. p. 393.

[2] Anat. pathol. Tom. I. Paris. 1829-35. XV. Livrais 6 et 7. Observ. Planche. II. Figs. 7 and 8.

[3] *Claessen* (loc. cit. S. 40) gives the following statistics of 262 cases of pancreas disease:

5	cases were new-born children.			
2	"	"	1 year old.	
20	"	"	from 1 to 10 years old.	
41	"	"	" 10 to 25	"
156	"	"	" 25 to 60	"
38	"	"	beyond 60	"

pression of the menses, mental depression, onanism, etc., have all and each been blamed. . The influence, however, of most of these causes is in the highest degree problematical. It is certain, nevertheless, that the abuse of alcoholic stimulants, and constitutional syphilis have considerable etiological importance in the causation of fatty disease of the pancreas and of chronic pancreatitis. Whether mechanical injuries, such as contusion in the region of the stomach or concussion of the abdomen, can give rise to carcinomatous degeneration, as has been frequently asserted, is not altogether impossible, though, in consequence of the deep and protected position of the organ, it is very doubtful.

Among the secondary diseases of the pancreas must be mentioned metastatic tumors and abscesses; also hyperæmia and chronic interstitial inflammation, the result of venous congestion, in chronic affections of the heart, lungs, or liver. The pancreas may also be attacked, through direct implication, by primary neoplastic, inflammatory, or ulcerative diseases of the surrounding organs (cancer of the stomach or of the liver, or ulcer of the stomach).

Treatment.

There is but little to report as to the treatment of pancreas diseases. It is evident that the development of a successful treatment must be slow in diseases which, like those of the pancreas, not only are so rare, but which also, even when present, are so difficult to recognize. So, in most cases which are said to have been cured by a certain treatment, comes the doubt as to the correctness of the original diagnosis. Again, in other cases where diseased pancreas can be diagnosed with considerable certainty, we have to deal with certain organ disturbances, which do not, as a rule, admit of any radical treatment, and in which only the carrying out of any symptomatic indications is possible.

The therapeutic worth of all those remedies described by physicians as specifics is entirely hypothetical. Among these may be mentioned preparations of iron (Eyting), oxide of bismuth (Hauff), Haller's acid elixir (Harles), alkaline ·carbonates (Urban), Friedrichshalle bitter-water (Eisenmann), foot-baths of aqua regia (Truempy, Annesley), and the like. Calomel has been recommended by various authors (Brera, Headland, Berlioz, Claessen), and in suitable cases it is well worthy a careful trial, especially if it should prove to be correct that calomel increases the functions of the human pancreas in the same way as it does that of dogs, which is proved by the large quantities of the digestive products of the pancreas (leucin and tyrosin) which are contained in fæces produced by the action of calomel.[1] It is as yet impossible to state the indications for its use in these diseases ; it is even probable, taking for granted its power of increasing the function of the pancreas, that this very condition of permanent irritation may be detrimental. In cases where a syphilitic origin is suspected, an energetic treatment with iodine or mercury is indicated (inunction or sublimation) ; with a scrofulous foundation or in general obesity, we must scrupulously adopt the remedies and dietetic restrictions which are suitable for these conditions. Occasionally, in cases of suspected chronic pancreatitis, a trial of mild purgatives is indicated, such as rhubarb, taraxacum, cream of tartar, sulphur, castor oil, senna, and mineral waters (Eger, Marienbad, Soden, Kissingen). In a case to be presently described, I obtained a complete and permanent cure by the use of Homburg water (Elizabeth Spring)— a case which, from the symptoms—fatty stools, epigastric pain, excessive emaciation—I ventured to diagnose as chronic pancreatitis. If the inflammatory symptoms should become prominent, cold compresses across the epigastrium, local bloodlettings by leeches to the epigastrium, or, still better, ad anum, together with derivatives and counter-irritation, are the remedies which must be relied on. For the pain, narcotics are indicated, either internally or externally (belladonna, opium, or morphia).

The attempt has frequently been made to supply to the patient suffering from this disease the pancreatic juice which in them is faulty, either in quantity or quality, and various methods for obtaining the active ferment (pancreatin) pure have been suggested, so that it might be used for therapeutical purposes,

---

[1] Comp. *Radziejewsky*, Archiv für Anat., Physiol., und wissensch. Med. 1870. 1. Heft. p. 60.

either in the form of a pill or in some other way. Especially the precipitate by alcohol from a watery extract of the pancreas, and called "pancreatin," has been used. The results obtained have varied, but in some cases undoubtedly seem to have brought about a good result.[1]

The simplest and best method is to use an infusion of pancreas, which will contain all the soluble principles of the gland. This is best prepared by macerating the gland recently obtained from a calf or a pig, and deprived of its surrounding fat, in four times its weight of water, at a temperature of 58.3° F. (25° C.). It must be allowed to macerate for two hours, and the temperature must never rise above 61.1° F. (30° C.). A reliable infusion can only be obtained from such glands as are taken while in a state of activity—that is, during digestion—which are then found to have an opaque, reddish appearance, and to contain the largest amount of active principles. The favorable results which have followed the administration of such infusions in infantile dyspepsia, with inability to digest starchy and fatty foods, speak strongly in favor of this proceeding, and justify its adoption also in diseases of the pancreas. The very remarkable case, described by Fles (l. c.), of a diabetic patient with atrophy of the pancreas, who ultimately died of phthisis, and who daily passed with his stools, not only a quantity of fat, but also a considerable quantity of undigested and unaltered muscular fibres, is here worthy of consideration (p. 570). A fresh calf's pancreas (sweetbread) was well beaten in a mortar, with six ounces of water, and strained; the so-obtained milky fluid was taken by the patient in separate doses, one after each meal, so that in this way an entire pancreas was consumed in the twenty-four hours, and although the previous diet, which largely consisted of bacon and fat meat, was continued, still, at the end of two days, all the fat, and in great part the undigested muscular fibre, had disappeared from the fæces. Each time the pancreatic infusion was left off, the fat and muscular fibres again appeared. The favor-

---

[1] Comp. *Langdon-Down's* case. Trans. of Clin. Soc. Vol. II. 1869. page 119. Schmidt's Jahrbücher. 150. Bd. p. 159. Centralbl. für die med. Wissenschaften. No. 38 1869. p. 608.

e effects of the daily use of the calf's pancreas on the general
lth were exceedingly marked ; the rapid emaciation seemed
be stayed, and the body to reassume its rounded proportions.
e quantity of urine and the amount of sugar voided still
ained entirely unaltered. The case we have just recorded
rits close consideration, and we may fairly hope that a similar
thod of treatment, if even unable to save life, may, by im-
ving the nutrition, at least prolong it.

II. Special Part.

Hyperæmia and Anæmia.

The pancreas, like other glands, is subject to physiological changes in its blood-supply, and this, in the estimation of pathological processes, must be carefully borne in mind. Thus, while fasting (period of rest), the pancreas is pale and bloodless; during digestion (period of activity) it is turgid and full of blood and of secretion. During the period of rest its venous blood is dark, but during the period of activity it is bright red and arterial in quality. Independently of these physiological conditions, anæmia may exist in case of general impoverishment of the blood, as after profuse hemorrhage, or in cases of continued secretory losses in marasmus from any cause. Passive hyperæmia may result from venous congestions, in consequence of heart, lung, or liver disease; in such cases often combined with evidence of interstitial connective tissue, hyperplasia, and consequent increase of volume and consistence of the organ. A diagnosis of these conditions is not possible.

Hypertrophy and Atrophy.

Cruveilhier, Traité d'anat. pathol. général. Tom. III. Paris, 1856. p. 87.—*Rokitansky*, Lehrbuch der path. Anat. 3. Aufl. 3. Bd. Wien, 1861. S. 308.—*Foerster*, Handbuch der spec. path. Anat. 2. Aufl. Leipzig, 1863. S. 215.—*Klebs*, Handbuch der path. Anat. Berlin, 1870. S. 536.

Hypertrophy of the pancreas, that is, not a simple swelling of the organ, but an increase in size from enlargement, out-growth, or new growth of glandular elements (true hypertrophy and hyperplasia), has not yet been proved to exist, and Cruveilhier entirely doubts its existence. At present, too, there are no sufficiently exact data as to the size and weight of the normal pancreas in relation to age and weight, so that we do not know within what limits the weight and volume of the normal pancreas may vary; we are, therefore, thrown back on a very approximative valuation for our present estimate. In many of the cases cited in the literature of this subject, as total or partial hypertrophy of the pancreas, it was more probably an enlargement or a swelling of the gland due to chronic inflammation or new growth.

Atrophy of the pancreas sometimes accompanies chronic cachexia and marasmus of various kinds. Sometimes it is found in extreme old age (senile atrophy,) and then, apart from its small size, it appears harder, granular, and of a brownish yellow, even of a light brown color (pancreas duriusculum, contractum). Secondary atrophy is sometimes caused by being pressed on by some neighboring swelling (aortic aneurism, cancer, indurated lymphatic glands), or by pressure from within (dilatation of the ducts, formation of cysts, chronic interstitial inflammation, new growths, lipomatosis). The atrophy may proceed so far that the gland-substance proper may entirely disappear, leaving only a tough, flaccid, cord-like piece of connective tissue in its place. Sometimes we find the lining epithelium of the atrophying gland in a state of fatty degeneration, in which cases the acini of the still existing portions appear of a yellowish color.

Those cases of atrophy of the pancreas, which are observed in diabetic patients, and which sometimes attain even the highest degree, with or without fatty degeneration, are of great clinical interest. We refer the reader to what has already been said (p. 574 et seq.), and repeat here that these cases are mostly secondary to the circulatory changes set up by the diabetes. We might be justified in diagnosing this condition, if, in addition to the symptoms of diabetes, were superadded others—such as fat and undigested muscular fibres in the fæces—and if the daily administration of a fresh calf's pancreas produced a favorable influence on these latter symptoms (p. 588). This diet, too, would be the most useful, and the most likely to improve the general nutrition of the patient, and by supplying the absent function of the pancreas might add a new lease to the patient's life, even if it did not cure the atrophy or the diabetes.

Acute Pancreatitis.

Portal, Traité de l'apoplexie. Paris, 1811.—*Harles*, Ueber die Krankheiten des Pankreas. Nürnberg, 1812. S. 36, 52.—*Schmackpfeffer*, Observ. de quibusdam pancreatis morbis. Diss. Hall. 1817. p. 19.—*Battersby*, Dubl. Med. Journ. May, 1824.—*Abercrombie*, Edinb. Med. and Surg. Journ. 79. Vol. 1824. p. 243.—Sammlung auserlesener Abhandlungen. 8. Bd. Leipzig, 1824. S. 663.—*Lerche*, De Pankreatitide. Diss. Hal. 1827.—*Bigsby*, Edinb. Med. Journ. No. 124. 1835.—*Gendrin*, Anat. Beschreibung der Entzündung und ihrer Folgen. Deutsch von *Radius*. 2. Bd. Leipzig, 1829. S. 191, 233.—*Mondière*, Arch. génér. de méd. Mai, Juillet, 1836. p. 265.—*Bécourt*, Recherches sur le pancréas. Thèse. Strassbourg, 1830. p. 33.—*Lawrence*, Med. Chir. Transact. Vol. XVI. Part. II. 1831. p. 367.—*Behrends*, Vorlesungen über prakt. Arzneiwissenschaft, herausgeg. von *Sundelin*. III. Bd. S. 332.—*Claessen*, Die Krankheiten der Bauchspeicheldrüse. Köln, 1842. S. 188.—*Loeschner*, Zur Pankreatitis. Weitenweber's Beiträge zur Medicin. Juli, 1842.—*Haller* and *Klob*, Fall von Entzündung des Pankreas. Zeitschrift der Gesellschaft der Aerzte zu Wien. Nr. 37. 1859.—*Oppolzer*, Ueber Krankheiten des Pankreas. Wiener med. Wochenschrift. Nr. 1. 1867.—*Klebs*, Handbuch der path. Anat. Berlin, 1870. S. 534.—*C. E. E. Hoffmann*, Untersuchungen über die path.-anat. Veränderungen der Organe beim Abdominaltyphus. Leipzig, 1869. S. 191.

Acute inflammations of the pancreas are either primary or secondary. We purpose to consider them separately.

I. *Acute Primary Pancreatitis.*

No doubt this is a very rare disease, and its existence has been altogether denied by some (Andral, Neumann). The earlier literature certainly furnishes no very convincing proofs of its occurrence, as the works, already referred to, of Harles and Claessen, well show ; but in the more recent clinical reports are to be found cases with *post-mortem* records (Loeschner, Haller, Klob, Oppolzer), which now leave no doubt that an acute primary pancreatitis may really occur. I will now briefly relate these cases, and add to them another one which has come under my own observation.

1. *Loeschner's case.*—A young man, æt. 26 years, a confirmed smoker and drinker, had suffered since his twenty-first year from occasional attacks of cardialgia and dyspepsia. On the 21st January he was seized with colicky pains in the upper

part of the abdomen, which during the next few days increased, and at last became constant, burning, and extremely agonizing; there was great anxiety, nausea, and vomiting, which, however, gave no relief. Obstinate constipation, and a slight degree of feverishness. In the course of a few days, there was great prostration, sunken face, tendency to collapse, headache, vertigo, cold sweats, constant thirst, thickly coated but moist tongue, and belching. The upper belly was distended, hot, and the seat of a continuous, violent, sometimes shooting, sometimes drawing pain, which attained its greatest intensity along the greater curvature of the stomach, shooting out on the right toward the duodenum, and on the left toward the spleen, downward towards the navel, and upward towards the shoulder-blade. Pulse, 75 per min.; small; persistent constipation. The mouth contained but very little saliva, which was viscid; extremities became cold; collapse; death. *Autopsy.*—The surroundings of the pancreas were dark red, livid, and here and there infiltrated with blood. In the head of the gland, some small, finely granular, yellowish exudations could be seen; the mucous membrane lining Wirsung's duct was darkly reddened.

2. *Haller and Klob's case.*—An old man, sixty-three years of age, previously healthy, had suffered during the past sixteen years with stomach troubles and vomiting. On his admission he was pale and cachectic, tongue coated, appetite gone; he vomits a thin-like stained fluid. Region of the stomach distended, tense, and painful on pressure; pulse 90; temperature somewhat raised; œdema of legs; aggravation of all symptoms, and death from acute collapse. On the same day autopsy. There were three perforations, as large as peas, on the posterior wall of the stomach, which formed the anterior wall of an abscess cavity into which these perforations lead. This cavity extended backward as far as the spine, to the left as far as the spleen, to the right behind the pylorus, and surrounded on all sides the pancreas, which was discolored, grayish, flaccid, and extensively infiltrated with pus. The authors considered this a genuine pancreatitis with sloughing and degeneration of the surrounding structures and perforating into the stomach.

3. *Oppolzer's case.*—A strong and previously healthy man was seized with violent cardialgia, which increased steadily in intensity. On admission, deathly pallor, great restlessness, frequent vomiting of a quantity of bile-like matter; repeated faintings, great pain, increased on pressure in the region of the stomach; constipation; high fever. Death within a few days. Intoxication could be excluded. *Autopsy.*—The pancreas was increased three-fold in size; on cutting into it, extravasated blood could be seen within the red stained acini. The surrounding bed of the pancreas was extravasated with blood.

4. *The author's own case.*—A lusty, well-nourished man, forty years of age, was seized with the symptoms of an acute general peritonitis. Very marked meteorismus and tenseness of the abdomen; pushing up of the diaphragm; dyspnœa; frequent belchings, and bilious vomiting. Belly very painful, especially on moving; constipation; high fever; dry tongue. Patient believes himself to have been taken ill but a few days ago with pains in the belly, and without any known cause. Death occurred three days after his admission without our being able to make out

clearly the cause of the acute peritonitis. *Autopsy.*—General sero-purulent peritonitis, especially marked in the upper part of the abdomen, where all the organs were matted together by fresh adhesions. The pancreas increased at least three-fold in size, strongly injected, and studded all over with hundreds of small abscesses, varying in size from a pin's head to a bean, and containing a thick, creamy, yellow matter. The abscesses which lay nearest to the surface appeared like pustules, of which many had opened into the abdominal cavity, and had evidently given rise to the peritonitis; atelectasis of both lower lobes of the lungs, but no important changes in the other organs.

The pathological anatomy of acute pancreatitis, as may be seen from the foregoing cases, consists in intense injection, firmer consistence, and enlargement of the gland to as much as three times its natural size; there also appears to be a tendency to hemorrhagic changes in the inter-acinose tissue and in the immediate neighborhood of the pancreas (Pancreatitis acuta hemorrhagica). During the suppurative stage, at the onset, numerous punctiform, and later on larger abscesses are formed, which may acquire a very large size and finally become confluent. As to whether the pus is formed in the manner described by Virchow for the parotid gland [1]—that is, within the excretory ducts or within the acini—or whether it is formed directly in the interstitial connective tissue, is not yet clearly established. Secondary peritonitis is set up by spread of the inflammation along the peritoneum, or by the bursting of some of the superficial abscesses. The transition of the inflammation into gangrene and peripancreatitic sloughing may be due to the previously mentioned hemorrhagic processes.

As yet we know nothing of the etiology of acute primary pancreatitis. Males are apparently more prone to it than females. Earlier authorities attributed, but with scarcely sufficient grounds, a predisposition to it in the scrofulous diathesis. As possible causes may be mentioned: the use of mercury, abuse of tobacco and alcohol drinks, and onanism. Mondière believes that pregnancy, and Schoenlein that suppression of the menses, may be of importance in its production. But all this is uncertain. That acute traumatic pancreatitis may result from contusion or a blow in the epigastrium will scarcely be doubted,

[1] Annalen des Charitékrankenhauses zu Berlin. 8. Jahrg. 3. Heft. 1858. S. 1.

though we do not happen to have any direct proofs in support of it.

Symptomatology.—In consequence of the very small number of cases at our disposal, we cannot claim for our symptomatological table either precision or completeness. But we can accept as almost certain that the disease begins either with a colicky or with a fixed and more continuous and deeply seated pain, commencing in the epigastrium, and shooting either towards the shoulder or towards the spine, and within a very short time becoming very intense. The pain is accompanied by great restlessness; præcordial anxiety, dyspnœa, tendency to faint, nausea, eructations, and the vomiting of a thin bile-stained fluid, which brings no relief, are seldom absent. The epigastrium is tense, bowels are costive, with more or less fever and evening exacerbations. There was no jaundice in spite of the swelling of the head of the pancreas (p. 579), in the cases at present known. The appreciation of a tumor by deep pressure will scarcely be possible on account of the pain which would be caused by such examination. In unfavorable cases the symptoms attain their greatest intensity within a few days, the pulse becomes small, suppressed and irregular, the extremities cold, the features hippocratic, and death takes place in acute collapse. How far we may accept a participation of the solar plexus, either from pressure of the enlarged gland upon it, or from spreading of the inflammation to it as an explanation of the peculiar nature of the pain and of the rapidly fatal collapse, we are unable to say, though a secondary irritation of these nervous structures is by no means improbable (p. 581). In some cases the pains spread over the entire abdomen, and we then get the symptoms of a general acute peritonitis.

We may venture to suspect acute pancreatitis, if, with the above symptoms, we are able to exclude pretty definitely acute inflammations of the other abdominal organs situated in that region. The absence of jaundice and of enlargement of the liver, the seat and primary starting-point of the pains, and in part also perhaps the anamnesis, may help to distinguish it from biliary colic. With a little care and attention it will be almost impossible to mistake it for acute gastritis, which latter disease is almost always produced by the action of corrosive substances. Nevertheless, according to the standard of our present knowledge of other diseases, the diagnosis of acute pancreatitis scarcely rises above the level of probabilities.

The possibility of recovery in the early stages of the disease cannot be altogether excluded. Cases also of a subacute nature occur; transitions into chronic inflammation with induration and swelling of the gland, and the formation of chronic abscess, also seem to occur, as the cases recorded by Claessen testify.

Therapeutics.—On account of the impossibility of a certain diagnosis, the treatment can only be symptomatic. Ice internally and externally; effervescing mixtures with narcotics to allay the sickness and the pain; leeches on the epigastrium, or, better still, to the anus. Derivatives through the intestinal canal by means of calomel, jalap, salines, etc.; sometimes drastic purgatives, such as colocynth, might be of real service in the early stages. Complete rest and antiphlogistic diet. On the supervention of collapse, analeptics and stimulants are indicated. It must be understood that these therapeutic suggestions are theoretical rather than the result of any practical experience. Should symptoms of an acute peritonitis set in, it must be treated accordingly.

II. *Acute Secondary Pancreatitis.*

In this group we must, first of all, treat of acute parenchymatous inflammation, the so-called parenchymatous degeneration, which has its analogue in the well-known acute parenchymatous degeneration of the liver, kidneys, muscles, etc., such as frequently occur in acute infectious diseases. This form of pancreatitis is found under similar circumstances, and corresponds histologically with the parenchymatous degenerations of the above-mentioned organs, without which it never seems to occur. The whole gland presents a swollen, tough, reddened condition, and is filled with turbid granular albuminoid contents. This affection appears to be extremely common in the acute infectious diseases; C. E. E. Hoffman was the first accurately to describe

this condition in typhoid fever, and Klebs speaks of its occurrence in acute general tuberculosis. I myself can testify to the
presence of this disease in the severer forms of typhoid and also
of pyæmia; and quite recently I found it in a case of double-
sided erysipelatous pneumonia in a young and strong man.[1]

In this case the whole pancreas was greatly swollen and reddened, both on its
external surface and on section; but in the head of the pancreas, where the swelling was most considerable, the cut surface presented a reddish gray appearance,
and the glandular structure in this part was indistinct, owing to the amount of
swelling of the acini. The microscope showed great enlargement of the gland-
cells and infiltration of their protoplasm, with an opaque, granular exudation,
which, on the addition of acetic acid and of potash, cleared up, leaving behind
but a few fat-molecules. Each cell contained two to three, some even as many as
five, large, round nuclei with nucleoli. At the same time, there was most marked
parenchymatous degeneration of the liver and kidneys.

The *diagnosis* of this affection of the pancreas is not at present possible. We can only suspect its presence if, in a severe
case of infectious disease, the clinical features of acute parenchymatous degeneration of the liver (acute swelling) and of the
kidney (albuminuria), together with enlargement of the spleen
and high fever, are present. It is possible that the intercurrent
jaundice, supervening in some very acute infectious diseases,
may be due to the pressure of an acutely inflamed (enlarged)
pancreas on the ductus choledochus. The treatment must be
guided by the nature of the original disease.

As a second form of acute secondary pancreatitis, we must
here mention metastatic abscess, the result of a circumscribed
purulent inflammation. It happens very rarely, and the diagnosis is impossible. We cannot say whether any, or what symptoms would result, and it can only happen perhaps once to find
it present in a body dead of some pyæmic or puerperal disease.

We ought also now to discuss another form of metastatic
pancreatitis, which affects the entire organ, with the view to
settle the question as to whether we are at present justified in
admitting the metastasis of a parotitis to the abdominal salivary
glands. The fact of a metastatic transference of a primary paro-

---

[1] Compare my Lecture on Acute Enlargement of the Spleen. Volkmann's Sammlung
klinischer Vorträge. No. 75. 1874. p. 579.

titis to the testicles, ovaries, breasts, and labia majora is well known and well recognized. Does an analogous metastasis to the pancreas take place, and is Mondière justified in including inflammation of the parotid as among the causes of inflammation of the pancreas?

We have already (p. 567) spoken against the admissibility of any existing vicarious and consensual alternation of function between the buccal and abdominal salivary glands. These conditions, however, do not concern the present question, and even if this alternation between the above-named glands in relation to their secretory processes could be established with sufficient certainty, we should not be able to deduce therefrom the possibility of a metastatic pancreatitis any more than we could exclude the latter because of the absence of the former. The metastasis of parotitis to the testis is a fact beyond all doubt, without there being any physiological relation between the parotids and the genital organs in a secretory or functional sense. The existence, therefore, of a metastatic pancreatitis in the above sense can only be determined in the future by observation at the bedside.

Some pathologists do, no doubt, speak of the occurrence of such metastases, e. g., Canstatt, in his chapter on Epidemic Mumps, but I have not been able to find any convincing data in the literature of this subject. The various reports are a little too vague; thus, Battersby's observation, that the symptoms of pancreas disease after the disappearance of a salivation became more pronounced; also the remarks by Andral and Mondière, that in the course of pancreas diseases one or other of the parotid glands swells up. The last-named author cites also the case, reported by Roboica, of a man with a severe parotitis, who, on the sudden disappearance of this disease, was as suddenly seized with a deeply seated pain in the epigastrium; this also quickly disappeared, but was followed by swelling of the testis; then the parotid again became affected. More precise is the case, communicated by Schmackpfeffer, of a pregnant woman, syphilitic, but otherwise strong, who, after her confinement, was treated by corrosive sublimate. The syphilitic symptoms disappeared, but an excessive salivation followed. As this decreased, a copious diarrhœa came on, with thirst, fever, anorexia, a feeling of anxiety, and burning in the epigastrium, together with a deeply seated pain in the gastric region, extending towards the right hypochondrium. The stools, of which there were thirty during the day, were yellowish, watery, and like saliva. Suddenly, one night, the diarrhœa ceased, and both parotids became painfully swollen, but there was no salivation. The pulse became small and intermittent, face anxious, with dyspnœa, and the patient died the following night in collapse. At the autopsy the pancreas was found swollen, reddened, very full of blood, and indurated. Both parotids were inflamed; there was a little serum in the pleural cavities; other organs healthy.

However little present experience goes to establish the existence of a metastatic pancreatitis, the possibility of its occurrence cannot be summarily dismissed, especially in view of the last-mentioned case. Future observation alone will have to decide this point, and perhaps an epidemic of mumps will afford the best opportunity of doing so.

Chronic Pancreatitis.

Gendrin, Anat. Beschreibung der Entzündung u. s. w. deutsch von Radius. 2. Bd. Leipzig, 1829. S. 213.—*Urban*, Hufeland's Journal, 1830. Nov. S. 87.—*Cruveilhier*, Anat. pathol. Tom. I. Paris. XV. Livrais. Observ. 6, 7. Pl. II. Figs. 7, 8.—*Lawrence*, Med. Chir. Transact. Vol. XVI. Part II. 1831. p. 367.—*Kirmsee*, Zur Lehre von der Entzündung des Pankreas. Allg. med. Zeitg. Nr. 70. 1838.—*Aran*, Arch. génér. de méd. Sept. 1846.—*Kilgour*, Lond. Med. Nov. 1850.—*Rostan*, Bullet. de la soc. anat. 1855. p. 26.—*Riboli*, Gazz. med. Sarda. Nr. 11. 1858.—*Klob*, Oesterr. Zeitschr. für prakt. Heilkde. VI. 33. 1860.—*G. Harley*, On Jaundice. London, 1863. p. 71.—*Oedmansson*, Virchow-Hirsch Jahresbericht für 1869. 2. Bd. S. 561.—*Rigal*, Gaz. des hôpit. Nr. 142. 1869. —*Nathan*, Med. Times and Gaz. II. Nr. 1052. 1870.—*Klebs*, Handbuch der path. Anat. Berlin, 1870. S. 559.—*Rokitansky*, Lehrbuch der pathol. Anat. 3. Bd. 1861. S. 254.—*Lancereaux*, Traité historique et pratique de la syphilis. Paris, 1866. pp. 318, 552.—*Birch-Hirschfeld*, Beiträge zur pathol. Anat. der hereditären Syphilis Neugeborener. Archiv der Heilkunde. 16. Jahrg. 1875. S. 166.—Consult also the treatises already cited, of *Schmackpfeffer*, *Dawidoff*, *Harles*, *Hohnbaum*, *Monlière*, *Décourt*, *Claessen*.

If we look through the earlier literature of diseases of the pancreas, we shall be easily convinced that much which has been described as chronic pancreatitis does not belong to this **category** at all. It is especially difficult to divest oneself of the **idea that** many of the cases which have been described as **induration** of the pancreas really come within the bounds of the **normal con-**dition, and that this organ, on account of its tough, granular condition, has often been described erroneously as **pathologically** altered, when such was not the case. On the other hand, it can-not be doubted that many of the glands described as " steatoma-tous " and " scirrhous " really belonged to the class of chronic inflammations. On these grounds, therefore, the earlier litera-ture must be carefully selected and studied before it can **serve** for the elucidation of this subject.

The most frequent form of chronic pancreatitis is the chronic interstitial inflammation, consisting of a hyperplasia of its inter-acinous connective tissue and consequent atrophy, even to the entire disappearance, of the gland-substance proper. This pro-cess has its analogue in cirrhosis of other glandular organs, such as the liver, kidneys, etc. Sometimes, during the stage of con-traction, there is closure of a smaller branch of the excretory duct, and so a secondary formation of cysts. The disease some-times attacks the entire gland, but with especial predilection the head ; sometimes only certain portions of it ; or it may show itself in the form of circumscribed, firm cicatricial bands and nodules.

Primary chronic interstitial pancreatitis, affecting the whole gland as a separate disease, is extremely rare. The secondary forms, however, are more common, and result, not unfrequently, from long-continued venous gorging, as in chronic heart, lung, and liver diseases. In these cases the changes scarcely ever at-tain such a degree as to produce complete cirrhosis, with destruc-tion of the glandular elements ; but we find, in varying degrees, tracts of connective tissue spreading in between the acini, and by their contraction giving to the gland a greater toughness, hardness, and a more granular appearance. Klob, on cutting into these tracts of thickened connective tissue, found here and there small white spots, from which little masses or molecules of chalk, sometimes fat-crystals, could be squeezed. Sometimes, in the hyperæmic forms, small interstitial hemorrhages are found, which become changed later on into masses of rust-colored pigment, or which form spaces containing a serous fluid, and bounded by hardened, rust-colored walls (apoplectic, hemorrhagic cysts).

With these cases produced by congestion must be classed also those in which the interstitial connective-tissue growth and atrophy are due to retention of the secretion through closure of the canal of Wirsung, with subsequent dilatation of the gland-ducts. In the latest stages of these cases the organ consists chiefly of connective tissue in which here and there the remains of the glandular structure can be recognized as small granules, yellowish in color, owing to their cells undergoing fatty degeneration. On section, the organ is found to be studded with cystoid spaces and beaded canals—the enlarged and dilated excretory ducts, filled with the retained secretion (Ranula pancreatica). The causes of the retention of the secretion may be of varied nature; among others, calculi, which stick in the canal of Wirsung or in the ductus choledochus, peripancreatitic swellings and adhesions, pressure from neighboring tumors, or diseases situated in the pancreas itself, especially in its head part, and the like. I will here relate a case in which an annular cancer of the duodenum was the cause.

A man, æt. 43, was taken into the hospital November 5, 1873. On examination, he was found very emaciated, with chronic jaundice and enlarged spleen. His liver was enlarged, smooth, and painless. We could not arrive at any more exact anatomical diagnosis. At the autopsy there was found in the descending portion of the duodenum a circular-shaped cancer, causing closure of the ductus choledochus, with considerable dilatation of the bile-ducts from retention of the bile. This dilatation extended even to the finer branches within the liver, which terminated in small cysts containing bile. The duct of Wirsung, which, in this case, opened separately into the duodenum, passed through the cancerous mass, and its terminal orifice was compressed by it. In consequence of this there was dilatation of the canal above the seat of constriction, and also a number of small saccular diverticula, filled with a clear fluid. The parenchyma of the gland was firmer and more granular than normal, the stroma increased in quantity and in toughness, and the acini in great part atrophied. It was evidently the pressure of the dilated vessels which had given rise to these interstitial inflammatory changes.

I am inclined to believe that a general, chronic, interstitial pancreatitis may result from excessive alcoholism (drunkards'

pancreas). It belongs to the same category as chronic interstitial inflammation and cirrhosis of the liver and kidneys, so frequently met with under similar etiological influences, and these
changes, as I have myself seen, may attain such a degree as to
warrant us to speak of cirrhosis, or of granular disease of the
pancreas.

At the autopsy on a drunkard, who, after long observation, died in my wards
of dropsy, asthma, and with symptoms of chronic asthenia, there were found chronic
fibroid myocarditis, well-marked granular kidneys, cirrhosis of the liver, and a
catarrhal condition of the stomach and duodenum, with hemorrhagic erosions, especially on the mucous membrane of the latter. The pancreas was rather large and
extremely tough and firm, feeling as though it were composed of cartilage-like
masses and nodules. Microscopic examination showed them, after the addition of
acetic acid, to be filled with cells having two or three nuclei, in which, however,
there was not the slightest appearance of any fatty degeneration. There had been
no symptoms during life at all suggestive of disease of the pancreas.

More frequent than a general pancreatitis are the forms of
localized chronic inflammation, the result of extension of inflammatory changes in some of the neighboring organs, such as peritonitis, retroperitonitis, affections of the lumbar vertebræ, etc.
In other cases it is the pressure of a neighboring tumor, or of an
aneurism of the abdominal aorta, or of the cœliac axis, or calculi
in the ductus choledochus at the point where it passes by, sometimes through, the head of the pancreas; or it may be neighboring ulcers and ulcerative new growths, which set up chronic irritation in that part of the gland which lies nearest to it, and
so lead to localized indurative changes. Most frequently it is
simple circular ulcer of the stomach or duodenum which, after
antecedent extension to the pancreas, and generally to the head
of the pancreas, invades its structure, so that the floor of the
ulcer is formed of the toughened pancreas tissue, and this,
spreading more or less into its substance, leads on to a fibroid
degeneration of the glandular elements of the organ. I remember
a case some time back of round ulcer of the stomach at the pyloric extremity, with stenosis and considerable hyperplasia, especially in the muscular coat, and in which this part of the stomach
was firmly adherent to the duodenum and head of the pancreas.
In fact, the head of the pancreas was converted into a hard cica-

trix-like mass, in which scarcely any remains of gland structure could be traced.

Especially worthy of mention are the cases due to constitutional syphilis. Our knowledge of syphilis of the pancreas is decidedly sparse, owing to its great rarity, but nevertheless we know that sometimes the entire gland, sometimes only portions of it, may be the seat of the disease; in these latter cases a local cicatricial mass, either with or without gummata, may be found. Rostan describes two gummata in the pancreas, with others in the muscles and in different parts of the body, in a man who had had chancres fourteen years ago. According to Rokitansky, in rare cases syphilitic masses are found in the pancreas along with similar growths in the liver, either with or without gummata. Lancereaux also affirms to have found the pancreas hard and indurated in several cases of visceral lues, and believes that these changes would be more frequently found if the pancreas were regularly examined after death. In newly born children and in the fœtus unmistakable evidence of degeneration of the pancreas in connection with hereditary syphilis, has been frequently demonstrated. To this class of cases certainly belong two which were reported by Cruveilhier in newly born children; in the first of these two cases (6. Observ.), which died shortly after birth, caseous inflammation of the thymus gland and amyloid swelling of the whole pancreas were found; the latter organ was adherent to the right kidney and supra-renal capsule, and on section it presented the appearance of a homogeneous, tough, yellowish white tissue, without any trace of acinous structure. Cruveilhier compared it to "tissu squirrheux." Oedmansson, among other changes in hereditary syphilis, found alterations in the pancreas, consisting of extensive fatty degeneration of the gland-cells and considerable interstitial hyperplasia, and Klebs describes several gummata in the pancreas along with syphilitic changes in the lungs, liver, and kidneys of a six months fœtus.

Very recently Birch-Hirschfeld has enriched our knowledge of this subject by the proof of the not unfrequent occurrence of interstitial connective-tissue hyperplasia in the pancreas in the hereditary syphilis of newly born children (thirteen times in twenty-five cases). In the most typical cases the organ closely resembled a fibroid structure, the acini were compressed, and their glandular endothelium atrophied. In the hyperplastic connective tissue lay a number of oval or spindle-shaped cells, in other places collections of round cells. The vessels were not numerous, but their walls were thickened.

I now append a case of well-marked disease of the pancreas in a case of congenital syphilis, which I saw some years ago.

On the 15th May, 1858, my colleague, Dr. Kussmaul, handed over to me for examination a still-born and very atrophied seven months fœtus. The epidermis in many places was peeled off, and the brown stained corium was exposed. The lower lobes of the lungs were unusually firm and voluminous; its tissue on section was seen to be composed of a mass of closely packed grayish white lobular infiltrations, smooth and dry on the surface, and of a somewhat caseous appearance. The microscope showed the alveoli to be infiltrated with masses of myeloid cells; these cells, mostly undergoing fatty degeneration, contained roundish or oval nuclei. The bronchi were filled with a creamy pus, which was undergoing fatty degeneration, and ciliated epithelium. The pancreas, and especially its head part, was much enlarged and very hard; it presented the appearance of a firm, almost cartilaginous and homogeneous amyloid mass, with a remarkably small supply of blood. The microscope showed chiefly connective-tissue hyperplasia, in which, on the addition of acetic acid, a small meshed hyaline stroma, containing connective-tissue corpuscles, became visible. Scattered throughout this stroma, but separated by broader bands of intercellular substance, lay a number of variously shaped collections of small nucleated cells, which were regarded as newly formed follicular structure rather than as the remains of the acini, inasmuch as they did not at all resemble pancreas gland-structure; neither were they undergoing any fatty changes. The newly formed cystoid cell-growths seemed to be analogous to the proliferating stroma of the kidneys in interstitial nephritis, or of the ovary in certain forms of ovarian tumors, and to proceed from the proliferation of the connective-tissue corpuscles. Hardened bands of new growth passed chiefly in the direction of the larger vessels far into the liver from the head of the pancreas, so that the latter was firmly adherent at the porta hepatis. It was impossible to trace the bile-ducts through this hardened mass, but they must undoubtedly have been closed, as the liver was distended with bile and of an orange-yellow color; the liver-cells were infiltrated with bile. The gall-bladder, the walls of which were thickened to 1''', contained a quantity of colorless slimy fluid, in which were found innumerable cylindrical epithelial cells. The wall of the duodenum was also thickened. In the lower part of the intestinal canal there was a large quantity of thick dark green meconium. In the upper part the contents were slimy and without any bile admixture. Spleen thickened and somewhat enlarged.

Our knowledge of chronic suppurative infiltration and abscess of the pancreas is very limited. Lieutaud has collected a series of cases from the earlier literature, but it is not very clear whether these cases were acute or chronic. Even modern literature is very poor in reliable cases. Chronic abscesses of the pancreas may perforate neighboring cavities (abdomen, intestine, etc.) or dry up into cheesy and, later, chalky masses. Chronic peripancreatitic suppurations, spreading from surrounding lymphglands and following the course of the connective tissue, may penetrate into the interior of the pancreas, so that the acini become surrounded by pus and separated from the stroma (dissecting suppuration). Concretions in the gland-ducts may give rise to suppurative inflammation in their neighborhood, analogous to liver abscesses brought about by gall-stones. Collections of pus, which resemble abscesses, but genetically differ from them, may result from closure of gland-ducts, causing cysts, the contents of which become purulent.

I do not venture to decide whether chronic parenchymatous pancreatitis without contemporaneous interstitial inflammation occurs as a primary or as a secondary condition. But I have shown in the case of the drunkard's pancreas (p. 602) that such a condition does obtain in connection with chronic interstitial inflammation. Nor do I venture to decide whether or not many cases of caseous degeneration of the pancreas, in combination with chronic swelling and caseous induration of the abdominal lymph-glands, in scrofulous and tubercular subjects, ought to be classed with chronic parenchymatous pancreatitis; perhaps the case by Aran, already mentioned (p. 578), ought to be classed here. These masses soften, and may perforate neighboring cavities (omentum, intestine, etc.) (phthisis pancreatica).

Symptomatology.—It is utterly impossible to give anything like a summary of the symptoms which characterize the various forms of chronic pancreatitis. Chronic disease spreading idiopathically through the whole gland, in the majority of cases, either remains latent, or fails to give rise to any symptoms characteristic of its presence. This is especially true in those cases which result from old-standing venous congestions, where the disease scarcely ever attains such a degree as to interfere much with the secretory function of the gland. And even in the cases where

this function is either partially or entirely destroyed, or where
there is obstruction to the outflow of the secretion into the intestine, there is frequently an absence of all distinctive symptoms,
and it is only in part of the cases that even single symptoms of
pancreas disease—fatty stools, for instance—are met with. If,
then, we consider how very seldom chronic pancreatitis occurs as
an isolated or primary disease, but rather in connection with organic alterations of the stomach, duodenum, peritoneum, liver, etc.,
etc., we shall easily conceive how great are the diagnostic difficulties, and how little justified we are in attributing emaciation,
a feeling of weight or pain in the epigastrium, pyrosis, vomiting,
increased flow of saliva, and the like, to disease of the pancreas.
The presence, however, of fatty stools, possibly intercurrent
mellituria, epigastric pain of a neuralgic character, especially an
appreciable and deeply seated swelling crosswise in the epigastrium, would be the symptoms on which the diagnosis of a chronic inflammatory disease of the pancreas could in some measure
be justifiably founded. It frequently happens that jaundice
comes on in the course of chronic pancreatitis, and when there is
no disease of the liver ; it is then due either to the enlarged head
of the pancreas pressing on the termination of the ductus choledochus, or to obstruction and closure consequent on contraction
during the later stages of the disease (p. 579). If the pancreas
press on the vena portæ, ascites may result ; if on the inferior
cava, œdema of the legs (Rigal) ; and if on the duodenum, we may
get the symptoms of intestinal stenosis (Nathan), so that in presence of such symptoms, by no means characteristic of pancreas
disease, its diagnosis is rendered all the more uncertain. In fact,
if the disease of the pancreas have been latent and of long standing, and have already attained a certain intensity, and then produce jaundice, ascites, or intestinal obstruction, the erroneous
diagnosis of disease of liver or of intestine could scarcely be
avoided.

This applies also to the partial forms of chronic pancreatitis.
The majority of these cases produce either indefinite symptoms
or remain absolutely latent, especially if the head of the gland
happen not to be affected ; but even though the disease be situated here, its position renders the objective proof of a tumor

almost impossible, and it is generally at the autopsy that the nature and locality of the disease is first made out. The pain, digestive troubles, vomiting, etc., depend on implication of neighboring organs, of which the changes in the pancreas are either the cause or the consequence. Even in cases characterized by fatty stools, mellituria, or by the presence of a tumor in the epigastrium, when the diagnosis of pancreas disease would be justified, its differentiation from cancer would again present further and serious difficulties. What we have to say concerning the cause of chronic pancreatitis, will be inferred from the preceding description of its various forms. It is impossible at present to speak with any degree of certainty as to its course and duration, owing to the want of sufficiently accurate clinical records; but doubtless there are greater differences in this respect in different cases. The prognosis would, as a rule, be an unfavorable one, especially in the later stages of the disease, if we judge from the analogy of other organs in a state of chronic interstitial inflammation. It is just possible that a return to the normal condition is possible in the earlier stages; but any doubts on this point are justified owing to the difficulty of the diagnosis; the cases in which recovery is believed to have taken place *ipso facto* possess but little worth.

In the year 1859, I was several times consulted by a shop-keeper, æt. 30 years, who had hitherto been healthy, and though active had yet lived a very regular life. For some months, and without any apparent cause, he had been subject to all kinds of 'dyspeptic troubles, especially frequent acid eructations, and also chronic diarrhœa. In the thin, yellowish gray stools might be seen, in considerable quantity, lumps large and small of tallowy fat. Especially obvious was the great emaciation, which had rapidly set in since the commencement of the disease, with sunken eyes and an earthy cachectic appearance. There was no jaundice, no pain in the epigastrium, but some tenderness on pressure. No appreciable tumor. The objective examination of the chest and abdomen gave negative results. The urine was free from albumen; unfortunately, it was not tested for sugar. The administration of the Elizabeth water (Homburg), after all other medicines had failed, brought about a complete and permanent recovery. Had we here really to do with disease in the pancreas? possibly with a chronic pancreatitis in the early stages? or was it a chronic gastric catarrh with participation of the duodenal mucous membrane, by which a temporary obstruction in the canal of Wirsung was brought about at the point of entrance into the intestine, and so retention of the gland-secretion?

The most important points in the treatment of chronic pancreatitis may be inferred from what has already been said (p. 586 *et seq.*), to which we refer the reader, in order to avoid repetition.

Morbid Growths in the Pancreas (Cancer, Sarcoma, and Tubercle).

Holdefreund, De pancreatis morbis. Diss. Hal. 1713.—*Rahn*, Scirrhosi pancreatis diagnosis. Diss. Götting. 1796.—*Schmackpfeffer*, De quibusdam pancreatis morbis. Diss. Hal. 1814.—*Urban*, Hufeland's Journal. 1830. 11. Stück. S. 87. —*Bécourt*, Recherches sur le pancreas. Thèse. Strasbourg, 1330. p. 58.—*Récamier*, Révue médic. 1830.—*Kopp*, Denkwürdigkeiten aus der ärztlichen Praxis. I. Bd. Frankfurt, 1830. S. 232. IV. Bd. 1839 S. 293.—*Suche*, De scirrho pancreatis nonnulla. Diss. Berol. 1834.—*Davidoff*, De morbis pancreatis observ. quaedam. Diss. Dorpat, 1833.—*Muehry*, Markschwammbildung im Pankreas. Casper's Wochenschrift. Nr. 10. 1835.—*Casper*, Einiges über den Krebs der Bauchspeicheldrüse. Ebendas. Nr. 28, 29. 1836.—*Bigsby*, Edinb. Med. and Surg. Journ. Nr. 124. 1835. p. 93.—*Bressler*, Die Krankheiten des Unterleibes. 2. Bd. Berlin, 1841. S. 274.—*Schupmann*, Hufeland's Journal. 1841. 92. Bd. S. 41.—*Claessen*, Die Krankheiten der Bauchspeicheldrüse. Köln, 1842. S. 274. —*Albers*, Einfacher Krebs des Pankreas. Medic. Correspondenzblatt rhein. und westfäl. Aerzte. Nr. 8. 1843.—*Schlesier*, Zur Lehre vom Skirrhus. des Pankreas. Med. Zeitg. des Vereins für Heilkde. in Preussen. Nr. 10, 11. 1843.—*Battersby*, Dubl. Journ. of Med. Sc. Vol. XXV. 1844. p. 219.— *Williams*, Med. Times and Gaz. Aug. 1852.—*Koehler*, Die Krebs- und Scheinkrebshrankheiten des Menschen. Stuttgart, 1853. S. 386.—*Haldane*, Assoc. Med. Journ. May, 1854. —*Bartrum*, Ibid. 1855.— *Willigk*, Prager Vierteljahrschrift. 1856.—*Frerichs*, Klinik der Leberkrankheiten. 1. Bd. Braunschweig, 1858. S. 146, 153.—*Da Costa*, Cancer of Pancreas. North Americ. Med. Chir. Review. Sept. 1858. p. 883. Schmidt's Jahrb. 107. Bd. 1860. S. 37.—*E. Wagner*, Fall von primärem Pankreaskrebs. Archiv der Heilkde. II. Bd. 1861. S. 285.—*Besson*, De quelques faits pathol. pour servir à l'étude du pancréas. Thèse. Paris, 1864.—*Roberts*, Brit. Med. Journ. Sept. 1865.—*Ancelet*, Études sur les maladies du pancréas. Paris, 1866.—*Boucaud*, Gaz. des hôp. Nr. 10. 1866.—*Luecke* and *Klebs*, Virch. Archiv. 41. Bd. 1867. S. 9.—*Paulicki*, Primäres Sarcom im Kopf des Pankreas. Allgem. med. Centralzeitung. Nr. 90. 1868.—*Klebs*, Handbuch der pathol. Anat. Berlin, 1870. S. 539.— *Webb*, Philadelph. Med. Times. II. Dec. 1871. p. 20.—*Gross*, Ibid. II. June, 1872. p. 354.—*Luithlen*, Memorabil. a. d. ärztl. Praxis. XVII. 1872. S. 309.—*Bowditch*, Boston Med. and Surg. Journ. July, 1872.—*Davidsohn*, Ueber Krebs der Bauchspeicheldrüse. Dissert. Berlin, 1872.

Our knowledge of growths in the pancreas is almost entirely confined to cancerous formations, and which, of all the heteroplastic cumors affecting the pancreas, are by far the most frequent. These growths possess but little clinical interest, partly on account of their great rarity (sarcoma, for instance), and partly because we are ignorant of any symptoms by which they may be distinguished.

The older records of cancer of the pancreas, such as those of Bonetus, Lieutaud, Heberden, can scarcely serve for the study of this disease, as many of the cases of obviously chronic induration are wrongly set down as cancerous. Later research, however, has established that not only is cancer the most frequent form of pancreatic new growths, but that it is also the most frequent form of primary disease of this organ. It generally appears as a compact scirrhus, with abundant stroma (Faserkrebs); less frequently as soft medullary cancer. E. Wagner has seen a case of cylindroma; Luecke and Klebs, a case of gelatinous cancer. Nevertheless, it is a relatively rare disease, especially in its primary forms, and it is a secondary and metastatic growth that we more frequently have to deal with. Willigk found only 29 cases in 467 *post-mortems* on cancerous patients, and Foerster mentions that he only saw 6 cases of cancer in the pancreas, and all as secondary growths, in 639 autopsies in all kinds of disease. As undoubted instances of primary cancer, we must mention the published cases of Muehry, Albers, Haldane, Webb, Gross, Luithlen, Roberts, E. Wagner, Bowditch, Davidsohn, Williams, and Frerichs. Primary cancer most frequently begins in the head, seldom in the body or tail of the pancreas, and appears as a roundish, knotty swelling, of variable size. From the original focus it may spread through the entire gland, converting it into a more or less uniformly knotty, uneven, tuberculated swelling, or it may give rise to separate, small tumors in different parts of the gland. According to Ancelet's table, of 200 cases of cancer of the pancreas, including both the primary and the secondary forms, the growth was confined to the head in 33 cases, to the body in 5, to the tail in 2, and in 88 cases the entire organ was implicated.

Neighboring organs are frequently affected by the pressure of the growing tumor. Thus we may get closure of the duodenum or of the pylorus, with consecutive dilatation of the stomach;

occasionally, as in Rahn's case, the cardiac end **may be com-**
pressed.   Petit [1] relates a remarkable case, in which the cancerous new growth so pressed the stomach against the **anterior wall**
of the abdomen as to give rise to symptoms of incarceration.   In
Récamier's case the infiltrated tail-end of the pancreas compressed the left ureter, and so caused a left hydronephrosis.
Should a cancerous growth in the head of the pancreas **press**
upon the bile-duct, jaundice would result ; or if upon the pancreatic duct, the secretion would be retained, with dilatation of
the ducts (ranula), and not unfrequently with the simultaneous
formation of concretions.   Sometimes the growth presses upon
the superior mesenteric artery and vein (Williams), or on the
splenic artery and vein (Sandwith), or on the vena portæ (causing
ascites) ; more frequently on the inferior cava (giving rise to
œdema of the lower extremities, etc.).   In rare cases, by compressing the aorta, it may give rise to epigastric pulsation and a blowing murmur, as in cases of aneurism of the abdominal aorta.

Primary cancer of the pancreas frequently attacks contiguous
structures and gives rise to secondary degeneration ; should it
spread to the stomach, duodenum, bile-duct and gall-bladder,
liver, vertebræ, kidneys, supra-renal capsules, peritoneum, or
elsewhere, we may have the most varied consequential disturbances, either from stenosis or from ulceration of the new growth
within the ducts or the organs themselves, so that it becomes
impossible, even in the dead body, to demonstrate with any certainty the original starting-point of the disease.   Ulceration of
the new growth into the stomach or duodenum may give rise to
hæmatemesis or to blood in the stools, just in the same way that
primary cancer might do (Muehry, Albers, Kopp).   Ulcerative perforation of neighboring blood-vessels (vena portæ, cava inferior,
art. splenica, art. coronar. ventric.), perforation of the softening
cancer into the abdominal cavity, and through the diaphragm
even into the pleural cavity, have been observed, and in the works
of Claessen and Ancelet we find cases and statements in support
of these possibilities.   In Battersby's case of primary cancer of
the pancreas pressing on the colon, there were symptoms of obstruction.

[1] Cited by *Ancelet*, op. cit. p. 130.

Secondary cancer is also more frequent in the head of the pancreas than elsewhere, and is generally due to propagation from a primary growth in the pylorus, duodenum, liver, or gall-bladder. More rarely the growth shows itself as an isolated, circumscribed mass, secondary to primary cancer in some distant organ. It might also possibly be the expression of a primary general carcinosis.

Causes.—All authors thus far agree that cancer of the pancreas is more frequent in men than in women, and that it occurs chiefly after the fortieth year of life; nevertheless evidence is not wanting of its occurrence at an earlier period of life. Of 37 cases collected by Da Costa, there were 24 males and 13 females, and Ancelet found in 161 cases that 102 were males and 59 females, and that the disease occurred most frequently from the thirtieth to the sixtieth year. In Bigsby's statistics of 28 cases, 16 were males and 12 females; of the men, fourteen were forty years of age and upward, and of the women, all had passed the fiftieth year of life. Statistics at present show nothing as to the part played by hereditary tendency in the production of this disease, and except as to age and sex we know nothing of the etiology of primary cancer of this organ. Neither are we able to say whether geographical influences or peculiarities in habits, food, or manner of living have any bearing on its production, nor whether traumatic influences, such as contusions, concussions, blows in the epigastrium, as indeed is conjectured by some, are in any way concerned in its onset.

Symptomatology.—The symptoms of cancerous disease in the pancreas are mainly those which have been indicated in chronic affections of this gland. In the majority of cases, the symptoms point to a more or less deeply seated organic lesion of one or other of the neighboring organs of the upper belly, such as their frequent participation in pancreatic affections would naturally lead us to expect; hence, we may get indications of either constrictive disease of stomach or of duodenum, or of chronic gastric catarrh, or of progressive liver disease with or without jaundice. Hohnbaum considers watery eructations or watery vomitings, great thirst with moist tongue, and extreme emaciation as especially reliable symptoms, but we must refer the reader to what has been said in the general part (p. 565 et seq.) as to the diagnostic value of these symptoms. Nor can we agree with Claessen, that vomiting is rarely present in cancer and rarely absent in chronic pancreatitis. We have already indicated that in consequence either of pressure on, or of the gradual ingrowth of the cancerous mass into surrounding structures, a series of the most varied symptoms may ensue, and that vomiting as a result of stenosis of pylorus or duodenum, hæmatemesis or blood in the stools, ascites and anasarca of the legs, as also jaundice, especially in the later stages of the disease, are frequent occurrences. Da Costa's own statistics show how commonly such complications are present. In 37 cases of cancer of the pancreas, vomiting, in consequence of concomitant disease of the stomach, was present 22 times, jaundice 24 times, dyspeptic difficulties 25 times, dropsy 15 times, either as anasarca or ascites. Whether there is constipation or diarrhœa depends on the presence or absence of complications with or consecutive changes in the intestinal mucous membrane. In his 37 cases, Da Costa found that obstruction occurred 19 times, and alternative constipation and diarrhœa 15 times. Fatty stools were observed in many cases, but although they were attentively looked for in all cases, they were frequently absent.

Pain in the epigastrium is an important sign in the diagnosis of cancer of the pancreas, and one which assumes a prominent position, partly on account of the frequency, not to say constancy, of its presence, and partly on account of its severity and obstinacy. In thirty-two out of the thirty-seven cases, Da Costa found it was mentioned as being unusually intense, and Claessen, after a careful comparison of a large number of cases, ascribed an almost diagnostic importance to this symptom. The pain is almost constant, with alternating remissions and exacerbations, frequently coming on in paroxysms and lasting even several days; they are of a decidedly neuralgic type, and suggest implication of the cœliac plexus (pressure, neuritis, or cancerous infiltration, cœliac neuralgia, p. 581). This pain may possibly depend on a chronic inflammation or secondary infiltration of the peritoneum. The patients complain sometimes of local pain, deep in the epigastrium, sometimes across the epigastrium, running either into one or other hypochondrium, generally the right, or shooting toward the back, or the sacrum, or the shoulder; at other times, the pain spreads from the upper belly over the entire abdomen. The position of the body has a decidedly modifying influence on the pain, and sometimes it increases so much when the body is upright that the patient prefers to preserve a flexed position forward.

A second and very important symptom is *an appreciable tumor*. This is more frequent in cancer than in chronic inflammation, since the enlargement of the gland in the latter affection would not easily attain the same extent as in the former disease. But the perception of the tumor, even in cancer, is only possible in the minority of cases. Da Costa appreciated it in only thirteen out of the thirty-seven cases, and in fifteen cases analyzed by Bigsby swelling was appreciable in only four cases. In the majority of cases, cancer attacks the head of the pancreas, which lies beneath the liver. It will, therefore, be easily understood why tumors are so difficult to get at, and why palpation, if at all feasible, only becomes so in the later stages, when the disease has spread to the rest of the organ, and when it has attained to a very considerable size. Occasionally there is only an increased resistance and a brawny induration in the epigastric region. A preliminary evacuation of the intestines by means of a purgative or clyster, and a fasting condition of the stomach, materially facilitate the perception of the tumor, the examination for which should be made in the knee-elbow position, or under chloroform, in order to relax the abdominal muscles. The size of the tumor, its hard, nodular surface, the possible presence of enlarged lymphatic glands in the neck, would materially support the idea of cancer. Doubtless, cancer of the stomach, of the liver, or of the omentum, might likewise give rise to epigastric tumors, so that one is here open to many sources of error.

From what has already been said, it will be seen how very uncertain is the diagnosis of cancer of the pancreas, and that it is only by the combination of a number of favorable circumstances, and with the help of the method of exclusion, that a correct diagnosis of this disease can be obtained. We should be justified in such a diagnosis if, in a patient of advanced years, we found a markedly cachectic habit, a continuous pain in the epigastrium, with an appreciable tumor in the region occupied by the pancreas, and when, at the same time, there were sufficient grounds for excluding the existence of primary disease of the surrounding abdominal organs. The supervention of fatty stools or of mellituria would assist in the diagnosis, though it would fail to give any absolute certainty to it, and, while the size of the growth would be of service in the differential diagnosis of chronic pancreatitis, its consistence and irregular surface would distinguish it from cystic degeneration.

The duration of the disease cannot possibly be stated, since it may undoubtedly begin imperceptibly and remain latent for some time. The special histological nature of the new growth, and its larger or smaller blood-supply, may, in some measure, influence its course, while the various complications (stenosis of intestines, jaundice, hemorrhage, etc.) would materially affect its duration. From Da Costa's tables it would seem that the symptoms, when once pronounced, seldom lasted more than one year, while in some cases the fatal termination occurred within a few months.

Sarcoma of the pancreas is infinitely rarer than cancer. It is just probable that in the earlier literature of this subject many of the cases given as "cancer" belonged to the sarcomata; but it is impossible to decide this now. At present we are acquainted with only one single reliable case of primary sarcoma of the pancreas; it is described by Paulicki, and was found to be of the small-celled variety; it was taken from the body of a young man, who had died of pulmonary and intestinal phthisis; it had not given rise to any noticeable symptoms during life. Sarcoma may, no doubt, occur as a secondary affection, but, nevertheless, I have not been able to find any well-authenticated case of this disease on record. The differential diagnosis of sarcoma and cancer is not possible, and what we have said for the one will probably hold good for the other.

Tubercle of the pancreas is very rare; when it does occur, it usually presents itself in the form of a more or less cheesy nodule, together with chronic tuberculosis and phthisis of the lung and intestine. That, however, which is generally described as tubercle seems rather to be of the nature of chronic caseous inflammation. As to the participation of the pancreas in general acute miliary tuberculosis, Klebs denies it, and seems never to have seen miliary tubercles in the pancreas in this affection; still, the statement requires confirmation. It is by no means necessary that tubercle in the pancreas should produce any definite symptoms, and hence its diagnosis during life is scarcely possible.

The treatment of these new growths, especially of cancer, must mainly be directed towards the symptoms it produces, and dietetic. The relief of the pain by narcotics, internally and hypodermically, keeping up the strength also, and so postponing as long as possible the fatal marasmus, must be the physician's chief aim. The daily administration of a calf's pancreas is well worthy a trial.

Cysts of the Pancreas.

A. Stoerk, Annus medicus. Vindobon. 1760. p. 245.—*Bécourt*, Recherches sur le pancréas. Thèse. Strasbourg, 1830. p. 56.—*Engel*, Oesterreich. med. Jahrbücher. 23. u. 24. Bd. S. 1841.—*Cruveilhier*, Traité d'Anat. pathol. Tom. III. Paris, 1856. p. 365.—*Parsons*, Brit. Med. Journ. June, 1857·—*Hoppe*, Virch. Arch. XI. 1857. S. 96.—*Gould*, Anat. Museum of the Boston Soc. Boston, 1847. p. 174.—*Klob*, Oesterreich. Zeitschr. für prakt. Heilkde. VI. 33. Bd. 1860.—*Rokitansky*, Lehrbuch der pathol. Anat. 3. Bd. 1861. S. 313.—*Virchow*, Würzburger Verhandlungen. II. Bd. 1852. S. 53. III. Bd. 1852. S. 368.—Die krankhaften Geschwülste. I. 1863. S. 276.—*Recklinghausen*, Virch. Arch. 30. Bd. 1864. S. 360.—*Wyss*, Ebendas. 36. Bd. 1866. S. 454.—*Pepper*, Centralblatt für die med. Wissensch. 1871. S. 156.—*O. Hjelt*, Schmidt's Jahrbücher. 157. Bd. 1873. S. 132.—*Curnow*, Transact. of the pathol. Soc. XXIV. 1873.—*Klebs*, Handbuch der pathol. Anat. Berlin, 1870. S. 547.

Cysts in the pancreas generally result from retention of its secretion, and subsequent dilatation of the excreting ducts ; they belong exclusively to the class of retention-cysts. They have seldom any other cause, though occasionally they result from hemorrhagic causes (hemorrhagic cysts). Concerning these latter, the most important points will be considered in the next paragraph. If the chief duct should be closed either at or near its termination in the duodenum, then we get dilatation of the duct in its entire length, and in its branches, and either an irregularly shaped mass, not unlike a bunch of currants, results, or a more uniformly rounded cyst, of the size of a fist, of a child's head, or even larger (Bécourt's case); or, in consequence of unequal dilatation of the branch ducts, there may be several larger or smaller cysts projecting prominently from the outer surface of the gland (Wyss' case). Virchow has given the name "ranula pancreatica" to all these and similar dilatations of gland-ducts leading on to the formation of cysts.

The surrounding gland-parenchyma may atrophy, from the increasing size of the cysts, or the walls of the cyst become thickened, and then gradually encroach on the gland-substance, through chronic interstitial growth and induration of the connective tissue. In this way, the entire gland-structure, even to its last acinus, may be completely destroyed. It is only in the smaller and recent cysts that the contents correspond, or nearly so, with the normal secretion. Later on, in old or large cysts, albuminoid or purulent degeneration not unfrequently takes place, or hemorrhage may occur, so that the contents assume a bright-red or chocolate-colored appearance (hæmatoma of the pancreas). Pepper has found numerous crystals of hæmatoidin in such a cyst. Hoppe, in a case described by himself, found the contents of a cyst to contain 0.12 per cent. of urea. Sometimes in old cysts concretions are deposited, which consist almost entirely of earthy salts—and, for the most part, combinations of lime.

The causes of retention of the secretions are manifold, sometimes within, sometimes without the gland. It may be due to the formation of calculi in the duct of Wirsung (Gould and Recklinghausen's cases); or to interstitial inflammation and hyperplasia of the connective tissue (Pepper's and Hjelt's cases); or to new growths in the head of the gland; or to catarrhal closure of the excretory duct at its entrance into the duodenum (Curnow's case). Among the outside causes must first be mentioned peripancreatitic indurations and adhesions, especially in the neighborhood of the head of the gland (Hoppe's case); then gall-stones in the ductus choledochus, pressing upon Wirsung's duct (Engel's case); and also benign or malignant tumors, large lymph-glands, and the like. In a case related by Virchow it was a villous tumor in the duodenum, and in a case which I have already related (p. 601) it was an annular cancer of the duodenum, which, by closing the duct, had so given rise to a retention of the secretion. Rarely could a displacement of the pancreas be expected, such as was the cause of retention in a case related by Engel, who found, in a woman æt. 60 years, that the tail of the pancreas formed a right angle upwards with the main duct of the gland.

The closure of the smaller branch ducts is mostly due to localized interstitial inflammatory thickening, giving rise to multiple, small, vesicular-like cysts, which may be found either in the substance of the gland or on its surface—the main duct being the while quite patent. Sometimes this closure of the small ducts may be due to catarrhal swelling of the lining membrane, or to a collection of stringy catarrhal secretion. The contents of these small cysts, which generally occur in groups, are sometimes bright and clear, sometimes opaque, yellowish, thickened, and mixed with fat-globules and cretaceous material similar to small abscesses, for which they may easily be mistaken. Klebs has described these changes as "acne pancreatica." We may here mention the case, described by Virchow, of a syphilitic woman, who had a gall-bladder fistula opening into the colon, and whose pancreas, enlarged and indurated, was covered with a light green, fatty substance, in small spots or nodules, which also spread into the substance of the gland. The duct of Wirsung was somewhat distended, and its branches were filled with a semi-liquid material, which, in addition to pus-elements, was found to contain a number of light albuminoid particles of hardened protein ; the walls of the ducts were yellow, infiltrated with fat, and in places eroded. The small white spots found on cutting into the thickened connective tissue, in cases of chronic pancreatitis, which result from obstruction in the vena portæ, as described by Klob, and from which molecules of chalk or tufts of fat-crystals can be expressed, seem to belong to the class of retention-cysts, with thickening and alteration of the contents.

The diagnosis of cysts in the pancreas will naturally be possible only in cases where the swelling has attained very considerable proportions. The chief point in favor of such a diagnosis would be the presence of a round or oval smooth-surfaced tumor, in which fluctuation could be appreciated, deeply situated and in the region of the pancreas. The small amount or entire absence of epigastric pain should be looked upon as excluding cancer, while the want of the cancerous cachexia and of extreme emaciation would confirm this view. The supervention or occurrence of fatty stools or of mellituria would assist in the diagnosis. Recklinghausen's two cases of "ranula" of the pancreas occurred in diabetic patients. If the tumor received any pulsatile movement from the aorta, an aneurism of the latter might easily be suspected. Our literature, indeed, contains a number of cases in which perception of even large cysts by palpation was not possible during life—cases, therefore, in which a diagnosis was not arrived at. If jaundice, from pressure on the gall-duct, or if pressure on the neighboring blood-vessels—which may occur just as in cases of cancer (p. 610)—or if peritonitis supervene, and so complicate the case, more especially when there are no symptoms to point specially to the pancreas, it would be utterly impossible to avoid an error in diagnosis. Large cysts sometimes open into the stomach or duodenum, and cause death in this way. This occurred in the case of a man—a drunkard, æt. 45 years—the subject of cirrhosis of the liver, whose death was caused by the bursting of hemorrhagic cysts of the pancreas into the duodenum, the symptoms being hematemesis and blood in the stools (Pepper).

The treatment must be of the symptoms as they arise, and by diet, with special attention to the points already alluded to (p. 586 et seq.).

Concretions in the Pancreas.

Lieutaud, Histor. anat. med. I. Longosal. 1786. p. 87 u. 312.—*Cawley*, Lond. Med. Journ. 1788. Sammlung auserlesener Abhandlgen. 13. Bd. Leipzig, 1789. S. 112.—*Portal*, Cours d'Anat. med. Tom. V. Paris, 1803.—*Elliotson*, Med. Chir. Transact. Vol. XVIII. London, 1833. p. 67.—*Bigsby*, Edinb. Med. Journ. Nr. 124. 1835.—*Schupmann*, Hufeland's Journal. 92. Bd. 1841. S. 41.—*Engel*, Oesterreich. med. Jahrbücher. 1841.—*Bécourt*, Recherches sur le pancréas. Thèse. Strasb. 1830. p. 69.—*Claessen*, a. a. O. S. 178.—*Gould*, Anat. Museum of the Boston Soc. Boston, 1847. p. 174.—*Virchow*, Verhandlungen der med. physik. Gesellschaft zu Würzburg. II. 1852. S. 53. III. 1852. S. 368.—*Henry*, Journ. de chimie méd. Mai, 1855.—*Fauconneau-Dufrèsne*, Traité de l'affection calculeuse du foie et du pancréas. Paris, 1851. p. 488.—*Recklinghausen*, Virch. Arch. 30. Bd. 1864. S. 360.—*Ancelet*, Loc. cit. p. 37.—*Klebs*, a. a. O. S. 544.—*Curnow*, Transact. of the Pathol. Soc. XXIV. 1873.

Calculi in the excretory ducts of the pancreas are much rarer than in the ducts of the salivary glands; they result in both cases from the precipitation of the inorganic constituents of the secretions. They are generally found in the chief duct—the canal of Wirsung—more rarely in the branch ducts also; they are sometimes embedded and encysted in one of the smaller branches of the duct, and then seem as if they were formed in the substance of the gland itself. Their color is mostly white or grayish white; sometimes dark, or even blackish; they are round or oval in shape, and very rarely branched; the surface may be either smooth or rough. Their size is equally uncertain, and may vary from the finest dust-like formations to the size of a hazel-nut. They may possibly attain to even a greater size, as, for instance, in Schupmann's case, where a calculus, weighing 200 grains, and measuring one and a half Paris inches long, and from five to six Paris lines in diameter, having a crystalline surface, with processes running into the smaller ducts, was found in the left extremity of Wirsung's canal. There may be either a single calculus or several, and even as many as twelve or more (Portal); in fact, the entire duct, and even its smallest branches, may be found full of small calculi (Elliotson, Curnow).

As to their chemical composition, like salivary calculi, they are found to consist chiefly of carbonate or phosphate of lime, or of a combination of the two.

Henry has described a peculiar concretion, which was found in the pancreas of a man who had died of cancer of the stomach. It was about the size of a walnut, roundish and hard, and was covered by a thick membrane; the interior presented several cavities, which were occupied partly with a white, milk-like fluid, partly with a chalky powder and with small yellow calculi, composed of phosphate of lime, mixed with a small quantity of organic matter. The exterior was coated with a mixture of phosphate and carbonate of lime. It is probable that this peculiar formation was the result of dilated ducts becoming encrusted, and that a simultaneous deposition of independent concretions took place within them.

Virchow describes small, microscopical, concentrically striped concretions, which he has found on two occasions in the pancreatic duct, consisting of insoluble, solidified protein substances.

These solid concretions are most likely to occur in cases where the outflow of the pancreatic juice is interfered with—in retention-cysts therefore. But it also seems probable, without any pre-existing cysts, that a catarrhal condition of the ducts may give rise to the concretions; and that they may also result from anomalies in the chemical composition of the secretion; and that these may then give rise to ranula by pressing on some of the ducts in their vicinity. In Recklinghausen's case a sac as large as a child's head had formed in this way, and in Gould's case, owing to plugging of the canal of Wirsung by a calculus at its point of entrance into the duodenum, a retention-cyst developed, which became so large that it could be distinctly felt through the abdominal wall.

The presence of a fixed calculus may give rise to chronic interstitial inflammation or to induration, wasting, and atrophy of the gland-parenchyma, and this may spread even to the entire gland (Engel, Elliotson, Curnow), or to acute irritation of surrounding structures, or to purulent inflammation (calculous abscesses). Portal's case deserves especial mention; his patient had suddenly died with symptoms of an aortic aneurism, and it was found that the pancreas, which contained twelve calculi, had so compressed the aorta against the vertebral column, that there was aneurismal dilatation above the seat of compression, while below it the aorta was narrowed and contracted to such a degree as hardly to admit the little finger. Together with calculous formations, there is sometimes associated a cancer of the pancreas (Schupmann) or cancer of neighboring organs, of the stomach, for instance (Henry).

The diagnosis of calculi is impossible. They mostly remain latent, having been found over and over again in the excretory ducts, in cases where their presence during life had never even been suspected. If, however, there should be any symptoms, they are mostly the result of complications, or of the consecutive disturbance which the calculi give rise to. They are the formation of cysts, chronic pancreatitis, or peripancreatitis, conditions which have already been described. In a series of cases, in which calculi were found in the pancreas after death, there had been mellituria, and in some cases also fatty stools. If the calculus be arrested just where Wirsung's duct enters the duodenum, it may at the same time press on the ductus choledochus and so cause jaundice (Gould).

Whether pancreatic calculi may be passed into the duodenum during a paroxysm of pain, and thus pass away with the fæces, in other words, whether "pancreatic stone colic," analogous to a bile-stone colic, ever occurs, is not proved by any direct observations, though it seems far from improbable that such is the case. It would be impossible almost to differentiate biliary colic, because the stone in its passage through the last part of Wirsung's duct would probably close the pars duodenalis of the ductus choledochus, and so give rise to jaundice.

The treatment will depend on the symptoms which arise, and for this we refer the reader to what has been said in the chapters on Cysts and Chronic Inflammation of the Pancreas.

Hemorrhages into the Pancreas.

A. *Stoerk*, Annus medic. Vindobon. 1760. p. 245.—*Portal*, Cours d'anat. méd. Tom. V. Paris, 1803. p. 353.—*Hooper*, Arch. of Med. II. 1861. p. 282.—*Klob*, Oesterr. Zeitschr. für prakt. Heilkde. VI. 33. Bd. 1860.—*Klebs*, a. .a. O. S. 549, 555.—*Zenker*, Tagblatt der 47. Versammlung deutscher Naturforscher und Aerzte in Breslau, 1874. S. 211.

Hemorrhagic processes in the pancreas are mostly due to passive hyperæmia, the result of organic disease in the lungs, heart, or liver, and then most frequently coexist with the chronic inflammatory changes which result under such etiological conditions (p. 600). The hemorrhagic spots are scattered through the actively growing connective tissue, which later on form round or oval pigmented masses, or spaces containing a colored serosity, and surrounded by thickened rust-colored irregular walls (Klob).

Large hemorrhagic masses may occur in the pancreas under other circumstances, perhaps in connection with pre-existing changes in the vascular system. These so-called apoplectic cysts which result from such hemorrhages, in view of their nature and cause, ought naturally to be distinguished from pre-existing retention-cysts, into which hemorrhage has taken place. The frequently quoted case of Stoerk's probably belongs to this category. A woman aged twenty-eight years, otherwise healthy, was taken with violent vomiting during the catamenial period ; the catamenia ceased, and a pulsating tumor appeared in the epigastrium ; there were fainting fits, palpitation, cold extremities, with a feeling of great distress. When the tumor had existed three and a half months, the violent bilious vomiting and diarrhœa recurred, and death from exhaustion resulted. At the autopsy the pancreas, weighing thirteen pounds, was found converted into a large sac containing blood, partially encysted. This hemorrhage came from a ruptured blood-vessel, which could be traced into the middle of the pancreas.

Especial clinical importance seems due to the hemorrhagic processes—which must be distinguished from those just described—in which the entire pancreas takes on a hemorrhagic condition, without any interstitial inflammatory changes or gross alterations being appreciable in the vascular system. According to Klebs, who recently drew attention to the subject, the whole gland is of a dark-red or violet color, the meshes of the interstitial tissue are filled with fresh or with altered blood, and the acini are tinged of a dead gray color, or with diffused blood-pigment. The hemorrhage may spread around the gland, more especially into the retroperitoneal connective tissue. Later on, the gland becomes soft and squashy ; the serous covering of its anterior surface sloughs, and masses of broken-down gland-substance get into the peritoneal cavity. Death sometimes occurs very suddenly in these cases, so that at times the peritoneum does not present any secondary changes at all. Klebs mentions a case, of which he himself made an autopsy, and where the sudden death could be ascribed to nothing else but the hemorrhage into the pancreas. It is doubtful whether an older case described by Portal can be classed with these.

Zenker has recently reported three cases of pancreas hemor-rhage, on account of its very puzzling nature and cause, in which death occurred very suddenly, and where the *post-mortem* ex-amination revealed nothing else to account for death. The first case occurred in a man aged forty-eight years, rather corpulent, who in the midst of perfect health awoke one morning with a feel-ing of malaise and inclination to vomit, and after a few minutes fell down dead. At the autopsy an extensive hemorrhagic infiltra-tion was found in and around the pancreas, with effusion of blood into the duodenum. The microscopic examination showed the pancreas to be undergoing fatty degeneration, so that scarcely a single acinus remained. The second case was that of a man twenty-eight years of age, also rather corpulent, who suffered from epilepsy, but was otherwise healthy. This man was one day picked up dead in a wood, in which one hour previously he had been seen at work. In this case also the most noticeable change was extensive hemorrhage into the pancreas with fatty degeneration of its tissue. There were no traces of violence any-where about the body. The third case was that of a very corpu-lent man—a drunkard—who was drowned. The evidence showed that this man, while standing near the water, was overtaken by sudden death, and fell into the water while in the act of dying. The autopsy showed a similar hemorrhagic infiltration of the pancreas with fatty degeneration as in the first two cases ; there was likewise effusion of blood into the duodenum. Perhaps, in all these cases, there was fatty degeneration of the pancreas, accompanied by fatty changes in the blood-vessels, which was the cause of these hemorrhages.

Zenker very justly points out that in these and analogous cases, the hemorrhage, on account of its very limited amount, cannot be the cause of the sudden death, and believes that for its real explanation we must think of nerve influences. In con-nection with this point, Zenker lays stress on the great venous hyperæmia of the semilunar ganglion, with perfect integrity of the nerve-cells and nerve-fibres, which was found in the second and third cases, and reminds us of Goltz's well-known "tap-ping experiment" (Klopfversuch), through which, by means of repeated tapping on the abdomen of a frog, diastolic arrest of the heart can be produced. But even if the heart was found flaccid in Zenker's second case, it does not seem to me to prove that the "tapping experiment" in any way explains the sudden death in cases of hemorrhage into the pancreas, because the very dilatation and overfilling of the collective abdominal vessels, which Goltz constantly found in these experiments as a sign of paralysis of the nervi splanchnici, and considered as explanatory of his experiment, are not even mentioned in Zenker's cases, and may have been altogether absent. We shall be better justified in ascribing this apoplectic form of death to pressure on the semilunar ganglion and solar plexus, brought about by the sudden swelling out of the pancreas by hemorrhage and consequent reflex disturbance of the heart's movements (reflex paralysis), which would remind the reader of the cases which have from time to time been published of sudden, even fatal, collapse in different diseases of the pancreas, in explanation of which I have drawn attention to the great sympathetic ganglia of the abdomen (pp. 581 and 595).

Cases such as those related by Zenker certainly merit great attention, and it must be an object with future workers to increase the statistical material by an addition of fresh cases bearing on this point. Probably, however, we are already justified in accepting the possibility of an apoplexia abdominalis pancreatica.

The diagnosis of hemorrhage into the pancreas is at present impossible, and consequently nothing can be said regarding its treatment.

Fatty and Amyloid Diseases of the Pancreas.

Bécourt, Loc. cit. p. 50.—*Handfield Jones*, Med. Chir. Transact. XXXVIII. 1855. p. 195.—*Rud. Maier*, Archiv der Heilkde. VI. 1865. S. 168.—*Friedreich*, Virch. Arch. XI. 1857. S. 389.—*Rokitansky*, Lehrbuch der pathol. Anat. III. 1861. S. 313, 369.—*Klebs*, a. a. O. S. 536.

A. Fatty Disease.

Two forms can be distinguished, lipomatosis and fatty degeneration. They may occur either separately or in combination.

In lipomatosis of the pancreas we have to do with a new growth of fat-tissue, proceeding from the inter-acinous connective tissue, and from the pre-existing fat-tissue, which is normally found in the gland. Occasionally an adipose tissue, which surrounds the gland, grows into it, and spreads through it in various degrees. In these cases yellowish bands and islets of fat-tissue can be seen among the acini, the continuous growth of which gradually leads to atrophy and even disappearance of the gland-cells of the acini. In the latest stages the whole organ is changed into yellow or yellowish white fatty lobules, and every trace of its earlier glandular structure is lost. The canal of Wirsung contains a fatty whey-like fluid. The above described changes are generally found as part and parcel of a general obesity, especially in drunkards, together with fatty liver, heart, and omentum, etc. R. Maier has described an exceedingly well-marked example of this disease.

Fatty degeneration of the pancreas consists of fatty degeneration, with destruction, of the gland-cells, analogous to fatty degeneration of other glandular organs. Handfield Jones was the first to describe this condition accurately. In the advanced stages of the process, the outward appearance of the gland is remarkably altered ; if the disease is not combined with interstitial hyperplasia of the connective tissue, the gland is soft, flaccid, and wasted ; the acinous structure is distinctly preserved, but the acini are pale, and of a whitish yellow color. Sometimes, owing to breaking down of the lining cells, the acini are filled with a fatty emulsion, which fills the ducts, and may even distend them (Rokitansky). After the discharge or absorption of these contents, the connective tissue of the gland remains as a flaccid band, beset here and there with the scanty remains of the acini, until at last it also becomes entirely atrophied. To this class of cases belongs a portion of the cases of atrophy of the pancreas already alluded to as being found in diabetes (p. 591), and in general marasmus (cancer, phthisis, and other chronic cachexia, senescence, etc.). As in the interstitial chronic inflammatory processes, so in lipomatosis of the pancreas, the secondary atrophy of the acini takes place after the manner already described in fatty degeneration, and also in morbid growths, cysts, and the like.   I have already (p. 575) related the case of a diabetic woman, in whom fatty degeneration of the pancreas went hand in hand with well-marked lipomatosis.

Finally, fatty degeneration is found in general obesity, especially, too, in drunkards, analogous to the fatty degeneration of the muscle of the heart under like circumstances; and if trophic changes in the blood-vessels be combined, we may here get a predisposition to the hemorrhagic processes described at p. 623. At all events, in the before-mentioned cases of pancreatic apoplexy, as described by Zenker, the fatty degeneration of gland-cells was always found along with general obesity.

B. Amyloid Disease.

This is only found in association with widely spread amyloid degeneration of other organs and tissues, and spreads, as I have shown, only along the blood-vessels of the gland—especially the small arteries and capillaries. The glassy particles which are sometimes found in the canal of Wirsung, and wrongly described by Rokitansky as "amyloid" formations, are really identical with the concretions described by Virchow as consisting of a firm protein substance (p. 620). Rokitansky's statement as to the occurrence of real amyloid degeneration confined to the pancreas alone has not yet been confirmed; neither have I ever succeeded in convincing myself of the existence of amyloid induration in the gland-cells, likewise described by this author. But in association with amyloid vessels we may get the most typical fatty degeneration of the gland-cells, such as I described in an excellent case occurring in a patient who had died of phthisis. In the present state of our knowledge neither fatty changes nor amyloid disease of the pancreas can be recognized during life.

The Accessory Pancreas.

Engel, Oesterreich. med. Jahrbücher. XXIII. 1841.—*Klob*, Wiener medic. Zeitschrift. N. F. II. Nr. 46. 1859. S. 732.—*Zenker*, Virch. Archiv. 21. Bd. 1861. S. 369.—*Montgomery*, The Lancet. VII. 1861.—*Rokitansky*, a. a. O. III. Bd. 1861. S. 291.—*Claessen*, a. a. O. S. 350.—*Wagner*, Archiv der Heilkunde. 3. Jahrgang, 1862. S. 283.—*Gegenbaur*, Archiv für Anat., Physiol., und wissenschaftl.

Medicin. 1863. S. 163.—*Hyrtl*, Ein Pankreas accessorium und ein Pankreas divisum. Sitzungsberichte der Wiener Akad. LII. Abthlg. 1. 1866. S. 275.— *Neumann*, Archiv der Heilkunde. 11. Jahrgang. 1870. S. 200.—*Klebs*, a. a. O. S. 531

A rarely occurring glandular organ, identical in structure with the pancreas, lying between the coats of the intestine, has been described as an accessory pancreas (P. accessorium, succenturiatum). The development of an accessory pancreas may be looked upon as a growing-out of the glandular layer of the intestine which takes place near the spot where, at an early period of fœtal life, the chief organ is developed, and which, by independent and further growth (development), becomes a separate gland. In consequence of the growth in length of the originally short and vertical intestinal canal, these double fœtal products become further separated, so that later on the accessory pancreas may be placed at a varying distance from the pancreas proper. The cardia on the one side, and the last coil but one of the ileum on the other, as the spot which gives passage to the ductus omphalomesentericus, and which is occasionally marked by the occurrence of a true diverticulum, may be given as the limits within which the occurrence of an accessory pancreas is possible.

The size of the accessory pancreas is always considerably smaller than that of the pancreas proper, and varies from that of a thaler (an English half-crown) to that of a pea. On section, the lobulated glandular structure is easily recognized, but the acini are smaller than those of the chief organ. These accessory structures are almost invariably smooth, flattened in shape, and correspond histologically with the gland proper. As a rule, perhaps always, they are provided with an excretory duct, which terminates on a small papilla in the mucous membrane, and empties itself into the duodenum. The accessory pancreas is always found between the intestinal coats, having its seat sometimes in the serosa, sometimes in the submucosa, or even partially in the musculosa, in which cases muscular fibres are found running between the acini. Accordingly as it is chiefly situated in the subserosa or in the submucosa, shall we best observe it as a flattened prominence towards the interior or towards the exterior of the gut.

These accessory formations are chiefly met with in the region of the jejunum, mostly near the duodenum and least often in the coats of the stomach. Klob, Wagner, and Gegenbaur have each had cases of this latter kind. In Kloh's case, the accessory pancreas was situated in the centre of the greater curvature between the serous and muscular coats; in Wagner's case, it was in the anterior wall near the lesser curvature, midway between the cardia and pylorus; and in Gegenbaur's case, near the pyloric end of the lesser curvature between the muscular and mucous coats. As to their position in the duodenum, there are two recorded cases: one by Engel, where the gland, as large as a half-crown piece, was situated below the head of the pancreas on the inner side of the descending duodenum, its duct opening into the canal of Wirsung; the other case, related by Zenker, where it was found on the convex border of the first portion of the duodenum, obliquely opposite the head of the pancreas. Zenker has described five cases in which the accessory organ appeared in the jejunum and ileum, in three of which the structure was found in the first loop of the jejunum; in one case somewhat lower down in the jejunum; and in the other case, a true diverticulum was found; it was 54 ctms. above the ileo-cæcal valve, was as large as a finger-stall, with a narrow, fatty mesentery, and buried in this fat there was an accessory pancreas near the extremity of the diverticulum. In another case, also described by Zenker, were found two accessory glands in the same gut, one 16, the other 48 ctms. below the duodenum. Neumann has reported a case in which the accessory pancreas was situated at the extremity of a diverticulum of the ileum, about two inches above the ileo-cæcal valve. Neumann believes, however, that this diverticulum was unconnected with the ductus omphalo-mesentericus, and resulted rather from the traction which the accessory pancreas exercised on the intestinal wall. I have twice found, at *post-mortem* examinations, accessory pancreas glands, which were situated high up in the duodenum—they presented themselves as oblong swellings, the long axis of which corresponded with that of the duodenum; they were placed exactly opposite the insertion of the mesentery. In one case, the growth, which was divided by a cross-furrow into two unequal portions, was fifteen Paris lines long by six broad, and projected about one and one-half externally and somewhat less internally ; it was chiefly situated in the submucosa, but a little also in the musculosa. Internally, a very small papilla of mucous membrane could be recognized, on which the delicate excretory duct opened. In my second case, the tumor was eight lines long by five broad, and was situated entirely in the submucosa ; an excretory duct could not be found.

Whether these accessory glands can be the starting-point of degeneration, or whether and how far they participate in diseases of the pancreas proper, is unknown.

We are not to confound these accessory glands with those anomalies, such as Hyrtl has twice observed and described as pancreas divisum. The pancreas was divided into two portions, which were connected together only by the branches of Wirsung's duct. In one case the separation corresponded accurately with the point at which the left gastro-epiploic artery crosses the pancreas, and in the other with the point where the superior mesenteric artery passes down behind it.

Here, too, we must mention Rokitansky's statement that an accessory spleen is not unfrequently embedded in the head of the pancreas, and also Klob's observation of the occurrence of a dark-red accessory spleen, as large as a bean, in the enlarged tail-end of a pancreas which was removed from the body of an idiot, who had died of atrophy of the brain.

Anomalies in the Position of the Pancreas.

Mondière, Arch. génér. de méd. Tom. XI. 1836. p. 50.—*Trafoyer*, Allgem. Wiener med. Zeitg. Nr. 29. 1862.—*Ancelet*, Études sur les maladies du pancréas. Paris, 1866. p. 9.—*Klebs*, a. a. O. S. 533.

The extremely rare occurrence of prolapse of the pancreas through penetrating wounds of the abdomen belongs to the domain of surgery, and the same may be said of the cases in which the pancreas, together with other organs, has constituted the contents of an umbilical or diaphragmatic hernia, or in which, after traumatic rupture of the diaphragm, it may have been displaced, along with the stomach, colon, omentum, or spleen, into the thoracic cavity.

More important for the physician, however, is the knowledge of the possibility of an invagination of the pancreas into the intestine. Mondière cites the case, observed by Baud, where in a man, twenty-four years of age, the pancreas, together with the duodenum and small intestine, had become invaginated into the colon. ..That bits of pancreas do slough off, and may be found in the stools, is proved by Trafoyer's unique case : the man had died of cholelithiasis, and in his abnormal-looking stools, in addition to gall-stones, Rokitansky found a considerable portion of the pancreas, in which the canal of Wirsung was still distinctly recognizable.

Foreign Bodies in the Pancreas.

Mauchart, De lumbrico terete in ductu pancreatico reperto. Diss. Tub. 1738.— *Lieutaud*, Histor. anatom. medic. Vol. I. Longosaliss, 1786. p. 312.—*Davaine*, Traité des entozoaires. p. 115.—*Engel*, Oesterr. med. Jahrbücher. XXIII. u. XXIV. 1841.—*Claessen*, a. a. O. S. 41.—*Klebs*, a. a. O. S. 553.

Our knowledge of the presence of foreign bodies in the pancreas is confined to the occurrence of round worms in the duct of Wirsung and its branches. Mauchart and Lieutaud have related examples in which ascarides had crept into and occluded the ductus pancreaticus. Among the cases found in the recent literature of this subject must be mentioned that related by Engel, in which several round worms were found in the pancreatic duct and its branches, and also in the gall-ducts, high up in the liver. Klebs once found in a dilated pancreatic duct three male and three female round worms ; the first pair was already turned half-way back again, but the other two pairs had their heads towards the left extremity of the pancreas. It is scarcely to be doubted in all these cases that it was a *post-mortem* occurrence, seeing that all secondary inflammatory changes were absent, and that during life there had been no symptoms at all pointing to such a condition.

THE DISEASES

OF THE

SUPRARENAL CAPSULES.

———

MERKEL.

DISEASES OF THE SUPRARENAL CAPSULES.

Anatomy and Physiology.—Bergmann, De glandulis suprarenalibus. Dissertat. Göttingen, 1839.—*Ecker*, Der feinere Bau der Nebennieren beim Menschen und den vier Wirbelthierklassen. Braunschweig, 1846.—*Koelliker*, Handbuch der Gewebelehre. Leipzig, 1855 u. 1867.—*Zellweger*, Untersuchungen ueber die Nebennieren. Dissert. Bern. 1858.—*H. Thompson Darby*, Anatomy, Physiology, and Pathology of the Suprarenal Capsules. Charleston Med. Journal. May, 1859.—*Luschka*, Der Hirnanhang und die Steissdrüse des Menschen. Berlin, 1860.—*Idem*, Anatomie, Bd. II.—*Moers*, Ueber den feineren Bau der Nebennieren. Virchow's Archiv. Bd. 29.—*Joesten*, Der feinere Bau der Nebennieren. Archiv der Heilkunde. 1864.—*Henle*, Zeitschr. für rationelle Medicin. Bd. 24. —*Holm*, Ueber die nervösen Elemente der Nebennieren. Wiener Sitzungsberichte. Bd. 53.—*M. Grandry*, Mémoire sur le structure de la capsule surrénale de l'homme et des quelques animaux. Journal de l'anatomie. 1867.—*Pfoertner*, Untersuchungen über das Ganglion intercaroticum und die Nebenniere. Zeitschrift für rationelle Medicin. Bd. 34.—*Eberth*, Article Suprarenal Capsules in Stricker's Histology.—*Morano*, Studio sulle capsule strumentuaii (Centralblatt. 1873. Nr. 53).—*v. Brunn*, Archiv für mikroskop. Anatomie. Bd. 8.—*Idem*, Göttinger Nachrichten. 1873. Nr. 16.—*Henle*, Handbuch der Anatomie. 1866. 2. Aufl. Eingeweidelehre.—*Brown-Séquard*, Comptes rendus. 1856.— *Idem*, Recherches expérimentales sur la physiologie et la pathologie des capsules surrénales. Archives générales, 1856. Vol. 2.—*Idem*, Comptes rendus. 1857. Tom. 44.—*Idem*, Nouvelles recherches sur l'importance des fonctions des capsules surrénales. Journal de physiologie. 1858. Tom. 1.—*Gratiolet*, Note sur les effets, qui suivent l'ablation des capsules surrénales. Comptes rendus. 1856. Tom. 43.—*Harley*, An Experimental Inquiry into the Function of the Suprarenal Capsules, and their Supposed Connection with Bronzed-skin. British and Foreign Med.-Chir. Review. 1858. Vol. 21.—*Idem*, The Lancet. I. 23. 1858.—*Philippeau*, Note sur l'exstirpation des capsules surrénales chez les rats albines. Comptes rendus. 1856. Tom. 43.—*Idem*, Ablation successive des capsules surrénales de la rat et des corps thyreoides sur les animaux, qui survivent à l'operation. Comptes rendus. Tom. 44.—*Schiff*, Sur l'exstirpation des capsules surrénales. L'union médical de Paris. 1863. Nr. 61.—*Seligsohn*, De pigmentis patholog. ac morbo Addisonii adjecta chemia glandul. suprarenal. Dissertat. inaug. Berolin. 1858.—*Vulpian*, Note sur quelques reactions propres à la substance des capsules surrénales. Comptes rendus. 1856.—*Vulpian et Cloez*, Comptes rendus. 1857. Tom. 45.—*Virchow*, Archiv für path. Anatomie. 1857. Bd. 12.—*Holmgreen*, Virchow and Hirsch's Jahresbericht. 1868. Bd. 2.—*Arnold*, Beiträge zur feineren Structur und zum Chemismus der Nebennieren. Virchow's Archiv. 1866. Bd. 35.—*Pincus*, Experimenta de vi nervi vagi et sympathici ad vasa, secretionem, nutritionem tractus intestinalis et renum. Dissertat. inaug. Vratislav. 1856.—*Budge*, Anatomische und physiolog. Untersuchungen über die Function des Plexus coeliacus et mesentericus. Verhandlg. der Leopold. Carol. Academie. 1860. Bd. 29.—*Adrian*, Ueber die Function des Plexus coeliacus et mesentericus. Eckard's Beiträge zu Anatomie und Physiologie. 1862. Bd. 3.—*Lamansky*, Ueber die Folgen der Exstirpation des Plexus coeliacus et mesentericus. Henle und Pfeuffer's Zeitschr. für rationelle Medicin. 3. Reihe. Bd. 28. 1866.—*Louis Schmidt*, Ueber die Function des Plexus mesentericus posterior. Dissertat. inaug. Giessen, 1862.—*Schiff*, Leçons sur la physiologie de la digestion faites au muséum d'histoire naturelle de Florence. Berlin, 1862. Vol. II.—*Rossbach*, Virchow's Archiv. 1872. Bd. 51.

The earliest memoirs and the more important later works on Addison's Disease are: *Addison*, On the Constitutional and Local Effects of Disease of the Suprarenal Capsules. London, 1855.—*Hutchinson*, Series Illustrating the Connection between Bronzed-skin and Disease of the Suprarenal Capsules. Med. Times and Gaz. Dec. 1855.—*Dechambre*, Peau bronçée. Gaz. hebdom. 1856. 6.—*Bouchut*, Maladies des capsules surrénales. Gaz. des hôpitaux. 1856. Nr. 49.—*Posner*, Bronzed-skin eine neue Krankheitsspecies. Med. Centr. Zeitg. 1856. Nr. 37, 38.—*Bamberger*, Krankheiten des chilopoetischen Systems. 1864. 2. Aufl. S. 662.—*Virchow*, Krankhafte Geschwülste. 2 u. 3 Bd. 1864. 1865. 1867.—*Oppolzer*, Klinischer Vortrag über Addison'sche Krankheit. Wiener medic. Wochenschrift. 1866. Nr. 81.—*Averbeck*, Die Addison'sche Krankheit. Erlangen, 1869.—*Rossbach*, Virchow's Archiv. Bd. 50. Heft 4, and Bd. 51. Heft 1. 1870; and Verhandlungen der physikal. med. Gesellschaft in Würzburg. Neue Folge II. Heft 1 und 2; daran anschliessend *Mueller*, Schweizerisches ärztliches Correspondenzblatt. Nov. 1871.—*Riesel*, Zur Pathologie des morbus Addisonii. Deutsches Archiv für klin. Medicin. 1870. Bd. 7.—*Laschkewitsch*, Wiener med. Jahrbücher. 1871. 3 (Formveränderung der rothen Blutkörperchen).—*Eulenburg* and *Guttmann*, Die Pathologie des Sympathicus auf physiologischer Grundlage. Berlin, 1873.

The notices of a great number of observed, isolated cases are referred to and collected in: Schmidt's Jahrbücher. Bd. 92, 95, 113, 115, 126, 142, 154, 155, 158, 160; in Averbeck's memoir; in Virchow's Krankhafte Geschwülste. Bd. II. S. 688-702, and Bd. III. S. 89-91; in Riesel's memoir; and in that of Eulenburg and Guttmann, pages 155-187.

Introduction.

The first indication of any form of illness resulting from disease of the suprarenal capsules is to be found in an instance recorded by Lobstein (De nervi sympathici humani fabrica et morbis, Paris, 1823), where, in the case of a female aged twenty-five, who had died of epileptiform convulsions, the post-mortem examination revealed tubercular degeneration of both suprarenal capsules and a remarkable thickening of the nerves passing to them. The matter first assumed importance, however, when, owing to Addison's well-known publication in 1855, the attention of the profession was directed to a definite form of disease, as having its anatomical basis in an alteration of the normal structure of the suprarenal capsules.

The works published since then on the diseases of the suprarenal capsules, and in particular on Morbus Addisonii, are so numerous that the mere recounting of all the observations collected during the twenty years that have elapsed, especially those bearing indirectly on the question, has become a tedious and unrequiting labor.

On glancing through them, what strikes us most forcibly is the fact that we have to do with the most completely different pathological processes, and that it would be a matter of extreme difficulty to discover and lay down a distinct set of symptoms as characteristic of each, for conflicting opinions may constantly be reduced to the consideration as to whether the disease which Addison described, and with which his name is universally associated, has to do with all the various abnormal conditions of the suprarenal capsules which have been actually observed and recorded as met with, in connection with the symptoms described by him, or whether it has to do only with particular forms thereof, or lastly, whether the condition of the suprarenal capsules is not after all only an accidental coincidence.

The cause of this confusion lies undoubtedly in the paucity of our knowledge as to the physiological significance of the suprarenal capsules, these bodies belonging to a class of organs concerning the functions of which, and the parts sustained by them in the general economy, there exists the utmost obscurity.

As soon as Addison had made the statement, that a certain set of symptoms were dependent upon a diseased condition of the suprarenal capsules, there arose a hope that from such a "*post hoc*" as this some insight might be gained into the physiological significance of these heretofore enigmatical organs. Unfortunately the results were but meagre; for the symptoms described as resulting from the diseased conditions were so general, and the diseased conditions themselves so frequently associated with anatomical changes elsewhere, that definite conclusions were only to be drawn with the greatest circumspection. Further, it was the very uncertainty as to the nature of the rôle sustained by these organs which induced men to look for the essence of the disease, not in any particular pathological change in these organs, but in the occurrence of any pathological change whatever.

While this is the aspect in which the question is regarded by some, by others, who look upon it from a different point of view, preponderance is given to the most essential and prominent symptom, namely, the discoloration of the skin; so that while the former speak of "Morbus Addisonii," the latter record cases of "bronzed skin," "melasma suprarenale," or "peau bronçée."

The appearance of Addison's memoir has not only stimulated to new investigations into the physiological significance of the organs in question, but has also given a fresh impulse to further investigation into the pathological anatomy of the various diseases by which they are attacked. We have become acquainted with chronic inflammatory processes, which are held to be the starting-point of the caseous degeneration so frequently met with; with tubercular and carcinomatous conditions; with fatty degeneration; with amyloid degeneration; and with apoplexy. And there is scarcely one of these various forms of degeneration that has not, at one time or another, been found accompanied by bronzed skin.

Brown-Séquard was the first to attack the physiological question suggested by the publication of Addison's views. He published the results of his experiments in 1856, according to which extirpation of the suprarenal capsules was quickly followed by death, which was to be ascribed to serious interference with the animal and vegetative functions. The facts which Brown-Séquard thought he had established, namely, the occurrence of death, accompanied by convulsions, and the rapid increase in the normal coloring matter of the blood, accorded too well with the phenomena of Addison's disease, not to give rise to the belief that the whole question had been solved by his experiments. Moreover, the following statement, made by Koelliker in 1854 (consequently before he knew of Addison's observations), tended to support this view: "I consider the cortical and medullary portions to be physiologically distinct. The former may be considered as belonging to the category of the so-called vascular glands, and doubtless is in some way related to the process of secretion ; while the latter, owing to its extraordinary richness in nerve-tissue, must be described as an appendage to the nervous system, in which the cellular elements and the plexus of nerves either react, one upon the other, in a manner similar to that obtaining in gray nerve-tissue, or else are actually directly connected."

Although important support to this view of Brown-Séquard's was afforded by the fact that he further believed he had discovered the cause of a certain epizoötic disease in rabbits, which is characterized by a remarkable increase in the coloring matter of the blood, to be an inflammation of the suprarenal capsules, still other investigators (Harley, Gratiolet, Philippeau) demonstrated that if the operation of extirpation was conducted with the greatest possible care, the life of the animal was not endangered, and that when the animal did die, its death was caused by the amount of injury done. Similar results were arrived at by Schiff, who did not observe particularly serious consequences follow either the extirpation of the suprarenal capsules or the destruction of the nerves passing to them. Similarly, also, Schmidt, Lamansky and Rossbach saw no special evil resulting from the removal of the plexus and its nerves. Still, in a large proportion of the experiments of these various authors, mention is made of profuse diarrhœa and of venous congestion of the stomach and intestines ; and, moreover, this observation is corroborated by other experimenters—Budge, Pincus, and Adrian.

Although some few investigators—Luschka more prominently than any other—have expressed themselves most strongly in

favor of the view of the suprarenal capsules being purely nervous organs, still the negative conclusion deduced from the negative result of these experiments cannot but be considered as
authorized, which Eulenburg and Guttmann have lately expressed thus: "We have no actually decisive proof that disease
of the abdominal sympathetic gives rise to the symptoms of
Addison's disease."

As soon as the fact was recognized by anatomists that at least
part of the suprarenal capsules was of a glandular nature—for
Koelliker has defined his view more accurately, and has established the existence of closed tubes in connection with a particular category of cells—it was natural that the immense development of pigment in the skin in Addison's disease should suggest
a chemical investigation of the suprarenal capsules.

Cloez and Vulpian announced in 1856-57 that the medullary
tissue of these bodies was colored rosy red by an aqueous solution of iodine, and green by chloride of iron. Virchow confirmed this statement, and further established the existence of
leucin, margarin, and myelin. Finally, Arnold demonstrated a
special coloring matter, which he separated out of alcoholic extracts, and to which he gave the name of suprarenin.

In connection with this it may be observed that Cassan, in
1789, starting with the idea that the suprarenal capsules were
actually "capsules," which under certain circumstances poured
their black contents over the skin, made the conjecture that in
the negro these bodies are considerably larger than in the white
—a conjecture which, however, still awaits confirmation.

The pigment found in the suprarenal capsules is, however, as
far as its nature is concerned, remarkably similar to that met
with in the rete Malpighii and in the choroid.

In contradistinction to these unsettled views, according to
which the suprarenal capsules are either nervous organs, or
glandules, or lastly, half-nervous and half-glandular, Henle and
v. Brunn take up a very definite position. With their statements
before us we can no longer doubt the enormous wealth of nerve-
tissue which these bodies possess; no other gland in the abdomen has such a number of ganglia, either in capsule or parenchyma, or such a fine plexus of nerves supplied to it. The

splanchnic nerve, the cœliac plexus, the upper lumbar ganglion of the sympathetic, the pneumogastric and the phrenic vie with each other in their supply of the suprarenal capsules ; and furthermore, the branches from the semilunar ganglion pass for the most part directly to these bodies, unaccompanied by any artery.

In the cortical as well as in the medullary portions there exist isolated tubes, limited by a basement membrane, containing coarsely granular, fatty cells, as well as rows of free, finely granular cells, which near the surface lie in groups separated by connective tissue. The meshes of the net-work of the tubes in the medullary portion are, to all appearance, destined during life to take up blood, and to serve as an intermediary part of the vascular system between the capillary net-works of the arteries and venous radicles passing through the cortex.

These observations, not made, as had generally been the case previously, on the lower animals, but on man, are decisive of the nature of the organs. The occurrence of tubes, which, moreover, are distinctly separable, and surrounded by a limiting membrane, prove the specific nature of their contents. v. Brunn argues: "From the relation of the cells to the blood-vessels we may conclude that they take up some constituent from the blood, alter this in some way, and return it again to the blood." He hereby distinctly decides in favor of these cells being gland-cells, although in his explanation he endeavors to define them as simply adventitious parts of the blood-vessels ; for the point in question is the nature of their function, and not as to whether the product they elaborate be destined to pass outward, or to re-enter the blood.

With such facts and theories as to the structure and function of the suprarenal capsules, we naturally find that authors are unable to arrive at any definite conclusion as to the essential feature of Addison's disease. Sometimes the balance is in favor of anæmia ; sometimes in favor of the discoloration of the skin ; and sometimes, again, in favor of the asthenia and the severe nervous symptoms. The first clear and comprehensive grasp of the whole matter is to be found in Averbeck's well-known book, where he, looking at the question in all its aspects, defines the disease as "a well-marked constitutional disease, exhibiting itself locally as a chronic inflammation of the suprarenal capsules, but in its essence consisting in a peculiar anæmic condition, always tending toward death, which is characterized by intense development of pigment in the cells of the rete Malpighii and in the epithelium of the mucous membrane of the mouth.''

Convenient and plausible as this definition may seem to be, it is not adequate ; for a large number of cases have been authenticated, where the well-known set of symptoms were exhibited in conjunction with other forms of disease of the suprarenal capsules, as may be seen from Averbeck's Table VII., as well as from many other works. On this account other pathological conditions were early sought for, and Addison retreated on the sympathetic nervous system, pointing out its intimate connection with the suprarenal capsules as a means of accounting for the great *prostratio virum.* A large number adhere to this opinion, and it has received corroboration from Oppolzer, Bamberger, and Virchow.

Here it may be mentioned that an important step further is taken by Rossbach ; for chancing on a case in which there had been severe nervous symptoms, together with a thickened and bronzed skin, and in which no degeneration of the suprarenal capsules was discovered, he ascribes all the complex phenomena of Addison's disease to the nervous system in general, and considers any relationship to the suprarenal capsules as merely to some special focus. Further, it may also be remarked that Williams, in a similar way, attempted to connect certain cases of melancholy with morbus Addisonii.

Riesel, in a most excellent work, has contended that we have to do with a lesion of the sympathetic nervous system which originates in the connection of this latter with the suprarenal capsules, an inflammatory process being set up in the connective tissue which surrounds the cells and fibres by such contact with these bodies, and that from the products of this inflammation there ensues (analogous to what occurs in the case of Goltz's Klopfversuch [1]) a paralytic condition of the vaso-motor fibres of the sympathetic, and consequently an imperfect distribution of

---

[1] The German title " Klopfversuch " is used in some of our English text-books. The experiment consists in arresting the action of the heart in diastole by a smart tap on the intestines.

blood, and that on this is to be saddled all the phenomena of the disease, the anæmia, the disturbance of the nutritive functions, as well as the bronzed skin, and a secondary affection of the blood.

Eulenburg and Guttmann, in their valuable book, "Die Pathologie des Sympathicus auf physiologischer Grundlage," place together nineteen cases in which the symptoms of morbus Addisonii were found associated with pathological conditions in the semilunar ganglion and sympathetic, while against these nineteen cases they place ten others, in which the sympathetic had been examined and found normal. No definite conclusion can be drawn from this until the number of accurate observations has been augmented, or until we are perfectly clear as to the part played by altered conditions of the sympathetic in other diseases.

Two works which have lately appeared afford some stepping-stones in this direction. While Eulenburg and Guttmann record, in cases of genuine morbus Addisonii, swelling and redness, four times; swelling simply, twice; redness simply, once; transformation into an albuminous mass, once; sclerosis, once; transformation into an adenoid mass, once; caseous degeneration, twice; fatty degeneration, three times; and atrophy of the nerves and ganglia similarly, three times, Lubimoff[1] has collected his records of 250 *post-mortems on bodies*, none of which, judging at least from the notes of the cases in his work, had died from morbus Addisonii. The examination of the nerve-trunks and ganglia of the sympathetic in these cases showed dilatations on the sides of the vessels and disease of their coats, fatty degeneration and cell-proliferation in the connective tissue, deposition of pigment, fatty degeneration and sclerosis of the ganglion-cells, and fatty degeneration of both medullated and non-medullated nerve fibres.

Pio Foa[2] similarly, in 140 *post-mortems*, enumerates instances of anæmia and hyperæmia, of pigmentary and fatty degeneration, and of abscesses and degeneration of the connective tissue.

---

[1] Virchow's Archiv. LXI. S. 145-207.
[2] Centralblatt. 1875. Nr. 14. S. 216; and Schmidt's Jahrbücher. 165. S. 245.

These observations in both instances were made on bodies which had died with every variety of disease and symptom, and thus distinctly disprove the idea that disease of the sympathetic and its ganglia is exclusively to be met with in morbus Addisonii ; as, indeed, owing to the small number of cases of which we have any accurate record before and after death, it would be impossible to exclude the chance, that the same condition in the sympathetic, which occurs in connection with other diseases as well as with degeneration of the suprarenal capsules, and which in the latter case js regarded as the *causa morbi*, may not after all lie within the limits of ordinary, physiological abnormity.

If we now bear in mind that a number of cases have been observed and recorded, in which the symptoms of Addison's disease have been but partially developed, and in which on postmortem examination no abnormity in the suprarenal capsules was found, so that even the term Pseudo-melanosis was employed to designate a distinct form of disease, and if we confront together all that has been stated above concerning the suprarenal capsules, both *pro* and *con*, positive and negative, fact and theory, we shall find that the question, whether in opposition to such facts the existence of a special form of disease of this kind can be upheld, is not unauthorized.

That such is authorized there is, in my opinion, no absolute proof. Nevertheless, such a number of well-observed cases have been established and recorded, in which the earlier symptoms of morbus Addisonii have been found in connection with disease of the suprarenal capsules, that the probability of a relation of cause and effect becomes almost a certainty. The ultimate proof can, however, only be afforded by physiology.

Furthermore, we are not without analogies in other diseases. I need only refer to a single instance. No medical man or clinical teacher doubts nowadays the identity of that form of disease which is described as resulting from multiple sclerosis of the brain and spinal cord, and yet cases certainly occur (I myself have seen two), in which, notwithstanding a most extensively distributed sclerosis, there was not a trace of anything abnormal exhibited in the phenomena of the central nervous system, more especially of the intelligence, beyond the mere paralysis of some isolated groups of muscles in the extremities.

Etiology.

In a form of disease, the exact nature of which is beset with so many obscure points, of which the pathological anatomy has not yet been worked out, where the earlier stages can scarcely be recognized, and which has been altogether so seldom observed, it will not seem strange if the etiology should appear to be the most obscure point of all. Want, anxiety, distress, unhealthy dietary, previously existing chronic gastric catarrh, old-standing constipation, exhausting diarrhœa, malaria, predisposition to cancer, mechanical injuries of the abdomen, as well as unavoidable alternations of heat and cold, are suggested as predisposing causes in the various cases by the different authors.

Some of the foregoing assume a certain importance owing to the fact that they are in the present day looked upon as predisposing to tubercle, and that by far the greatest number of cases of morbus Addisonii are found to be associated with a tubercular affection of the suprarenal capsules.

Four out of my five cases were tubercular, and Averbeck's tables contain but fifty-one undoubted instances of the uncomplicated disease, and in thirty-six of these tubercular, scrofulous, and caseous degeneration was met with, while the statements in the remaining nineteen cases in Table I. leave it doubtful as to what the form of disease actually was, and in forty-nine out of the fifty-six complicated cases in Table II. tubercular and caseous affections were found in other organs.

From the exceedingly small number of accurate observations, we can, of course, make no definite statement as to hereditary predisposition. All that can be gleaned on this point consists in a few slender statements to the effect that in one case a parent, in another a cousin, was said to have died of the same or a similar disease.

The majority of the cases were males ; Averbeck gives the relation of 1.74 men to 1 woman, and in my five cases there was no female. The disease occurs most frequently in the prime of life, from the ages of fifteen to forty-five, no instance having as yet been recorded as occurring before ten or after sixty.

So far our records refer only to the Caucasian race.

As regards the frequency of Addison's disease, Averbeck has collected 126 published cases which occurred during the decade beginning·in· 1850, and further records do not tend to raise this average.

From the 1st January, 1867, to the 31st December, 1874, I treated 14,217 patients in the medical department of the hospital here, and amongst these were five cases of morbus Addisonii, verified by post-mortem examination, giving therefore an average of 0.35 per thousand; while in addition to these, during the same interval, twenty-one instances of unilateral disease of the suprarenal capsules, occurring without any of the other phenomena of morbus Addisonii, were met with in the course of the various post-mortems, the cases in which they were found being generally tubercular, thus giving an average of 1.4 per thousand.

Symptoms.

The earlier stages of Addison's disease have never come directly under observation. This, however, is no more a reason for denying the existence of the disease than the circumstance that the later stages are often obscured by complications, and that thus the general aspect of the whole is rendered indistinct. Owing to this fatality, the disease in question is mixed up with a great many others, especially those arising out of chronic pathological conditions in those internal organs which cannot be considered as actually essential to life.

The first and most prominent symptom of which the patient complains to his physician is anæmia and debility. We are told by the patients almost always (even in the so-called acute cases) that their malady is of long standing, extending back months, or even years. The phenomena of the earlier stages are readily recalled afterwards if the patient is in a condition to relate them, and is not prevented from so doing by loss of memory. There are generally found to be weariness throughout the whole body, which comes on so insidiously that the patient first becomes aware of it when attacked by some other illness, or when any unusual circumstance calls for increased mental or bodily exertion. Still, there are occasionally cases where the gradual loss of power is readily observed by the patient, and it is his perceiving this that induces him to seek medical advice. There are often associated with this tearing, dragging pains in both hypochondria (frequently more intensely in the right), along the back, in the sacrum, and especially in the joints. I have seen these pains in the joints, which resemble most closely the arthritic neuroses of a hysterical individual, reach such a pitch that the disease has been mistaken for acute rheumatism, as the slightest movement was accompanied by the most intense pain. The absence of any swelling or alteration in the shape of the joints quickly clears up the mistake, and this all the more quickly as sensibility on pressure is not increased over the joints themselves, while it is very considerably intensified in the hypochondriac, lumbar, and dorsal regions.

While these symptoms remain tolerably constant, or are subject to but slight variations, the dyspepsia which universally occurs is not so constant, and sometimes intermits. Cardialgia, which sometimes has no connection with the repletion of the stomach, and sometimes, on the other hand, comes on immediately after a meal, is often associated with distention of the abdomen, especially of the stomach, eructation, loss of appetite, nausea, and more or less vomiting. In a great many cases frequent or even intercurrent diarrhœa is met with, and occasionally (more particularly in the earlier stages) constipation. Patients remain in this condition for a long time, during which there are generally apparent changes for the better, until at last, impelled by increasing weakness, they seek advice. The objective phenomena discoverable are then found to be but slight compared with the symptoms complained of by the patient.

While the fat of the body is well preserved, especially in uncomplicated cases, there is generally a considerable loss of muscular power ; and this is evidenced by a slight tremor in the hands, as well as by an inability to squeeze, and a tendency to tiredness on very little exertion.

If in a certain sense we can speak of these symptoms as constituting a prodromal stage, we find subsequently in what will be the second stage the occurrence of remarkable symptoms in the circulatory system. We observe—apart from complicating circumstances—an exceedingly soft, small, weak, and generally rapid pulse, weak cardiac impulse, and a want of sharpness, or even faint casual murmurs here and there, in the case of all the valves, as also in the larger vessels. In most of the cases we have, resulting from the weak action of the heart, a remarkable paleness of the skin, sometimes amounting to cyanosis. In connection with the respiratory organs—so long as there are no complications—there is nothing to be observed beyond a somewhat quickened respiratory rhythm. The temperature is generally somewhat under the normal ; very occasionally slight evening exacerbations are observed, but these never attain to any magnitude. The dyspeptic symptoms generally increase ; constipation and diarrhœa alternate one with another, but in no way do they present any peculiar or characteristic phenomena. The excretion of urine proceeds normally. The urine contains, as a rule, no abnormal constituent (in very occasional cases albuminuria is recorded). Thudicum demonstrated in a single case an abnormity in the coloring matter of the urine (diminution of the uromelanin), accompanied by diminution of urea. Up to the present time we have no confirmation of this interesting observation.[1] The excretion of urine is in no way altered. The examination of the abdominal organs gives us similarly no positive result. The liver and spleen (excluding, of course, complicated cases) are neither enlarged nor painful.

According to some investigators, there is an increase in the white corpuscles of the blood, while, according to others, there is a remarkable decrease, and others, still, record the remarkably small tendency in the red corpuscles to form *rouleaux*. Laschkewitsch, of Charkow, has lately published the result of an observation by which he has established a peculiar property of the red blood-corpuscles. In blood taken during life the blood-corpuscles were seen in active cleavage, just as was observed and

---

[1] *Huber* (Deutsches Archiv f. klin. Med. I 635 ; and IV. 615) mentions also an occurrence of a remarkably concentrated (hochgestellten) urine.

depicted by Friedreich[1] in a case of nephritis and pseudo-leucæmia. In this case, in which, amongst other symptoms, there was
an increasing brownish discoloration of the skin, there was unfortunately no confirmation by post-mortem examination. This
observation receives not unimportant corroboration from two
others (made post-mortem), which will be subsequently related.

Along with these subjective and objective symptoms, there
occurs another—the most constant and most remarkable of all
—namely, an important alteration in the tegumentary surfaces.
This consists in a more or less distinctly marked discoloration of
the skin, which begins as a light dusky gray, and passes on to
dark brown; it at first attacks those parts of the body exposed
to the light—namely, the face and hands—either as a mottling,
or diffusely, or occasionally in streaks. Parts which naturally
have a tendency to pigment, as the areola of the breast, the genitals, and the folds of the axilla, color most intensely, as do also
old cicatrices and parts exposed to mechanical irritation, such as
the rubbing of clothes. On the mucous membrane of the lips and
cheeks there also occur irregular bluish or blackish spots. The
sclerotic, the nails, the palm of the hand, and the sole of the foot
remain meanwhile perfectly clear. For months long the aspect
of an uncomplicated case remains unchanged; then, however,
the evidences of a more intense anæmia gradually make their
appearance, sometimes coming on quickly, and sometimes more
slowly. The debility becomes more and more marked, the loss
of muscular power increases, the gastric symptoms become
worse, there is almost complete loss of appetite (in opposition to
this, Kussmaul records a case in which there was an insatiable
appetite, which, however, is distinctly an exception to the rule),
while painful deglutition and distention of the stomach utterly
weigh the patient down. Then profuse diarrhœa, comes on,
which wastes the patient's strength, and later on, nausea, and
vomiting — often uncontrollable—of watery, dark, bile-colored
material. Then are superadded severe nervous symptoms. If a
peculiar affection of the head, which often in the earlier stages
amounts to severe headache, should have produced some dul-

---

[1] Virchow's Archiv. XLI. 3, 4. S. 395.

ness of the sensorium, the patient will now frequently suffer from actual fainting fits, a difficulty in collecting his thoughts, and weakness of memory. Most remarkable of all are the attacks of faintness and severe fits of dyspnœa which occur when the patients, who find lying in bed intolerable, attempt to sit up. In certain cases we observe slight muscular twitchings in some small groups of muscles, while in others epileptic seizures, which often occur in an isolated manner in the earlier stages of the disease, but become more and more frequent towards the close of the scene. In other cases, again, there ensue general convulsions, with confused consciousness, and Broadbent relates a most interesting case of choreic attacks.

Hand and hand with these severe symptoms, or even sometimes in advance of them, proceeds the discoloration of the skin. It passes from a light dusky brown through grayish yellow and grayish brown to intensely dark bronze-color, so that the patients become successively ashy gray, darkly icteric, mulatto, and even copper colored (one of our patients, who, during his illness, used frequently to come to the hospital, was known by the inmates of the house by the nickname of "Turko"). These "blackened" men present a very remarkable appearance with their strikingly white sclerotics, which give them a very different aspect from that of a jaundiced patient. The nails remain likewise white; the palms of the hands and the soles of the feet not completely so, but often present a brown, mottled appearance. Cicatrices do not exhibit any uniform behavior; they often remain particularly clear, while in other cases they become more darkly colored; this fact being always observable, that those parts of the skin which are naturally darker than others exhibit a more intense discoloration. Further, the spots on the mucous membrane of the mouth, namely, on the lips and cheeks, generally become intensified and larger.

It must be observed that the discoloration of the skin, more particularly in this well-marked form, is not constant, in so far that, according to the observations of most careful investigators, it appears in certain cases distinctly to diminish. Severe cerebral symptoms, or most intense, gradually increasing exhaustion, usher in the end in uncomplicated cases.

This is the course of events in by far the greatest number of uncomplicated cases. There occur, however, occasionally cases which present a very different aspect, and in which matters run a much more acute and tumultuous course.

We find in such cases that the patient, who sometimes is said to have been a considerable time out of health, but more generally is supposed to have become ill suddenly, has taken to his bed with symptoms of intense prostration. Loss of flesh is always observable. The patient does not speak above his breath, he can hardly hold himself up, his extremities tremble on being raised, and his head is confused; tongue and lips are dry, and covered with sordes; the pulse is small and frequent, and the temperature is up to 104° F. There is generally distention and meteorism of the abdomen, and diarrhœa. In a word, there are all the phenomena to make one imagine that the case is one of enteric fever, were it not for the absence of rose-spots and enlargement of the spleen. There came under my own observation a case of this kind in private practice, which was believed to be one of typhoid fever until the post-mortem examination revealed the truth. In a minority of the cases this condition leads rapidly to death; the intensity of the symptoms remains the same, the fever continues, and exhaustion sets in. In the majority, on the other hand, the temperature comes down, the patient becomes somewhat better, and there succeeds to this apparently stormy invasion, a long course of events which are hardly, if at all, distinguishable from those related above.

It stands to reason that this description of the disease, drawn from its most general aspect, should be essentially modified by the occurrence of complication with other diseases. Pulmonary consumption especially, which is by far the most frequent complication of Addison's disease, so mixes itself up with the peculiar characteristics of the latter, that we are often induced to look upon the double set of symptoms as almost inseparable. Similarly certain modifications are necessarily produced when we have to do with secondary cancer.

Pathological Anatomy.

In by far the greatest number of cases of Addison's disease we find caseous masses of various sizes which, beginning in the medullary portion, grow into the cortical, extending as far as the capsule, and exciting in this a proliferation of the connective tissue, which leads to thickening and sclerosis. The following is Virchow's[1] most accurate description of these masses: "The development of the tubercular masses begins in this case, as is the rule in others, in the medullary tissue. On making a section through the suprarenal capsule we observe occasionally in the middle of the medullary portion the first stages of the development, in the form of small gray nodules: These gradually increase in size, become caseous, amalgamate with one another, and thereby produce the caseous masses. It not unfrequently occurs that this process is but partial, and that both internally and externally some normal tissue remains, while all in the centre has become metamorphosed. Again, the process may proceed by the development of new nodules, not only in the medullary, but also in the cortical portions, around the circumference of the original mass, with which they subsequently blend. In this way, gradually every trace of proper tissue disappears, and we have nothing left but a firm caseous mass, which reaches the surface on one or both sides, or even occasionally includes every atom of the organ. As a rule, however, in such extensive disease as this, we do not meet with a single uniform mass, but the whole thing appears lobular, or nodulated, corresponding to the various original foci. These masses have, therefore, an irregular shape, proportionally thicker than the normal form of the organ, they attain occasionally a very considerable size, namely, that of a plum or small hen-egg, and possess a firm or even hard consistence."

There was an attempt made at the outset, by Addison, to describe these masses as the growth of a scrofulous degeneration, while other investigators, Wilks, for example, regarded them as the product of a chronic inflammatory process.

---

[1] Krankhafte Geschwülste. II. S. 689.

My own observations have shown me, in cases where the entire structure had not been broken down into a mass of detritus, that it consists in a proliferation of small cells, lying in a fine reticulum which includes giant-cells (Riesenzellen) in great numbers. I have never seen any appearance which so forcibly reminded me of Schueppel's drawings, as in tuberculosis of the suprarenal capsules. If we take into consideration along with this that undoubted beginnings have often been observed as small, miliary, translucent nodules, occurring in the medullary portion; and further, that well-marked pulmonary tuberculosis and phthisis is a very frequent concomitant of this disease, we shall be justified, even without actually asserting giant-cells to be characteristic of tubercle, in describing the process in question as tubercular.

There are some cases in Table I. of Averbeck's work in which a "sero-albuminous" (serösalbuminösen) condition of the suprarenal capsules is spoken of, but in these cases, however, in so far as they appear to have been carefully observed, there is further mention of caseous matter having been found, so that a doubt must arise as to whether the shrivelling and calcification are not to be regarded as occurring in the product of a tubercular process.

Schueppel[1] has published an accurately observed[2] and recorded instance of a chronic inflammatory condition of both suprarenal capsules occurring in a case of Addison's disease, in which, according to this author's view, the idea of tuberculosis cannot be entertained. The left suprarenal capsule was the size of a walnut, and was sharply defined from the surrounding fat. It consisted of a fine light-gray translucent mass of cicatricial tissue, in the interior of which some caseous irregularly formed parts lay scattered. There was not a trace of the normal tissue of the suprarenal capsule to be found, and this body, together with the kidney and the tail of the pancreas, was firmly agglutinated to the descending colon. There was a stricture of the intestine at this spot from a cicatrized circular ulcer. Schueppel considers that the inflammatory process began in the intestine, and spread

---

[1] Archiv der Heilkunde. XI. p. 87.   [2] By *Averbeck*, l. c. p. 20.

by contact outward to the suprarenal capsule. Further, the right suprarenal capsule in this case was described as a hard light-gray mass, the size of a damson, of firm cicatricial consistence, in the interior of which were several irregular, caseous, firm nodules, which attained the size of a small pea. Schueppel, in this case, connects an interstitial proliferation of tissue in the left testicle, and a few caseous masses in the right, with the disease of the suprarenal capsules.

A second condition of the suprarenal capsules, which has been established in many cases of undoubted Addison's disease, is the occurrence of hemorrhages into the tissue of these bodies, which may be so severe as to swell one of them up into a tumor the size of a child's closed fist. I give here, as a prototype, the description which Zenker gave me in one of my own cases:

"The left suprarenal capsule enormously thickened, 5 centimetres long, up to 1.5 thick. Cortical layer mottled, light yellow and dark brown, normal in thickness. In the position of the medullary portion, a material, thick, somewhat uniform, dark cherry-colored, in parts passing into reddish brown, brittle, and beset by spaces the size of a pin's head, which, on pressure, exuded a thin red sanguineous fluid. The microscopic examination of this red material showed everywhere a thick, finely reticulated net-work of fibrin (swelling up with acetic acid), which was thickly beset by an exceedingly fine, molecular mass. Here and there, in connection with diffuse yellowish coloring, were found very beautifully formed hæmatoidin crystals, sometimes small and sometimes large. The fine molecular mass showed the following peculiar constitution: First, a small number of easily recognizable, as yet slightly altered, colored blood-disks (without, however, the bi-concavity); next, smaller, distinctly yellow, more spherical corpuscles. Passing downward in the scale, increasingly small, sharply but palely contoured granules (the larger distinctly yellow), down to the very finest molecules, are met with. Between these there occur vast numbers of little bodies, which most closely resemble the rod-shaped, dumb-bell (bisquitförmige) forms, which ensue on the addition of urea to frogs' blood; then others, similar to these, with smaller particles partially separated by constriction; then whole chains of granules, and these in direct connection with distinct, yellow blood-corpuscles, and possessing identically the same optical properties as the isolated granules. The usual forms met with in retrograde metamorphosis of the blood-corpuscles (namely, with little particles sitting on them) are not met with at all. The cells in the cortical portion, corresponding with the color, in parts overladen with fat, in parts with little or no fat, brownly pigmented."

Whether, in this case, there was any disease of the walls of the vessels, must remain undecided. I wish to remark, however, that this and a similar case, which, nevertheless, did not produce the symptoms of Addison's disease, reminded me, by their coarse anatomical appearances, of many conditions met with in struma. Virchow[1] describes a form of undoubtedly strumous tumor of the suprarenal capsules, which, moreover, has been observed in connection with Addison's disease; and he states concerning these tumors that they occur diffusely, or uniformly distributed throughout the entire organ. They may be limited to particular regions, and appear in the form of smaller or larger nodules. These nodules may be of the same sulphur or lemon yellow as the normal cortical substance itself; they may be intensely brown or olive-green, like the pigmentary zones, or they may present a more reddish gray appearance.

New formations in the suprarenal capsules form a fourth category, which is less frequently met with, and which comprises carcinoma, sarcoma, and echinococcus.

An exquisite example of isolated sarcoma of the suprarenal capsule, occurring in conjunction with chronic pneumonia and tubercular meningitis, was met with in dispensary practice (Polyklinik) in Erlangen, and communicated to me by Professor Zenker. The skin was light brown, and was said to have been at one time darker. The case had been so obscured by the severe complication that it would hardly be possible to say that there had been any definite diagnosis. The red blood-corpuscles exhibited the same indentations and the various forms of constriction described above; still, this observation is not altogether to be relied on, as the preparation, when it came into my hands, was not absolutely fresh, and therefore processes of decomposition could not be entirely excluded.

But few examples under this head have been recorded, and still fewer when the disease has been primary. In Averbeck's

[1] Krankhafte Geschwülste. III. p. 91.

Table VII. there are but two instances in which the occurrence of primary cancer of the suprarenal capsules had been established.

These various forms of disease of the suprarenal capsules occur, in the vast majority of cases of morbus Addisonii, on both sides; and but few instances are known in which the symptoms as a whole were well marked where there was disease in but one suprarenal capsule. As a constant concomitant must be mentioned the occurrence of sometimes slighter, sometimes more considerable swelling of the follicular and Peyer's glands in the intestine, and further, a somewhat less amount of swelling in the mesenteric and retroperitoneal glands, which are often found in a state of caseous degeneration or even completely broken down.

The spleen is sometimes said to be swollen, and sometimes normal; still the rule distinctly is, that nothing abnormal is found, for most of the instances where enlargement is recorded occurred in complicated cases, or where there had been suppuration of the suprarenal capsules. Equally little evidence exists of anything pathological in the liver. The entries which the post-mortem records contain, concerning the liver and spleen—at one time, large; at another, small; at one time, the parenchyma light colored; at another, dark; at one time, soft; at another, firm — show most distinctly that we can make no statement whatever as to the constancy of any one of these conditions.

Next in order of importance is the condition met with in the sympathetic nervous system.

It is necessary at the outset to draw attention to the fact that the deposition of pigment in ganglion-cells, and even in connective-tissue cells, has been observed in connection with every pathological process; and further, that its occurrence can all the less be taken as evidence of any pathological change, as it is observed in healthy conditions, occurring in all normal newly born children, and increasing quickly in old age. The same is the case with fatty degeneration, which is recorded in some cases. Some observers speak of an "exudative" process in the ganglion-cells without describing it any further. The conditions to which most importance is to be attached are proliferation of the connective tissue, excessive hyperæmia, and dilatation of the vessels, which latter appears to occur rather frequently, and, moreover, has been observed not only in Addison's disease, but also in other conditions (I shall only recall Zenker's case of fatal hemorrhage of the pancreas). The brain and spinal cord present nothing characteristic anatomically.

Among the changes met with in the blood, in a number of cases, a remarkable thinness of the fluid and deficiency in fibrin has been established, and in a few, excess of the white blood-corpuscles. Buhl and Laschkewitsch lay stress upon the absence of the tendency in the red blood-corpuscles to form *rouleaux*. Mention has already been made of the peculiar cleavage-process and alterations in form which they exhibit. As far as the organs of circulation are concerned, atrophic conditions frequently occur, and in some cases fatty degeneration of the heart is mentioned; in some few cases the remarkable smallness of the heart is especially emphasized.

As in life, the most prominent phenomenon in the corpse is the discoloration of the skin, which assumes every shade, and occurs either in a circumscribed manner or as a profuse mottling, or—as in the most fully marked cases—as a uniformly dark bronze color. It is always darkest in those places where pigment normally exists, as in the folds of the axilla, the areolæ of the breasts, the genitals, and in those places where the clothes fit tightest, as round the waist. There occur, not unfrequently, isolated, remarkably dark, or even blackish brown, disseminated spots [1] which look almost like nævi. Cicatrices exhibit a varying behavior; in the cases that I have seen they were more darkly colored, and a similar condition has been observed by others, while in some isolated cases they are described as remaining uncolored.[2] Microscopic examination demonstrates nothing pathological in the epidermis and cutis of the colored parts beyond the deposition of granular pigment, which for the most part occurs in the deeper layers of cells of the rete Malpighii, and, in the most intense cases, in the papillary region of the cutis, even in the connective-tissue cells, and occasionally in a dotted manner over the course of vessels and nerves.

---

[1] *Addison* depicts a beautiful example in Plate X.

[2] In a case of bronzed skin, without disease of the suprarenal capsule, the cicatrices remained uncolored (Deutsches Archiv f. kl. Med. X. S. 205).

A lesser degree of pigmentation, occasionally diffuse, generally dotted or streaky, occurs irregularly in the epithelium of the mucous membrane of the lips and cheeks (especially corresponding with the edges of the teeth), while the conjunctivæ and the nails may be said to be absolutely free from pigmentation, and the skin of the palm of the hand and of the sole of the foot almost so. The pigment itself is not in any way distinguishable from other pigment, especially that occurring in the cortex of the suprarenal capsules and in the choroid.

Pigmentation of internal organs[1] does not occur any more in the best-marked examples of Addison's disease than in other cases, and particular stress must be laid on the fact that the entire pigmentation, even of the skin, differs in no way anatomically from the pigmentation in other cases. The skin of an individual who has died of Addison's disease is generally smooth, not slaty, and in many (uncomplicated) cases there is a remarkably good supply of fat in the subcutaneous areolar tissue. I have seen this only in one (uncomplicated) case; and I believe that the condition of the fatty tissue depends in reality on the duration of the disease and on complications. The occurrence of swelling in the intestinal and lymphatic glands, along with a well-developed panniculus adiposus, has reminded me of what we so often find in post-mortems on rickety children.

Herewith concludes all that can be said properly to belong to the pathological aspect of morbus Addisonii. Anything further must be regarded as a complication, or, at least, not directly bearing upon the symptoms of the disease. Waldeyer's[2] case, in which, in connection with intense pigmentation, he discovered masses of bacteria in the skin, in the various internal organs, and also in the suprarenal capsules, need only be mentioned here for the sake of completeness; it receives no support from Marowski's[3] case, in which a similar condition was observed during life, without, however, any further confirmation being afforded by the post-mortem.

---

[1] Such depositions of pigment as Addison describes in his Case IX., and depicts in Plate VII., are not recorded elsewhere. The case was one of tubercular peritonitis!

[2] Virchow's Archiv. LIII. 4. S. 533.

[3] Deutsches Archiv f. kl. Med. IV. 5, 6. S. 465.

The principal and most important complication is pre-eminently chronic, caseous inflammation, and tuberculosis of the lungs and of the other internal organs connected with them; which, with its resulting conditions—most prominently phthisis —produces the well-known phenomena.

Significance of the Symptoms and Essential Features of the Disease.

Addison has omitted to sift the symptoms of the disease which he has described, by the aid of post-mortem examination, and to connect them individually with the pathological conditions thereby disclosed, excluding the phenomena which must be referred to complications. A considerable number of the subsequent workers accept Brown-Séquard's experiments, and the anatomical investigations of Luschka and Koelliker. Averbeck refers all the symptoms to a constitutional malady, to an alteration in the constitution of the blood, which must have its cause outside the organism, and hence, therefore, in an infectious disease.

Risel has most studiously attempted to balance the phenomena of the disease with the results of pathological anatomy, and it is essentially his idea that, from the standpoint of both my own observations and what is recorded in the literature of the subject, I am induced to adopt.

If we separate all that is secondary and which must be referred to complications, there remain three groups of symptoms which may be regarded as constituting the characteristic phenomena of morbus Addisonii.

These are, first, those of the digestive tract; secondly, those of the nervous system; and thirdly, those which must be referred to alterations in the constitution of the blood.

With regard to the phenomena presented by the organs of digestion, the most important are the dyspepsia, the vomiting, and especially the constipation and diarrhœa.[1]

---

[1] As a curiosity may here be mentioned S. *Gilliam's* (Philad. Med. and Surg. Reporter. XXIV. June, 1871) attempt to refer the entire complex set of symptoms to degeneration of the glands of the stomach.

If we remember, as was already mentioned, that most experimenters observed profuse diarrhœa to follow the extirpation of the semilunar ganglia, that hyperæmia, extravasations, and the formation of ulcers throughout the entire intestinal tract, have been recorded as the sequences of this operation, and that these do not occur if the same operation upon the peritoneal cavity be performed without injury to the nerves ; if we consider, in conjunction with this, that a lesion of the principal abdominal ganglia of the sympathetic, whether a progressive inflammation or simple irritation, is very naturally suggested ; and that, on the other hand, in those cases in which our attention is directed to these organs, pathological conditions can, in many instances, be established ; we shall not consider it a hazardous conclusion to ascribe these gastric symptoms to irritation, and perhaps also paralytic conditions, of the abdominal sympathetic. The swelling of the mesenteric glands offers no difficulty to this view, when we consider the influence of the long continuance of the hyperæmia and intestinal catarrh, and also the fact that caseous degeneration of the suprarenal capsules is the condition by far most frequently found in our cases. The very inconstancy in the phenomena, and the sudden occurrence of the serious symptoms, are best explained by these etiological considerations, which allow us at one time to accept simple hyperæmia as the exciting cause, and at another, the irritation produced in the nerves passing directly to the ganglia by the progressive disease in the suprarenal capsules. The vaso-motor property of the abdominal plexuses of the sympathetic, the existence of which can no longer be doubted, explains many other vague phenomena, as, for example, alterations in the sexual functions,[1] the cardialgia, and the pain in the sacrum and back. We learn from Goltz's well-known "tapping experiments" (Klopfversuche) how comparatively slight a mechanical irritation to the abdominal viscera suffices to excite a disturbance in the vaso-motor functions of the abdominal nerves and ganglia. The dilatation of the vessels which ensues is said to be sufficient to withdraw one-half the entire mass of blood from the circulation. Ought not, therefore,

---

[1] Mentioned by some reporters.

the direct irritation of the nerves, in which these vaso-motor fibres are known to lie, be capable of producing the same effect? This view, moreover, explains not only the phenomena presented by the digestive organs, but also in part those which occur in connection with the circulation, especially the weakness of the heart, the small, wretched, rapid pulse which results primarily from the diminished quantity of blood passing through the heart, and secondarily, from the impoverished condition of the heart arising from the same cause. Herewith accords also the fact that the smallness of the heart is expressly mentioned in the records of a large number of post-mortems, and also that fatty degeneration of the muscular tissue of the heart is often found. The paleness of the skin and the low temperatures, occurring in cases in which a general well-marked poverty of blood does not exist, can without difficulty be referred to the same cause.

To no less a degree may a large number of the severe cerebral and nervous symptoms be attributed to a determination of blood to the abdomen, such as results from an irritation and subsequent paralysis of the abdominal ganglia. Fainting and nausea, vertigo and headache, dyspnœa, occurring particularly severely when the patient attempts to raise himself up into an upright position, are phenomena which we often meet associated, as here indicated, in persons who are suffering from anæmia of the brain, resulting from loss of blood ; which I, moreover, have seen most strikingly exemplified in some cases of violent gastralgia, in which no loss of blood had taken place. I remember two cases in particular, with most violent cardialgia, and intense pain extending from the region of the stomach into both hypochondria and to the sacrum, in which no indication could be discovered of any disease of the stomach, but in which the most gentle efforts to change from the horizontal into the vertical position immediately occasioned giddiness and a feeling of faintness, together with paleness of the face and an imperceptibly small pulse. With complete rest and a tonic treatment, all these symptoms disappeared in eight days, and I do not hesitate to ascribe them likewise to an irritation of the abdominal ganglia, which was immediately followed by dilatation of the vessels and determination of blood to the abdomen.

While these phenomena are but transitory in cases of this kind, they are characterized in the disease in question by their very stability, which, towards the end, gives place only to a gradual increase in the symptoms, and now and then is interrupted by most violent fits of recrudescence. In other words, we are not here concerned with transient irritation and consecutive paralytic phenomena, but with a progressive organic disease—a process of actual degeneration.

The dyspnœa which ensues on assuming the vertical position may be referred to anæmia of the medulla oblongata from mechanical causes (weakness of the heart), and the quickening of the pulse, also, would be produced by increased excitation of the excito-motor nerve of the heart. These ideas, borrowed from Risel's comprehensive physiological essay, accord so fully with what I have myself observed in my few cases, that I cannot hesitate to accept them as the explanation of the symptoms.

As a phenomenon connected with the nervous system, the frequent violent pain in the joints must particularly be mentioned. This is closely analogous to hysterical arthritic neurosis, as in both instances, up to the present, at least, no local pathological conditions have been found. Erb (vide Vol. XI. of this Cyclopædia) mentions that irritation of abdominal organs, according to the experience of Esmarch, Stromeyer, and Sims, must particularly be regarded as frequently the source of these neuroses, so that in this case, also, the idea of irritation of the sympathetic, from disease of the suprarenal capsules, is not to be repudiated.

In none of these cases, in which great loss of blood is to be regarded as the cause of such symptoms, and in which we observe other severe disturbances of nutrition, do we find the remarkable discoloration of the skin so constant as it is in morbus Addisonii. While Averbeck retreats upon an infectious idea of the whole disease, Risel would attribute the discoloration to an abnormal distribution of blood in the various vascular regions, and an imperfect supply of oxygen to the tissues, which is further borne out by the weakness of the heart and a frequently observed atheromatous degeneration of the vessels (a condition which I have not observed). Still, Risel evidently feels that, in spite of the influence of light on the skin, these arguments will not suffice, for he also speaks of an alteration in the red blood-corpuscles, of a "secondary, not fully understood change in the blood, which probably gives rise to the bronzed skin."

If the discolorations of the skin were attributable, as many seem inclined to think, simply to the lesion of the sympathetic, it ought to occur much oftener; for pathological conditions of the sympathetic are, as we have already seen, not so rare as might be imagined; and I myself have seen, in a case of slowly growing carcinoma, the semilunar ganglia firmly embedded in a cancerous mass, without a trace of bronzed skin. But it certainly will not do to deny all significance in this respect to the nervous lesion, for though dark and often remarkable pigmentation of the skin is frequently seen (apart from melanæmia and Vogt's "gipsy-color" [Vagantenfärbung]), the phenomena of depression and anæmia, in the degree at least that is characteristic of Addison's disease, are wanting, unless these cases are otherwise complicated. The affection of the sympathetic is certainly not sufficient to explain the emaciation, the wretchedness, and the debility of the patient. It explains certain essential phenomena of the disease very adequately, but not the gradually increasing general wretchedness nor the ultimately not less important anæmia. And, as bearing on this question, I claim—if as yet not actual importance—at least some attention for the condition of the red blood-corpuscles met with in the three cases alluded to, which, in connection with Thudicum's preliminary and as yet isolated examination of the urine, tend to throw some light upon the diseased state of the blood. The trio of symptoms, the intense anæmia, the nervous depression, and the discoloration of the skin, are most simply explained in connection with those pathological processes, which, on the one hand, interfere with the functions of the suprarenal capsules, and thereby indirectly affect the properties of the blood, and which, on the other hand, both in a reflex manner react upon the general nervous system, and also directly affect the tissue of the sympathetic nervous system by propagating a diseased condition per contiguitatem.

It may be urged in opposition to this, that we not unfrequently find degeneration of the entire parenchyma of the suprarenal capsules (particularly amyloid) without the coexistence of the symptoms of Addison's disease; still to this we may reply that similar degeneration of other organs is often well borne for a considerable time, provided it does not exceed a certain limit, and also that amyloid degeneration of the suprarenal capsules has hitherto only been seen in connection with similar degeneration of other organs, which latter gave the general aspect to the disease, and which doubtless, in some cases at least, were primary. Bearing upon this, the requirement of a certain chronicity in the disease as a conditio sine qua non for the occurrence of the complex set of symptoms (which Virchow, for this very form of degeneration, rejects as unauthorized), appears to me to be authorized; for the suprarenal capsules are undoubtedly the last of all the abdominal viscera to be attacked by amyloid degeneration, —at all events I have never seen a case where they were the only organs affected. We cannot regard the symptoms as depending upon the extent of the degeneration, for there are occasional examples in which small nodules, even in one suprarenal capsule, have been observed in connection with fully developed morbus Addisonii.

All ambiguity arises out of our inadequate knowledge of the physiological significance of the suprarenal capsules. Anatomy having definitively spoken (and this, in my opinion, is not unimportant), it remains for physiology to decide the question.

Diagnosis.

If we find indications of the severe nervous symptoms just described, of remarkable anæmia, which cannot be explained by any organic disease, combined with considerable discoloration of the skin, the diagnosis of morbus Addisonii, if not actually certain, is at least authorized. The slow course of the disease further confirms the diagnosis, if there be no complications. Where complications exist, especially those of pulmonary consumption, the diagnosis can never attain to anything beyond probability; and I have found for myself that it is only too easy to make mistakes. This difficulty of diagnosis, as already stated, gives no actual ground for denying the coincidence of the pathological conditions found in the suprarenal capsules with the observed and often described set of symptoms of morbus Addisonii, or for regarding such coincidence as merely accidental. A belief in the connection between the pathological conditions met with after death and the symptoms occurring during life takes undoubtedly a form equivalent to mathematical probability.

From the foregoing may be deduced all that can be said concerning a differential diagnosis. It is only possible in entirely uncomplicated cases, in which the most conspicuous symptom, the discoloration of the skin, is not wanting, and this is to be distinguished more or less from other pigmentary deposits in the skin by being darker on the face and hands than on the body ; by the existence of still darker spots throughout the dark skin, while the conjunctivæ and nails remain quite white ; by the skin continuing smooth and shiny, and not becoming slaty ; and by the subcutaneous areolar tissue retaining its fat for a lengthened period.

The small, weak, rapid pulse, the weak heart's action in general, the gastric disturbances, the vomiting and diarrhœa occurring without apparent cause, the intense, general asthenia, the general feeling of faintness, which later on is particularly increased if the patient attempts to rise from his bed, the various neuroses, especially of the joints, the pain in the sacrum, and the absence of other organic disease, or abnormal conditions in the blood, all tend to put us on the right track, but still any certainty is only that which may be derived by the method of exclusion. What the value of a more thorough investigation of the blood and the urine may be, remains to be proved.

Prognosis.

An absolutely fatal prognosis must always be made. In all those cases which are recorded as having been cured there exists a doubt as to the accuracy of the diagnosis, and among the cases in Averbeck's Table V. there is not a single one which does not admit of another interpretation of the symptoms, even without our questioning in the slightest the accuracy of any of the statements there made. Proofs do seem to exist of certain symptoms decreasing in the course of the disease, most of all the discoloration of the skin; still, in all the accurate records to which I have had recourse, death ultimately ensued as the result of the degeneration of the suprarenal capsules.

In the majority of cases, after a more or less chronic course, death is caused by pulmonary tuberculosis, while in uncomplicated cases it occurs as the result of exhaustion.

Treatment.

Experience teaches us that patients get on best with perfect rest. This gives the first and most important indication for treatment. Whenever it can be done, therefore, the first thing is to get the patient free from all occupation and anxiety. Along with this as generous a dietary as possible must be given, which ought to comprise plenty of meat, eggs, and milk. The insufficiency of the muscular tissue of the heart demands stimulants under all circumstances, and these are best given in the form of good, strong wine. Good beer, also, and, under certain circumstances, the stronger alcoholic forms—in particular, old brandy—must not be withheld. In treating the gastric symptoms, we must proceed in the manner described in the various handbooks—still, the exhibition of stimulating medicine is generally attended with good results—and, above all, we must avoid strong purgatives, whereas gentle saline aperients are generally of much service. It will appear, from the course here laid down, that preparations of iron and quinia are not to be withheld; and opiates and morphia, also, are often productive of beneficial effects, which must not be lost sight of.

By the very variety of the conditions met with in the suprarenal capsules, it is most distinctly shown that treatment in by far the greatest number of cases must merely be to palliate symptoms; and that we cannot as yet expect much from any efforts directed against the source of the disease itself.

Definite corroborative observations are wanting to show how far the much-recommended iodide of potassium and galvanism have had any effect in this way in producing a cure. However, in the meantime, they must be tried.

Further Diseased Conditions of the Suprarenal Capsules.

If the description of the disease just given comprehends all phenomena which may be recorded as occurring during life and which may be referred to pathological conditions of the suprarenal capsules found post-mortem, and if thereby the entire clinical history of diseases of the suprarenal capsules is exhausted, in that part, also, which treats of the pathological conditions met with in Addison's disease, almost everything is contained which has ever been observed in the way of alterations in the suprarenal capsules and their parenchyma.

To complete the account of the latter, however, must be mentioned the following :

Abnormal Development and Imperfections.

The few cases are recorded in *Rokitansky*, Pathol. Anatomie. III. S. 381.—*Averbeck*, Addison'sche Krankh. S. 90.—Schmidt's Jahrbücher (*Meissner*, Ueber Pigment-krankheit). 142 u. 154.

Complete absence of the suprarenal capsules is only observed in very imperfect monstrosities. Cases in which one or both of these bodies are said to have been absent are recorded, but they are not sufficiently described to allow us to feel fully convinced of the carefulness of the observation.

It occurs much more frequently—although still rarely—that the suprarenal capsule is found lying in the same capsule with the kidney, being bound to the cortical portion of the latter by firm connective tissue.

Not unfrequently, also, there occur accessory suprarenal capsules, varying in size from a millet-seed to a pea, sometimes in the immediate neighborhood, and sometimes actually embedded in the tissue of the normal suprarenal capsules. I once saw a suprarenal capsule formed out of a great conglomeration of small accessory bodies, each of which, on section, presented the appearance of a very small normal suprarenal capsule.

Atrophy.

Rokitansky, Path. Anatomie. III. S. 381.

It occurs in old age. Rokitansky describes the atrophied suprarenal capsule as shrivelled, tough as leather, the cortical portion dirty yellow, the medullary substance wasted, or the body throughout rusty brown, barmy yellow, and readily broken down.

We may here recall the condition in which the organs, on being taken out, are found to be very friable, forming a sac with dirty, dark colored, half-fluid contents—a condition which, although it originated the name of " suprarenal capsules," must be looked upon only as a post-mortem appearance.

Hemorrhages.

Averbeck, Addison'sche Krankheit. S. 91, 92.—*Fiedler* (Archiv der Heilkunde. XI. 1870).—*Ahlfeld* (Ibid. S. 491).—*Rokitansky*, L. c.

These, apart from what has been already said in the pathological anatomy of morbus Addisonii, have been observed most generally in newly born children, in whom they have produced a fatal loss of blood. Fiedler describes two cases, in one of which a severe extra- and intraperitoneal hemorrhage had caused the death of a child four days old. In the position of the right suprarenal capsule was found a tumor the size of a hen-egg, which proved to be a hemorrhagic suprarenal capsule, the cells of the tissue of which were found to be affected with intense fatty degeneration. Similar fatty degenerations with slighter hemorrhages are described by Fiedler in a second case. (By the rapid way in which death ensues we are again struck by the similarity to Zenker's hemorrhage of the pancreas.)

Here we are almost led to conclude that we have to do with congenital

Syphilis,

in connection with which Virchow has found similar conditions.

Hutchinson's test case (Med. Times and Gaz. Dec., 1855,) belongs to this category.

—*Baerensprung*, Die hereditäre Syphilis. Berlin, 1864.—*Hecker*, Monatsschrift für Geburtskunde. 1869. 33.—*Huber*, Deutsch. Archiv für klin. Med. V. 2. 1869.—*Virchow* (Krankhafte Geschwülste. II. S. 431; and Archiv. XV. S. 315).

In addition to this form of fatty degeneration, which v. Baerensprung and Huber confirm, gummata are described in congenital syphilis by Virchow and Hecker.

We do not possess any further definite information as to how syphilis subsequently attacking the suprarenal capsules is indicated clinically, or how it is anatomically manifested.

According to Baerensprung and Huber, the suprarenal capsules are found on inspection to be considerably swollen, hyperæmic, and beset with granules or spots, small, white, miliary, and the size of a poppy-seed, which traverse the cortical substance in the form of radiating striæ. These spots and granules are found to be masses composed of nuclei and young cells. In another case (a syphilitic child nine days old, affected with sclerosis), Hecker records a peculiar cartilaginous consistence of the suprarenal capsules, and a uniform gray infiltration of the parenchyma.

The only animal parasite observed in the suprarenal capsules is

Echinococcus,

and that (Heller, Diseases from Migratory Parasites. Vol. III. of this Cyclopædia, p. 589) only in two cases.

To one of these (Davaine's) I was unable to obtain access. Huber reports the other (Deutsch. Archiv f. klin. Med. Bd. IV. S. 613; and V. S. 139) as a multilocular echinococcus, and he describes the symptoms occurring in this case as those of morbus Addisonii, without, however, discoloration of the skin.

DISEASES OF THE BLADDER.

———

LEBERT.

.

DISEASES OF THE BLADDER.

Rufus, Ephes., De vesicæ renumque morbis. Paris, 1754.—*S. Olivier*, Traité des malad. des reins et de la vessie. Rouen, 1731.—*Zuber*, De vesic. urin. morb. Argent. 1771.—*M. Troja*, Ueber die Krankheiten der Nieren, der Harnblase u. s. w. Aus. d. Italien. Leipzig, 1738.—*J. P. Frank*, Oratio de vesica urinali, etc. Paris, 1786. —*P. J. Desault*, Traité des maladies des voies urinaires, etc. Bichat. Paris, 1798.— *F. A. Walther*, Einige Krankheiten der Nieren und Harnblase, Vorsteherdrüse u. s. w. denen Männer im höheren Alter ausgesetzt sind. Wien, 1806. —*J. Howship*, Practical Observations on the Diseases of the Urinary Organs. London, 1807.—*H. Johnstone*, Observations on Stone, Diseases of the Bladder, Prostate, and Urethra. Edinb. 1806.—*J. Th. v. Soemmering*, Abhdlg. über die schnell, und langsam tödtlichen Krankheiten der Harnblase bei alten Männern. Frankf. 1822.—*M. Nauche*, Des maladies de la vessie chez les personnes avancées en âge. Paris, 1810.—*Chopart*, Traité des maladies des voies urinaires. Paris, 1821.—*Robert Bingham*, Practical Essay on Diseases and Injuries of the Bladder, etc. Lond. 1822.—*M. E. Lallemand*, Observ. sur les maladies des voies urinaires. Paris, 1824.— *W. Coulson*, On Diseases of the Bladder. Lond. 1828.—*B. Brodie*, Lectures on Diseases of the Urinary Organs. London, 1832.— *L. A. Mercier*, Recherches anat. path. et thérap. sur les maladies des organes genito-urinaires. Paris, 1841.—*R. Willis*, Urinary Diseases and their Treatment. Lond. 1838.—*W. Acton*, A Practical Treatise on Diseases of the Urinary and Generative Organs. London, 1851.—*H. Rosenmüller*, Chron. Leiden der Harnwerkzeuge u. Extr. uvæ urs. frig. par. Rhein Monatsschr. Juli, 1850. S. 411.— *Ditto*, Abtreibung von Stein und Gries durch die Elisab.-Quelle zu Kreuznach. Rhein. Monatsschr. Juli, 1850. S. 413.—*Kraemer*, Trichiasis cystina, Medic. Correspond. Bl. bair. Ærzte. 1850. H. 18.—*Ricord*, Catarrhe vesical intense, action avantageuse des injections de nitrate d'argent à haute dose. Gaz. des Hôpitaux. 1850. No. 14.—*L. Macdonell*, Observations on the Treatment of Chronic Cystitis. Monthly Journal of Medical Science, May, 1850. p. 478.—*D. Pointe*, Traitement médic. des douleurs produites par les calculs vésicaux; efficacité des extraits combinés d'opium et de bellad. dans ce traitement. Gaz. des Hôpitaux, 1849.—*E. Gradowicz*, Semen lycopod. gegen Blennorr. vesic. Medizinische Zeitung. Russlands, 1849. Februar.—*Rayer*, Recherches sur la pilimiction (trichiasis des voies urinaires). Gazette Médicale. 1851. No. 31.—*Pitha*, Krankheiten der männlichen Genitalien und Harnblase. Erlangen, 1864.—*Lebert*, Krankheiten der Harnblase. Handbuch der praktischen Medicin. II. Bd. 791 et seq. 4. Aufl. Tübingen, 1871.

I. Defects of Development of the Bladder.

Vogler, Bemerkungen über Harnblasenvorfall nebst zwei Beobachtungen dieser Missbildung und einem Anhang über angeborenen Mangel beider Augäpfel. Magazin für die ges. Heilkunde in Preussen. LXIII. N. F. XXI. Bd. 3. H. 1844.—*Argenti*, Absence of the Bladder. Memor. della med. contemp. Sept. 1844.—*T. H. Starr*, Case in which Urine escaped by the Navel. Lond. Med. Gaz. Jan. 12, 1844.—*Edward Daniell*, Cases of Malformation of the Bladder. Provincial Medical and Surgical Journal. 1846. p. 451.—*Mr. Thomas Paget*, Case of Patency of the Urachus. Extraction of a Ring-shaped Calculus, formed upon a Hair in the Bladder, through the Umbilicus. Med. Chir. Trans. Vol. XXXIII. 1850. p. 293.—*Braun*, Abnorme Lage der Harnblase. Rhein. Monatsschrift. October, 1851.—*Buehrlen*, Extroversio Vesicæ. Würtemb. Corresp.-Bl. 30. 1852.—*B. Dulley*, Malformation of the Genital Organs and of the Bladder. Lancet, June 26, 1852.—*Chance*, Two Cases of Extroversion of the Bladder, with Remarks on the Mode of Origin of such Malformations. Lancet, Dec. 11, 1852.—*Hafner*, Prolapsus vesicæ urin. congenitus cum inversione. Würtemberg Corresp.-Bl. 40. 1853.—*Roux*, Ectopia vesicæ. Autoplastic Operation. L'Union, 114, 115. 1853.—*Daniel Ayres*, Operat. der Blasenektopie. Verhandl. der Gesellsch. f. Geburtsh. Berlin, 1859. S. 195.

As most of the malformations of the bladder are of more interest anatomically than clinically, we shall treat of them briefly here. Absence of the bladder, the ureters opening into the urethra, is of very rare occurrence, and invariably fatal. Absence of the anterior wall of the bladder, with a corresponding defect in the abdominal wall, the symphysis, and often of the urethra and penis, or rudimentary development of the same, is much more frequently met with, and is compatible with viability. In these cases the posterior wall of the bladder is visible as a red, swollen surface of mucous membrane, depressed backward so as to form a cavity, or, as is not unfrequently the case, bulging forward, the openings of the ureters being very conspicuous, and the urine seen to escape from them constantly drop by drop. That this inversion of the bladder—ectopia vesicæ—is compatible with long life is evident from the fact that a number of cases on record occurred in adults, and I have myself seen this anomaly in an old woman at the Salpêtrière Hospital in Paris.

In other cases the bladder is closed anteriorly, but is deficient behind, and communicates with the rectum or vagina; congenital recto-vesical or vesico-vaginal fistula.

Very rarely the bladder is bifid, an occurrence easily explained by the presence of a septum, which, as in the case recorded by Blasius, may divide the bladder into two wholly distinct sacs, each having a ureter opening into it. Diverticula from the bladder are, commonly, non-congenital, and occur in consequence of various diseases.

Ayres' successful autoplastic operative procedure for ectopia vesicæ, and the cases of recto-vesical and vesico-vaginal fistula, which have not unfrequently been operated on with good results, show that surgery can deal successfully with these malformations. For details, we must refer to special works on surgery.

II. Hernia of the Bladder.

In its simplest form this is met with as a mere protrusion of the mucous membrane through the urethra, which may increase to a partial or complete prolapse of the bladder (cystocele, Blasenbruch). In other cases a portion of the bladder prolapses at one of the usual seats of hernia, as cystocele inguinalis, cruralis, perinealis, ischiadica, foraminis ovalis, and, in women, as cystocele vaginalis and cruralis. It is but rarely that hernia of the bladder is congenital; mostly it results from violent exertion, injuries, excessive straining in micturition, and occasionally it follows pregnancy when the labor has been a difficult one. The hernia vesicæ may be associated with pre-existing ordinary hernia, or may occur alone. In the first case, as a rule, adhesions gradually form between the bladder and the other viscera and the sac, and the flow of urine may thus be much impeded, stagnation of urine, irritation of the bladder, the formation of stone, or even septic poisoning, resulting. Very rarely the prolapsed portion of the bladder may become strangulated. When the urine is retained, the tumor naturally increases in size, and diminishes when the urine is evacuated; as the tumor fills, the efforts at micturition increase, and the same result is produced when the tumor is compressed. By the use of a catheter, not only may the diagnosis be rendered certain in doubtful cases, but the prolapse may be reduced by pressure, and the bladder may be retained in its place by a suitable bandage. In women, a pessary may keep the bladder in its place. If replacement is impossible, owing to adhesions, a suspensory bandage must be worn, and the urine evacuated by pressure or the use of a catheter. In very rare cases herniotomy may be necessary to relieve strangulation.

If the bladder prolapses through the urethra in females—as sometimes happens, in rare cases, in young girls, owing to the urethra being very large, and allowing the bladder to extrude as a red, fungoid tumor—thorough replacement is generally sufficient to effect a cure, or, if not, we may follow Lowe's example, and cause the urethra to contract by cauterizing it after each renewed protrusion, and thus prevent any further prolapse of the bladder.

III. Inflammation and Catarrh of the Bladder.

(Cystitis, Catarrhus Vesicæ.)

J. Mueller, De Inflam. Vesic. Urin. Altd. 1703.—*F. Hoffmann*, De exulcer. vesicæ. Hal. 1724.—*C. Vater* (*Volck*), Ulceris vesicæ origines, signa et remedia. Hal. 1709.—*Arnaud*, Plain and Easy Instructions on Diseases of the Bladder, etc. Lond. 1763.—*Ivermann*, De vesic. urin. ejusque ulcere. L. B. 1763.—*Tomlinson*, The Medical Miscellany. London, 1774.—*Zuber*, De vesic. urin. morh. Argent. 1771.—*Pohl*, De abscessu vesic. urin. Lips. 1777.—*Sommerer*, De Cystitide. Vienn. 1782.—*M. Troja*, Lezioni int. ai mali della visica orin. Nap. 1785. —*F. Gerber*, D. de cystitide chron. Hal. 1823.—*G. Pitsch*, D. de vesic. urin. inflam. Greifsw. 1823.—*D. Bianchi*, D. de cystitide et de ischuria. Patav. 1823. *Berdt*, Cystitis im Encycl. Wörtb. Berl. 1833. Bd. IX. S. 92.— *W. Coulson*, Two Lectures on Stricture of the Urethra, with Observations on Inflammation of the Bladder. Lond. 1833.—*Naumann*, Handb. d. m. Kl. Bd. VI. p. 194.—*Eisenmann*, Die Krankheitsfamilie Rheuma. Bd. III. S. 463.—*Begin*, Im Univ.-Lex. Bd. IV. p. 537.—*Arming*, Im Gräfe u. W. Journ. Bd. XXV. H. 1.—*Cumin*, In der Uebers. der Cyclop. Pract. Med. Bd. I. p. 554.—*Sprengler*, in Schmidt's Encycl. Bd. III. S. 260.—*Civiale*, L. c. p. 452 et p. 48.—*Budd*, Case of Extensive

Ulceration of the Bladder. Lond. Med. Gaz. 1841. Nov. 26th.—*G. King*, Gangrene of the Bladder. Dublin Med. Press. 1841.—*Lynch*, Cystitis in Consequence of Injury to the Spinal Cord. Dublin Journ. 1841. March. p. 118.— *Courty*, On the Use of Injections of Balsams in Chronic Vesical Catarrh. La Clinique. 1. Juin, 1842.—*Baumgaertner*, Injections of Nitrate of Silver into the Bladder. Journ. de Conn. Méd.-Chir. Eerr. 1843.—*Leydel*, Der Blasencatarrh u. seine Behandlung mit Zugrundelegung der Civialischen Abhandlg. n. fremd. u. eig. Erfahrungen dargestellt. Dresden u. Leipzig. 1843. Arnold. gr. 8. S. 199. —*Cossy*, On Certain Affections of the Bladder after Typhus. Arch. Gén. Sept. 1843.—*Seydel*, Die natürl. Heilwäss von Vichy als ein wicht. mittel gegen Unterleibsübel, Harnbeschwerden u. s. w. Nach den französ. Originalquellen, sowie eigen. Beobacht. u. Versuchen dargestellt. 2. mit einem Nachtr. Vermehrte Auflage. Dresden u. Leipzig. 1844. Arnold. 8. IX. u. S. 109.—*Deberey*, Treatment of Chronic Cystitis by Caustic Injections. Journ. de Conn. Méd.-Chir. Avril, 1845.—*W. H. Colborne*, Case of Chronic Inflammation of the Bladder. Provincial Med. Journ. No. 47. Nov. 1845.—*Hutin*, Vesical Catarrh. Incontinentia urinæ. Annal de Thérapeut. Méd. et Chir. par Rogretta. Avril. IV. No. 1. 1847.—*Duvivier-Goeury*, Nouveau traitement du catarrhe chronique de la vessie, par la méthode des injections et la méthode spéciale. 1848. Paris. Hebrad. J. B. Baillière. 8. 80 pp.—*Ricord*, Severe Vesical Catarrh. Excellent Results from the Use of a Concentrated Solution of Nitrate of Silver. Gaz. des Hôp. 14. 1850.—*Prieger*, Chronische Leiden der Harnwerkzeuge u. Ext. uræ ursi frig. parat. klin. Monatsschr. Juli, 1850.—*Lemnistre-Florian*, Constant Irrigation with a Solution of Salt in Chronic Cystitis. Gaz. des Hôp. 1847. 48.

Inflammation of the bladder, vesical catarrh, may have an acute or a chronic course, and we shall describe each separately.

Acute Inflammation of the Bladder, Cystitis Acuta.

A. Cystitis Mucosa Acuta.

Eliology.

Acute cystitis in the simplest cases is the result of injury in the region of the bladder from pressure, blows, contusion, or fracture of the pelvis, more particularly of the pubes; the latter is very rarely a cause. Professional unskilfulness in passing a catheter, for instance, may lead to irritation of the bladder. This also results not unfrequently, as may easily be understood, after the first "sitting" in lithotrity. The irritation of the bladder

set up by the long-continued pressure of the head during difficult labors is generally of a transitory character ; when the pressure has been very long continued, however, and artificial aid
has been rendered, I have seen gangrene, followed by the formation of large vesico-vaginal fistulæ, result. Displacements of the
bladder and vesical calculi are more likely to cause chronic than
acute inflammation of the bladder.

Chemical irritants, in unsuitable combinations, or in too strong
solutions, injected into the bladder to check bleeding, etc., etc.,
may directly cause acute inflammation. In this category comes
the remarkable irritation set up by cantharides applied in the
form of blisters. The cantharidine becomes absorbed and is
excreted by the kidneys, but only excites its characteristic irritation and inflammatory symptoms when it is carried by the
urine into the bladder and brought in contact with the mucous
membrane. Long-retained, decomposing urine is very irritating,
chiefly owing to the formation of carbonate of ammonia, and in
this way neglected retention of urine, such as is observed in
cases of severe typhus, is very injurious ; hence the rule to see
that such patients are induced to pass water several times in the
day, or, if necessary, that the catheter be used.

A chill, or getting wet through, especially during sweating,
and long-continued wetting of the feet, will excite acute vesical
catarrh. The acute vesical irritation, occasionally very severe,
though transitory, set up by new, imperfectly fermented beer
and by all sorts of beverages of bad quality owes its origin
probably to chemical irritation. Acute cystitis also sometimes
develops secondarily in the course of infectious diseases with
various local complications, but, curiously, at certain times more
frequently than at others. For instance, on one occasion I saw
acute vesical catarrh develop secondarily in a series of cases of
typhoid fever at Breslau, and I have at various times observed
it in articular rheumatism. When inflammation attacks the
bladder by extension from other parts, it is generally from without inward, as, for instance, from disease of the urethra, prostate, vagina, or uterus. In other cases, however, an acute inflammation of the mucous membrane of the pelvis of the kidney,
whether of spontaneous origin or set up by the presence of cal-

culi, is transmitted along the ureters to the bladder. Inflammation spreading from without may also be conveyed from the peritoneum and its various processes to the external layers of the bladder and its connective-tissue covering, as pericystitis. Lastly, in a series of cases we may see acute vesical catarrh arise without any obvious cause, spontaneously, and we may be disposed, as was especially the case formerly, to regard the disease as of a rheumatic or gouty character, generally, however, without sufficient reason.

Symptomatology.

Acute cystitis may begin suddenly, with fever, severe pain, frequent desire to pass water, and marked derangement of the digestive functions, or the patient's general condition may be but little, or not at all, affected, whilst the local symptoms attract most attention. The pain and sense of pressure and tightness in the lower part of the abdomen over the region of the bladder may be constantly present and aggravated at intervals, in paroxysms, or may be felt principally during micturition, being entirely absent or only insignificant at other times. In proportion as the cervix and trigonum vesicæ are affected, the difficulty in making water will be more severe and constant, and the pains will radiate from the hypogastrium to the inguinal or even to the sacral region, the perineum, and the testes and glans penis (in men). The pain complained of spontaneously will be greatly increased by pressure, especially on the hypogastrium and perineum, and (in women) on the fundus of the bladder through the vagina. The frequent desire to pass water is particularly distressing, only a little urine escaping each time, with considerable pain and spasm, and complete retention may ensue. Even when the difficulty in passing water is but moderate, the patients are not completely relieved after attempts at micturition, for they still feel as if they wanted to pass water. This condition is called tenesmus vesicæ, strangury. The urine thus voided with great pain and by drops at a time, or, at any rate, in small quantity, is generally thick, of a dark reddish color, and sometimes contains blood. If complete retention ensues, the bladder gradually becomes more and more distended, and can be felt as a rounded tumor, giving a dull sound on percussion, rising higher and higher above the pubes. The tenesmus vesicæ occasionally becomes communicated to the rectum ; all the pelvic organs may participate in the painful sensations. If the pain and desire to pass water are less violent, they subside with the act of micturition, but only to return subsequently. If the turbid, high-colored urine is allowed to stand, a layer of mucus, sometimes tinged with blood, quickly settles at the bottom, as a rule, and an examination with the microscope reveals in it a number of white blood-corpuscles (mucus or pus-corpuscles). It is very rarely that blood is present in any large quantity. Albumen is present only when the urine contains a quantity of mucus, cells, and blood, and is most marked in cystitis from cantharides ; a form of cystitis which for this reason was formerly regarded as a nephritis.

In very acute cases fever is present, and not unfrequently also in cases in which the local symptoms are not very severe. Occasionally the fever is ushered in by a shivering fit ; I have observed this several times in connection with cystitis following on the application of blisters. As a rule, the fever, which may be absent altogether, is associated with a moderate increase of temperature, 100.4°-102.2° F. (38°-39° Cent.), and moderate frequency of pulse, 92-100, the fulness and tension of the arteries being but slightly more than normal. If cystitis comes on in patients affected with fever, it may be sufficient to raise the temperature after it had already begun to fall, as in typhus, for instance.

In addition to the usual symptoms of gastric disturbance associated with fever, such as thirst, loss of appetite, and tendency to constipation, there are often nausea, retching, and even severe vomiting, which also occurs, as is well known, not unfrequently in other affections of the urinary organs. The amount of fever depends usually on the intensity of the inflammation ; in not a few cases, however, it seems to be associated with some special predisposition.

If we are compelled to make use of the catheter in consequence of retention of urine and increasing distention of the bladder, it will be found to give rise to much pain, even when skilfully passed and the instrument is a flexible one. In many cases, also, pain is complained of when passing a motion, so that, if a mild laxative, such as castor oil, is not administered occasionally, the patient, in order to avoid pain, neglects to evacuate the bowels, and distention of the abdomen, meteorismus, and increased pressure on the bladder follow. In rare cases, and more especially in vesical irritation following on the internal use of large doses of cantharides, which, as is well known, is regarded, though erroneously, as a remedy for impotence in the male, we may observe the irritation spread to the external genitals, and even produce priapism, a symptom often described in connection with poisoning by cantharides since the time of Ambroise Paré. In this form we also often see portions of false membrane in the urine ; their passage is accompanied by violent tenesmus vesicæ, and they are occasionally tinged with blood. Also in connection with croupo-diphtheritic processes attacking other parts, croupous cystitis becomes developed in the form of pseudo-membranous diphtheria, and then large fibrinous masses of exudation may be thrown off, and, after previous blocking of the bladder, may be passed gradually with great difficulty and straining. The bladder may also participate in diphtheritic puerperal processes.

Progress and Result.

As a rule, the disease only has a rapid course, terminating within a few days when it is due to some accidental irritation, such as an injury, or to badly fermented beverages, or cantharides. In these cases usually the pain diminishes, the fever abates, the quality of the urine improves, and the patient makes water easily in the course of a few days, and a cure results in four or five, or, at most, eight days. In other cases, in which the disease progresses favorably towards recovery, it nevertheless lasts for one or two, or even several weeks. In these cases there is almost invariably very great improvement in the second week, resulting in recovery in the third or fourth. In other cases the cure is imperfect, the fever abates, the pain diminishes or wholly subsides, but there is still too frequent desire to pass water, and the urine remains abnormal in quality for a long time. The cystitis, instead of being acute, has become chronic. In rare cases gangrene ensues. This is especially liable to occur in typhus, if prolonged retention has been overlooked, and in those cases in which there seems to be some inherent tendency for inflammation to terminate in gangrene. In puerperal women, gangrene of the bladder is generally due to long-continued pressure of the child's head on the bladder, but also in normal labors puerperal cystitis may now and then terminate in gangrene. We must also mention as one of the results of cystitis, complete suppression of urine accompanied by all the signs of uræmic poisoning, fever of a typhoid character, and even death, if, as a result of the cystitis, the openings of the ureters have become blocked. I have some doubt, however, as to the possibility of cystitis alone, without any complication, setting up any such symptoms.

B. Inflammation of the Submucous and Subserous Connective Tissue and of the Structures surrounding the Bladder. Cystitis Submucosa, Subserosa, Parenchymatosa, Pericystitis, Paracystitis.

Though inflammation of the mucous membrane is by far the most frequent form of acute cystitis, any of the other anatomical structures may be the seat of inflammation. The symptoms, then, however, are much more severe, especially when the submucous tissue is affected. Whilst the white corpuscles poured out on the free inner surface of the bladder and mingling with the urine relieve to some extent the parts from which they come, submucous and subserous purulent localized or diffused infiltration causes much more serious complications on account of the comparatively narrow space within which it is confined. The walls of the bladder, thickened by infiltration, rigid, hypertrophied, adherent and contracted by pericystitis are, on the one hand, rendered much less capable of expelling the urine, and, on the other hand, the bladder can contain but a small quantity of urine, so that the continued secretion of urine leads to an excruciating sense of pain over the whole vesical region and to frequent, almost constant attempts to pass water, which is only voided in very small quantities, often guttative, and as a consequence the glans, the prepuce, the whole penis, and the scrotum become excoriated. If an abscess in the submucous tissue bulges considerably into the interior of the bladder it may, if situated in the posterior or lateral walls of the bladder, considerably obstruct the flow of urine from the ureters and so cause regurgitation of the urine to the kidneys, whilst a similar collection in the neighborhood of the neck of the bladder may block up the opening of the urethra and lead to complete retention of urine. The pain and desire to pass water remain constantly; the sense of pressure in the neighborhood of the bladder and deep in the pelvis, steadily increasing and constant, radiates to the lumbar, sacral, and perineal regions, and even more distant parts. Attacks of shivering occur irregularly in the course of the fever and, together with the typhous state of the patient which often develops very rapidly, indicates suppuration or absorption of the constituents of the urine. Complete loss of appetite, intense thirst, frequent retching and, not unfrequently, obstinate vomiting ensue. If the abscess bursts into the cavity of the bladder, the pain and attempts to pass water diminish, the fever abates, the rigors cease, the pus escapes with the urine, which is voided more copiously and easily, pus continues for a time to be constantly, or at intervals, mixed with the urine, until finally the bladder heals by cicatrization.

Both the subserous and the submucous abscesses may also, however, burst externally; in rare cases into the peritoneum, setting up rapidly fatal peritonitis; much more frequently into the cellular tissue surrounding the bladder, giving rise to the well-known symptoms of infiltration of urine, inflammation, intense congestion, œdematous swelling of the ano-perineal region, followed by bursting of the abscess in this situation or into the rectum or vagina, and the escape of urine through the fistulous openings subsequently remaining. Inflammation may also spread widely around the rectum in consequence of this infiltration of urine. In other cases, fistulæ may form at the side of the pubic symphysis. Pus may also deeply undermine the cellular tissue in the peritoneum and give rise to gravitating abscesses. It is well known that death may ensue within a few days or weeks under such circumstances, preceded by typhous symptoms with coma, extreme prostration of strength and high fever. By appropriate treatment, however, the regular use of the catheter to draw off the urine, the dangerous symptoms may pass away, the fever subside, and complete recovery gradually follow, or one or several urinary fistulæ, which may subsequently be successfully treated, may be left.

If, on the other hand, we have to deal with adhesive peri- and paracystitis, either as a primary affection, or, what is more common, as an extension of inflammation from the cellular tissue of the pelvis, from the iliac fossæ, or from the neighborhood of Douglas's pouch; the febrile symptoms are unimportant, and there are scarcely any symptoms due to pressure, but the bladder, owing to adhesions of neighboring organs, is much less able to contract, so that the urine is voided with increasing difficulty ending in retention, which, however, is not important, owing to the ease and painlessness with which catheterization can be effected in these cases. If the paracystitis ends in suppuration, either primarily or by continuation from suppuration in the cellular tissue, especially of the right iliac fossa, the abscess may become evacuated through the bladder, the pus escapes with the urine, the suppuration soon ceases, and recovery follows. In other cases evacuation takes place through the bladder and the rectum, recovery also resulting subsequently. In other cases, which are happily rarer, but of which I have several times observed examples, the site of the opening of the abscess into the bladder becomes converted into a fistula, so that pus continues to pass into the bladder for a long time and is evacuated with the urine. In one case which I treated in Paris, in association with Louis and Velpeau, the fistulous opening was probably small, a considerable quantity of pus escaping with the urine from time to time, and then ceasing for days or weeks. As a rule, these abscesses in the neighborhood of the bladder end in death, preceded by gradual wasting and hectic, but in some cases the suppuration gradually diminishes and recovery follows. Under the head of diagnosis I shall return to some of these points.

Pathological Anatomy.

It is but rarely that opportunity is afforded of observing acute cystitis in those who have died quickly from other diseases. It is then seen that the mucous membrane is intensely congested over its whole surface, or only partially in a punctiform manner, or in streaks, or with ecchymoses. Usually it is much altered in structure, softened and thickened. The few closed follicles at the entrance of the bladder are sometimes, especially at the centre, the seat of a partial injection. On the free surface of the mucous membrane of the bladder we find either a more or less muco-purulent fluid, or even pseudo-membranes. The inflammation may also be of a more diphtheritic character; if so, a finely granular exudation will be infiltrated in the mucous membrane, and will lead later to abrasions or deep ulcerations. Occasionally we may demonstrate a submucous purulent inflammation with perforation inward or outward, and, as already mentioned, infiltration of urine. More rarely, gangrene has resulted either from long-continued retention of urine in typhus, or after prolonged pressure from a bulky fœtal head during delivery. The anatomical characters do not present any special features.

Diagnosis.

This is usually easy. The violent pains in the region of the bladder, associated with fever and the mixture of mucus, pus, or blood, easily distinguish acute vesical catarrh from vesical spasm, in which the pain and straining may be almost as severe, but the quality of the urine remains unchanged, or may for a time only most probably be more watery and clearer than in the normal condition. It is difficult to recognize parenchymatous vesical abscess, as there are no special signs to indicate it; and intense fever, a more protracted course, and increased difficulty in passing water rather indicate submucous suppuration; it is only the escape of large admixtures of pus which renders the diagnosis certain, whilst at the same time a marked improvement gradually ensues. If, however, a quantity of pus and mucus had previously been mixed with the urine, all signs of bursting of the abscess would be wanting. The symptoms of pericystic infil-tration of pus, such as pain, swelling, doughy œdema, etc., are much more readily recognized, especially when the abscess is situated between the front of the bladder and the symphysis pubis. If the abscess is situated laterally or posteriorly, the pain and sense of fulness are felt more deeply, the bladder is much more impeded in its efforts to expel the urine, and the phlegmonous swelling can be detected either about the fundus of the bladder through the abdominal wall, or deeply placed at the sides, or through the perineum, or from the rectum. If, on the other hand, the bladder is so compressed by the surrounding suppurative inflammation that only a small quantity of urine can be retained in it, the diminution in the capacity of the blad-der is discovered, on passing a catheter, by the small amount which can be withdrawn, and after the urine has been drawn off the tumor continues undiminished in size. If the abscess burst into the bladder, the signs before mentioned avail for diag-nosis, and fluctuation may be detected in the perineum, rectum, or vagina, of the abscess present in either of these situations.

Prognosis.

In ordinary cases of acute inflammation of the mucous mem-brane of the bladder, the prognosis is of a hopeful character, as cystitis, when uncomplicated, is not attended by any danger. The kind which is set up by chemical irritation generally passes through its course quickly and favorably, and if in poisoning from cantharides death ensues, the vesical irritation, as a rule, has but little share in the result, and only secondarily. The cystitis, also, which comes on secondarily in the course of severe acute diseases, usually ends in recovery in a few days or two or three weeks. On the other hand, the course of acute vesical catarrh may become protracted and it may take on the chro-nic form. This occurs most frequently when the cause of the cystitis is not of a transitory character — for instance, stricture of the urethra, the presence of foreign bodies in the bladder, etc.

Here the existing disease has predisposed to a protracted course. If, however, by appropriate treatment we can remove the cause, the prognosis becomes much more hopeful. Deeply situated in. flammation of the bladder, with suppuration, is always a source of great anxiety and danger, whether it is situated in the sub. mucous and subperitoneal connective-tissue layers of the bladder, or occurs in the form of pericystitis. A vesical abscess bursting inwardly may quickly end in recovery; but it may burst out. wardly, and pericystic suppuration, whether primary or second. ary, if it be peripheral, is always an extremely critical condition, as it may lead to infiltration of urine and a septic-typhoid state, which is not unfrequently fatal, or may be the starting-point for long-standing urinary fistulæ. Diphtheritic inflammation of the bladder is always very dangerous; gangrene, invariably fatal.

Treatment.

We must invariably aim, in the first place, at removing the cause. Chemically irritant remedies or beverages, such as young, imperfectly fermented beer, must immediately be countermanded, and we must also avoid using any more blisters if vesical irrita. tion has followed the application of cantharides. If the inflam. mation of the bladder was preceded by gonorrhœa, we should be very cautious in the use of balsamic remedies directed against this disease. If the disease has originated from causes which cannot for the moment be removed, we should be very cautious in ex. ploring the bladder, especially with the catheter.

If the acute cystitis is moderate in its severity, soothing remedies, rest, and low diet will often be sufficient to effect a cure. Lying in bed is always very advantageous, as the pain is not unfrequently increased by the sitting or standing posture, or on moving about. Under the head of soothing drinks, we may mention marsh-mallow, or linseed or hemp-seed tea, or almond emulsion, and also cow's milk, half or a whole cupful every two or three hours, as sole nourishment. Warm fomentations or poultices over the abdomen relieve the pain more, as a rule, than cold applications, though the latter are more grateful and useful to a few patients, and should, therefore, be cautiously tried. If the pain does not subside, morphia or opium is most advantageous, the former every three hours in doses of .077 gr. (0.005 gramme), the latter in doses of a grain or a grain and a half (0.06-0.1) daily in mucilage or almond emulsion, about five ounces (150.0), so that .15 gr. (0.01) of extract of opium is given per dose, that is, one or two tablespoonfuls every hour or two hours. In many cases, emollient enemata of linseed tea and oil afford great relief; and we may also profitably order, especially at night, a small enema of three and a half ounces (100 grms.) of water with ten drops of tincture of opium, which ought to be retained. Still more certain in their action under these circumstances are suppositories of hydrochlorate of morphia and cocoa butter, the proportion varying from one per cent. to fifteen per thousand. It is only when the pain is very violent and persistent, and the inflammation very intense, that we order leeches (10 to 12) to be applied to the hypogastrium, or, still better, though certainly less conveniently, to the perineum, or, in women, to the labia majora. The remedies which have been reported to act as specifics, such as herniaria glabra, herba chenopodii, semen lycopodii, have no such effect, and must, therefore, be banished from our list in the treatment of acute cystitis. Lukewarm hip or immersion baths, at a temperature of 80.6°-82.4° F. (27°-28° C.) are useful in proportion to the length of time for which the bath is continued. At first, half an hour is sufficient, but the duration may be increased to an hour or two hours, and the bath may be repeated a second time in the course of the day. Warm injections into the bladder, which have been so much recommended in many quarters, and especially by Brodie, cause more injury by the necessary introduction of instruments than the presence of soothing fluids in the bladder for a short time does good.

If there be a copious muco-purulent sediment, when the intensity of the inflammation has abated, an astringent may be administered and none acts better, under these circumstances, than tannin. We shall recur to this point under the head of Chronic Vesical Catarrh.

If the urine is voided in small quantity, or wholly retained, and warm baths and sedatives have not had the desired effect, the cautious passage of a soft wax bougie into the bladder will sometimes cause the urine to flow. If, however, it is absolutely necessary to use a catheter, the greatest caution should be exercised, and the instrument should be flexible and without any stylet. Lasserre's catheter is particularly adapted for such cases. If infiltration of the neck of the bladder, dependent on its great sensitiveness, remains after an attack of gonorrhœa, the systematic passage of a wax bougie will greatly diminish the excessive sensitiveness which tends to keep up the inflammation.

If an abscess forms, we have no means of accelerating its bursting. As soon, however, as any suspicious, reddened, doughy patch of infiltration makes its appearance externally at the lower part of the abdomen, in the groin, or in the perineum, we take care to provide a free outlet for the pus. In doing this, however, we do not incise deeply, at once, but cut carefully layer by layer, examining from time to time as to whether we are not too near the bowel or peritoneum or bladder, or the commencement of the urethra. It is only when distinctly fluctuating abscesses present themselves in the perineum that we can proceed in the ordinary way. Otherwise, after we have laid bare the abscess, we pass a catheter, determine the position of the neighboring organs and then make a small puncture and, if pus comes, enlarge the opening sufficiently to give exit to the pus. Fluctuating abscesses projecting into the vagina or rectum may be tapped with a fine exploring trocar. If, however, the diagnosis is doubtful, it is better to abstain from even this procedure. Gravitating collections of pus and abscesses in dependent positions are also to be opened early. The usual consequences of the infiltration, such as urinary fistulæ, etc., are to be treated on general surgical principles. A septicæmic condition associated with extensive infiltration of urine, and a high state of fever should be combated by large doses of quinine, decoction of bark with acid, and if collapse is threatened, musk and wine, whilst surgical treatment is not neglected. Unfortunately, however, the best remedies are often quite powerless under such circumstances.

Chronic Vesical Catarrh, Chronic Inflammation of the Bladder.

Etiology.

Men are much more liable than women to vesical catarrh. In the young and middle-aged, it is met with much less frequently than after the forty-fifth year; in the old it is most frequent of all. In early life, it is due, not unfrequently, to an extension of inflammation along the urethra from a neglected gonorrhœa, or extension takes place from a suppurative pyelitis not unfrequently set up by phosphatic concretions forming in the kidneys. In advanced age, vesical catarrh is sometimes idiopathic, and at other times a complication of various affections of the uropoietic system. It is common after long-continued and frequently repeated chills, and in those who are liable to gout and hemorrhoids; it is very difficult, however, to explain the causative connection between them. Repeated excesses and a too luxurious mode of life predispose to the disease. Any impediment to the flow of urine, owing to permanent stricture of the urethra or enlargement of the prostate, may give rise to a very obstinate vesical catarrh, unless the urine is regularly and completely drawn off. The urine first of all contains a little mucus, this leads to the production of a ferment by which a portion of the urine becomes converted into carbonate of ammonia, which is a source of constant irritation to the bladder, and in this way an obstinate catarrh is excited. The chronic irritation of the bladder which develops in cases of paralysis, arises in a precisely similar manner, whether the paralysis is idiopathic or the result of some disease of the central nervous system and associated with paraplegia. Irritation of the bladder from repeated attempts at lithotrity may also give rise to obstinate vesical catarrh, which will be persistent in proportion to the extent to which the bladder has been previously irritated by the foreign body.

Symptomatology.

We have already explained that chronic vesical catarrh may develop out of the acute form. In the majority of cases, however, the disease commences insidiously and slowly either in the course of various diseases of the kidneys, prostate, or urethra, or as a complication of some other affection of the bladder. In a considerable number of cases, however, vesical catarrh develops as an independent affection. These are the very cases in which the unimportant character of the symptoms in the early stage becomes a cause of intractableness later, as the catarrh has, to a certain extent, already gained firm footing before it gives rise to symptoms which cause a medical man to be consulted. The local pains are but slight. For a long time the patient is simply conscious of a certain amount of uneasiness in the vesical region, in the hypogastrium, and in the perineum. The increased frequency of attempts at micturition indeed soon become troublesome, but the urine, necessarily voided in small quantities, is still of tolerably normal appearance. As the disease progresses, all these symptoms increase in severity. The region of the bladder and the perineum are the seat of frequent pains, accompanied by various spasmodic symptoms and vesical tenesmus if the neck of the bladder be inflamed. The patients are compelled to micturate frequently, but pass only a small quantity of urine each time, and are especially troubled with urgent desire to pass water after taking food or after drinking, and also at night, only exceedingly small quantities of urine being voided each time, sometimes accompanied by a burning sensation in the urethra and irritation of the glans. The examination of the urine is of the greatest importance. It often becomes cloudy very early. Its specific gravity will not be markedly increased. Generally, it is feebly acid, neutral, or alkaline, and often has an offensive odor; from time to time blood may be present, and forms a reddish layer superimposed on the general sediment, or gives to the whole quantity of urine a more or less brownish red tinge. The most characteristic feature, however, is the usually tolerably copious muco-purulent sediment which separates in a tolerably thick layer from the turbid urine, and, as a rule, adheres firmly to the bottom of the vessel. Occasionally the whole of the urine has a somewhat ropy, syrupy consistence if ammonia has become fully developed. We can always produce this condition by agitating the purulent urine with caustic ammonia and allowing the mixture to stand for some time, when the fluid will become of an almost gelatinous consistence. In addition to this sufficiently conclusive experiment, we should always make a microscopic examination. For we find apparently thoroughly purulent urinary sediments which really consist almost entirely of earthy phosphates, especially the ammoniaco-magnesian phosphate, lithic acid, and mineral substances, and therefore are not dependent on the vesical catarrh. We may also easily fall into error if we merely examine the urine chemically, as we may be alarmed by the constant presence of albumen, and inclined to diagnose disease of the kidney when none exists. The presence of a number of pus-cells, together with large pavement epithelial cells from the bladder, is important as an aid to diagnosis, as in association with pus coming from the kidney we generally find the much smaller, oval, or cylindrical kidney epithelial cells, and, in morbus Brightii, the well-known casts. The characters, therefore, which are discoverable on a minute examination of the urine are of the greatest importance. Not unfrequently, the urine contains a number of bacteria. Sometimes a thick, muco-purulent mass is voided, either at the commencement or at the termination of the act of micturition, and may give rise to symptoms of dysuria.

When the disease has lasted for some time, the pain diminishes as a rule, but the urine continues to be voided very frequently. Sometimes we can feel the bladder through the hypogastrium and also through the rectum as a round, globular tumor, owing in a great measure to the thickening of the walls. This would occur more frequently were it not that the bladder often retains but small quantities of urine, and its cavity becomes considerably contracted. As a rule, the digestive organs also suffer in vesical catarrh. The appetite becomes impaired, digestion is slow and imperfect, and there is more or less obstinate constipation. Many patients suffer from sickness. Owing to this mal-assimilation and the daily drain from the formation of pus, the general system suffers. The patients have a pale and sickly appearance, the bodily strength and weight slowly diminish, but the disease rarely leads to a truly hectic febrile condition. If the vesical catarrh is not dependent on some other disease which it is difficult to cure, though it certainly belongs to the class of intractable diseases, yet it does yield to appropriate treatment after several fluctuations, often only after the lapse of many months, and in many patients it may become habitual, improving in the summer and being aggravated in the winter. Relapses and exacerbations from time to time into acute cystitis are not unfrequent. Decided improvement is accompanied by a gradual diminution in the quantity of pus in the urine, and, finally, the latter ceases to be present at all. The painful sensations also disappear. The urine can be retained for a longer period. Digestion improves and the strength returns. The patients can also again bear long-continued exertion, whilst at the height of the disease this often occasions such pain that the patients are compelled to avoid any great exertion for weeks and months at a time. Vesical catarrh is certainly not of itself fatal, but if complicated with other diseases it may hasten the fatal event by enfeebling the constitution. It may, however, directly cause death if in the diphtheritic form, or if perforation occur into the peritoneal cavity or the cellular tissue of the pelvis or perineum.

Pathological Anatomy.

In chronic catarrh, the mucous membrane is usually slightly swollen, thickened, congested, and, after the disease has existed for some time, of a slate-gray color. The bladder contains some purulent urine, which not unfrequently abounds in earthy phosphates. In consequence of increased nutrition the mucous membrane and the submucous tissue may become hypertrophied, so indeed may the whole bladder if the disease has existed for some time, and there is some mechanical impediment to the flow of urine. The hypertrophy of the mucous membrane may be localized to certain portions, and thus polypoid excrescences may be formed which may have a branched or dendritic appearance. The hypertrophy of the walls is sometimes more apparent than real, as, if the bladder can retain but little urine, it becomes very contracted and small, which makes the coats seem thickened. If the bladder is capacious and hypertrophied, with thickening and hyperplasia of the muscular tissue, the internal surface of the distended bladder has a somewhat trabecular or reticulated appearance. The mucous membrane not unfrequently prolapses into the depressions of this vesical network and presses the muscular bundles asunder, and thus diverticula result, in which, subsequently, calculi may be found which are detected with great difficulty during life, and which it is still more difficult to treat by operation. In some cases, which are fortunately rare, the diseased mucous membrane gradually becomes covered with diphtheritic ulcers, constantly increasing in size, a form which usually ends fatally either by perforation, owing to the destruction of the tissue of the bladder becoming deeper and deeper and peritonitis being set up, which is rapidly fatal, or infiltration of urine occurs into the cellular tissue of the pelvis and perineum, leading to widespread inflammation, sometimes followed by considerable sloughing of the cellular tissue, and resulting in urinary fistulæ. Chronic cystitis, like the acute form, may be more or less localized, attacking, for instance, chiefly the fundus, or, more usually, the neck and its neighborhood, being not unfrequently associated with chronic urethritis or stricture of the urethra. If, under these circumstances, the stricture, instead of being cured, gives rise to increasingly severe effects, the cystitis, at first confined to the trigonum vesicæ, may spread over the whole of the bladder, along the mucous lining of the ureters, and from thence to the kidneys. Enlargement of the prostate, causing considerable impediment to the flow of urine, may produce similar results, and so indeed may any stagnation of urine.

Diagnosis.

Chronic vesical catarrh is not difficult to recognize as a rule. The sense of uneasiness in the neighborhood of the bladder, the frequent desire to empty the bladder, and the thick, purulent urine, leave scarcely any room for doubt, and a microscopic examination of the urine, at least from time to time, will be an additional aid. It is of greater importance to estimate whether the vesical catarrh is idiopathic or the consequence of diseases of the urethra or prostate, and especially whether a foreign body, such as a calculus, is present in the bladder, which, of course, can only be ascertained by careful examination with a catheter (or sound). It is also important to differentiate spasm of the bladder, which is also attended by pain and frequent micturition, but the quality of the urine remains normal. In polyuria also, it is true, the urine is voided frequently, but without any pain or purulent sediment.

Prognosis.

This is always doubtful; but it is certainly only exceptionally that there is any danger to life. For instance, in the diphtheritic form and also in all cases in which perforation occurs externally as such, patients not unfrequently succumb, owing to some septicæmic, perhaps bacteric, infection. Usually, however, the disease is rather troublesome and very intractable than dangerous, even when it is purely idiopathic and without any complication. The prognosis in relation to the occurrence of a complete cure is just as doubtful in cases where some mechanical cause exists which cannot be removed and whose consequences do not yield to our skill, as happens in other cases ; whilst, on the other hand, in paralysis of the bladder, and in hypertrophy of the prostate with retention of urine, all the symptoms improve as soon as catheterization is practised regularly and thoroughly. Such cases are so far satisfactory that they improve much sooner with regular emptying of the bladder than idiopathic cases of vesical catarrh, however appropriately treated. The same applies to long-neglected stricture of the urethra. If the stricture is sufficiently and permanently dilated, the symptoms produced by the stricture also quickly improve.

In idiopathic vesical catarrh the prognosis is the more hopeful the earlier the patient comes under care, and especially if he follows the rules of diet and hygiene prescribed. In young and middle-aged patients, and in those of good constitution and in a good state of health, the prognosis is more hopeful and treatment more effectual than in those who are advanced in years, enfeebled, or out of health. When chronic cystitis has been set up by foreign bodies or lithotrity operations, it generally wholly passes off in from two to six months after the removal of the exciting cause. At an advanced age, or when pyelitis, or a considerable enlargement of the prostate ·is present, or when the constitution has become much enfeebled from other causes, or when there is a tendency to chronic catarrhal affections in general, it may be very difficult or impossible to effect a cure. We must be content with transitory occasional improvement.

Treatment.

Our first aim must be to remove the cause. Strictures of the urethra must be dilated, foreign bodies must be removed, retention of urine from enlargement of the prostate or paralysis, etc., must be treated by the regular use of the catheter in order to relieve the irritation of the bladder, set up secondarily. Such patients must also be carefully protected against any sudden chill.

As regards diet, a copious supply of milk is especially indicated, and it may be mixed with acorn-coffee, or chocolate, or cocoa, according to the patient's taste, and taken in the morning. At other times, fairly nutritious, especially animal food, is to be preferred to any other. Coffee, tea, and beer are to be wholly prohibited for a time, or only allowed in small quantities. If the patients complain of thirst, unirritating drinks, such as almond emulsions, or hempseed-tea, or good, pure drinking-water, are to be recommended, whilst the artificial waters containing much carbonic acid irritate the bladder and increase the desire to micturate. Light white, or, still better, light red wines containing tannin, such as Rhine wine or Bordeaux, are the most suitable. When the digestive organs sympathize, as is usually the case, fatty substances are to be avoided in the preparation, etc., of food, and indigestible vegetables in the form of roots or leaves must be countermanded; whilst fruits, raw or cooked, may be recommended in reasonable quantity. For this reason the use of grapes in the autumn may be serviceable sometimes. We take care that the patient's habitation is dry and surrounded by good, pure air, and that for some part of the season he goes into the country, or to the hills, or the seaside. The clothing must be warm, and the rain, wind, and even the cool morning and evening air must be avoided, whilst gentle exercise at other times is usually to be much recommended. If the flow of urine in the usual posture is impeded by enlargement of the prostate or abnormal position of the uterus, this may often be remedied by making the patient try to pass water in some different posture.

Lukewarm baths of water simply at first, and, later, salt-water or sulphur baths, relieve the vesical uneasiness and desire to pass water; and later on we may recommend daily sponging with cold water, cold hip-baths, and river- or sea-bathing as soon as they can be borne. A number of mineral waters enjoy a certain amount of deserved repute in the treatment of chronic vesical catarrh. Among the mildest which may be drunk at home, the natural Seltzer water, and also that of Bilin may be strongly recommended. In France they use more particularly the natural springs of Vichy, and also the springs of Evian and Amphion, which are also employed in Switzerland adjoining. Residence there, in a mild, sheltered, and beautiful situation on the southern [northern?] shore of the Lake of Geneva, is justly much sought after by such patients. Among the most advantageous mineral waters for use in chronic vesical catarrh is the water of Wild-ungen. Any of these waters may be given as a curative means in doses of two or three glasses every morning or in the course of the day, at or between meals. Among the watering-places to which I send such patients, unless I send them to climatic health resorts, I prefer Ems to any other in the milder cases and in the more painful forms, whilst in the more severe cases I prefer to send them to Karlsbad. Wildungen is also to be strongly recommended. Among the remedies used as curative drinks, lime-water deserves special mention, from half a pint to a pint and a half (half a litre to a litre) being administered daily, either alone or mixed with milk; and later, in obstinate cases, tar-water may be substituted in a similar way.

I have practised local bloodletting in the neighborhood of the bladder, or in the perineum, more sparingly from year to year, and it is only strictly adapted to cases in which the symptoms have become very urgent, owing to acute exacerbation in other-

wise vigorous patients, the pain being severe, the desire to pass
water very troublesome, etc. Even in such cases we first of all
try lukewarm, long-continued baths, warm poultices, oily embrocations, preparations of opium, especially morphia administered hypodermically, internally in clysters or in suppositories.
The preparations of cannabis indica, acting as narcotics, sometimes exercise a soothing influence on the troublesome symptoms
to which vesical irritation gives rise, the tincture being given in
doses of five or ten drops several times a day, and the extract in
doses of half a grain or a grain (0.03–0.05) several times daily.

We have already seen that among the mineral waters which
can be recommended as useful, the alkaline occupy a prominent
place. They are especially indicated so long as the urine is not
alkaline. Bicarbonate of soda is also decidedly useful if the
case is not too far advanced. I generally order from one to two
drachms daily (4.0–8.0), either in the form of a mixture, or,
when sufficiently diluted with water, as a drink which will often
successfully take the place of a dearer mineral water. It is
especially in the cases of chronic inflammation of the vesical
mucous membrane that the use of astringents is indicated. An
old remedy, which has been popular since the time of De Haen,
is bearberry-tea. We infuse from two to four drachms (8.0–15.0)
of uva ursi in thirty-five ounces (a litre) of water and let the
patient drink it, after it has been sweetened, in the course of
the twenty-four hours. Subsequently we administer the more
active astringents. Of these, the most preferable is alum, half a
drachm or a drachm (2.0–4.0) being given daily in solution in
five ounces (150.0) of water, with an ounce (30.0) of raspberry
syrup, one or two tablespoonfuls of this mixture being taken
every hour or every two hours. The alum may also be administered in the form of alum-whey as a drink. Still more active is
tannin, which is also thrown off by the kidneys and reaches the
bladder. It may be given in gradually increasing quantities of
from seven and a half to thirty grains (0.5–2.0) daily, in solution
or powder, in doses of from three to five grains (0.2–0.3). It sur-
passes all other astringents, such as the preparations, decoction,
extract, etc., of rhatany, formerly so much in vogue; catechu,
extract of cascarilla, and the weaker vegetable astringents, such

as tormentil, buchu, etc. The preparations of iron are not adapted for employment as astringents on the mucous membrane of the bladder, for they neither come in contact with the interior of the bladder nor are they absorbed as astringents. The preparations of bark, on the contrary, exercise a beneficial influence on the mucous membrane of the kidneys and bladder when in a state of chronic irritation. Formerly, in these cases, I used the decoction of cinchona or the extract in solution, and also the tincture of quinoidine in doses of from 25 to 30 drops, thrice daily. In order to keep the quinoidine in solution when mixed with water, a little hydrochloric acid must be added to the tincture, 1 part to 15. Of late years, when wishing to use bark in the treatment of vesical catarrh, I have almost invariably employed the hydrochlorate of quinine thrice daily, in doses of three or four grains (0.2–0.3), with the addition of from a twelfth to a sixth of a grain (0.005–0.01) of cannabis indica in each pill, and a grain or a grain and a half (0.06–0.1) in the course of a day. The astringent red wines, such as Bordeaux, Burgundy, Rhone wine, the red Rhine and Hungarian wines, Assmanshäuser, Erlauer, etc., are to be recommended to be taken at meal-times in the more atonic and protracted forms of the affection.

Among the alterative remedies, the balsams have always been in good repute. One of the simplest of these is a decoction or infusion of fir or juniper tops, from two to four drachms (8.0–15.0) in one to two pints (½–1 litre) of water being taken in the course of the day. An infusion of buchu or matico leaves, with their essential oils and bitter extractive matters, have been recommended. The most efficient, however, are balsam of copaiva, turpentine, and oil of turpentine. We give the balsam of copaiva in doses of half a drachm or a drachm (2.0–4.0) daily, either in gelatine capsules, or in an emulsion with from two to four drachms (10.0–15.0) of liquorice. Balsam of Peru is also given in emulsion; I have, however, but little experience of its use. Venetian turpentine, on the contrary, either alone or in combination with camphor and lupuline, I have frequently prescribed, in order to allay the constant desire to pass water, and the spasmodic symptoms. The following is the formula for the pills: ℞. camphoræ, gr. xx. (1.25), lupulinæ, ℨi. (4.0), terebinth. venet.,

℈ii. (8.0), extract. glycyrrh., q. s., ut fiat pil. cxx. Consp. D. S.,
from two to six pills to be taken thrice daily, and gradually
increasing to ten pills. The oil of turpentine is best given in the
form of capsules. We must also here mention tar-water, of
which several tablespoonfuls may be given daily, either alone or
in combination with a balsamic syrup—balsam of Tolu, for example. Oil of cade in capsules has also been recommended of
late.

If, while the local symptoms improve, the constitutional con
dition seems to deteriorate, if the patient is feeble and sinking,
then we must administer quinine wine, the milder preparations
of iron, such as the lactate or citrate, and the tinctures of ferrated apple extract, or of acetate of iron ;[1] or some chalybeate
water, water containing pyrophosphate of iron, with milk, may
be taken in the morning; or Pyrmont, Schwalbacher, or St.
Moritzer water at meal-times ; or the water-cure may be tried in
the summer at some chalybeate spring—by preference, among
the hills. The more purely irritating remedies, such as tincture
of cantharides, have, indeed, been recommended, but we have no
certain evidence of their good effects. Counter-irritants, applied
to the neighborhood of the bladder, in the form of blisters, fric-
tions with croton oil, etc., may assist internal remedies in not
very advanced cases.

As in every other affection of the bladder, so in vesical catarrh, we watch carefully whether the bladder is emptied regularly and completely ; and if this be not the case—as, for instance,
more especially where the bladder is hypertrophied and enlarged
—we draw off the urine regularly for some time, because, otherwise, not only will some of the urine, but also the muco-purulent
sediment be left. Moreover, the longer the urine remains stagnant in the bladder, the more the contractile power of the bladder is interfered with ; whilst, on the other hand, we quickly see
the bladder regaining power to contract within a short time after
we begin to use the catheter. I am now (Dec., 1873) treating, in
consultation, a boy seven years old, in whom, for a long time, a
severe vesical catarrh existed, with thick, purulent sediment, and

---

[1] Special preparations of the German Ph.

the bladder often remained partly filled in spite of the partly involuntary escape of large quantities of purulent urine. When the catheter was first used, the urine could only be made to flow by exercising strong pressure over the region of the bladder, while, later, it quickly came in a full stream, and the bladder permanently recovered its power of contracting. The best instrument for drawing off the urine is a thoroughly well-cleansed silver catheter, or else one of Lasserre's. We should frequently wash the catheter, outside and inside, with a two per cent. solution of carbolic acid, and we may also keep it in such a solution constantly. Catheterization is necessarily connected with the employment of injections, and it is well, after the very first withdrawal of the urine through the catheter, or in obstinate cases, even when the use of the catheter is not otherwise necessary, to inject a solution of tannin, of the strength of from five to fifteen grains (0.3–1.0), in an ounce and a half (50.0), gradually increased to a three per cent. or still stronger solution every two or three days at first—later, every day. The injections must remain in the bladder for at least five minutes, and more effect is produced if the whole of the fluid is not withdrawn again through the catheter. Injections of nitrate of silver, which have been so much praised, must be used cautiously, most suitably in the proportion of a grain (0.05) to from four to two ounces (100.0–50.0) of water, and even of this only a small quantity should be injected at first. Solutions of zinc are also sometimes useful. If the injections are well borne, we may, in many cases, increase the strength considerably. On the other hand, I am not in favor of cauterizing the mucous membrane of the bladder with Lallemand's porte caustique, as has been recommended in many quarters. It is evident that those who are not practised in the use of the catheter must not undertake such a mode of cure, which requires much patience and skilfulness. Rightly employed, however, surgical procedures may greatly aid the dietetic, hygienic, and medicinal treatment.

Neuroses of the Bladder.

Although spasm is probably the most frequent affection in neuroses of the bladder, and even neuralgia and hyperæsthesia, especially of the neck of the bladder, are chiefly troublesome, owing to reflex spasm, yet neuralgia may exist without any spasm. We may, however, treat of hyperæsthesia, neuralgia, and spasm together, while atony, paralysis of the bladder, and retention of urine must be dealt with separately, from a practical point of view.

Spasm of the Bladder, Cystospasmus—Hyperæsthesia and Neuralgia of the Bladder, Neuralgia Cysto-urethralis.

Here, also, we will quote a few bibliographical references.

Campaignac, Considérations sur les névralgies des organes genito-urin. et de l'anus. Journ. hebdom. de médecine. T. II. p. 396. 1829.—*Vidal (de Cassis)*, Bulletin de Thérap. 1848. Août.—*Lagneau*, Traité pratique des malad. syph. I. p. 130.—*Neucourt*, Névralgie uréthrovésicale. Archiv gén. de méd. 1858. Juli. p. 30.

Spasm of the bladder, cystospasmus, and its accompanying distressing sensitiveness and pain, hyperæsthesia and neuralgia vesicæ, are especially located at the neck of the bladder, and consist in a more or less consciously distressing irritation of the motor nerves by the sensitive nerves of this region, those muscles being more particularly affected which expel the urine, and hence the frequent desire to pass water and the various difficulties attending it.

Etiology.

The sensibility of the bladder in its normal state is comparatively slight. The reflex irritation, which stimulates the bladder to empty itself, is not attended by the slightest sensation of discomfort. Bad habits, however, may disturb the equilibrium. Not a few men, for instance, are accustomed to pass water more frequently than is necessary, and thus increase the sensitiveness of the neck of the bladder, and though not to such an extent as would justify us in terming it a pathological condition, yet to such a degree that a desire to empty the bladder is felt when it is but partially filled. As a rule, such a condition may be traced to a rapid fall of temperature and a comparatively slight amount of clothing, and then becomes customary. Repeated sexual indulgence, especially in men, increases the frequency of the desire to pass water, and the old saying, "Raro mingit castus," though it has many exceptions, is repeatedly confirmed by observation. On the other hand, many, especially girls and women, accustom themselves to empty the bladder but seldom, a practice which mostly entails no ill-consequences, but, if carried too far, may be the starting-point of many troubles.

Setting aside cases in which foreign bodies are present in the bladder, or some disease exists, we meet with spasm of the bladder in the hypochondriacal and hysterical, and in very nervous persons in general, in whom mental excitement, excessive sexual indulgence, the incautious use of cantharides, and the unskilful introduction of catheters, will sometimes act as exciting causes. Occasionally, also, it is met with in connection with onanism and spermatorrhœa. Other exciting causes are: drinking copiously of young, sour wine or young beer, a chill, and sitting on damp, cold ground. Spasm of the bladder is sometimes connected with some disease of the rectum—fistulæ, fissures, ulcers, hemorrhoids, etc. The spasm may, lastly, be a symptom in connection with other neuralgic affections and various cerebro-spinal diseases.

Spasm of the bladder may be met with in children, but is most frequent in adults; sometimes being more prevalent in women, and sometimes in men. If the former are more predisposed to it on account of greater nervousness, still, in the latter, the normal anatomical relationships of the urethra, its opening into the bladder, etc., are not without great influence in predisposing to spasmodic as well as other urinary affections.

Symptomatology.

The heightened sensibility of the bladder, and especially of its neck, and the spasmodic symptoms caused by it, have their seat and starting-point in the lumbar and sacral plexuses, branches

of the ileo-scrotal nerve also participating. From the sacral
plexus, branches are distributed to the rectum, bladder, perineum,
and penis, and this circumstance explains the radiation of the
pains from the bladder and urethra to the surrounding parts,
and inversely from these to the bladder and urethra. . Pure neuralgia, without any reflex spasm in the urethra or at the neck of
the bladder, is rarely met with alone, and then, as a rule, I have
found it associated with ileo-scrotal neuralgia. Usually, however, the pain either passes by unnoticed, or shows itself first of
all as an uncomfortable sensation before the passage of urine, or
as soon as the reflex action is obeyed. Amongst the first group
we must enumerate increasing intolerance, especially of the neck
of the bladder, for the normal irritation of the urine, even a small
quantity of urine exciting painful and severe vesical tenesmus
with muscular contractions affecting the detrusor urinæ and
sphincter vesicæ alternately, and thus causing the stream of
urine to come in jerks, with frequent interruptions, slowly,
and with much trouble and pain, while as yet the capacity of
the bladder remains normal, as is shown directly the spasm disappears. But besides this abnormal exceedingly frequent desire
to pass water, there are also present various neuralgic pains or
other very distressing sensations in the hypogastrium and in the
ano-perineal region. The bladder is very sensitive to the introduction of any kind of instruments ; yet I have several times
observed that on introducing a soft wax bougie the unpleasant
sensations were very considerable at first, as soon as I reached
the neck of the bladder, but quickly ceased to be felt, so that the
bougie was allowed to be retained for five minutes or more without exciting any special inconvenience. The neck of the bladder
is much more sensitive to the introduction of a metal catheter.
The urine itself in cases of simple spasm of the bladder is usually in a normal condition. It contains neither blood, nor mucus,
nor pus ; on the contrary, it is often remarkably pale, like urine
in spasmodic conditions generally. In exceptional cases and
usually at first, spasm occurs at each attempt to pass water ;
later, and in many cases from the first, the urine is now and then
voided naturally, whilst at other times painful paroxysms occur,
and sometimes the urine escapes involuntarily. Severe constrict-

ing pains are felt, more especially at the end of micturition, and spread to the urethra, glans, testes, clitoris, thighs, loins, and inguinal region, or may even extend upward to the epigastrium or the lowest ribs. Tenesmus of the rectum even, with involuntary evacuations, may occur. In severe paroxysms and in very irritable individuals, the pains may occasionally be accompanied by great excitement, anxiety, nausea, and vomiting, or even clonic convulsions, the pulse being small, and the body covered with a cold sweat. Such attacks may last from a few minutes to half an hour or more, and usually subside when the urine flows. The patient is deprived of sleep, owing to the necessity for frequently passing water. In many patients, these attacks occur but seldom; in others frequently, even daily; in the worst cases almost at each act of micturition. Then the patients become exceedingly irritable, hypochondriacal, and melancholic, and their condition is truly a very pitiable one. Heat, fatigue, sexual excitement, and an incautious use of the catheter aggravate the symptoms. The course of the disease, as a rule, is very irregular, in many patients extending continuously or with interruptions over months or years, while the affection may subside spontaneously much more quickly, or may end in cure as the result of appropriate treatment.

Diagnosis.

If we disregard secondary spasm of the bladder, we shall find that as a primary affection it is chiefly distinguished from the inflammatory diseases of the bladder by the absence of any admixture of blood, mucus, leucocytes, and pus, or the various kinds of crystals with the urine; in a word, by the absence of any abnormal constituent. The urine is normal, and it is only the act of expulsion which is disordered. Moreover, this is effected in a very irregular manner, with distinct paroxysms and groups of paroxysms, and with very unequal, sometimes long, sometimes short intervals between them. There is no pain on pressure over the bladder, and, what is of importance, there is no fever. There is often a much greater resemblance to the symptoms of stone in the bladder, and it is all the more important to examine very carefully with this similarity borne in mind, since the difficulty experienced in introducing the catheter, owing to the considerable spasmodic irritation excited, may all the more easily mislead, because the bladder contracts on the catheter and offers a certain amount of resistance to the instrument. Velpeau states that three instances were known to him in which lithotomy had been performed in cases of neuralgia of the bladder. The stoppages in the stream of urine, the fixed pain in the neck of the bladder, and the associated pains in the rectum, penis, and extremity of the glans also occur, indeed, with calculus. Civiale, Velpeau, and others, relate cases in which the patients have complained of a sensation as if a hard foreign body were pressing on the neck of the bladder or urethra; so that, properly speaking, only an examination with a metal catheter can settle the point, and even this, as we have seen, does not always lead to a correct diagnosis. Symptomatic spasm of the bladder may be distinguished from the idiopathic form by the easily recognized symptoms of the primary disease in or independent of the urinary organs. The nervous, hypochondriac, or hysterical constitution of the patients may also afford some help in diagnosis.

It is obvious that we are not here dealing with the diagnosis of the great disturbance and even interruption to the flow of urine occurring in ischuria, which has its seat more especially in tonic spasm of the sphincter, while in dysuria spastica, properly so called, the detrusor is chiefly affected, the sphincter is only affected secondarily, slightly, and transitorily, and then the flow of urine is not impeded, it is only interrupted. Though, therefore, strangury may be associated with spasm of the bladder, ischuria is to be all the more dealt with separately, because it is comparatively much more frequently connected with paresis and paralysis of the bladder than with mere spasm. It is quite true that, in spasm of the bladder, strangury may exceptionally in isolated cases and for a short time increase to ischuria, but only as a transitory symptom of secondary importance, while in atonic and paralytic conditions of the bladder the ischuria is a prominent feature, and I have already mentioned that, clinically, spasm of the bladder must be treated of apart from paresis and paralysis of the bladder.

Prognosis.

Spasm of the bladder is not at all a dangerous disease, but is painful and harassing in the highest degree. According to its course, it may be divided into an acute, a subacute, and a more chronic form. The acute and subacute forms are the more hopeful as to prognosis, and if due to some special cause, such as the drinking of badly fermented or stale beverages, subsides as soon as the cause ceases to act. Even when the subacute form is aggravated into violent and frequent paroxysms, owing to the highly nervous condition of the patient, it is a slighter malady and ends more quickly in cure than is the case in the chronic protracted form when the attacks are less frequent and less violent. Nevertheless, this even admits of thorough cure, on the one hand, by appropriate treatment and dietetic and hygienic regulations, and, on the other hand, even when the disease offers great resistance to appropriate treatment, by the lapse of time, as is the case in all other neuroses. As a rule, even in these obstinate cases, the duration does not exceed a year, and those having a much longer duration, or which are quite incurable, form rare exceptions. I have heard Velpeau relate that a patient, who had for long suffered from spasm of the bladder and presented all the symptoms of stone, was at last subjected to lithotomy and completely cured, though no stone was found—a method of cure which is certainly not worthy of imitation.

Treatment.

Here, also, we must seek as far as possible to remove the cause, and with this object we urge the patient to avoid sexual excesses and onanism. Not only are any complications which may exist in the urinary organs to be dealt with, such, for instance, in the first place, as slight strictures of the urethra, which are not unfrequently present, but also complications external to the urinary organs, diseases of the rectum, such as hemorrhoids, catarrh, spasm of the sphincter and fissures, especially diseases of the female genitals, etc. Special treatment has for its object, first of all, the mitigation of the paroxysms; and secondly, the removal

of the disease itself. In the treatment of the paroxysms, lukewarm baths are often found very soothing, the patients being
allowed to remain in them for half an hour or longer. Many
patients will be able to pass water freely in the bath, though
much troubled by spasmodic dysuria when out of it. Sedatives
and antispasmodics are fully indicated. The most efficient are
preparations of opium. The quickest to afford relief is a subcutaneous injection of hydrochlorate of morphia, containing from
one-sixth to one-fourth of a grain (0.01–0.015). A suppository of
from one-sixth to one-third of a grain (0.01–0.02) of hydrochlorate
of morphia and fifteen grains (1.0) of cacao butter placed as high
up as possible in the rectum after the bowel has been emptied,
acts more slowly, but influences the spasm of the pelvic organs
more directly. Clysters of from two to three ounces (80.0–100.0)
of water with fifteen drops of tincture of opium act in a similar
manner after the bowel has been previously emptied. If these
plans cannot be conveniently carried out, we may administer extract of opium internally, in doses of a grain or a grain and a
half (0.06–0.1) in an almond emulsion, a tablespoonful being
given every hour, and the patient may drink an infusion of valerian alone, or in combination with an infusion of orange flowers.
Among the remedies which very much relieve some patients,
either alone or in combination with opium, we must mention lupuline, in doses of three or four grains (0.2–0.3) several times a
day, with or without from half a grain to a grain and a half
(0.05–0.1) of camphor and the preparations of cannabis indica,
the extract in doses of a grain and a half (0.1) daily, the tincture
in doses of ten to fifteen drops, thrice daily. As the way in
which individual remedies act varies greatly in nervous people, it
is well to have a certain amount of choice, so that we may either
employ the remedies singly, or combined to suit the varying
necessities of the case.

This method of treating the attacks of spasm obtains in the
acute form with very frequent paroxysms, and may be supplemented occasionally by warm poultices, or, if the patients bear
them well and seem relieved by them, by (cold) moist applications to the perineum and the lower part of the abdomen. If
the paroxysms are very frequent and severe, the inhalation of

chloroform is recommended, and I have frequently of late found the hydrate of chloral very advantageous in doses of from seven and a half to fifteen grains (0.5–1.0) several times repeated, especially at night. If the difficulty in passing water increases to complete retention, the careful introduction of an elastic (by preference, a Lasserre's) catheter not only empties the bladder, but also allays the irritability of the neck of the bladder. In this, and also in the more protracted form, I have also several times succeeded in effecting rapid, marked, and occasionally permanent improvement, or even a cure, by the regular introduction of soft wax bougies, which I allowed to remain in for a few minutes each day. I have only lately learnt that Willis, and subsequently Civiale, had previously recommended this plan, which has also of late been much praised by Pitha. The spasm is relieved in the same way as that affecting the œsophagus in spasmodic dysphagia.

In the chronic form special attention must be paid to the regulation of the diet. We recommend bland, nourishing food, a copious supply of milk, animal food, fresh vegetables, ripe fruit, etc., but forbid all irritating beverages, such as tea, coffee, beer, wine, and especially water containing carbonic acid. We also enjoin the avoidance of all sexual excitement. In reference to the application of electricity, and especially of the constant current, a metallic catheter introduced into the neck of the bladder being brought in connection with one pole of the apparatus, and the other pole being applied to the perineum, there are no sufficient data available, but its employment would seem thoroughly reasonable in obstinate cases. Of internal remedies the most efficient are: quinine, at first in large, and subsequently in smaller doses; small doses of arsenic, one-sixtieth of a grain (0.001) of arsenious acid in pill three or four times daily, alone, or in combination with quinine (a grain of muriate of quinine (0.05) in each pill) and bromide of potassium, systematically employed, whilst preparations of opium, cannabis, lupuline, and camphor are only suitable occasionally during aggravations of the paroxysms, or employed in small doses in combination with the remedies above mentioned. I have frequently seen benefit result from the systematic use of tepid sulphur baths containing three and a half ounces (100.0) of potassium sulphide. Alkaline mineral waters, such as those of Vichy, Bilin, Wildungen, Selters, Griesshübel, etc., may be taken in the chronic form of the disease. Sometimes a change of locality, residence among the hills, sea-air, and the use of tepid and subsequently cold sea-baths, are exceedingly beneficial. Neucourt recommends clysters of turpentine and iodide of potassium as a specific. Niemeyer advises the administration of balsam of copaiva in obstinate neuralgia of the neck of the bladder following gonorrhœa. In such cases I have found the careful introduction of wax bougies very efficacious. Wendt and Soemmering recommend the juice of the mesembryanthemum crystallinum. The number of remedies which have been recommended is altogether very great, but the chief, in addition to the use of sedatives during the paroxysms, are the cure by means of wax bougies, the internal administration of successive doses of quinine, alone or in combination with arsenic, bromide of potassium, and externally the use of warm and then of cold baths, which we may always employ first of all in the form of the easily prepared hip-bath, before trying complete immersion.

Ischuria, Atony, Paresis and Paralysis of the Bladder, Retention of Urine.

Behrend, Geheilte Lähmung der Blase. Casp. Wochenschr. Nr. 29. 1839.—*Mr. F. Hale Thompson*, On Idiopathic Irritable Bladder. Clinical Lecture. Lancet. March 30, 1839.—*Civiale*, On the So-called Nervous Affections of the Neck of the Bladder. Bull. gén. de thérap. L. 7. 8. Avril, 1841.—*Leroy d'Etiolles*, On Neuralgia and Rheumatism of the Bladder, and on the Diagnosis of Commencing Enlargement of the Prostate Gland. Journ. d. conn. méd. prat. Avril-Mai, 1842.—*Lafoye*, Retention from Paralysis of the Bladder Cured by Nux Vomica. Journ. d. méd. d. Bordeaux.—*Schniewind*, Ueber die Anwendung des Secale cornutum bei Blasenlähmung. Medic. Zeitung. v. V. f. H. in Preussen. Nr. 45. XII. 1843.—*Steinbeck*, Enuresis paralytica. Casp. Wochenschrift. Nr. 24. 1844. —*Jacksch*, Secale cornut. gegen Blasenlähmung. Prag. Vierteljahrsschr. II. Jahrg. I. (V.) Bd. 1845.—*Roux*, Neuralgia of the Bladder Simulating Calculus. Gaz. d. hôp. XX. No. 34. 1847.—*Michon*, Treatment of Paralysis of the Bladder by Galvanism. Gaz. d. hôp. XXII. 22. 1849.—*Seydel, a.* Beiträge zur Erkenntniss und Behandlung der Krankheiten des uropoetisch. Systems. *b.*

Fall von Blasenlähmung. Journ. f. Chirurg. IX. 1. 1849.—*Lecluyse*, Paralysis of the Bladder Cured by Injecting Strychnia into the Bladder. L'Union. 52. 1850.—*Pavesi*, Paralysis of the Bladder Treated by the Injection of Infusion of Tobacco. Gaz. Lombard. 41. 1852.—*P. G. Huth*, D. de Ischuria. Altd. 1703.— *G. Albrecht*, D. de Ischuria. Gött. 1767.— *Murray*, Dissert. de paracentesi cystid. urin. Upsala, 1771.—*Morgagni*, Epist. anat. 42.—*Schwarze*, Lotii suppressio unde? Marb. 1790.—*Plaquet*, De ischuria cystica. Tübing. 1790.— *Lentin*, Beiträge. Bd. III. S. 37.—*J. Wagner*, D. de ischuria vesicali atque vesicæ paracentesi. Argent. 1799.—*Ronn*, Bemerk. über die Harnverhaltung und den Blasenstich. A. d. Hol. Leipzig, 1796.—*Heinlein*, Bemerk. über die Ischurie. Herbst Jahrb. d. deutsch. Med. u. Chir.—*Paletta*, Neue Sammlung auserles. Abhandlung. Bd. XI. S. 515.—*Moulin*, Nouveau traitement des retentions d'urine, Paris, 1824.—*Civiale*, Op. cit. Vol. III.; De la stagnation et de la retention d'urine.—*Chelius*, Von der Zurückhaltung des Harns. Handbuch d. Chirurg. 7. Orig.-Aufl. Heidelb., 1852. Bd. II. S. 143.—*Schneider*, Retentio urinæ. Casp. Wochenschrift. Nr. 12. 1839.—*Troussel*, Case of Retention of Urine, with Practical Remarks on the Cure of Enlargement of the Prostate Gland. Revue méd. franç. et étrang. Mars, 1840.—*Bierbaum*, Traumatische Urinverhaltung, Blasenstich, Urinfistel. Med. Ztg. v. V. f. H. in Preussen. Nr. 38. 1840.—*Kaiser*, Ueber den Nutzen von Liq. ammon. anis in Dysurie. Hufeland's Journ. N. 12. 1840.—*Lasiauve*, On Various Cases of Retention. L'Expérience. Nos. 193, 195. 1841.—*Lerche*, Urinverhaltung aus ganz eigenthümlichen Ursachen. Med. Ztg. v. V. f. H. in Preussen. Nr. 35. 1841.—*Combal*, Bericht aus Caizergnes' med. Klinik. Ein Wort über Harnverhaltung im Allgemeinen. Ueber die Symptome und Diagnose der organ. Harnverengerungen. La clinique. I. Août et Septr. 1842.—*G. D. Dermott*, A New Method of Treating Retention of Urine. The Med. Times. October 1, 1842.—*Pétréquin*, A Remarkable Case of Retention of Urine. L'Examinateur méd. T. II. No. 22. 1842. —*Deville*, On a Case of Retention of Urine. Rev. méd. franç. et étrang. Juin, 1842.—*Cotta*, On Ischuria Senilis. Gazette med. del. Prof. Panizza. Nos. 11, 12. 1842.—*Dr. Kingsley*, On the Use of Ergot of Rye in Retention of Urine. Dub. Med. Press. April 26, 1843.—*Ross*, Retention of Urine Cured by Incising the Urethra. Journ. d. conn. méd. chir. Janv. 1844.—*Wittke*, Ueber Urinbeschwerden der alten Männer. Med. Ztg. v. V. f. Heilk. in Preussen. Nr. 38. 1844.— *Stendel*, Fall von Ischurie. Würtemb. med. Corresp.-Bl. Bd. XIV. Nr. 24. 1844. —*Mr. George Todd*, Retention of Urine Produced by Collection of Gray Peas in the Rectum. The Lancet. April 19, 1845.—*Salomon*, Tödtlicher Ausgang einer Harnverhaltung. Casper's Wochenschrift. No. 25, 1845.—*Canuti*, Disease of the Liver. Retentio urinæ. Bull. delle scienze med. di Bologna. Majo. Gingeo, 1845.—*Dr. Hargrave*, Cases of Hydrocele. Retentio urinæ, etc. Dub. Med. Press. No. 357. November 5, 1845.—*Landerer* and *Steege*, Volksmittel der Türken, Griechen, Walachen, und Serben. Tabakspfeifensaft gegen Urinverhaltung. Med. Ztg. v. Petersburg. III. Jahrg. Nr. 35. 1846.—*Bednár*, Beitrag zur Ischuria neonatorum. Zeitschr. d. k. k. Gesellschaft d. Aerzte zu Wien.

Febr. 1847.—*Drude*, Urinverhaltung bei einem dreijährigen Knaben. Zeitschr. d. nordd. Chir. Ver. I. Bd. 3. Hft. 1847.—*Bazonni*, Case of Ischuria. Gaz. méd. del. Panizza. Tom. VI. Nr. 8. 1847.—*Sainmont*, Ergot of Rye in Retention of Urine. Gaz. des hôp. X. 80. 1848.— *W. M. Fairbrother*, Case of Retention of Urine. Lancet. August 12, 1848.—*Dicenta*, Fall von Entartung der Prostata durch Hypertrophie verbunden mit Urinverhaltung. Würtemb. Corresp.-Bl. XVIII. 7. 1848.—*F. Hahn*, Ueber die Verhaltung und den unwillkürlichen Abfluss des Urins, welche durch die Vergrösserung der Vorsteherdrüse bedingt ist. Würtemb. Ver. Zeitschr. I. 2. 1848.—*Stanelli*, Langwierige Harnverhaltung. Pr. Vereinszeitschrift. XVII. 27. 1848.—*Blandin*, Retention of Urine. Annal. de thérap. Sept., Oct., Déc., 1848, Janv., 1849.—*Dr. W. S. Oke*, Total Suppression of Urine Lasting for Seven Days. Prov. Med. Journ. 1849. p. 259.—*Dr. J. C. Hall*, Cases of Suppression of Urine. Lancet. June 2, 16, July 7, 1849.—*Hahn*, Harnverhaltung mit tödtlichem Ausgange. Würtemb. chir. Vierteljahrschrift. III. 2. 1850.—*Milton*, On a New Method of Applying Caustic in the Treatment of Stricture. Lond. Medical Gazette. July 4, 1851.—*Mercier*, Mode of Operating in Retention in Old Men. Gaz. d. Paris. 50, 51, 52. 1852.—*Kerlé*, Merkwürdiger Fall von Ischurie. Hannov. Corresp.-Bl. II. 22. 1852.—*Coeck*, Surgical Operations for Retention of Urine. Med.-Chir. Trans. 1852; Dubl. Med. Press. May 12, 1852.—*L. A. Basset*, De la retention d'urine, ses causes, ses effets, son traitement. Paris, 1860.—*Toucher*, Sur les causes de la difficulté de cathétérisme dans les cas de retention d'urine, suite de cystite du col. Revue de thérap. méd.-chir. 1860. Dec. 15.—*B. Holt*, On Certain Errors in the Diagnosis and Treatment of Retention of Urine. Lancet. 1863. Feb. 21. —*Th. Bryant*, On Stricture, Retention, etc. Guy's Hospital Reports. VIII. Third Series. 1862. p. 147.

We have already treated of ischuria as the manifest symptom of spasmodic dysuria, and have noted that it is an uncommon occurrence. We now deal with ischuria in the sense of retention of urine apart from spasm.

Etiology.

Atony, paresis, or paralysis of the bladder consists, at first, in a tardy, prolonged, imperfect contraction of the longitudinal and oblique muscular fibres of the bladder and of the detrusor urinæ muscle; this subsequently increases, and ends, at last, in absolute inaction. In consequence, the urine remains in the bladder much longer than is the case normally, and is only partially, at last not at all, voluntarily voided, a condition which may lead the practitioner, if not on his guard, to be deceived by the involuntary escape of a small quantity of urine, and, if neglected, causes great distention of the bladder, pressure on the neighboring parts, and decomposition of the urine remaining stagnant in the bladder, which may not only set up vesical irritation and catarrh, but may also possibly result in absorption of ammonia and its tedious, dangerous consequences. If the relaxation of the sphincter vesicæ is not merely secondary and caused by the continuous pressure of the quantity of urine, instead of the slight overflow in small quantities, there may be a constant, incomplete, involuntary passage of the urine — a condition of which we shall treat more in detail under the head of Enuresis.

Apart from the paresis and paralysis of the bladder dependent on some central cause, and therefore coexistent with disease of the brain or spinal cord, we meet with the most highly pronounced forms of local paresis and paralysis of the bladder, principally at an advanced age, and much oftener in men than in women; in the latter, however, occasionally in youth and middle age in the form of hysterical paralysis; rarely in children, in whom, however, I have several times observed it in connection with hysterical neuroses. Paralysis of the fundus of the bladder is more common than of the neck.

Another, though unfrequent cause, is a disregard of the desire to empty the bladder. This may be due to narcosis from drunkenness, or may occur in the course of diseases which strongly affect the sensorium, such as typhus and typhoid, in which, therefore, we must see that the patient's bladder is regularly emptied several times a day. We not unfrequently, however, meet with this disregard of the desire to void the urine associated with the perfect retention of consciousness. The calls of nature are either utterly disregarded or incompletely satisfied for want of time; or, in young girls and women, from a sense of false shame, the urine is not voided for many hours, until, after constantly increasing desire, retention ensues at the very moment an opportunity offers for affording relief, or, in rare cases, incontinence may follow. Weakness of the system generally, and especially of the genitals locally, marasmus, exhaustion following on long and severe illnesses, may lead to paresis and paralysis of the bladder. Sometimes a similar effect is produced by over-irritation of the genitals from sexual excess or onanism. Tight strictures of the urethra or considerable enlargement of the prostate may afford material obstruction to the flow of urine, and, subsequently, may cause weakening of the bladder in consequence of over-straining; a portion of the urine remains behind, and atony and paralysis of the bladder result by degrees. We have already mentioned the effect of interrupted nerve-conduction in diseases of the central nervous system. But, besides chronic diseases of the brain and spinal cord, we must also bear in mind that acute traumatic mischief, such as concussion and contusion of the brain, spinal cord, etc., may produce the same effects. Also injuries to the bladder and urethra may seriously interfere with micturition. Apart from spasmodic ischuria, in which, in consequence of severe spasm of the bladder, complete spasmodic retention may occur, the common paralytic form may come on rapidly, unexpectedly, suddenly, and then, either only for a time or recurring at steadily diminishing intervals, and gradually becoming permanent. Retention, coming on suddenly, may also from the first be permanent. More frequently, however, instead of the paralysis setting in suddenly or after various paroxysms, it comes on gradually. The patient first of all complains that he can only make water slowly. The urine at first merely comes in drops, and only by degrees in full stream; the desire to pass water is soon felt less frequently and only when the bladder has become greatly distended, and passes off quickly again if not soon attended to. Subsequently the urine no longer escapes in a full stream, or this is feeble, sluggish, and frequently interrupted. The stream of urine is more rectangular. In still more advanced cases of paralysis, the urine flows away now and then, or uninterruptedly, guttative, and has a disagreeable ammoniacal odor. This occurs more especially when the sphincter has yielded to the pressure exercised on it by the constantly distended bladder. It is of greater importance from the fact that the urine is not completely voided, and the bladder is liable to become irritated into a condition of catarrhal inflammation if timely interference is not practised. In these cases the region of the bladder should invariably be examined, and will be found to be the seat of a rounded tumor, giving a dull note on percussion.

Paralysis of the sphincter and of the detrusor gradually ensues, and the urine then flows away uninterruptedly, true incontinence of urine existing. In rare cases, prolonged incomplete evacuation of the urine may lead to uræmic and ammoniacal symptoms, and may thus endanger life. Sopor, convulsions, paralysis, vomiting, etc., may form a pseudo-cerebral group of symptoms. If the cause can be removed, the retention of urine and consequent atony are capable of cure. If, however, we have to deal with a more primary paralysis in old people, or if, at the same time, other paralytic conditions exist, the affection is, as a rule, incurable. Retention, which has been overlooked, may prove fatal owing to severe vesical catarrh, or even gangrene of the bladder, and, sooner or later, by uræmic infection.

Diagnosis.

Dysuria and cessation of the stream of urine form most important symptoms, rendering it necessary to investigate the cause. The involuntary dribbling of the urine may easily mislead and prevent one's suspecting paralysis of the bladder; an error can easily be avoided, however, by paying attention to the history, and more especially by examining over the region of the bladder, which, indeed, should never be neglected. If the urine is not drawn off by the catheter, the bladder remains fully distended, reaching far above the pubes, or even as high as the navel, and may be felt as a rounded tumor of elastic consistence, though some urine dribbles away. I have not unfrequently seen the bladder allowed to remain distended for months, so that, at last, a condition of uræmia and ammoniæmia became developed by infection, the patient showing a tendency to sopor, deranged appetite, frequent vomiting, even urinous odor, and paralytic symptoms. When the case has reached this stage, the regular use of the catheter cannot avail, the patient succumbs to the progressive infection. If, however, the continuous distention of the bladder be recognized in good time, the urine regularly withdrawn, and obstructions such as strictures dealt with, I have repeatedly had the satisfaction of seeing such severe affections result in complete recovery. For purposes of diagnosis, examina-

tion with the catheter is necessary in all these diseases, either in
the erect posture or while the patient is lying down ; in the latter
position it is often necessary to press over the region of the
bladder strongly with the hand in order to empty the bladder
completely.

Prognosis.

In cases of transitory atony, or of retention of urine, in
young or middle-aged patients, in the hysterical affections, in
the neuroses of childhood and of women, the prognosis is favorable.   Also in patients of the male sex who have a fair amount
of vigor, we see that if appropriate treatment, such as the regular emptying of the bladder and proper hygienic measures
be adopted in good time, a complete or almost complete cure
may result.   Others complain for long of tedious and somewhat difficult micturition, but retention of urine does not occur,
and it is quite exceptional for the bladder to become distended
once, and then only temporarily.   The prognosis in cases of
spasmodic ischuria also is good, as the attacks are usually of a
temporary character, isolated, and associated with an otherwise
healthy condition of the muscular structure of the bladder.
The inflammatory ischuria, which we occasionally meet with in
connection with very acute gonorrhœa, catarrh of the neck of the
bladder, or acute abscess of the prostate, is also transitory.   In
stricture of the urethra and calculus vesicæ the prognosis partly
depends on appropriate treatment and removal of the cause.   If,
however, the muscular structure of the bladder has already
become severely and permanently affected, it is possible that
a certain degree of improvement will follow the dilatation of the
stricture, lithotrity, etc.   If an affection of the brain or spinal
cord exists, the prognosis is good when the condition depends
on some acute mischief set up by injury, such as concussion of
the brain or spinal cord.   In chronic central lesions, however,
when the retention has come on gradually, the bladder symptoms improve but seldom with the disappearance of the primary
disease, and still less frequently while the central disease persists.   If paralysis of the bladder and retention of urine come

on at an advanced age, a cure may still take place, and I have several times met with such cases in old men; but they are the exception, and incurability the rule. Those cases are the worst and the most deceptive in which the urine dribbles away involuntarily in association with paralysis and distention of the bladder. If this condition is neglected, as so often happens, from carelessness in old people, or for want of attention to treatment, there is added to the doubtful character of the paralysis that of general and progressive poisoning. Indeed, I have several times noticed that when, after the lapse of some time, the bladder is at last regularly emptied, the patient loses strength and succumbs even more rapidly in comparison, especially in old age.

Treatment.

As a prophylactic measure, we cannot sufficiently urge the importance of satisfying the desire to relieve the bladder as soon as it arises, especially when hours have elapsed since the last occasion, and the patient has not acquired the bad habit of emptying the bladder on the slightest impulse thereto. When the patient is in bed he should only make water in a kneeling position, because when lying on the back the bladder is incompletely emptied. If retention comes on and is not relieved spontaneously within a few hours, or after the use of poultices, warm baths, etc., a catheter should be passed and the bladder emptied, and this should be repeated as often and for as long a period as the bladder is not completely relieved spontaneously, or is only partially so. In simple atony of the bladder, the plan proposed by J. L. Petit, that the patient should press the cold chamber utensil firmly against the thighs and scrotum, is to be recommended, and another device, which is of some value owing to the sudden sensation of cold produced, consists in dipping the hands in cold water. Otherwise, we can treat weakness of the bladder best by cold general sponging, cold lotions to the abdomen, and cold hip-baths. If the latter are not well borne, lukewarm aromatic baths may be substituted. Aromatic beverages, also old wines, preparations of ammonia with camphor, friction

over the region of the bladder with an ammonia-camphor lini.
ment, to which oil of turpentine may be added, may prove of
great service combined with a tonic regimen and a strict hygiene.
If we have to deal with neurotic or hysterical paresis, or paraly.
sis of the bladder, it is well to order cold or warm baths, accord.
ing as they suit the patient best or seem more efficacious, and,
internally, lactate of zinc, quinine, arsenic, valerian, castor, assa-
fœtida with camphor, and preparations of ammonia in various
combinations. In hysterical paralysis, electricity may be of the
greatest service, whilst I have found it of little use in simple
paralysis of the bladder. I have several times seen patients who
have simulated paralysis of the bladder and have refrained from
passing water till the bladder was fully distended. If we have
satisfied ourselves that no real disease exists, it is better apparently not to take much notice ; the patient will commonly find it
advisable to empty the bladder regularly again. In the hospital
at Zurich I had a hysterical young woman under care, who
required the attendance of the medical officer several times in
the day and often during the night, in order to pass a catheter.
I effected a cure in this case by simply ordering the nurse to
pass the catheter when required.

The first time that a catheter is passed, in a case of retention,
the bladder should be emptied gradually, with interruptions,
in order to give the distended viscus time to contract slowly.
If the bladder is very much distended, and if we can only
empty it by firm pressure over the region of the bladder, the
patient must not only shortly after obey any desire to pass
water, but the catheter must again be used, if the bladder has not
been relieved, or only incompletely so, in the course of the next
four or six hours. So long as the paralysis remains unchanged
the bladder must be relieved three or four times in the twenty-
four hours, either by the practitioner, or the patient, or a relative, or a skilled and experienced nurse. When the medical man
himself does not pass the catheter, an elastic one without a stylet, or Lasserre's, should be used and passed slowly, carefully,
without any force, and only after special instructions being
given by the practitioner. The plan of leaving the catheter
in has great disadvantages. It is difficult to fix it, great irrita-

tion is set up in the bladder and urethra, and an elastic instrument spoils very quickly. At the commencement of my career,
when fresh from Dupuytren's school, I often used to leave an
instrument in the bladder for a long period, but I have given up
the plan, as a rule, for a long time. In exceptional cases, however, when it is very difficult to introduce a catheter, owing to
tight stricture or other obstruction, and it is impossible to obtain
repeated skilled attention, the catheter may be left in, but not
longer than for two or three days. Under these circumstances
a soft, elastic Nélaton's catheter of vulcanized caoutchouc, such
as is used for the drainage of pus, is well adapted. The instrument, however, should not be pushed farther than the neck of
the bladder. If, during catheterization, the urine begins to flow
by the side of the catheter, it is time to urge the patient to expe-
dite the expulsion of the urine by voluntary efforts, in order
gradually to improve the contractile power of the bladder. The
same end may be served by the introduction of wax bougies,
which are allowed to remain for a few minutes. It is best not to
remove them until the patient experiences a desire to micturate,
which not unfrequently ensues spontaneously, under the influence of this stimulus. Pitha recommends this plan strongly,
and adds that the treatment by bougies is essentially aided by
the voluntary efforts of the patient, by repeated attempts to pass
water in various positions favorable to the escape of the urine,
by violent movements of the lower extremities, bending the
trunk and the hips, walking about quickly, etc.—aids which
the patients themselves are very ingenious in varying. We are
careful, however, to prevent the bladder becoming over-distended in spite of these imperfect attempts at emptying it, and
pass a catheter from time to time.

In well-marked paralysis of the bladder, injections of cold
water, after the urine has been drawn off, are sometimes useful,
and if the bladder is very insensible to stimulus the temperature
may be steadily lowered almost to that of ice. This treatment
should be supplemented by cold douches over the region of the
bladder, perineum, or sacrum, and by cold enemata, cold hip-
baths, or, in short, by rational hydropathy.

Of internal remedies, we find those are most recommended

which act as stimulants, as is supposed, on the spinal cord and on the motor nerves of the bladder. For a long time I have been convinced that preparations of nux vomica exercise no specific influence whatever on any motor paralysis. In paralysis of the bladder I have not found either the extract of nux vomica or strychnia of any efficacy, nor the celebrated ergot and its preparations. Balsams, such as balsam of copaiva, Peru, or tolu, oil of turpentine, rock oil, etc., upset the stomach without improving the condition of the bladder; cantharides inflames the mucous membrane without in the least stimulating the muscular structure beneficially. The same may be said, also, of stimulating and astringent injections into the bladder, by which much harm and scarcely any good may be done. The sole stimulant acting directly on the bladder, which is attended by any good result when the central nervous system is healthy, consists in the application of electricity and galvanism; this is supported by very competent authorities, such as Michon, Monod, Duchenne, Meyer, and others. By introducing a metallic catheter into the bladder, and another into the rectum, or placing the other pole on the sacrum, we may send a powerful electric or galvanic current through the neck of the bladder. Stimulating embrocations, vesicants, etc., are, as a rule, of no service.

Internal treatment in cases of localized paralysis of the bladder must be directed chiefly to improving the general condition and strengthening the constitution, and with this object in view, especially in the chronic form met with in old people, we prescribe a good, nutritious diet, tonics, such as preparations of quinine and iron, country air, mountain air, residence at the seaside, or at a watering-place which, in addition to a chalybeate water rich in carbonic acid, also contains good peat-baths; such as Schwalbach, Franzensbad, or Cudowa; or where the influence of the chalybeate spring is assisted by the pure air of an elevated mountain region, as at St. Moritz in the Engadine. During residence at the seaside, we shall also often find baths useful, at first tepid, and subsequently cold. Any catarrh of the bladder complicating the case is to be treated most carefully. If the urine constantly dribbles away, the greatest attention to cleanliness must be enjoined, and the patient should wear a properly contrived portable urinal made of vulcanized caoutchouc, and we should see it properly secured. It is also important to take care that these patients have their bowels opened regularly, and we may assist nature by cold enemata, magnesia, cathartic effervescing powder, compound liquorice powder, or pills of aloes and jalap.

Enuresis and Incontinence of Urine.

C. D. Distel, De incontinentia urinæ. Vitenb. 1697.—*J. Hirschfeld*, De incontinentia urinæ post-partum diffic. Argent. 1759.—*J. P. Nonne*, D. de enuresi. Erf. 1768. —*B. Ritter*, in Graefe und Walt. Journ. Bd. XVII. H. 4. S. 272.—*Naumann*, Handb. der med. Klinik. Bd. VI.—*Devergie*, Incontinence of Urine and its Rational Treatment by Injections; übers. v. Mueller. Leipz. 1840.—*Sprengler*, in Schmidt's Encycl. Bd. III. S. 278.—*Froriep*, Notiz. 1843. H. 545.—*Willis*, L. c. p. 366.—*Duffin* und. *Lay*, Heilung der Enur. noct. durch Cauterisat. der Urethra mit Brechnuss und Eisenmoor behandelt. Boerhave. Dcbr. 1838. S. 200.—*Ramaugé*, On Congenital Incontinence of Urine. Journ. d. conn. méd. Octb. 1839.—*Mercier*, Mémoire sur la veritable cause et le mécanisme de l'incontinence, de la retention et du régorgement d'urine chez les vieillards; lu à l'Institut—Académie des sciences—le 10 Juin, 1839.—*Froriep*, Neue Bebandlungsweise der .Incontinentia urinæ und der Enuresis. Froriep's neue Notiz. Nr. 545. 1843.—*Gottschalk*, Fall von geheilter Enuresis. Hamb. Zeitschr. f. d. g. Mediz. Bd. XXIV. H. 3. 1843.—*Ruettel*, Nächtliches Bettpissen. Med. Corresp.-Bl. bair. Aerzte. Nr. 47. 1844.—*Delcour*, On the Use of Nitre and Benzoic Acid in Nocturnal Incontinence of Urine. Gaz. des hôp. Nr. 149. 1845.—Journ. f. Kinderkrankheiten vor Behrend und Hildebrand. 3. Jahrg. 4. Heft. 1845.—*Robert*, Incontinentia urinæ. Annal. de Thérap. méd. et chir. p. Rognetta. Nr. 2. 1845.—*Gerdy*, Incontinentia Urinæ in Children. Annal. de Thérap. méd. et chir. p. Rognetta. IX. année. Août, 1849.—*Roux*, Incontinentia urinæ nocturna. Annal. de Thérap. méd. et chir. p. Rognetta. IV. année. Juli, 1846.—*De Fraene*, Incontinentia Urinæ Nocturna Cured by Benzoic Acid. Journ. de méd. de chir. et de pharm. de Bruxelles. Juin. IX. année 1846. —*Kemerer*, On Incontinence of Urine. Journ. des conn. méd.-chir. Avril, 1846.— *Maurab*, On a Means of Mitigating the Irritating Quality of the Urine and on the Irritation of the Integument set up in Incontinence of Urine. Revue méd.-chir. Malgaigne. Fevr. 1847.—*Guérand*, Flying Blisters in Nocturnal Incontinence. Ann. d. Thérap. Septb. et Octb. 1848.—*Heidenreich*, Zur Heilung des Bettpissens der Kinder. Norrd. med.-chir. Ztg. IV. 21. 1848.—*Morand*, Treatment of Incontinence of Urine by Belladonna. Journ. des conn. méd. Fév. 1849; Bull. de thérap. Mars, 1849.—*Chassaignac*, Case of Incontinence of Urine Treated by Galvanism. Gaz. des hôp. 1849. 149.—*Demeaux*, On the Cauterization of the Neck of the Bladder with Nitrate of Silver in Incontinence of Urine in Young People. Gaz. des hôp. 9. 1851.—*Panel*, Strychnin gegen Harnincontinenz. Journ. v. Bord. Sept. 1852.—*Halsey*, Successful Treatment of Incontinence of Urine remaining after Lithotomy by Sulphuric Acid. New York Medical Journal. Jan. 1852.—*Aug. Millet*, Du traitement de l'incontinence nocturne (Ferrum et Secale Cornut.) Bullet. de thérap. LXIII. 8.—*Denaux*, De l'incontinence d'urine nocturne. Bullet. de la soc. de méd. de Gant. 1860.— —*Th. Clemens*, Liquor ferri muriat. oxydati, ein treffliches Mittel gegen Enuresis nocturna. Duet. Klinik. 1861. 14.—*Hedenus*, Ueber Enuresis nocturna. Ibid. H. 35.—*Roeser*, Incontinenz in Folge eines angeblichen Fehlers der Harnrohr. Arch. f. klin. Chirurg. 1863.—*Bois*, Injections sous-cutanées (Strychnin) c. enures. infant. Gaz. méd. 1863. 52.

We have already treated of incontinence of urine as a symptom of paralysis of the bladder where the bladder is constantly distended and partly overflows. We have now to speak of two other conditions: of complete incontinence, and of the form met with in children, at night more especially—the so-called enuresis nocturna.

Etiology and Symptomatology.

In its more chronic form, inability of the sphincter vesicæ to contract is either incomplete and occasional, or more permanent, with continuous overflow of urine. If the atony is but slight, the contractile power in general may be retained, but the patient has to empty the bladder directly any desire is felt, or else the urine flows away involuntarily. This may be called an active form and the former a passive incontinence, and these may be accompanied by various spasmodic symptoms, and hence we have enuresis spastica as a third form added to the active and passive. In the fourth form, enuresis nocturna, we have lastly, to some extent, a narcosis of the sphincter. The patient is not fully conscious of the desire to empty the bladder, and this is therefore gratified without precaution and immediately, and as a consequence the bed is wetted. Enuresis paralytica is either associated with other symptoms of extensive paralysis, or is of a more local character. Besides the enuresis met with in connection with insensibility in deep sleep, all forms of sopor, narcosis, or even intoxication, may be associated with temporary enuresis;

hence the involuntary escape of urine which occurs in severe cases of typhus and typhoid conditions of all sorts. Moreover, mechanical obstructions may prevent the closure of the neck of the bladder or render it imperfect, such, for instance, as congenital defects of the prostate and neck of the bladder, epispadias, induration, thickening, rigidity, or incrustation of the walls of the bladder, especially of the trigone, associated with diminution in the capacity of the bladder, concretions and foreign bodies, which are fixed in the bladder and partially blocked up, inflammatory swelling and hypertrophy of the prostate, excrescences and carcinoma at the neck of the bladder, compression of the bladder by neighboring tumors and organs, such as the pregnant uterus, inversion or dislocation of the bladder, with displacement and stretching of the neck, and the like, may induce incontinence—enuresis mechanica. The neck of the bladder may also be directly paralyzed as the result of contusion, wound, excessive mechanical dilatation (by surgical instruments), tearing, ulceration, or even owing to rheumatism (Froriep).

The nocturnal incontinence of children arises occasionally from indolence, and is merely a bad habit; another time it is a consequence of sleeping very deeply and soundly; we must also admit, however, that not seldom an extraordinarily obstinate form of the affection is met with in connection with an otherwise healthy constitution, as a local atony associated with increased sensitiveness of the neck of the bladder. Boys are more frequently affected than girls, and grown-up persons far less frequently than children. Unhealthy children, with pasty complexions, and those affected with scrofula or rickets, suffer much more frequently than strong, healthy children. The tendency to it may be increased for a time by indigestion, drinking freely in the evening, insufficient clothing, and more especially by inattention to emptying the bladder regularly before the child goes to sleep, in the course of the night, and the first thing in the morning. It is doubtful whether the irritation of worms has really any influence, such as has been asserted. Any imperfect paralysis or atonic condition, any condition of irritation or spasm, without remote or local organic changes, is capable of complete cure, but may occasionally last for a long time. The

nocturnal incontinence of children ceases on the average about
the tenth or twelfth year, or, even in obstinate cases, steadily
becomes less and less frequent, and disappears at puberty. The
casual enuresis of young children of three or four years of age,
previously insufficiently attended to, is usually quickly and
easily curable by careful attention.

Diagnosis.

The diagnosis is not of itself attended with any difficulty ; one
need only invariably examine the region of the bladder thoroughly in order to ascertain whether the bladder is empty, since,
if this should not be the case, the incontinence is only a symptom of retention, and has a wholly different significance to the
form we are now considering. Seeing, therefore, that enuresis,
or incontinence, is easily recognized, its diagnosis from other
affections requires less notice than the question of the causes
which determine its origin, continuance, or aggravation.

Prognosis.

When the cause can be removed, the prognosis is favorable,
as a rule ; in old people, however, it is less so, as in them the
affection is generally due to paralysis or deep-seated disease of
the urinary apparatus. The enuresis nocturna is quite susceptible of cure, but is not unfrequently a very obstinate malady ;
it commonly, however, disappears spontaneously, especially at
the time of puberty.

Treatment.

The removal of the cause is especially important in diseases
and obstructions materially interfering with the normal retention
of the urine. In children, as well as in adults, atonic conditions
often lie at the foundation of the insufficient control over the
passage of the urine, and, in these cases, preparations of bark
and iron, especially, and the aromatic baths recommended by
Lallemant, are strongly indicated. We infuse three ounces

(100.0) of aromatic herbs in from eight to ten pints (four to five litres) of boiling water, and pour this infusion, with the herbs, in the bath, the temperature of which should not exceed 92.75° F. (27° R.), and by preference should be 88.25-90° F. (25-26° R.). Lallemant added a certain quantity of brandy to the bath, for which we may substitute one or two glasses of strong spirit for each bath.   In enuresis nocturna we allow the children but little fluid in the evening, cover them up warmly at night, and take care that they are encouraged to pass water before getting into bed and during the night.   Trousseau's advice, that we should urge the patients to hold their water as long as possible during the day, in order to diminish the sensitiveness of the neck of the bladder, may be useful under certain circumstances, but when abused may lead to ill results.   We also avoid roughness, chiding, or chastisement, as they are quite useless, or only to be employed in exceptional cases.   Niemeyer's proposition to give non-irritating (indifferent) remedies, so that the patients may go to sleep confidently, and only be awakened by the desire to pass water, is not worthy of being recommended seriously, as most children suffering from nocturnal incontinence go to sleep untroubled, without any such manœuvre, and after it, nevertheless, wet the bed.

Among the narcotics which are administered with the view of diminishing the sensitiveness of the neck of the bladder, and thus aiding the sphincter in resisting pressure, belladonna and its preparations, atropine, etc., have been especially recommended by Bretonneau and Trousseau.   We order a sixth of a grain (0.01) of extract of belladonna, or $\frac{1}{120}$ gr. (0.0005) of atropine, every evening at bedtime, and may, in some cases, increase the dose carefully ; we shall have, however, to continue the treatment for months.   I have also employed belladonna in children for this affection on various occasions—hitherto, however, with doubtful success.   The same applies to stramonium, henbane, etc.   Lupulin, in doses of three or four grains (0.2-0.3), at bedtime, is sometimes useful.   The preparations of nux vomica have also been much lauded, and we may administer the tincture of the seeds, in gradually increasing doses, several times a day, from three to five minims or more at a time.   It is well, also, to combine with this double or treble the dose of the tincture of ferrated apple-extract. The preparations of ergot have been recommended in several quarters, but I have not had any special experience with them. The preparations of iron have been much praised, and are, in fact, of great value where atony is one of the chief causes of the malady. The action of the iodide of iron has appeared to me to be exceedingly efficacious, in a series of cases, in the form of Blanchard's pills, of the syrup of iodide of iron, and especially in the form of the syrup which I have recommended. I dissolve a drachm (4.0) of sulphate of iron with forty-five grains (3.0) of iodide of potassium in an ounce (30.0) of cinnamon-water, filter, and mix with five or six ounces (150.0–180.0) of simple syrup or syrup of orange-peel, and let the patient take a dessert- or tablespoonful two or three times a day, one being taken at bedtime. Tannin is the sole astringent which is of any use, and must be given for a long time in increasing doses. We may administer it in powder, as a syrup, or in pills. We may also allow such children to take a little good red wine, containing tannin, at meal-times. We have already mentioned that aromatic baths are of service, though I prefer cold baths if they can be borne, and in the form of hip-baths, at first merely consisting of several dips, and later as a continued local bath, lasting from five to fifteen minutes. At favorable seasons of the year, when possible, I order river- and sea-bathing. I have no particular experience of the use of electricity, but physicians who are fully deserving of credit speak well of it. As it entails the introduction of a catheter, which is then connected to one pole, the plan can be carried out at an earlier age in girls than in boys, in whom we must wait till the time of puberty, and shall then meet with considerable difficulties. The same applies to the introduction of bougies. All the various mechanical means of compression are useless and inapplicable, as a rule.

In cases of incurable incontinence later in life, a proper urinal should be worn day and night.

Hypertrophy of the Bladder.

Though hypertrophy of the bladder is mostly secondary to some other disease, we must, nevertheless, once more mention the chief facts concerning it. It may be associated with dilatation or contraction of the bladder; in the former case diverticula may form between the muscular fasciculi, which are separated from one another, and may become the seat of the formation of calculi which are very difficult of diagnosis. The most important causes of hypertrophy of the bladder are: obstructions to the passage of urine, calculi, concretions wedged in the neck of the bladder, prostatic or urethral calculi, hypertrophy of the prostate, compression of the neck of the bladder or of the urethra by cancerous or other new growths, and strictures of the urethra. Chronic catarrh of the bladder, however, or indurations of the connective tissue surrounding the bladder, may lead to hypertrophy of the bladder, owing to obstruction to the flow of urine. It is only very exceptionally that I have met with it in boys before the age of puberty; as a rule it only occurs in men advanced in years.

The distended bladder may attain enormous dimensions, but may be capable of great diminution if there be a thorough evacuation of the urine, and it is rare to find the bladder reach three or four fingers' breadth above the pubes, when empty or moderately filled, and without there being any obstruction to the outflow of the urine. When the bladder is filled, percussion and palpation naturally give much more certain indications; even in the empty state, however, it may be detected if of considerable size. The bladder feels remarkably hard, and presents most resemblance to a tumor above the pubes when hypertrophied, at the same time that it is diminished in capacity — a condition which I have more especially observed in those forms of catarrh of the bladder in which the patients have accustomed themselves to pass their urine in small quantities and very frequently. Partial hypertrophy of the bladder is but seldom primary, being commonly secondary to other local affections.

It is evident that we cannot cure hypertrophy of the bladder when once well established; but we can alleviate, if not entirely obviate its unpleasant consequences by removal of the causes—strictures, stones—and by the regular emptying of the bladder. A girdle constricting the region of the bladder, an apparatus similar to the ceinture hypogastrique, may mechanically prevent much distention, and facilitate contraction of the bladder, which we may also assist by the administration of tonics and strengthening food. In contraction of the bladder, with too frequent micturition, it is most important that the patient should voluntarily assist the medical man by resisting as much as possible the too frequent desire to pass water. We may diminish the irritability of the neck of the bladder by the introduction of bougies, aided by narcotics and lukewarm hip-baths, and, at a later stage, by injections of water in steadily increasing quantities, and retained for some time in order to increase the capacity of the bladder.

Hemorrhage from the Bladder—Hæmaturia Vesicalis.

Civiale, On the Treatment of Hæmaturia. Journ. d. conn. méd. Mars, 1842.—*Foucquier*, On the Various Kinds of Hæmaturia and their Treatment. Journ. des conn. méd. Mai, 1842.—*Leroy d'Etiolles*, On Copious Hæmaturia and on the Means of Removing Coagula from the Bladder. Journ. des conn. méd. Dec. 1842.—*Van Wageninge*, Hæmaturia hæmorrhoid. mittelst Kali jod. gestillt. Boerhave 1843.—*Leney*, Case of Hæmaturia. Med. Times. No. 229. 1844.—*Wehle*, Fall von chronisch. periodisch. Blutharnen. Med. österr. Wochenschr. Nr. 51. 1844.—*Melchior*, Hæmaturia et Metrorrhagia nach Anwendung des Morph. acet. Med. österr. Wochenschr. 49. 1847.—*Rayer*, Endemic Hæmaturia in the Tropics. Annal. d. thér. Nov. 1847.—*Gerdy*, Cystorrhagia. Annal. d. thér. Dec. 1847.—*Rognetta*, Cauterization of the Mucous Membrane of the Bladder: a. In Hæmaturia; b. In Hæmaturia Complicated with Spermatorrhœa, Impotence, and Paralysis. Annal. d. thérap. Août, 1848.—*Mercier*, The Method of Removing Coagulated Blood from the Bladder. Gaz. de Paris. XVIII. 21. 1848.—*Leroy-Dupré*, Marked Urethrorrhagia Cured by the Use of Cold and Astringents. Gaz. de Paris. XIX. 6. 1849.—Fr. and Not. IX. 5.—*Hughes*, On Hemorrhage from the Urethra and Irreducible Omental Hernia. Dublin Med. Journ. May, 150.—*Pizzorno*, Cure of Hæmaturia by the Use of Balsam of Copaiba and Cubebs after Various other Remedies had been tried in vain. Gaz. med. ital. fed. Lomb. 13. 1851.—*A. Legrand*, Quelques mots sur l'hématurie, etc. Union méd. 1860. 144.—*A. Mercier*, Note sur l'hématurie, qui suit le cathétérisme dans les cas de retention, etc. Union méd. 1860. 3.

Hæmaturia, properly speaking, is only exceptionally vesical in its origin, and is, therefore, usually rightly treated of under the head of hemorrhage from the kidney. Bleeding may occur directly from the bladder in consequence of injury, such as a wound, rupture, squeezing, concussion, laceration by instruments, pressure, kick, blow, or fall on the buttocks. Violent horse-exercise, ulcerations of the mucous membrane of the bladder in consequence of calculi, etc., may also bring it about. So, also, very severe catarrh of the bladder, or tubercle or vascular papillomata, or carcinoma of the bladder may set up by no means inconsiderable hemorrhage. The same applies to the irritation induced by cantharides. Varices of the veins of the bladder, the so-called vesical hemorrhoids, are exceedingly rare, but may undoubtedly cause hemorrhage from the bladder. The same may be said of all forms of scorbutic or hemorrhagic morbid conditions, and, besides the common form of scurvy, we meet with it in hemorrhagic small-pox more especially, and, more rarely, in hemorrhagic scarlet fever and typhus.

The blood may either escape in a fluid form, or, by coagulation, obstruct the flow of urine considerably; and this is the case more especially when there is a stricture or hypertrophy of the prostate, and it is necessary to empty the bladder by means of the catheter, an operation which is by no means easy of execution under these circumstances, as the clots frequently block up the opening in the catheter, and must be washed away by injections or by cleaning the catheter. For this reason it is well in such cases to select a large catheter with a large circular opening in it. We treat this hemorrhage as a symptom by the application of bladders of ice to the hypogastrium and perineum, or by the administration internally of alum or tannin, and we may also inject a three or five per cent. solution of the latter into the bladder. Now and then oil of turpentine administered internally may be very useful. In extreme cases Lallemant has practised direct cauterization of the bladder with nitrate of silver with success.

Calculus Vesicæ.

The affections due to the presence of stone in the bladder belong properly to the domain of the surgeon, and I shall not give any account of any technical procedures. I shall, however, mention shortly the symptoms set up by calculus vesicæ, as I have found that practitioners, as a rule, have a very imperfect knowledge on the decidedly important question of the diagnosis of this affection.

As, with the exception of the calculi which form around foreign bodies introduced into the bladder, the greater number of vesical calculi have descended from the kidney, a detailed account of the concretions met with in the urinary passages may also come under the head of Diseases of the Kidney. In the account here given, I shall follow Pitha's excellent description. One important clinical distinction is as to whether the stone is movable or fixed. Small concretions may remain unnoticed for a long time. This not only applies to small, smooth concretions, but also to large, immovable ones lying in a diverticulum of the bladder. The symptoms, therefore, may vary very much. Among the subjective ones may be mentioned the sensation of a foreign body in the bladder, the situation of which varies according to the position of the body. Much more frequently, the patients complain of pain in the neck of the bladder and in the fundus, on walking, standing, or sitting, when passing a hard motion or when the body is shaken during riding in a vehicle, or on horseback, etc., and which passes off after resting either on the back or on the belly. Not unfrequently, transitory hæmaturia accompanies the attacks of pain excited by shaking. Pain at the end of the glans penis or along the whole urethra is a remarkably frequent symptom. Less frequently, swelling of the prepuce occurs. The dysuria, increasing sometimes to strangury, which is caused by stone in the bladder, generally comes on at the end of micturition during the expulsion of the last few·drops, and the signs of irritation of the neck of the bladder then persist for some time longer. We must also note the stoppage of the stream of urine, which not unfrequently occurs quite suddenly, followed by renewed easy flow when the position of the body is altered. The patients often experience a sensation as if a foreign body falling in front of the neck of the bladder caused this stoppage. If the stone becomes wedged in the neck of the bladder, but without completely blocking it, either ischuria or enuresis may follow ; whilst, if a larger stone is wedged in the neck of the bladder, causing obstruction to the flow of urine, complete retention results. Besides these symptoms which have their seat at the neck of the bladder, radiating pains, very unpleasant sensations, spasmodic contractions in the rectum, vagina, testes, neighborhood of the kidneys, perineum, or thighs, burning sensations in the soles of the feet, in the heels, or in the elbows, may be present, occurring mostly in paroxysms. When many movable stones exist in the bladder, they may, in exceedingly rare cases, give rise to a distinct sensation, or even an audible noise when they strike against one another during efforts in walking, riding, jumping, etc.

Without underrating the value of these signs, a stone can only be detected with certainty by a careful exploration with a metallic catheter or sound. We then feel with the instrument the resistance caused by the stone and the hardness of its surface, and by striking the instrument against the stone we elicit a distinct, clear sound ; at the same time we form an impression as to the situation, mobility, form, size, and number of the concretions. In addition, an examination of the urine not unfrequently reveals the presence of gravel, or, if this is absent, of crystals which resemble the chief constituents of the stone. Nevertheless, small, or even moderately large, very movable stones may elude even the most careful examination. The same happens when large concretions are present, if they are situated deeply in the fundus of the bladder, and hid by a hypertrophied prostate, or embedded in a niche in the bladder, which is difficult of access. Encysted calculi, having only a small portion projecting into the interior of the bladder, may easily escape detection with the sound. This is especially liable to happen when the sounding is attempted with an unsuitable instrument, such as a catheter with a large curve. The sound should have a short, abrupt curve, like that of a lithotrite or a Mercier's sound, in order that it may

move freely and easily in the bladder, and be able to reach easily
every part of its inner surface.

It is important also to know that the stone may occasionally
be situated at the anterior (upper) wall of the bladder, above the
symphysis, so that a sound passed along the lateral and posterior walls merely would fail to touch it. If the search along the
posterior (lower) wall has been without result, we must turn the
point of the sound upward towards the symphysis, and carefully
explore the whole of the anterior wall of the bladder. During
lithotrity we frequently have the opportunity of demonstrating
this remarkable and, at first sight, unaccountable situation of
the stone. The walls of the bladder in its empty state lie, as is
well known, in contact, so that they closely surround the calculus lying between them, and especially when there is spasm. In
this state of affairs the rough, tuberculated, or even branched
surface of the stone may easily so penetrate into the muscular
network, that it may be partially or completely ensnared and
held fast by the muscular fasciculi, and therefore, after the
anterior wall has been lifted away by injection of water, may
remain hanging from it, or, indeed, wholly encysted in it. If we
then fortunately turn the lithotrite upward (forward) and touch
the stone, it is often difficult to seize it, because only a small
part of it is uncovered ; and if we succeed in catching it, it seems
more or less fixed, so that one can only release it by lever-like
movements of the lithotrite. Small stones may in this way be
quite covered up by the muscular structure, and wholly out of
reach of detection. On this account, therefore, in doubtful
cases, the examination must be frequently repeated and in various positions of the patient, standing, lying down, on the side,
on the belly, with a full and with a partially emptied bladder,
before a definite opinion can be given as to the presence or absence of a calculus. Occasionally, it is necessary to supplement
the instrumental examination of the bladder by means of the
forefinger passed into the rectum, and by exercising pressure on
the abdominal wall. Large stones at the fundus of the bladder
may sometimes be distinctly felt per rectum, and in thin individuals we may press the stone from the hypogastrium towards the
rectum, and so grasp it between the thumb and forefinger. Cel-

sius's method of performing lithotomy depends on the possibility of hooking and pressing down the stone towards the perineum by the forefinger passed into the rectum.

For evident reasons, I shall not enter here either into the etiology or prognosis and treatment of stone in the bladder; this short sketch will, however, it is hoped, avail to show how important it is, even for the medical man not engaged in surgical practice, to be acquainted with the diagnostic features of calculus vesicæ.

The Presence of Hairs in the Bladder—Trichiasis Vesicæ, Pilimictio.

It is probably known to but very few practitioners that hairs may occasionally be passed with the urine, and that even when one recognizes with the greatest care all sources of error and deceit and wholly leaves such cases out of count, still a series of cases of pilimictio remain which have been well observed. Out of the whole number of cases the records of which are scattered here and there, I only know of two modern treatises on the subject: one is by Rayer and the other by myself, and both are contained in the Comptes Rendus des Séances et Mémoires de la Société de Biologie. Rayer's article, of which I make a short abstract below, deals only with the subject of Trichiasis of the Urinary Passages, and will be found in the second volume of the Proceedings (Paris, 1851), whilst my own is contained in my detailed Treatise on Dermoid Cysts, in the fourth volume of the Proceedings of the Paris Biological Society (for the year 1853).

The hairs which are met with in the urinary passages may either have been developed there, or have sprung from dermoid cysts which have opened into the bladder, or may have been introduced from without.

I. Trichiasis of the Urinary Passages Developed Intrinsically.

(It seems to me very doubtful whether this is a primary affection.) It is very rarely met with, and all cases in which the urine was not passed in the presence of the medical man, and those in which it is not certain that the hairs were real, must be wholly disregarded. Real hairs have been detected in normal urine, in urine mixed with blood, mucus or pus, and sometimes among gravel. Hairs may also be met with on the surface or in the interior of calculi. The passage of hair with the urine may be either painless, or accompanied by the various well-known inconveniences.

We know nothing positively as to the etiology of trichiasis as an independent affection. It has been observed in both sexes, and at various periods of life. We know very little, also, as to the state of the mucous membrane of the pelvis of the kidney and of the bladder in such cases, as no record has been made on the subject. It is, therefore, very uncertain and improbable that there is such a condition as idiopathic trichiasis vesicæ.

II. Trichiasis Due to the Bursting of a Dermoid Cyst into the Bladder.

In spite of the authority of Rayer and of other observers who mention the affection, it seems to me that the cases of simple trichiasis in which no deception occurred also belong to this second category. The cases on record in which hair was voided with the urine, and in which subsequently the communication with a dermoid cyst was demonstrated, all occurred in women. As a rule, the presence of the dermoid cyst was indicated during life by the existence of a tumor in the neighborhood of one or other ovary, or, if situated more deeply, the cyst may be detected by examination through the vagina or rectum. As dermoid cysts contain fat and fragments of bone and teeth, as well as hair, these may be voided at the same time. Both before and after the perforation of the cyst, we also observe symptoms of inflammatory irritation. I quote the following from my Treatise on Dermoid Cysts, pp. 249–52 :

1. Delpech[1] reports the case of a woman, aged twenty-four, who, when pregnant for the second time, complained of pains in the region of the bladder. The urine contained hair, which the

---

[1] Observation de pilimiction (Clinique chir. de Montpellier. T. II. p. 521. Paris, 1828).

husband picked out with a hook. Delpech subsequently removed a hard substance from the bladder, and great improvement followed. Two months later, when a similar attack recurred, Delpech removed a portion of bone and skin, covered with hair, from the bladder, and found a socket in the bone containing a molar tooth. The extraction was only effected after incising the urethra ; a complete cure resulted.

2. In Marshall's[1] case the patient was a woman, aged forty, who had frequently suffered for four or five years from pain in the abdomen, with progressive enlargement of the abdomen. Frequent purulent leucorrhœa was also present. Subsequently repeated attacks of retention of urine occurred, until, on one occasion, the patient voided, with great pain, some pieces of bone, one being more than an inch long. She became emaciated and marasmic, and finally died. At the post-mortem a communication was found between the bladder, which was distended, and a dermoid cyst of the ovary, containing pus, fat, a good deal of hair, and five teeth.

3. Laney's[2] case was a very remarkable one. The patient was a woman, aged thirty-three, and the mother of three children. A short time after her last confinement she noticed a painful tumor in the lower part of the abdomen on the left side. The urine deposited a muco-purulent sediment. The tumor burst externally, and discharged pus, along with some hair, part of which was long and matted together. At the end of four months, urine came through the fistula ; and through the urethra, urine, pus, hair, gravel, and, on one occasion, a substance like bone escaped. Subsequently a calculus developed. Larrey enlarged the fistulous opening and partly removed the tumor. He also cut across the opening communicating with the bladder, and removed the calculus. The patient was completely cured.

4. Hamlin,[3] an American physician, on making a post-mortem examination of the body of a woman aged twenty-four, who died

---

[1] Arch. gén. de méd. T. XVIII. p. 282. 1828.

[2] Kyste pileux de l'ovaire, compliqué, etc. (Mém. de l'Acad. de méd. T. XII. ; et Arch. gén. de méd. 3 Série. T. XV. p. 510. 1842.)

[3] Observations sur des cheveux trouvés dans l'intérieur de la vessie. Bull. de la soc. de l'Ecole. No. 4. p. 58. 1808.

during her first confinement, found a very offensive mass, mixed with hair, in the bladder. The latter communicated with a cystic tumor of the right ovary, containing hair, fat, and a bony substance.

5. Phillips'[1] case was that of a woman aged thirty, who had often suffered since childhood from attacks of dysuria. Two years previously obvious signs of inflammation of the bladder had appeared; pains in the hypogastrium, distention of the bladder, and increasing dysuria, and a tumor could be felt which reached upward as far as the liver. Then acute peritonitis set in, and carried off the patient. At the post-mortem examination, in addition to a hemorrhage in the peritoneal cavity, a large ovarian cyst was found, containing a good deal of sebaceous matter and hair matted together. In the bladder similar substances were found, together with a portion of bone, and an incisor tooth. The cyst communicated with the bladder by three openings of rather large size.

6. Delarivière[2] records the case of a woman aged fifty-eight, who had complained for seven years of a sense of weight in the abdomen, and of frequent and urgent desire to pass water. Micturition was painful and increasingly difficult. The catheter drew off highly purulent urine. Finally, severe gastro-intestinal catarrh set in, of which the patient died. At the post-mortem examination the bladder was found to communicate freely with a cyst, and contained a small convoluted mass of hair and several pieces of bone.

Though as yet no case of a similar character has been recorded in a man, there is no reason why such should not occur, as dermoid cysts of the lower part of the abdomen are met with in men, but much more rarely.

III. Introduction of Hairs into the Bladder from Without.

This happens but rarely; occasionally, however, hairs introduced from without have, undoubtedly, been found in the centre

---

[1] Med.-chir. Trans. Vol. II. p. 527.

[2] Journal de méd. et de chir. de Vandermonde. T. X. p. 516. Janvier, 1759.

of calculi in women when no dermoid cyst was present. Rayer quotes a case in which a hair from the pubic region reached the bladder through a fistula. It is possible, also, for hairs to be carried into the bladder along with instruments, and it is in this way that Rayer accounts for some of the cases in which he found hairs with fragments of stone removed by the lithotrite.

New Growths in the Bladder, and Especially Cancer of the Bladder.

Mendalgo, Carcinoma vesicæ. Giornal di Venezia. Maggio. Junio, 1839.—*Douglas*, On Tumours of the Bladder. Lond. Med. Gazette. Feb. 4, 1842.—*Contini*, A Large Scirrhous Tumor of the Bladder. Annal. med.-chir. dell Metaxa. Vol. 9. Settemb. 1843.—*Vaché*, Treatment of Fungating Polypus of the Bladder. L'Expérience. Nr. 327-330. Oct. 1843.—*Bulley*, Fungus Hæmatodes of the Bladder. Medical Gazette. Oct. 31, 1845.—*Hiltscher*, Carcin. medull. cranii, gland. lymph. et vesic. urin. Oest. med. Wochenschrift 46. 1847.—*Kesteven*, Fungus of the Bladder. Lond. Med. Gazette. Oct. 12, 1849.—*Fuchs*, Colloid-geschwulst im Corium mit Durchbohrung der Darmwand und der Urinblase. Nederb. Weekl. Octb. 1851.—*R. V. Gorham*, Case of Fungus Hæmatodes of the Bladder. Prov. Med. Journ. Aug. 1851, p. 431.—*Lebert*, Traité des maladies cancéreuses. Paris, 1851. *Koehler*, Die Krebs- und Scheinkrebskrankbeiten des Menschen. Stuttgart, 1853.—*Savory*, Polypus of the Bladder. Med. Times and Gazette. July 31, 1852.

Etiology and Pathological Anatomy.

Owing to the variety presented by the new growths occurring in the bladder, nothing definite can be said in relation to age and sex. While carcinoma develops, as a rule, at an advanced age, polypoid growths are met with in youth and middle age. Little is known as to the ultimate causes of most of the new growths. Under the head of inflammatory diseases will come tubercular inflammation of the bladder, which, as is also the case with most inflammations and new growths, attacks chiefly the cervix and trigonum vesicæ. As a rule, tubercular disease of the bladder is associated with extensive implication of the urinary or of the genito-urinary organs. It is evident that it is not a mere ordinary inflammation, but a disease of mal-nutrition, and dependent fre-

quently on a peculiar predisposition. As in other parts of the
genito-urinary tract, tuberculosis of the bladder is usually attended with incrustation, the mucous membrane is infiltrated
diffusely and up to the surface, and small deposits and granula-
tion-like foci of disease may occur in other parts of the mucous
membrane or beneath it.

Polypoid growths from the mucous membrane are met with
both in the healthy bladder and after chronic inflammation.
They may be either pedunculated or sessile, and may consist
either of simple hypertrophy of the mucous membrane, or have a
papillary, dendritic structure, resembling that of villous cancer,
and may then attain the size of a hazel-nut or walnut. The
branching outgrowths of connective tissue, covered with epithelium, correspond to manifoldly-branched vessels. In rare cases
they may be cast off spontaneously. Villous cancer may be
distinguished from these dendritic outgrowths by the truly carcinomatous structure of its framework, which also penetrates
into its branches, by its attaining relatively much greater dimensions, and by its being accompanied occasionally by carcinomatous deposits in other parts of the vesical walls, in adjacent
organs, or in distant parts. Most frequently cancer of the bladder is met with in the form of a soft, copiously cellular medullary growth, originating in the submucous connective tissue,
confined to the region of the neck of the bladder, and gradually
spreading more and more towards the middle and fundus of the
bladder. The new growth then projects considerably into the
interior of the bladder. The hard and colloid forms of cancer
are rarely met with in the bladder. On the whole, the bladder
is one of the localities in which cancer develops least frequently
as a primary disease. Ulcerations occur now and then in the
ordinary medullary cancer at a late stage, but rarely in the villous form. The bladder is seldom enlarged in cancer ; as a rule,
it is rather diminished in capacity. The mucous membrane is
generally in a state of chronic inflammation, and cancer also
gives rise to various forms of calculi. In one case I found very
fine phosphatic faceted stones in the bladder. In another case,
medullary cancer had extended along the urachus to the umbilicus, which subsequently became ulcerated. In addition to its

occurring primarily, cancer of the bladder may be met with, and, indeed, commonly as a secondary affection, in consequence of disease of adjacent organs, and especially of the uterus. Sometimes it occurs secondarily, but discontinuously; and sometimes as the result of direct extension of carcinomatous growths in the neighborhood into the bladder.

Symptomatology.

Tubercular inflammation, as a rule, differs but little from other forms of cystitis. Small, vesical polypi do not give rise to any special symptoms, and large dendritic growths produce the same local phenomena as cancer of the bladder. Moreover, whatever form of cancer may be present, the symptoms will be very similar, but if the growth be situated so as to block up either of the openings into the bladder, or if it be copiously supplied with blood-vessels so as to give rise to hemorrhage, the symptoms may be modified. As a rule, the disease is latent at its commencement; in simple papillary growths it may occasionally be so for a long time. It occurs after the fortieth year in persons who have never suffered from any other affection of the urinary passages, and among the earliest symptoms is a frequent desire to pass water, accompanied by pains in the hypogastrium or perineum, or even spreading more widely. When the tumor is liable to obstruct the urethra during micturition, the stream may be suddenly interrupted and then again flow freely if the patient changes his posture, and on this account many patients make water more easily in a particular position. If, on the contrary, the tumor spreads more and more towards the urethra, and if it is not merely that a few villous growths now and then obstruct it, the difficulty of micturition steadily increases. By degrees the urine comes to be voided only drop by drop, and, at last, retention ensues. The pains, which at first were chiefly felt in connection with micturition, are felt at other times, and occasionally occur in violent paroxysms, last for hours almost without any cessation, and spread to the lumbar, sacral, and inguinal regions, or even down the thighs. If the bladder is somewhat enlarged and the coats hypertrophied, it can be felt as

a rounded, globular tumor behind the symphysis pubis without
our being able to detect the cancer itself by palpation. In one
case which came under my notice, I could feel a hard cord passing from the bladder to the navel, and diagnosed it to be the
urachus infiltrated with cancerous growth. At the commencement, the urine is normal; later, it becomes at times thick and
purulent, and then mixed with blood, which occasionally is met
with in considerable quantity. When the disease has progressed
insidiously, I have several times found that hæmaturia was the
first symptom. This leading to the introduction of a catheter,
portions of tissue on several occasions were brought away in the
openings of the instrument, and, when examined microscopically,
were shown to be of a cancerous nature or derived from a villous
growth. In other cases, fragments of cancer-tissue are not unfrequently voided with the urine, and may be easily recognized
as such on microscopic examination. In one such case which
came under my observation, the medical man in attendance
could not at first believe the diagnosis I made, based on a microscopic examination; but, subsequently, it was completely verified
by the autopsy. The blood is but rarely present in any great
quantity in the urine, and is sometimes quite fluid and sometimes
coagulated; the patient may, however, be much exhausted by
the frequency of the hemorrhage. Examination by means of the
catheter is sometimes not attended by any certain result, but
may, however, be the means of detecting the presence of a soft,
fungoid mass in the bladder, and may also prove of service by
noting the amount of pain or hemorrhage excited by its use, or
by its bringing away portions of tissue. Occasionally we may
examine the tumor more thoroughly per rectum than by any
other means. In rare cases, in women, the growth may so
spread along the urethra that we may actually see it. As the
disease progresses, the digestion becomes impaired as a rule,
there is loss of appetite, dyspepsia, constipation, or diarrhœa;
sometimes cancerous deposits may be developed in other organs.
The patients lose strength, emaciate quickly and markedly,
have restless or sleepless nights, and become pale and cachectic
in appearance, their skin having a yellowish, straw-colored tint;
sometimes, also, œdematous swelling of the feet and legs comes

on, and the patients die either from extreme exhaustion or from an acute thoracic affection, peritonitis, or even uræmia, if the vesical openings of the ureters are obstructed. In many cases of cancer of the bladder the patients die in about six months or a year, but, on the average, they live from one to two years, and, in rare cases, several years.

Diagnosis.

It is not, as a rule, attended by any considerable difficulty. The sudden onset of pains in the region of the bladder, frequent desire to pass water, frequent attacks of hæmaturia, the rapid and marked deterioration of the system generally, the combined results of palpation, use of the catheter, and examination per rectum, and, also, the microscopic examination of fragments voided with the urine or entangled in the catheter, render the diagnosis a matter of certainty as a rule.

Prognosis.

This is always very unfavorable. No case has been known to terminate otherwise than fatally. We can only hope for a somewhat longer duration so long as the general constitution seems comparatively slightly affected. Repeated hemorrhages or any other complication will hasten the fatal event.

Treatment.

Though surgeons of an early period, such as Lecat and Covillard, and those of modern times, as Civiale, and, following his example, Pitha and others, have been able to remove tumors from the bladder by operation, of late with the aid of lithotrity instruments, and though it seems probable that Chassaignac's excellent invention, the écrasement linéaire, may prove of great service here, yet success, as a rule, only follows operative procedures in cases of growths from the mucous membrane, pedunculated, polypoid, or other outgrowths. But, on the one hand, carcinoma of the bladder is, as a rule, not of a pedunculated character, nor even is villous cancer usually, and, on the other hand, such growths can neither be completely removed nor is there much prospect of permanent relief; therefore, our treatment is limited to palliative measures. By the very careful introduction of a catheter we may combat the symptoms of dysuria; by the methodical use of bougies, we may even prevent further complications when it is to be feared that the opening into the urethra may gradually become more and more obstructed by the increase of the tumor. If the catheter is plugged by clot or portions of the cancerous growth, the escape of the urine may be facilitated by washing out the catheter with cold water. Pain may be relieved by lukewarm baths, emollient or narcotic poultices and liniments, and, more especially, by the use of preparations of opium internally or in the form of clysters, or of suppositories of morphia, a plan which I often adopt. The patients should be freely supplied with nourishment, and the cachectic, marasmic condition must be combated by tonics. If hemorrhage from the bladder persists, the use of tincture of iron, ergotine, the infusion of ergot, alum, tannin, or, in short, any of the remedies previously mentioned as efficacious in hæmaturia, is indicated, and also cold applications externally or in the form of clysmata, or the application of a bladder filled with ice to the hypogastrium, if the bleeding is considerable. The treatment, in general, consists in carefully dealing with individual symptoms.

DISEASES OF THE URETHRA, INCLUDING GONORRHŒA.

This chapter will be chiefly taken up with the consideration of gonorrhœa, which is one of the most important affections with which medical men have to deal. The defects of development of the urethra are of more interest from an anatomical and surgical point of view than from that of clinical medicine. The simple inflammatory affections of the urethra, with the exception of the mode of origin, the specific infection, so closely resemble the slighter forms of gonorrhœa that we need only deal with them briefly. Tumors of the urethra need but a very secondary consideration. In short, both in the male and female sex, the discharges from the genitals of a purulent or muco-purulent character and arising from infection are the most important subject of consideration.

Congenital Defects of the Urethra.

In this short description, I shall follow the account given by Pitha. The cases in which the urethra is absent, or very incompletely developed, or in which a portion of it, of the pars spongiosa or of one wall, usually the lower, is deficient are extremely rare. Mere defects are well known, which are named epispadias and hypospadias, in which the opening of the urethra is situated farther back, or too low, whilst the anterior part is either deficient or imperforate, or consists of a mere groove, generally ón the under surface of the penis. A portion, only, of the glans may be imperforate, or the whole of it, or the meatus may lie still

further back and underneath, or there may be no perforation
whatever and the urine may flow through an abnormal fistulous
opening in the abdominal wall. Pitha in one such case saw a
patent urachus supply the place of an imperforate urethra. The
cases of double urethra reported are very obscure ; in several of
them, the appearance seems to have been due to false passages
which had remained permanently open; yet, such a good observer
as Vesalius is said to have seen a man whose penis had two urethral canals, one for the passage of the urine and the other for
the semen—a fact which was certainly difficult to establish with
certainty, and must remain of no value when based simply on the
patient's statement. Abnormal shortening or lengthening of the
urethra is seen not unfrequently, but the cases in which there is
much abnormal lengthening are rare. Pitha treated two cases
of stricture in which a catheter twelve inches in length did not
reach the bladder, and it was necessary to push the penis back
as far as possible before the bladder could be reached. In cases
of hypertrophy of the prostate, the prostatic portion may be considerably increased in length. As regards changes in the calibre
of the urethra, now and then, the normal enlargements at the
fossa navicularis and the bulba may be wanting, or may be
enormously increased, or there may be abnormal contractions or
dilatations at other parts, and it has also been observed that the
mucous follicles (sinus Morgagni) have had very wide orifices,
and lateral depressions of considerable size have been found near
the openings of the ejaculatory ducts. Very considerable congenital contractions of the pars nuda urethræ occur occasionally,
whilst, in other cases, there may be very considerable dilatation.
Comb-like elevations or valvular folds of the mucous membrane
of the urethra may narrow or deform the capacity of the urethra
in various ways at different parts, especially in the neighborhood of the caput gallinaginis or close to the opening into the
bladder.

The curve of the urethra may also vary, having occasionally
a zigzag course ; in children and old people the opening into the
bladder may be situated very high up. In other cases it may
lie very deeply near the rectum. The corpus spongiosum urethræ
is occasionally very thin. Ruysch describes a case in which the

urethra passed along the dorsum of the penis. Haller once saw the urethra open in the inguinal region.

Simple Inflammation of the Urethra.

Inflammation of the connective tissue—periurethritis—is rare. Primary urethritis mucosa, independent of infection, strictures, or foreign bodies, or tubercle of the urethra, is also an unfrequent disease, and occurs, for the most part, only in patients who have previously suffered from gonorrhœa or from infection. Its supposed connection with gout or hemorrhoids seems to me doubtful.

Circumscribed periurethritis has its seat either anteriorly or in the perineum; it is seldom that this inflammation spreads extensively along the urethra. The compression produced by it may cause impediment to the flow of urine—dysuria. Either the induration disappears or suppuration follows, and such abscesses need opening early, as they otherwise are very liable to burst into the urethra, and be followed by infiltration of urine or the formation of fistulæ. Periurethritis generally comes under the notice of the surgeon, as it commonly results from injury, mechanical causes, operations, etc.; but it may also coexist with contagious gonorrhœa.

Simple inflammation of the mucous membrane is mostly transitory and catarrhal in character, accompanied by but little pain or discomfort in micturition, and a clear and slight mucous discharge often results from excess in Baccho et venere, and, as a rule, when it is clearly not due to infection, subsides spontaneously in a few days. This simple catarrh may, however, last a long time, and, occasionally, may be very intractable. We ought always, under such circumstances, to examine very carefully as to whether there is any ulcer of the urethra present. It seems doubtful to me whether a merely idiopathic urethritis can take on a croupous character, and, in addition to a purulent secretion, also excite the formation of fibrinous membranes. Disregarding all traumatic causes, the presence of foreign bodies, irritation of the urethra by instruments, such as bougies, catheters, lithotrites, and also that form of inflammation which often arises apparently spontaneously, and which is due to an ulcer or a stricture of the urethra, simple idiopathic inflammation of the urethra is an unimportant and transitory affection. Its prognosis, therefore, is favorable, and its cure, as a rule, easy, within a few days or one or two weeks, by means of a bland diet, the avoidance of irritating drinks, a copious supply of milk, and absolute sexual and bodily rest. It is somewhat more obstinate when chronic contagious gonorrhœa has existed previously. We then administer internally, and also in the form of injections, tannin, or alum, or the balsams—especially balsam of copaiba in capsules. The treatment, in fact, is the same we shall have to detail when dealing with chronic intractable gonorrhœa—the so-called gleet.

Tubercular Inflammation of the Urethra.

I have but seldom had an opportunity of observing this rare and little known disease, and of verifying my diagnosis by post-mortem examination. The urethra may not only contain a few granulations, as is not unfrequently the case in tuberculosis of the genitals, but may also be affected to a much greater extent in its deeper parts toward the prostate and the neck of the bladder, and may even be actually coated and infiltrated with tubercle. Tubercular cystitis, especially affecting the neck of the bladder, is generally present at the same time. In addition to a slight discharge from the urethra, which has developed gradually without any infection, symptoms of dysuria, set up by the irritation of the neck of the bladder, present at the same time, become developed, and are the more marked, as, in addition to the increased desire to micturate, a considerable impediment is offered to the escape of the urine. We then ascertain that, for a long time, the patients have not been able to pass water in a full stream, and that the quantity has been steadily diminishing. We are astonished to find that we cannot reach the bladder with an ordinary catheter; in short, we soon find that there is great and extensive contraction of the urethra, which only yields slowly and incompletely to dilatation or even to incision. It is not only reasonable, but also established by a series of observations, that, at last, under such circumstances, retention, infiltration of urine, urinary fistulæ at the root of the penis or in the perineum, or even rectovesical fistulæ may result. I saw the most striking instances of this affection in Ricord's clinique, in Paris, and also, from the same source, at the Anatomical Society of Paris. Ricord's pupils also, especially Dufour, have published important observations on this subject.

It is obvious that the prognosis in cases of tubercular disease of the urethra is unfavorable. Not only is there a general disposition to tuberculosis or extension of tubercular disease through-out the genito-urinary organs, but also, in the majority of cases, tubercular disease of the lungs has either made its appearance previously, or does so subsequently. The patients who came under my notice, and a few whom I have seen subsequently in the department for venereal diseases in the Zurich Hospital, were all of them emaciated, much out of health, and cachectic. Dufour only describes cases in which he obtained a post-mortem. Could we even suppose that tubercular urethritis may remain for a long time as a mere local disease, like tubercular disease of the testis, with which it is so closely related, but of which there is not any evidence forthcoming as regards the urethra, yet this affection of the urethra would be quite incurable. Owing to the irritation of the urinary secretion, which will be voided the more frequently in proportion to the irritation of the neck of the bladder present, the inflamed mucous membrane will be kept in a constant state of disease, and the more so as in these situations the tubercular infiltration is not usually eliminated, but, on the contrary, steadily increases in quantity, and on this account not only excites catarrhal inflammation in the adjacent healthy mucous membrane, but also affords an increasing impediment at the deepest part of the urethra to the flow of urine, and the most appropriate local surgical treatment only suffices to check in some measure the retention of urine.

It would lead us too far if we were to enter here into the details of the treatment of tubercular urethritis. In relation to the general treatment we must refer to that of tuberculosis in general, and the local treatment is precisely that adapted for contraction of the urethra and obstinate discharge, to which we shall return later and deal with fully.

We shall now discuss the chief subject of this section.

Contagious Purulent Discharges from the Genitals and their Consequences.

Gonorrhœa and Gonorrhœal Affections.

The name "Tripper," "Clap," in use for this disease, has always seemed to me unfortunate, as being unscientific and not sufficiently expressive. So long ago, therefore, as the first edition of my Handbook on Special Pathology and Therapeutics, I advocated the adoption of the designation "Pyorrhœa of the Genital Organs." By the addition of the word "contagious" ("ansteckend") one expresses the most important clinical character of the disease, as well as its anatomical seat. I have specially avoided using the term "Urethral Pyorrhœa," because in the greater number of cases it does not hold good for the analogous disease in the female sex. In the male sex, however, we may use the expression, "Urethral Pyorrhœa," as all extensions and consecutive diseases, as well as the primary seat of the affection, are connected with the urethra. If we do not wish to prejudge the question of infection in the name given to the disease, we may designate the gonorrhœal affections by the term given in my Handbook—"Venerismus pyorrhoicus."

A Short Historical Sketch.

I have always opposed the monstrous view that syphilis is a modern disease, originating at the close of the middle ages or the commencement of modern times, and, on the other hand, have shown on what a slight foundation the theories are supported which for long were believed to substantiate this view. Except the diseases which have arisen in consequence of new branches of industry, prisons, external bad influences of all sorts not previously existing, most maladies have originated at such a very remote period of time as to be beyond the scope of history ; though, for instance, yellow fever first became known in Europe on the discovery of America, and Asiatic cholera early in the present century, the companions of Columbus found yellow fever existing in the Antilles on their first settlement. And now that we have a better knowledge of Sanscrit literature, we learn that cholera has been endemic in India for a period reaching as far back as the historical records of India, and therefore for thousands of years.

So in reference to gonorrhœa, if would appear that it was known to the Israelites at a very early period, for it is alluded to in Leviticus.[1] Not only was any one suffering from a discharge from the urethra, declared to be unclean and condemned to devote seven days after he was cured to purification, but also his bed, his chair, and his horse, were declared to be unclean. In the eighteenth century syphilis began to be recognized more and more as a special disease, but general confusion existed between gonorrhœa of the mucous membrane of the genitals and true chancres, Fernel, Fracastore, and others confounding them together. The origin of these affections from infection was also not well established. Paracelsus was the first to start the supposition that they only arose from contact, especially during coitus, but might be inherited. The latter statement of course would apply only to syphilis itself. It is only in the second half of the eighteenth century, that we find, in the work of Balfour,[2] that a real advance is made, for he held that contagious gonorrhœa was a thoroughly distinct affection from chancrous syphilis—a scientific fact now placed beyond all doubt. Unfortunately, soon afterwards the immortal John Hunter[3] caused this fact to be disputed for a long time. In his praiseworthy experiment of inoculation of the discharge from the urethra he must unfortunately have met with one of those rare and exceptional cases in which a urethral chancre was the cause of the discharge, and therefore the result of the inoculation was the production of a chancre, followed by the symptoms of constitu-

---

[1] Chap. 15, verses 1-13.
[2] Dissertatio de Gonorrhœa Venerea. Edinburgh, 1767.
[3] Treatise on the Venereal Disease. London, 1786.

tional syphilis. It is greatly to be regretted that so discriminating an experimenter as he was should not have repeated his inoculations of gonorrhœal matter; he would soon have recognized the error and danger inherent in his conclusion, formed without any foundation from his isolated inoculation, and would have saved science from great mistakes, and many patients suffering from gonorrhœa from unnecessary doses of mercury. It was reserved for the celebrated Scotch surgeon, Benjamin Bell,[1] to definitely establish the distinction between contagious pyorrhœa and chancrous syphilis, and by experiment. Two young individuals were experimented on by scarifying the skin of the glans and prepuce with a lancet, and then applying charpie dipped in gonorrhœal pus to the places for forty-eight hours. In one, a purulent discharge followed from the glans, with small erosions which quickly healed; in the other, some of the pus penetrated into the urethra and set up an obstinate gonorrhœa. A series of experiments were then made, amounting to a considerable number in all, and the distinction between the two affections was firmly established. For many years, however, Hunter's doctrine of identity retained its hold on the minds of physicians, and led to the adoption of fresh indefinite names, such as pseudo-syphilis, gonorrhœal blood-poisoning, and gonorrhœal scrofula. I was myself taught in this wholly unsatisfactory and indefinite way in my young days, and only obtained clear and satisfactory views on the subject from Ricord in Paris, in 1834. He showed both experimentally and clinically that simple gonorrhœa of the urethra has nothing in common with syphilis, so long as there is not a chancre actually present in the urethra; the chancre may be a simple, soft, non-infecting one, and possibly followed by suppurating buboes, or an indurated one followed by constitutional syphilis—points which he further illustrated by personal and very varied experiments. He also established the important fact that a negative result after inoculation was not in itself sufficient evidence to exclude the existence of a chancre, because the latter may be in the stage of simple, non-specific granulation, and may, therefore, not furnish any infectious secretion. There

---

[1] Treatise on Gonorrhœa Virulenta and Lues Venera. London, 1793.

is only one point, which is still accepted by many very competent physicians, in which I am not in accord with Ricord's teaching—that is, the denial of any peculiar specific contagious element in gonorrhœa. According to his theory, mere urethral or vaginal catarrh suffices, but I am convinced that this is untenable. Great merit attaches to Ricord for having demonstrated almost completely the mode of propagation of gonorrhœa in both sexes, and the total clinical dissimilarity between it and syphilitic infection.

It is unnecessary to give more exact historical details here, and I now pass on to describe the disease.

General Observations on Venerismus Pyorrhoicus.

Before we describe the special characters of gonorrhœa in the two sexes we will briefly mention those which are common to both.

Nature of the Disease.—In the first place, we must again insist on the absolute distinction between true gonorrhœa and true syphilis, as regards their symptoms, the localities attacked, their consequences, complications, and mode of progress ; the former never producing suppurating buboes, nor being followed by constitutional syphilis. If a soft or a hard chancre exists within the urethra, the discharge is no longer a primary affection, but a secondary consequence of the syphilitic ulcer, due entirely to its special localization. This purely symptomatic pyorrhœa, moreover, does not lead to the same consequences which we so often see in primitive gonorrhœa. If it happens, as is not unfrequently the case in practice, that a patient has both gonorrhœa and chancre at the same time, each of these affections has arisen from special and distinct contagion from its own source, either from the same person, who was affected at the same time with gonorrhœa and a chancre, or from two different individuals, who each communicated the disease from which they suffered. I have given careful attention to this subject for forty years, and the whole of my experience is opposed to the idea that gonorrhœa and chancre can proceed from the same source. It is quite true that one person may get a superficial chancre, and another a urethral chancre, by infection from the same source; but the same true syphilitic ulcer never excites in one person a similar chancre and in another a primary gonorrhœa of the urethra without any ulcer. Neither does a true gonorrhœa at one time give rise, by infection, to a chancre, and at another to gonorrhœa. It multiplies simply what it contains within itself—the germ of infecting gonorrhœa—which, to judge by its effects, differs wholly from that of true syphilis. It is an invariable rule that when suppurating buboes or infecting syphilis has followed simple contagious gonorrhœa, the primary syphilitic ulcer or primary infecting tubercle has been overlooked. How easily this may occur, as regards the inner surface of the prepuce, especially at its lower part, if it be tight; how easily an ulceration at the base of the glans may escape observation, especially if balanitis exists; how easily, also, such may fail to be noted on the pudenda unless careful search is made. This may occur still more easily if, in addition to gonorrhœa of the genitals, a primary syphilitic ulcer existed near the anus, or in the mouth, or on the finger, as so often happens in the case of medical men and midwives.

Contagious gonorrhœa is, therefore, essentially distinct from syphilis. Of those who maintain their non-identity some consider that gonorrhœa is a simple inflammation, and others assert it to be a specific morbid process. The first say that urethral pyorrhœa may occur in men from mere excess in coitus, from drinking immoderate quantities of beer, or from having connection with a woman who merely suffers from leucorrhœa, or who is menstruating at the time. Really, this only shows that the urethra may be the seat of catarrhal inflammation set up by irritation of various sorts, and, as a rule, passing away quickly and without ill-consequences, but not at all that every pyorrhœa is a simple catarrh. Without speaking too lightly of the female sex, I hold that any argument as to the morality, and any conclusion based thereon as to the healthiness of any woman yielding to the wishes of a strange man, are not very trustworthy. It often only shows that the conceit and vanity of men themselves are not in the least diminished by their own visible disease. I am, therefore, certainly of opinion that gonorrhœa depends on a specific principle, which is communicable by contact. On the one hand, I have always observed that women only catch gonorrhœa from men when the latter undoubtedly have gonorrhœa, of which I often had certain evidence as a medical man. On the other hand, I have pretty constantly found that women who have infected men have led gay and dissolute lives, though sometimes very secretly, the fact being better known to the circumspect physician than to the lover. Many women affected with gonorrhœa, who had previously suffered from leucorrhœa, have asserted to me positively that they could tell exactly when the leucorrhœa was converted into gonorrhœa. Though this may not be always possible, especially when the female urethra is intact, still we have an important aid in the infection of men having connection with such a woman. I have treated many respectable women suffering from fluor albus, and have never known their husbands to be affected with a true gonorrhœa in consequence of it alone. At the most, and very exceptionally, they have had a transitory and insignificant catarrh. There is exceedingly little force in the argument that the seasoned husband may escape, while the lover is affected. Where such a thing happens at all, it seems to me, on the contrary, much more probable that the intervention of a third individual affected with gonorrhœa has conveyed the disease to the woman and through her to the lover. And where a woman gives gonorrhœa to her lover she also generally conveys it to her husband, unless she is able by various means to prevent his having any intercourse.

It is therefore in the highest degree probable that there is a specific contagious element inherent in gonorrhœal pus, but the microscope and chemical analysis are, however, just as unable to detect it as in the case of a chancre. We may suppose that some sort of fungoid specific germ may be developed in the deeper part of the urethral mucous membrane, and set up a contagious inflammation, but the fungus may not be evident, except rarely, in the secretion. It would be highly desirable if we could examine the diseased mucous membrane itself at an early period.

That this specific pyorrhœa depends on some peculiar agent may be gathered from its course. For, if we regard most of the consequences of gonorrhœa as inflammations in continuity, and the ophthalmia as a direct transference, yet the latter sometimes appears at a time when direct transference could not occur, and if even then a local, though certainly scarcely demonstrable, infection is suggested, there still remains the rheumarthritis gonorrhoica, which has a decidedly peculiar character, and can neither always be regarded as articular rheumatism complicating the gonorrhœa, nor be explained by continuation of the inflammation or local infection. A denial is a very easy solution of the difficulty.

We arrive, therefore, at the two following conclusions :

1. The venerismus pyorrhoicus depends on a peculiar contagious element, different from that producing a chancre.

2. The whole class of these affections represents a distinct group of diseases, etiologically, clinically, and therapeutically.

Anatomical Characters.

In spite of the definite peculiarities of these affections, their anatomical characters are not by any means specific. Chiefly affecting mucous membranes, gonorrhœa has all the characters of ordinary inflammation of mucous membrane ; it begins near the surface where the contagious secretion is first applied, and thence spreads towards the interior of the body ; it is attended by redness, with scattered or more general hyperæmia, swelling of the mucous membrane, considerable increase in the secretion of mucus, with the addition of many wandering leucocytes, and in severe inflammation there are also red corpuscles; subsequently the swelling, hyperæmia, increased mucous secretion, and escape of leucocytes diminish, the superficial epithelium desquamates, and the secretion of mucus gradually abates—such are the anatomical characters, and they are those of any catarrhal inflammation. Neither is there anything very peculiar in the inflammation by continuity which attacks the glands opening on the surface of the mucous membrane, and which may result in abrasions and ulcerations which may share with the localized fungoid outgrowths of the mucous membrane in producing subsequent contraction. Moreover, the extension of the inflammation to other tissues than mucous membranes—as, for instance, from the vas deferens and the vesiculæ seminales to the epididymis ; in women, extension to the large sebaceous glands of the labia and Bartholini's vulvo-vaginal glands ; in men, to the large conglomerate glands of Mery, or the glands of Cooper—simply follows the ordinary laws governing extension of inflammation by continuity in general. I have frequently taken the greatest trouble to find some specific material by microscopic examination ; but even the highest magnifying power and the best immersion lenses detected only ordinary pus-cells, cast-off epithelium, and fine granules, and the microscopic fungi present here and there do not differ from those met with on the surface of any mucous membrane exposed to the air. This does not in any way show, however, that there is no such specific germ which must be sought for especially in parts not in contact with air, as, for instance, deep in the mucous membrane and in the interior of the epididymis. We find just the same in diphtheria, where the fungoid elements on the mucous membrane do not show any special peculiarities, but, owing to the mode in which they make their appearance and their action in distant internal organs, distinctly point to a fungoid infection. Whilst in the male subject gonorrhœa enters at the urethra, and is specially located there, in women it attacks much larger surfaces and various structures, and for this reason gonorrhœa in the female is the exception instead of the rule, the vulva being the starting-point of the gonorrhœal inflammation as a rule, and the mucous membrane around the orifice of the os uteri occasionally, though usually when the disease attacks this part and the mucous membrane of the uterus generally, it does so by extension. Gonorrhœal ophthalmia, which is so dangerous to vision, is very instructive in relation to the specific nature of the disease. Ordinary catarrh is one of the most frequent maladies, and when inoculated on the conjunctiva merely produces, at the most, a slight and transitory catarrh. Just as in trachoma, inoculation only gives rise to trachoma, so the gonorrhœal secretion, when applied to the conjunctiva, excites the well-known dangerous gonorrhœal ophthalmia, which may permanently injure one or both eyes in the course of a few days.

Symptoms and Course.

The course of the disease is no less characteristic. There is a stage of incubation, which lasts, as a rule, for one or several days, but may vary in duration from a few hours to six or eight days, or longer. During this time the gonorrhœal germs, which, while in small quantity, were not pathological, have probably increased till, by sufficient multiplication, they have set up disease in the mucous membrane. The different phases presented by the symptoms also correspond to this gradual increase; at first there is considerable sexual excitement, turgescence of the external genitals, and mucous secretion, and, before long, decided pain, redness and swelling of the mucous membrane, muco-purulent secretion, according to the locality affected, great sensitiveness of the urethra to any irritation, pain on micturition, and painful coitus. The secretion of mucus steadily increases to marked secretion of pus, and is not unfrequently mixed with blood; the quantity of secretion may also be very considerable in both sexes. As a rule, the symptoms increase during the first eight or ten days, remain about as long at the maximum of severity, and then gradually diminish until they disappear, which happens in favorable cases at the end of three or four, usually, however, only at the end of six or eight weeks, unless a slight mucous discharge remains for a still longer period. As a rule, the gonorrhœal inflammation especially spreads along mucous surfaces, ducts of glands and their corresponding glands; not unfrequently the lymphatic vessels share in the extension of the inflammation, and the submucous connective tissue and even the adjacent lymphatic glands may become swollen, the inflammation of the adjoining connective tissue possibly entailing very important consequences.

Etiology.

We have already remarked above that though simple irritation may excite a catarrh of the mucous membrane resembling gonorrhœa, yet, as a rule, sexual intercourse with some infected person is the cause. Where, however, the disease has become chronic, or where the sequelæ which are difficult to cure, such, for instance, as strictures of the urethra, or growths from it, remain, any irritation of the genitals may set up an acute gonorrhœa. Women suffering from simple leucorrhœa, even with granulating or spreading ulcers of the neck of the uterus, do not communicate gonorrhœa. It is erroneous to conclude, with Ricord, that the more purulent the secretion, the more contagious it is. In many women suffering from fluor albus, pus-cells in considerable quantity may be detected without any infection occurring; the virulence depends solely on the intensity and quantity of the specific gonorrhœal poison; the mucous membranes of the urinary and genital organs, and also the ocular conjunctiva, appear especially obnoxious to this poison, whilst the gastro-intestinal mucous membrane is much less capable of infection.

Whilst I believe it to be quite certain that gonorrhœa depends on a specific contagion, yet I willingly admit that its action may be modified by a number of accidental circumstances. We are well aware that the gonorrhœal contagion does not always excite gonorrhœa; it may dry up, or by ablution or micturition may be quickly washed away after coitus. On the other hand, the chances of infection may naturally be much increased by disproportion in the size of the genitals, small female or large male organs, by long continuance of coitus, or by a quick repetition of it, etc.

Diagnosis.

It is of the first importance not to place too much reliance on the statements of the patients; vanity, hypocrisy, interest, and shame have great influence on them; on the part of the medical man, however, tact and discretion are very necessary in these matters, as otherwise he may be the means of seriously disturbing domestic peace and family happiness. In the male, the diagnosis of ordinary gonorrhœa is not usually attended with difficulty; we must, however, examine as carefully as possible whether a chancre is not concealed by the prepuce, or whether there is one just within the urethra, and, for this purpose, the lips of the meatus must be carefully separated. If any suspicion exists as to the presence of a chancre, inoculation is indicated; the simple gonorrhœal secretion does not produce any pustules when inoculated on the individual affected, whereas such will be produced if there is a urethral chancre; a negative result, of course, is of much less diagnostic value than a positive one.

In the female, the diagnosis is often not by any means easy; urethral gonorrhœa is much less common in them than in men, and, if a woman knows she is going to be examined, she passes water previously and washes the urethral secretion away. I have repeatedly been told by women suffering from contagious gonorrhœa that even when they were at the time suffering from muco-purulent leucorrhœa they could nevertheless appreciate the exact period at which the gonorrhœa came on, and Ricord's vast experience has led him to the same conclusion; the change to the contagious affection being marked by symptoms of acute irritation, great sensitiveness on sexual intercourse, and acute purulent vulvo-catarrh. If the urethral affection is absent, as is so often the case, there is no certain sign; one rather arrives at a moral conviction that gonorrhœa is present than at an absolute certainty, and, in such cases, I am very cautious in giving my opinion either in a court of law or in private practice. In all such matters it is very difficult to arrive at the truth. A husband, for instance, complains that his wife has infected him; the wife may actually have caught gonorrhœa from a third party; and, at the same time, it is just as likely that the husband, having had intercourse with other women, has caught the disease from another source, and his wife may accuse him as justly as he can accuse her.

Prognosis.

This is favorable, as a rule, and most so in the so-called gonorrhœa of the glans—balanitis—which, when present alone, is due either to simple irritation or venereal ulceration. Gonorrhœa of the female genitals is, as a rule, not by any means difficult to cure, and also is comparatively seldom followed by ill-consequences, whilst urethral gonorrhœa in the male has not only a decided tendency to be intractable and become chronic, but owing to the strictures which are liable to result from it, to the possibility of an extension of the inflammation to the epididymis, or of a transference of gonorrhœal matter to the eye, it is a more serious affection. I have frequently heard patients say that they had rather have had an attack of constitutional syphilis which could be cured by mercury or iodine, than a gonorrhœa followed by a scarcely controllable gleet, or a stricture of the urethra defying all methods of dilatation, and have silently agreed with them. Double epididymitis may be followed by sterility owing to obliteration of both vasa deferentia, of which I have seen instances. I would strongly urge a young practitioner never to treat a case of gonorrhœa too slightingly.

General Treatment.

Notwithstanding that so much has been written as to the prophylaxis of venereal diseases, there is little or nothing of any efficacy in preventing contagion, except protecting the penis by a condom from contact with the virulent secretions of gonorrhœa or syphilis. Efficient supervision and frequent examination of prostitutes may do much to check these diseases, but, on the one hand, many may become infected between any two examinations, and, on the other hand, the number of women and girls who cannot be subjected to examination is considerable. It would lead me too far to go into further details on this important subject of hygienic measures. The chances of infection are diminished by avoiding roving and excess in venere, and the quick repetition of coitus with any woman who is even suspected. Careful ablution and micturition soon after coitus may wash away the infecting mucus. All astringent lotions and injections, of which we shall speak further by and by, are of no use as prophylactic measures, and may even very much aggravate the disease. The fact that the chances of contagion are diminished by circumcision applies more particularly to chancrous than to gonorrhœal infection, and cannot be recommended as a preventive measure.

We have but little to say, also, in regard to special treatment. We have long ceased to entertain any prejudice which would lead one to believe it possible to cure gonorrhœa too quickly; rest, low diet, the avoidance of any sexual excitement, and the local application of cold are most suitable in the early stage of irritation; whilst later, balsams and astringents, internally and in the form of injections, as soon as the inflammatory symptoms have subsided, must be perseveringly employed. Further details will be given when treating of the affections separately.

Urethral Pyorrhœa in the Male, Gonorrhœa in the Male.

The affection which is met with by far most frequently is pyorrhœa urethralis, urethral clap, gonorrhœa, chaude-pisse, blennorrhœa; pyorrhœa of the rectum, due to unnatural connection, is comparatively rare. Urethral pyorrhœa or urethral clap, in the male, is characterized by a muco-purulent or distinctly purulent discharge from the urethra, accompanied by more or less severe scalding, and usually caused by intercourse with a suspected person.

Etiology.

As regards acute gonorrhœa, we must refer to what we have already said in our general remarks on pyorrhœa. We shall only remark here that, though we are convinced that in by far the greatest number of cases gonorrhœa springs from gonorrhœa, originates in contagion, and spreads in the same way, there are also special predisposing causes of its development. Among these are: tedious or long-continued intercourse with a woman suffering from gonorrhœa, several repetitions of coitus at short intervals, excess in venere, and, at the same time, indulgence in spirituous liquors, especially drinking much beer, eating a quantity of asparagus, or taking very warm baths. Any one who has once had gonorrhœa is very liable to have it again. The occurrence of gleet is favored by incomplete treatment, neglect of the requisite temperance and dietetic regimen during the acute stage, bad external hygienic conditions, over-fatigue, especially from rid-

ing, chronic dyscrasiæ of all sorts, repeated attacks of gonorrhœa previously, and especially slight, scarcely noticeable commencing stricture of the urethra, chronic inflammation of isolated
urethral glands, and chronic circumscribed inflammation and
swelling of the mucous membrane at the commencement of the
urethra, which I have often observed to be a cause of gleet. I
have very often, also, noticed that patients have protracted their
gonorrhœa for a long time by pressing on the glans and urethra
several times a day, in order to squeeze out drops, by this means
continually irritating the urethra; and I have often quickly
cured the gleet by instructing the patient to desist from this
mischievous manipulation. It is also important for the young
practitioner to know that the introduction of even the softest
bougie excites an increased discharge. This is, however, but
transitory, and the gleet may not infrequently be cured by appropriate treatment of the same sort.

Symptoms.

From one to two, rarely from four to six, but it may be even
eight days or more after the suspected intercourse, the patient experiences a voluptuous sensation, with sexual excitement, and tendency to seminal emissions, followed by itching of the glans, and
the lips of the meatus are stuck together by viscid mucus. The
meatus soon becomes slightly irritated, swollen, and congested.
The tickling sensation and itching become converted into a pricking or burning pain, the swelling increases, micturition becomes
painful, and sets up a burning sensation in the fossa navicularis
which lasts for some time, and the urine, as it flows, brings away
muco-purulent flocculi from the urethra. An opaque discharge,
at first of a yellowish gray color, and then yellowish green, and
consisting of pure pus, now begins to come from the urethra.
At the end of the first week the pain, scalding, and greenish
purulent discharge have usually reached a considerable intensity, and, at the same time, the lips of the meatus are red,
swollen, and very sensitive. Occasionally the anterior surface of
the glans is reddened, and inflammation of the lymphatics occurs, with swelling of the inguinal glands. Young, powerful,

plethoric patients not infrequently have a slight amount of fever. Sometimes the whole prepuce becomes œdematous. The patient has but little rest at night, being excited by voluptuous dreams, and sleep being interrupted by painful erections and emissions. The sensitiveness and pain in the urethra gradually spread backward to the level of the scrotum, and micturition is attended with difficulty, and the stream is diminished ; the patient cannot sit without discomfort, and defecation is attended by agonizing pain. In the majority of cases, however, the various painful symptoms begin to abate as early as the second week, and disappear, as a rule, in the third ; the purulent discharge, however, remains copious, and in some patients erection is attended by pain for some time. From the fourth to the end of the sixth week the discharge gradually diminishes, becomes less purulent and more mucoid, and either disappears entirely, a complete cure resulting, or becomes transformed into a chronic gleet, which is a blenno-pyorrhœa rather than a purely purulent one ; of this we shall speak later. Gonorrhœa may vary in character according to the constitution of the patient, the degree of its severity, and, especially, according to the complications present. We will now deal more in detail with the different forms.

1. Slight, Superficial, Sero-Purulent and Mucous Gonorrhœo-Catarrh.

Though this slighter form is not by any means strictly defined, since the epithelial and mucous catarrh may pass into the deeper purulent form, and, inversely, a gonorrhœa which commences acutely and with purulent discharge frequently changes into the slighter form, yet the latter represents a special type, which may either be developed primarily and as a first attack, or, in some cases, may follow on previous repeated attacks of pyorrhœa with relaxation of the mucous membrane. The primary superficial form of gonorrhœa is distinguished from that which appears at a later period and secondarily by its being located in the fossa navicularis, while the secondary form is situated in the membranous and prostatic portions of the urethra. In the slighter form of gonorrhœa, the inconveniences are less severe, micturition is attended by little, if any pain, the mucus squeezed out from the meatus is viscid, of a greenish yellow rather than yellowish green color, and contains desquamated epithelium and a comparatively small quantity of leucocytes. The discharge is comparatively slight and glues the edges of the meatus together, which are then separated each time the urine is voided, but without any pain. When examined on a glass slide, or in a watchglass, the secretion is seen to contain many threads and flocculi of mucus. We do not, however, by any means always regard this slighter form of gonorrhœa as easily curable; in favorable cases, it may, it is true, disappear in a few days, but is, not unfrequently, very obstinate, and may, as has already been mentioned, become aggravated into the more severe form, which, however, may sometimes have the effect of accelerating the cure. Not unfrequently a concealed urethral chancre coexists with this form, and may be followed by its special ill-consequences. The slightest form of this primary gonorrhœa is just as contagious as the most severe form.

2. Inflammatory Pyorrhœa.

This is characterized from the first by much greater severity; the persistent sense of uneasiness, and the discomfort in micturition, increasing to dysuria, being very troublesome. The mucous membrane at the entrance of the urethra is so greatly swollen, that it bulges over the opening; the copious discharge consists almost exclusively of pus-cells, and has a yellowish green or greenish color, and, occasionally, owing to admixture with blood, may for a time be of a dirty yellowish brown tint. Micturition is not merely very painful, but also, in the more severe cases, an insufficient quantity of urine is voided in an interrupted, fine stream, and, in the most severe cases, the bladder may even remain incompletely emptied for days. In other cases, the frequent desire to pass water, owing to spasm of the neck of the bladder, may be very distressing. The quantity of the purulent secretion is considerable; its reaction is feebly alkaline, and it contains microscopic fungi. The inflammation may spread outward on the surface of the glans and along the inner surface of the prepuce, while the outer surface is œdematous, and the constant swelling of the corpora cavernosa keeps the whole organ enlarged and in a state of incomplete erection. In this form of inflammatory gonorrhœa, which is mostly met with in young and vigorous individuals, the patients complain of a sense of great discomfort, depression, languor, loss of appetite, and, not unfrequently, there is at first slight fever. If anything, the nights are worse than the days. Sleeplessness, pain, and dysuria are accompanied by frequent and painful erections, which are more troublesome than in the daytime, and are not unfrequently followed by painful emissions. By absolute rest and mild diet, especially a milk diet, these extremely troublesome symptoms begin to abate considerably in the second or, at latest, in the third week, and we then have the symptoms above mentioned of the usual form of gonorrhœa. Micturition steadily becomes less painful, the discharge diminishes and becomes more fluid, and a cure results, as a rule, at the end of six weeks. After the slightest excesses, however, or even without them, relapses not unfrequently occur, and the cure may be incomplete, a chronic intractable slight discharge remaining.

Amongst the more important symptoms met with in individual cases, may be mentioned the hemorrhagic or black gonorrhœa, in which there is a large quantity of blood mixed with the discharge, a form which is rarely observed here. Great inconvenience may arise also from isolated submucous, periurethral patches of inflammation, which may spread to the corpora cavernosa, and either terminate in resolution if not very severe, or go on to suppuration, and if incisions are not made early may lead to very troublesome urinary fistulæ. Cicatricial indurations remaining in the cavernous tissue may subsequently permanently interfere very considerably with the normal erection of the penis. During the inflammatory stage of the gonorrhœa, erection may not only be exceedingly painful, owing to stretching of the inflamed mucous membrane or inflammatory exudation, but, in consequence of the latter condition, may give a peculiar curve to the organ when in a state of erection, the so-called chordee, which may affect one side only, or the whole penis may be curved. This condition disappears, as a rule, with the inflammatory stage. Permanent ill-consequences may arise from the prevailing idea that chordee may be removed by a blow from the edge of the palm held flat. The rapid disappearance of the chordee under such treatment can only be due to considerable lacerations.

Among the symptoms which indicate that the case has taken a favorable turn may be mentioned the so-called gonorrhœal threads, which may be seen to float as whitish streaks of various lengths if we mix the discharge with water when the secretion has become very much diminished in quantity and of a seromucous character; they are also present in the urine. They consist of cells undergoing retrograde metamorphosis held together by mucus. We shall speak of gleet in detail further on.

Anatomical Changes.

The above-mentioned symptoms of inflammation of the mucous membrane have their starting-point in the fossa navicularis, and steadily spread from here backward almost as far as the opening of the urethra into the bladder; and as early as the second or third week the membranous and prostatic portions of the urethra are affected, though the subjective symptoms are throughout referred to the fossa navicularis. Anatomically, it is of great importance, in reference to sequelæ, as to whether the part of the urethra where the bulb passes into the membranous portion is affected, for, owing to the numerous glands situated in this part, as well as farther forward, close to the entrance of the urethra, the mucous discharge may be protracted, and in consequence of ulcerations and the formation of cicatrices strictures may subsequently occur here or in the membranous portion. They may also result from localized outgrowths of the mucous membrane, being followed by indurations.

Chronic Pyorrhœa—Gleet.

That the anatomical changes just mentioned are of great importance in reference to this disease is obvious. The pain has disappeared, the discharge has lost its purulent character, but nevertheless there is still a mucous secretion which may contain some pus-cells from the urethra, especially in the morning, and the lips of the meatus are adherent in the morning before the urine is voided for the first time.   The patient's curiosity induces him, not only in the morning, but also several times in the course of the day, to squeeze the urethra to see whether any mucus will escape.   This frequent squeezing is often the means of protracting the urethral gonorrhœa, and we must strongly urge the patient to discontinue the practice entirely.   As a rule, if there is no stricture, the urine is voided easily and normally, and the only pain complained of will be an occasional pricking sensation in the neighborhood of the fossa navicularis, or in the deeper portions of the urethra, or in the perineum, and occasionally in the anus.   All these symptoms may be aggravated for a time by dietetic or sexual irregularities, over-fatigue, etc., and temporarily also, now and then, by seminal emissions.   If this intractable catarrh is situated in the deeper portion of the urethra, it may not unfrequently be aggravated by indiscretion on the part of the patient in drinking and sexual intercourse, and occasionally without any demonstrable cause, into an acute purulent catarrh, and these are the cases in which, if no deep-seated changes exist, the gonorrhœa, which has again become acute, is more quickly cured than would otherwise have been the case.   Occasionally this sort of catarrh may even be so aggravated as to take a croupous form, which is described by Zeissl[1] as follows: "A patient, whose urethra would seem to have returned almost to its normal state, suddenly complains of a severe tickling sensation in the perineal portion of the urethra. The discharge, which had previously become mucous, nearly disappears, but micturition is attended with more difficulty, and the stream of urine becomes smaller.   If we pass a moderate-sized bougie along the urethra in such a case, and subsequently after the removal of the bougie inject a syringeful of water, the fluid injected into the urethra will bring away with it, at one time or another, clear white membranous masses more than an inch long, which to the naked eye do not resemble the hyaline

---

[1] Lehrbuch der Syphilis. 2. Auflage. Erlangen, 1871. Bd. 1. S. 24.

epithelial tubes undergoing fatty degeneration previously mentioned, but band-like or cylindrical, firm masses of fibrine, which are due to the fact that a fibrinous exudation has occurred on the free surface of the mucous membrane, and, therefore, on the epithelium. The band- or tube-like firm masses, of which we are now speaking, cannot be drawn out into threads by stretching, but tear short off. When acetic acid is added, they swell up and become transparent like fibrine, while it is well known that mucus is made opaque by the addition of acetic acid and coagulates into threads. These croupous affections, according to our experience, are mostly situated in the membranous portion of the urethra, and appear to be set up usually in consequence of the injection of strongly irritant fluids, such as a solution of corrosive sublimate. We reported such a case in the year 1852,[1] and exhibited the band-like membranous masses at the same time. In the same year also Hancock[2] published a similar observation."

As a rule, a few drops of discharge collect in the urethra during the night, and escaping upon the linen leave behind colorless, or grayish yellow, or yellowish green, small, stiff spots; while in acute gonorrhœa the linen is stained to a much greater extent with yellowish green pus, or, not unfrequently, with brown, sanguineous spots. While in acute gonorrhœa a few drops of pus may always be seen to escape from the meatus on the slightest pressure being applied to the anterior part of the urethra, this only occurs to a very slight degree, and not by any means constantly, in gleet. In the daytime, also, only a drop escapes at a time. It is quite a mistake to call this discharge, which escapes drop by drop, goutte militaire, for, though it is an uncivil and intractable disease, yet it does not occur at all more frequently among soldiers than among civilians. This disease is extraordinarily intractable, lasting not unfrequently for months, and occasionally for a year, or several years; some patients even are never quite cured, though it may disappear for a time, and the discharge may have lost its purulent and infectious character.

[1] Zeitschr. des Ges. der Aerzte zu Wien. 1852. Heft 1.
[2] On the Anatomy and Physiology of the Male Urethra, etc. London, 1852.

Diagnosis.

Both the acute and chronic forms of gonorrhœa are easily recognized in the male subject. Gonorrhœa of the glans, balanitis, is distinguished from gonorrhœa of the urethra by the fact that in the first the discharge is confined to the space around the glans, and that no pus escapes when the urethra is squeezed. The whole course of the disease differs from that of a simple catarrh, which may in some cases develop without any sexual intercourse, and in the others after moderate and untainted intercourse, and usually disappears quickly. The same occurs when the gonorrhœa is in great measure due to a disproportionately large penis or violent efforts to enter a small vagina. Rest for a few days and cold applications suffice usually to cure the malady quickly. The diagnosis from a urethral chancre is assisted by the fact that the latter is frequently situated at the commencement of the urethra, and may often be directly exposed to view by separating the lips of the meatus. If this cannot be accomplished, then inoculation when it is successful, the detection of an induration in the course of the urethra, and especially the existence of the characteristic, painless, indurated, and swollen inguinal lymphatic glands, and the appearance of characteristic syphilitic symptoms, will enable the medical man in the great majority of cases to arrive at a correct diagnosis. The absence of any positive result after inoculation is not conclusive evidence as to the absence of a urethral chancre. The most important and trustworthy evidence in such cases, therefore, is disease, painless enlargement of the inguinal glands, in the first place, and then by degrees of many of the superficial lymphatic glands. Lastly, in gleet, it is always necessary to ascertain whether there is any stricture of the urethra, or outgrowths from it present, conditions which may be mostly recognized by there being some, though it may be slight, difficulty in making water, and by the stream being diminished in volume.

Prognosis.

Usually the prognosis in cases of gonorrhœa is not by any means unfavorable. It is well, however, to speak cautiously to the patient. It not unfrequently happens that a patient, for naturally special and urgent reasons, is anxious that the medical man should cure him in a few days. The practitioner must, however, represent to the patient with tact and caution that this is un-- likely to occur. Other patients, who will not press for so speedy a cure, will want to know how long the disease will last, or how long it will be necessary for them to abstain from intercourse without fear of communicating the disease. On all these points it will be necessary to speak very cautiously. The slightest attacks of gonorrhœa are often those which last the longest and are the slowest in yielding to treatment. It not unfrequently happens that with the best possible treatment a gonorrhœa will appear to be quickly cured, but will then, when incompletely cured, remain stationary or even become chronic. On the other hand, the practitioner must not hold out too little prospect of speedy relief, or else the patient will simply go to another medical man. Tact and caution, as well as professional knowledge, are, as a rule, highly necessary in the prognosis of all venereal diseases. A first attack of gonorrhœa, coming early under treatment, in a young, vigorous male, who will assist medical treatment by abstinence and attention to diet, admits of the most hopeful prognosis. The inflammatory forms are more hopeful than the cases in which the disease is insidious and atonic. When there have been previous attacks of gonorrhœa, the subsequent attacks are generally less severe, but intractable. Among the complications, the most important are extension to the neck of the bladder, and abscesses in the course of the urethra and in the prostate, as they may cause the disease to be very much protracted. Permanent indurations of the corpora cavernosa are particularly troublesome, as they lead to persistent malformation of the penis and a state of incomplete erection. In chronic gonorrhœa the prognosis as to duration is particularly doubtful, but it is not so difficult to cure if there be no signs of stricture. The latter is a very serious complication, owing to its intractability and the tendency to relapses. Lastly, it is important to bear in mind that gonorrhœa alone is never followed by symptoms of constitutional syphilis, and that it is very rarely that a careful practitioner will meet with a concealed chancre which cannot be detected. There is, of course, a great difference between non-recognizable and non-recognized ulcers of this sort.

Treatment.

We have already discussed the question of prophylaxis in gonorrhœa with sufficient detail. Another equally important question is that of the abortive treatment. Here let me say that according to my experience there is no sort of evidence that we have it in our power to make any actually specific gonorrhœa abort. It has, indeed, several times happened to me to cut short an attack, to the great delight of the patient, but I was not in a position to determine whether in these cases I had to do with simple or specific pyorrhœa, though discharges were caught from women quite competent to excite gonorrhœa. The treatment which I usually employ in these cases is at least quite safe. The patient being kept perfectly at rest and under strict regimen, I order the following to be injected thrice daily :

> ℞. Acidi tannici.............. ℥ ss. (2.0)
> Zinci sulphatis............ gr. xv. (1.0)
> Aquæ destillatæ........... ℥ iv. (120.0)

In order to avoid any staining of the clothes, the penis should be wrapped in linen after the injection, and should also be carefully wiped dry.

Internally, I order, at the same time, moderate doses of cubebs or balsam of copaiba. On two occasions I have seen a gonorrhœa so treated quickly checked ; not unfrequently this method has seemed to do no good whatever, but I have never seen it do any harm.

The method recommended by Debney, Ricord, and others, of injecting nitrate of silver in large doses, from ten to fourteen grains (0.6–0.9) to an ounce (30.0) of water, is employed in the following way : the patient having previously passed water, the penis is put slightly on the stretch, and the injection made; severe pain very quickly follows, and spreads along the spermatic cords; at the end of an hour the pain abates; micturition is then accomplished with difficulty, and there escapes at the same time a white membrane, resulting from the cauterization, and at the end of twenty-four or forty-eight hours the pain and the gonorrhœa should both have disappeared. Theoretically this method is quite satisfactory, since caustic fluids, such as nitrate of silver, often quickly produce a change for the better in acute and recent inflammations of mucous membranes. But this plan is not unfrequently followed by deep-seated, phlegmonous inflammation of the urethra, severe pain, and sanguineo-purulent discharge,—in short, by all the signs of intense urethritis; if, therefore, we can by this means deprive gonorrhœa of its specific character, yet we substitute generally a more troublesome and dangerous malady than that which we had to treat. We must bear in mind, further, the practical rule that different mucous membranes resist the nitrate of silver in very different degrees; whilst the mucous membrane of the mouth, throat, nose, larynx, and female genitals, and the conjunctiva, especially when severely affected with gonorrhœa, will bear even concentrated solutions of nitrate of silver quite well, the urethra and the mucous membrane of the bladder, especially, are very sensitive to its influence; I therefore regard this plan as a dangerous one, and consequently consider several repeated injections of this sort, or cauterization with Lallemand's porte-caustique, as still less advisable.

At the very commencement of an attack of gonorrhœa I have seen very good results follow the use of cold, in the form of cold applications around the penis, or, more particularly, in the form of injections with cold, or ice-cold water, every two or three hours. I have also often succeeded in allaying the scalding during micturition by instructing the patient to pass his urine while his penis was under cold water.

Each year I become more convinced that under a moderately strict regimen gonorrhœa yields more readily than if one is too lenient on this point: milk, mucilaginous drinks, or broths, fruit which has been cooked, greens, a small quantity of white meat, bread, potatoes, also in small quantity, form the most appropriate nourishment, especially during the first fortnight. Subsequently we may allow more substantial and more animal food. Coffee, tea, beer, beverages containing carbonic acid, Seltzerwater, champagne, and, among vegetables, asparagus, especially, are to be avoided. At a later stage wine, and especially good red wine, in small quantities, may be allowed, but sparkling wines are to be avoided ; in addition, the bowels must be carefully kept open, partly by fruit and vegetables, partly by clysmata, mild electuaries, cold infusion of senna, or compound liquorice powder, composed of sulphur, senna leaves, sugar, anise, and liquorice-root, the three latter being added to improve the taste, while saline purgatives are never to be administered in gonorrhœa. The most complete rest, especially in the recumbent posture, as little movement as possible, and the use of a properly fitting suspensorium, which does not exercise any compression, and especially not posteriorly, are greatly to be recommended. For the painful nocturnal erections and emissions I usually order two or three of the following pills, to be taken in the evening :

> ℞. Camphoræ,
> Lupulini......... āā gr. xxx.–xlv. (2.0–3.0)
> Ext. opii........ gr. ivss. (0.3)
> Ext. glycyrrhizæ. q. s.
> u. f. pil. xxx.

Bromide of potassium, also, in doses of from eight to fifteen grains (0.5–1.0), taken at bedtime, gives many patients a better night's rest. For any of the other painful sensations complained of, the extract or tincture of cannabis indica or of belladonna, or small doses of opium, may be ordered with advantage. The most important internal remedies we possess for the treatment of gonorrhœa are cubebs and balsam of copaiba.

Cubebs is, comparatively speaking, much milder in its action and is better borne by the stomach, but is decidedly inferior to the balsam of copaiba in curative power. As is well known, it contains cubebine, oil of cubebs, resin, and extractive matters ; the two former, prepared separately, and also the ethereo-alcoholic extract, have been tried in gonorrhœa, but according to Clarus [1] are not specially efficacious. I have myself always used cubebs in powder, and at a very early stage, beginning with small doses of thirty grains (2.0) thrice daily in half a glass of eau sucrée, increasing the dose daily by thirty grains (2.0) till the patient takes two (8.0) or even three drachms (12.0) three times a day. It is only in exceptional cases that any eruption on the skin or irritation of the stomach and intestines occurs; the drug should then be discontinued, and also if no improvement follows after the larger doses have been given for eight or ten days. The urine of such patients has a peculiar odor, and the same may be detected in the breath; the odorous substance is unknown, and it has also never been shown whether it or some other substance is the effective agent in the cubebs; this much only is certain, that both cubebs and balsam of copaiba act by virtue of some peculiar substances which are either formed solely in the organism, or are only modified, pass out with the urine, and impart to it a curative power on the specifically inflamed urethra. Ricord also recommends the combination of cubebs in the doses above given, with alum in powder in doses of from twenty to thirty grains (1.25-2.0) thrice daily in moist wafers, a draught of water being taken afterwards.

The balsam of copaiba is obviously the most important of all the remedies administered internally—one might call it a specific for ordinary gonorrhœa—but it is not well borne by the stomach and intestinal canal, and, if continued for a long time in large doses, is liable to excite symptoms of cardialgia, and, at first, severe purging. If this is only slight, without any special disturbances of the system generally, its influence is beneficial rather than otherwise. I have never found that the balsam of copaiba has had the influence on the brain attributed to it by Ricord,—that is, of producing a state of congestion only passing off on the discontinuance of the remedy; but I have repeatedly met with the peculiar eruption, which is sometimes of a roseolous character and sometimes greatly resembles measles, or is more like urticaria or lichen urticans. It is accompanied by severe itching,

---

[1] Handbuch der spec. Arzneimittellehre. Leipzig, 1856. S. 1028.

is situated chiefly in the neighborhood of the joints and on the extensor surfaces, sometimes on the neck, and disappears in a few days if the remedy is discontinued. That even distinguished dermatologists should confound this eruption with roseola syphilitica is certainly a wilful, I might say, a malevolent mistake. The balsam of copaiba also imparts a peculiar odor and a special curative power to the urine. When applied locally to the urethra, it irritates and makes matters worse. Pereira states that he employed the ethereal oil in doses of from ten to twenty drops in gonorrhœa with good results.

On account of its unpleasant taste and disagreeable odor, the balsam of copaiba has been administered in very various ways. Many medical men, regardless of improving the taste, order it in doses of from twenty to forty drops or more thrice daily in a solution of sugar. The best way of disguising the taste is, undoubtedly, to use gelatine capsules; these, however, are much too dear for hospital and any but well-to-do patients; of the well-known Mothe's capsules, I administer from two to six or more thrice daily. Each capsule contains about four and a half grains (0.3) of the balsam; they are made up with gelatine or gluten. It would certainly be very desirable in practice to have capsules so constructed that one could pour ten or fifteen drops into one of them, close it with a cover of gelatine, and then let it be swallowed, such, for instance, as I saw in Paris, which one could buy in the form of small boxes consisting of two shell-like portions; the capsules are quickly dissolved in the stomach, and the copaiba is absorbed. For hospital practice, I have prescribed a very simple formula, in which the taste of the copaiba is fairly disguised, and which is well adapted for private use among poor patients; it is as follows:

> ℞. Copaibæ............. ℨ i.-ij. (4.0–8.0)
> Extracti glycyrrhizæ.. ℨ ij.-iv. (8.0–16.0)
> Aquæ destillatæ...... ℥ vi. (180.0)

Of this mixture the patient takes from three to six tablespoonfuls or more daily. We may also order the daily dose in a mixture specially prescribed, beginning with a dose of half a drachm (2.0) daily, and increasing it to two drachms (8.0) daily.

If the copaiba purges severely or causes indigestion, a grain (0.06) of extract of opium may be added. At first, I made the balsam into an emulsion with powdered gum or mucilage before mixing it with the water and the liquorice, but I have since found that the latter alone forms an excellent mixture. Another plan which can be recommended is that suggested by Simon, in which half an ounce (16.0) of the balsam of copaiba is mixed with half a drachm (2.0) of tincture of orange-peel, and from twenty to thirty drops of the mixture given thrice daily in a glass of Madeira or gin. Many attempts have also been made to make the balsam semi-solid by the addition of magnesia, and then to form a capsule with a thin layer of gum ; this is the composition of the so-called Raquin's capsules, which I used a good deal in my practice in Paris and with a good result, in doses of from four to eight thrice daily. Of great repute in France and Germany is also the well-known Chopart's mixture, which has the following composition :

> ℞. Copaibæ,
> Syrupi tolutani,
> Aquæ menthæ piperitæ,
> Alcoholis .... āā ʒ i. (30.0)
> Spiritus ætheris nitrosi.......... ʒ ss. (2.0)
> A tablespoonful to be taken two, four, and six times daily.

In this form, however, the balsam is much more unpleasant to take than in the formula which I have recommended.

Balsam of copaiba has also been ordered in various ways in the form of electuaries, which have this advantage, that one can prescribe them in a cheap form and let them be taken enclosed in wafers ; it is also well, however, at the same time to add a small quantity of an ethereal oil, especially oil of mint which will mask the disagreeable odor, especially when eructation occurs. Balsam of copaiba and cubebs may be ordered together in pills or electuaries, and this combination is to be specially recommended if cubebs alone is not efficient, and copaiba alone in large doses is not borne. Trials with the individual constituents of copaiba have not been attended with any satisfactory results, neither has the use of matico. In obstinate cases, if copaiba is not borne, it is much more useful to order alum or tannin internally in increasing doses, amounting at last to large doses of as much as half a drachm (2.0) or more daily.

As in inflammatory affections of the eye the acute inflammatory element must subside considerably before we can have recourse to the undoubtedly useful local application of collyria; so also in gonorrhœa of the urethra, under similar circumstances, the use of injections is of manifold service; one might say they are indispensable. The india-rubber syringes employed must be quite air-tight, the injection should be made slowly, and we must begin with small quantities. It is well to give an injection of water for cleansing purposes merely before using a medicated one; the latter should gradually be left in longer and longer, from a quarter of a minute to several minutes, the opening of the urethra being closed. Injections which are made slowly penetrate more effectually and more deeply than those which are made quickly. The injections should at first be unfrequent, but should gradually be increased till they number from three to six in the day.

It has already been mentioned that of late I have found cold-water injections of great service in the early stage of gonorrhœa, from four to six being given in the day, and I have never seen any of the ill-results follow their use, of which many practitioners have been afraid.

So soon as the gonorrhœa ceases to be attended by pain and severe scalding, I order injections of tannin, which is better borne by the urethra than any other astringent in gradually increasing doses of from four to fifteen grains (0.3-1.0), or even thirty grains (2.0) in an ounce (30.0) of water, at first only every evening, and subsequently morning and evening, the injection being most suitably made with a syringe of hard rubber, or, in the absence of one of these, with a blunt-pointed glass syringe. The tannin is not completely dissolved, even if the solution is made with hot water; but it is quite probable that its efficacy depends on the fact that the tannin remains in direct contact with the diseased mucous membrane; the burning sensation caused by the concentrated mixture is but transitory and soon passes off. If the remedy does not act quickly, as sometimes happens in old and neglected cases, I add from two to four grains (0.12-0.3) of sulphate of zinc to the ounce (30.0). Ricord recommends a combination of sulphate of zinc with acetate of lead in the following form :

> ℞. Zinci sulphatis,
> Plumbi acetatis.............. āā gr. xx. (1.25)
> Aquæ rosæ.................. ℥vi. (180.0)

If the urethra is very sensitive I add from one to four grains (0.1–0.3) of extract of opium to the injection. Zeissl recommends an injection of fifteen grains (1.0) of alum with four grains (0.25) of sulphate of zinc in four ounces of water. He frequently substitutes acetate of zinc in somewhat larger doses for the sulphate. We may also vary the mode of using the astringents from time to time.

It is only in very intractable cases of gleet which resist the tannin and zinc that I use the nitrate of silver, and then in increasing doses of from one to two grains (0.06–0.12) to the ounce (30.0) of water, which generally excites a burning sensation. If the discharge is more copious and more purulent subsequently, it is well to desist for a few days, and it is not by any means rare for the gonorrhœa to disappear then entirely. In obstinate cases I have now and then derived great benefit from the use of a solution of corrosive sublimate employed cautiously in small doses of from half a grain to a grain (0.03–0.06) in six ounces (180.0) of water.

If gonorrhœa resists all these remedies, there are still certain other injections which have been employed empirically, and which we will mention; and, on the other hand, we must not neglect to make a careful exploration in order to ascertain whether a commencing stricture is not the cause of the intractability ; if so, dilatation with a sufficiently soft wax bougie is the best plan to be adopted ; of this we shall speak later when dealing with strictures of the urethra.

Of the empirical injections, we must specially mention that of port wine diluted, recommended by Simon. Ricord recommends diluted aromatic wine, also a solution of forty-five grains (3.0) of tannin and alum in three ounces (90.0) of rose water and the same quantity of Roussillon wine. Various solutions of copper and iron have·been recommended, but they are not of any special benefit.

If the patient has already used various kinds of injections without avail, we often succeed best by abstaining from their employment, or, at the most, merely ordering an injection of cold water once daily, advising the patient not to squeeze the penis or draw it forwards, recommending hip-, river-, or sea-baths, and administering balsams, astringents, or tonics internally. After an interval, balsam of copaiba will often be found of service again, but should it not be well borne, I prescribe one or two pints of tar-water with from an ounce to four ounces (30.0–120.0) of syrup of tolu in the course of the day, or order the latter with a decoction of uva ursi of the strength of two drachms (8.0) to sixteen ounces (500.0) of water. The *decoctum turionum pini* has obtained celebrity as a drink. Finally, if we have to do with feeble or scrofulous individuals, or those whose constitutions have been enfeebled by excesses, the best treatment often consists in substantial, tonic food, especially meat, with good racy wines, Burgundy, port, or Madeira, change of air, residence among the Alps or at the sea-side, and, lastly, the internal administration of quinine and preparations of iron in the form of two or three pills thrice daily, each pill containing one grain (0.06) of quinine and the same quantity of the lactate of iron with extract of gentian. The following formula of Ricord's is very worthy of notice:

R. Syrupi tolutani.............. ℥ xvi. (500.0)
Ferri citratis................. ʒ ij.–iij. (8.0–12.0)
A tablespoonful to be taken four times a day in a glass of tar-water.

Cod-liver oil, sulphur-baths, and salt-baths may be of service under certain circumstances. In short, the practitioner in these cases does not so much adhere to a methodical line of treatment as devote careful attention to thoroughly investigated local and general indications. In several cases of late years I have met with very good results from sea-bathing in intractable gleet not dependent on stricture.

We have previously mentioned a number of troublesome inflammatory complications, which require special modes of treatment.

When the penis is curved and in a state of spastic erection, chordee, the pills of camphor, lupulin, and extract of opium, previously mentioned, are very serviceable, also clysmata of camphor and opium, about four ounces (120.0) of camphor emulsion, containing 0.36 gr., with twenty drops of laudanum for a clysma, or a hypodermic injection of morphia; also, if the persistent use of cold locally is of no service, general, long-continued, lukewarm baths may be tried; the forcible rupture of the bow-like curvature, however, is an utterly objectionable plan. If the patient has already tried it, as is not unfrequently the case in France, hemorrhage from the urethra is easily produced, and may require the application of cold, or of pressure by means of a gum-elastic catheter introduced into the urethra.

The medical man cannot be too careful as to the treatment of dysuria, or retention, if it exists; he cannot use the catheter too early. A copious supply of mucilaginous drinks, emulsions of lactucarium and opium, repeated and long-continued lukewarm baths are to be most strongly recommended, and the patient must be advised as to the need of considerable patience. If these means are not successful, we must introduce a gum-elastic catheter, one of Lasserre's by preference, with extreme care and gentleness. If we cannot reach the bladder without using force, we must then try soft wax bougies, and the attempt is often followed by the flow of urine being renewed; as a last resource, the bladder may be punctured.

Treatment of Chronic Pyorrhœa.

The treatment of chronic pyorrhœa is a matter of far greater difficulty and importance, and the reasons for this, as we have already pointed out, may be very various. We ought never to take such a case in hand without at once making a careful examination with a bougie; and this examination should be repeated several times in the course of the treatment; we may either use a soft wax bougie of sufficient consistence, or an elastic conical one, such as Lasserre's. If, on introducing a bougie of moderate size, pain is produced at a particular spot in the pars membranacea, we may suspect the existence of a catarrhal ulcer or follicular erosion, but can only be certain that such is the case if we find mucus or pus, though it may be in but slight quantity, in the fluid which escapes after slowly and carefully injecting the urethra with pure water. The microscope may reveal the presence of débris of tissue, as well as of mucus and epithelial cells, and leucocytes. If we find little clots of blood washed away by each careful injection, they would suggest the presence of exuberant granulations, which may spring from a small ulcer or from localized outgrowths from the mucous membrane. In rare cases of croup of this part of the urethra, according to Zeissl, we may wash away tubular portions of membrane. For the most part, however, these ulcerations and granulations only give rise to discharge during the first few months, as they subsequently cicatrize and contract, and cause stricture of the urethra. The latter is a much more frequent cause of protracted gonorrhœa, of intractable gleet, than any one who has not had much experience in the matter would imagine. The introduction of bougies constitutes the only effective treatment in such cases. If we find an obstruction in the deeper part of the urethra, where the most troublesome strictures are generally situated, which one cannot overcome by any amount of perseverance, we shall have not only discovered the seat of the cause of the gleet, but also the calibre of the bougie, which finally passes the obstruction, enables us to estimate the degree of constriction present. We must always avoid forming any opinion as to the existence or non-existence of a stricture from the merely vague statements of the patient as to the mode in which the stream of urine passes.

If, on examination, we find evidence of the existence of simple ulcerations or granulations, we should introduce a bougie daily, and leave it in for a short time, and then inject a solution of tannin, or zinc, or copper, the *cuprum aluminatum* (*lapis divinus*) being the most suitable form of the latter, in the proportion of from three to five grains (0·2–0·3) to three ounces (100·0) of distilled water or rose-water. Zeissl also recommends an injection of from six to eight drops of the solution of chloride of iron to three ounces (100·0) of water, and also emulsions of insoluble, astringent metals, in the proportion of half a drachm (2.0) of bismuth or oxide of zinc to three ounces (100-0) of water, and well shaken up. Under such circumstances, I prefer the strong solutions of tannin, previously mentioned. In intractable cases, in which there are probably granulations, Zeissl also recommends the introduction of a bougie, which has been previously dipped in a solution of gum and then coated with powdered bismuth. He advises a similar method of treatment, also, when croupous membranes are formed, and he injects a solution of from one and a half to three grains (0.1–0.2) of chloride of zinc in four ounces (120.0) of water. All the astringent injections before mentioned may be employed one after the other in such cases. Tannate of lead must also be specially mentioned. It is formed by adding fifteen grains (1.0) of acetate of lead, with eight grains (0.5) of tannin, to four ounces (120.0) of water. As in using injections it is difficult to avoid leaving more or less conspicuous stains on the linen, it is well, after the injection and after the penis has been properly washed, always to have the glans and anterior part of the urethra wrapped in a piece of linen, so as to avoid leaving any such.

Not only is dilatation the sole treatment available when stricture is at the foundation of the continuance of the chronic discharge—and we must here avoid being misled by the increased discharge which occurs at the commencement of the cure by bougies—but also, without any stricture being present, the careful use of bougies may result in the cure of gleet when injections have utterly failed. We shall enter into detail as to the question of dilatation when dealing with the subject of stricture. Of course, while the discharge continues we must let hygienic measures go hand in hand with the local treatment. Beer and beverages containing carbonic acid must be especially avoided, and also excesses of any sort, or any over-fatigue, and great moderation as to sexual intercourse must be enjoined. Warm baths are but rarely of service; cold hip-, river-, or sea-baths are much more beneficial. Of internal remedies, the balsams, capsules of copaiva, etc., may be serviceable at different times; but when remedies have to be continued for a long time, I prefer the astringents which pass off by the urine, alum and tannin, which certainly

deserve more notice in the treatment of pyorrhœa, and are well
borne for a long time in comparatively large doses.

Balanitis, Balanopyorrhœa, Balanopostheitis, Catarrh of the Glans and Prepuce, Gonorrhœa of the Glans.

The prepuce is already predisposed to become irritated on
account of the frequency with which it is covered and made
dirty by the secretions of the sebaceous glands of Tyson, especially when the requisite attention is not paid to cleanliness,
which, indeed, is very difficult, if the prepuce is narrow. Gonorrhœa of the glans is usually rather a seborrhœal catarrh of the
glans. It is well known that all these conditions predispose to
the occurrence of chancres in this region. It is quite true that a
purulent balanitis often occurs in patients affected with gonorrhœa, but it is exceptional for this to be caused solely by
virulent gonorrhœal secretions, for we never meet with balanitis
attended by copious secretion and following on gonorrhœa in
those who have been circumcised. It partakes rather of the
nature of a simple inflammation set up through the gonorrhœal
discharge from the urethra getting under a tight foreskin.

The patients complain of severe itching, even burning, in the
region of the glans, and frequently of great sexual excitement.
Externally, the prepuce is slightly reddened and swollen, sometimes œdematous, while internally, distinct sero-purulent discharge mixes with the sebaceous preputial secretion. Subsequently, ulcerations occur here also not unfrequently. The odor,
which naturally is very disagreeable, is made still more so by
the inflammation, and a spreading lymphangitis may be developed. As a rule, however, the secretion of pus diminishes by
appropriate treatment, and after from eight to fourteen days a
cure follows. In rare cases, however, adhesions occur between
the prepuce and glans, and in one case of the sort I had a great
deal of trouble to remedy them by operation. In still rarer
cases, I have seen gangrene of the prepuce occur, but as far as
my experience has gone, this has invariably resulted favorably.

It is obvious that when there is a tight foreskin, there may
be no little difficulty experienced in discovering whether the

balanitis is of a simple character or set up by a syphilitic ulcer. The simple erosion may be distinguished at the first glance from a soft or hard chancre, but if any doubt remains, inoculation will settle the point; an erosion will not be followed by any result, while a chancre will produce another chancre. If the prepuce is a very tight one, avoid circumcision if there is any probability that there is a syphilitic ulcer present. Dilatation by means of a sponge-tent, changed in a few days and replaced by a larger one, is the most convenient means of getting the foreskin back.

In simple balanitis, the prognosis is very favorable. The

Treatment

is comparatively simple. Careful and repeated cleansing, and the introduction of a strip of linen or charpie dipped in cold water or lead lotion, between the glans and the prepuce, suffices in average cases; whilst, if the secretion is more abundant, an astringent fluid (a solution of salts of lead or zinc, alum, tannin, or nitrate of silver) must be injected four or five times daily between the glans and prepuce, and the charpie or lint placed between the glans and the prepuce should be dipped in the same solution. When the prepuce is tight, we combine the dilatation by means of sponge-tents with the use of astringents. In obstinate cases, we may cauterize the whole of the inner surface of the prepuce and the glans with a stick of nitrate of silver, or with a concentrated solution. If the inflammation is severe and acute, we wait awhile before applying astringents, and envelop the penis, laid against the abdomen, in compresses dipped in iced water and frequently renewed. If the disagreeable odor and fetid discharge indicate that gangrene is threatened or commencing, we must not hesitate to slit up the whole prepuce. Under certain circumstances also, if the glans is still constricted in spite of slitting up the prepuce, circumcision may be necessary. Paraphymosis should be reduced at once, and if this cannot be done without operation, we must pass a director from before backward beneath the constriction and then divide the latter, which can generally be accomplished without difficulty.

Inflammation of Lymphatics and Lymphatic Glands in Consequence of Gonorrhœa.

All the secondary consequences of gonorrhœa result more or less from extension of the inflammation, and when such cannot be demonstrated, the etiological connection between the gonorrhœa and the disease in some distant part is often doubtful.

Inflammation of the lymphatics to a slight extent is a very common occurrence in pyorrhœa. More rarely we meet with lymphangitis, properly so-called, in the form of painful swelling and red streaks in the course of the lymphatics, which on the dorsum of the penis follow the blood-vessels; parts so affected are very painful on pressure, on movement, and during erection. As a rule, these symptoms disappear in from eight to ten days, or somewhat later. The lymphangitis may, however, extend as far as the inguinal glands, which then become swollen and painful; but only extremely rarely, in scrofulous or tubercular subjects, or in others whose constitutions have become very much enfeebled, does suppuration occur.

In a few cases, some weeks or months after an attack of gonorrhœa, I have observed a number of enlarged lymphatic glands in the inguinal region on one or both sides, in the form of small, painless, movable glandular tumors of the size of beans, which have gradually disappeared. I have never seen tubercular degeneration take place; the enlargement of the glands invariably disappears after some time. The observation of such glandular swellings very probably gave rise in former times to the extravagant notion of there being a gonorrhœal scrofula.

The ordinary forms of gonorrhœal lymphangitis yield to rest and cold applications, and the swelling of the lymphatic glands mostly disappears spontaneously; in the intractable cases of enlargement of the lymphatic glands I have seen good results follow methodical treatment with iodide of potassium. I prescribe it in the form of pills, each containing a grain and a half (a decigramme), with a sufficiency of liquorice, and I order from one to three or four (the dose being increased by degrees), to be taken thrice daily.

Inflammation of the Submucous Connective Tissue and of the Periurethral Glands.

We have already seen in how many ways inflammation of the mucous membrane may extend to the submucous tissue and possibly suppuration ensue. It is obvious that such collections of pus must be opened early. The same also applies to suppurative inflammation of Cowper's or Meny's glands. The ducts of these glands are first of all affected by inflammation in the bulbous and membranous portions of the urethra. The inflammation then extends to the parenchyma of the glands and the surrounding connective tissue, and a lobulated or uniform circumscribed tumor makes its appearance in the perineum between the anus and the scrotum; it is painful, renders it difficult for the patient to sit down, excites dysuria owing to pressure on the urethra, and causes pain on defecation. When the disease has attained this degree of severity, suppuration usually occurs, and it is of the greatest importance to provide a free outlet for the pus by incision, as, otherwise, the abscesses may easily burst into the urethra and infiltration of urine occur, and even be followed by symptoms of pyæmia. Few of the secondary consequences of gonorrhœa require such prompt surgical interference, while delay may entail most unpleasant results. We must also take care that an opening which has been made early enough is kept open as long as suppuration lasts. In the slighter cases, rest, the application of cold, and the use of sedatives suffice to effect a cure.

Induration of the corpora cavernosa is fortunately rare, but is an extremely troublesome complication; it is not painful *per se*, but may be attended by ill-consequences, owing to the fact that a portion of their cavernous structure may become filled up with indurated cell and cicatricial tissue, in consequence of which the blood required to produce erection cannot gain entrance to this part, so that the penis does not become straight, but, according to the seat of the partial induration, the glans is curved upwards or downwards when erection occurs, while if the whole circumference of the upper part of the corpora cavernosa be in a state of induration, the penis is only capable of erection at its lower part, and the upper part hangs down quite flaccid. It will be easily understood that, under these circumstances, incapacity to effect intercourse may result. I have never myself, however, observed such a condition, but it has been several times described, and especially by Ricord. According to the latter, in such cases, while the posterior part of the penis is fully capable of erection, the anterior portion of the glans hangs down flaccid and like a flail; and it is difficult in such cases to decide whether the absurd plan of rupturing the curve was not the cause of the permanent induration of the corpus cavernosum.

Inflammation of the Prostate, Prostatitis, and Swelling of the Prostate in Consequence of Gonorrhœa.

The ducts of the prostate become affected by the gonorrhœal secretion, and either a slight attack of catarrh is set up in them, or the inflammation spreads to the substance of the gland and its connective-tissue elements; when the latter occurs, suppuration often follows.

Catarrh of the Prostate.—When the discharge is of a simple, sero-mucous character, a tenacious, clear fluid of a light yellow color is effused several times daily into the urethra, and leaves yellowish stains on the linen. Zeissl calls attention to the fact that in these patients, at the end of micturition, urine always trickles drop by drop, and that the lips of the urethra subsequently are never so dry as is the case in a healthy individual. Pressure of any sort on the prostate, even that occurring during defecation, causes a momentary expulsion of this fluid. In its simplest form this catarrh of the prostate forms a urethral catarrh which is often very intractable, especially if the patient's mode of life be unsuitable. Hemorrhoidal enlargement of the veins in the neighborhood of the prostate and anus renders the condition more intractable. Owing to very urgent desire to pass water, or to the introduction of instruments, hemorrhage may occur. At a later period, the secretion in the ducts may become inspissated, concretions may form, and so cause swelling of the prostate, which, if long continued, may lead to hypertrophy—a starting-point by no means unfrequently of senile hypertrophy of the prostate. The catarrh may also easily spread from the ducts to the neck of the bladder. If this catarrh is complicated with stricture of the urethra, pseudo-intermittent feverish paroxysms, which Zeissl associates with the thrombosis, phlebitis, and periphlebitis of the plexus urethræ et vesicæ venosus described by Virchow, may occur from time to time.

Suppurative Prostatitis, in contrast to the form just described, is an acute disease, and severe throughout its whole course. Painful swelling of the prostate rapidly occurs, whilst the gonorrhœa ceases for a time. A constant sense of pressure, often increasing to pain, a tumor which may be felt from the rectum, or even in the perineum, considerable dysuria, the impossibility of sitting, and the necessity of lying with the legs outstretched, characterize this painful affection. Defecation becomes so agonizing that the patient wilfully abstains from relieving the bowels. The dysuria may increase to absolute retention. At the same time a state of fever, which is often ushered in by a rigor, is developed, and in many patients is not by any means inconsiderable. After these severe symptoms have lasted three or four, or even six or eight days, a considerable discharge not unfrequently takes place suddenly, owing to the abscess or abscesses in the prostate having opened into the urethra. Occasionally the practitioner may open such an abscess involuntarily while passing a catheter to relieve an attack of retention. All dysuria naturally disappears with the bursting of the abscess; the urine still contains pus for a time and then returns to a normal state. If other abscesses form, the disease may become protracted, but will be less severe than at first. More rarely, an abscess dependent on periprostatitis set up by gonorrhœa may burst externally in the perineum, and may be unattended by the ill consequences which otherwise result. It is remarkable that under these circumstances, though pus escapes freely into the urethra, yet usually no infiltration of urine results from the establishment of the discharge. It is rare for an abscess to open into the rectum, and is a much more troublesome occurrence; an abscess may burst very exceptionally into the urethra and into the rectum at the same time, and then, of course, owing to the more extensive disturbance which occurs, a urethro-rectal fistula, or even infiltration of urine, may result.

Prognosis.

The prognosis in the sero-mucous form of catarrh of the prostate is not by any means unfavorable as to the severity of the symptoms, but the question of duration is more doubtful, for the disease may last a very long time. Abscess of the prostate runs an acute course, but generally ends in recovery. If a rigor occurs at the commencement, it generally indicates suppuration. The bursting generally gives relief, and is soon followed by recovery ; and if, in consequence of rather extensive suppuration, a considerable portion of the tissue of the prostate is sometimes destroyed, this is not attended by any very ill result, while the swelling of the prostate which remains after the slighter, transitory catarrh of the prostate is not only intractable, but, if not relieved, is very liable to be followed later in life by troublesome permanent enlargement of the prostate and its consequences. The more serious import of bursting of the abscess into the rectum has been already mentioned. In the cases of tubercular disease of the prostate which I have observed, I could not trace any connection between it and past gonorrhœal inflammation of the prostate.

Treatment.

The thorough, methodical treatment of the gonorrhœa of the urethra is essentially the sole prophylactic. On the slightest indication of inflammation of the prostate we must enjoin complete rest, the horizontal position being maintained constantly, and an unirritating and scanty diet. The severe pains will be best relieved by prolonged and repeated lukewarm hip or immersion baths, and in the intervals by the application of warm poultices to the ano-perineal region. Among the sedatives which may be required to mitigate the pain, we may first of all try the milder ones,—tincture of cannabis Indica, or of belladonna in doses of from eight to twelve drops every two or three hours, or suppositories of butter of cacao containing one-sixth grain of extract of belladonna, the same quantity of morphia being substituted for the latter if no relief is produced ; we may also administer a sub-cutaneous injection of morphia in such cases once or even twice daily. The cure will be expedited by the inunction of mercurial ointment into the perineum. The regular evacuation of the bowels is to be insured by castor-oil or enemata of oil. If retention occurs, the catheter must be used with care ; the best instrument is a Lasserre's catheter, and if difficulty is experienced in reaching the bladder, the catheter may be left in. For the fever, we give acid drinks, lemonade, small quantities of very much diluted phosphoric acid, etc. The local abstraction of blood, formerly in such repute, has too transitory an effect to be of service save in exceptional cases.

If doughy infiltration with redness, indicating suppuration, shows itself externally, a sufficiently free opening should be made as early as possible. Bursting of the abscess into the urethra requires no special treatment, whilst if the abscess opens into the rectum, lukewarm water should be thrown up after each evacuation of the bowels in order to wash away any fecal matter lodged in the opening.. Any other consequences must be treated by surgical means.

If a chronic catarrh of the prostate results, unless this is owing to stricture, which must be treated by dilatation, astringents must be ordered internally and locally, followed by the preparations of iron, and to complete the cure, chalybeate mineral waters, residence in the country or amongst the hills or at the sea-side, and sea-baths, with nourishing or unirritating diet, must be recommended.

Inflammation of the Spermatic Cord and of the Epididymis, Epididymitis Pyorrhoica.

This mode of extension of the inflammation is one of the most frequent results of gonorrhœa; it spreads from the prostatic portion of the urethra to the vas deferens, and then usually quickly involves the epididymis, and but rarely and very exceptionally remains confined to the spermatic cord. As a rule, it occurs in connection with neglected gonorrhœa, or in cases in which hygienic conditions have been much neglected, though the treatment in other respects may have been appropriate. Extension of the inflammation to the vesiculæ seminales, which we may feel to be swollen and painful on pressure, on examining per rectum, is an occasional complication, and possibly a more frequent one than is generally believed, of the epididymitis. As a rule, only one side is affected, but it is not at all an unfrequent occurrence for the side which escaped at first to be subsequently involved. The development of the affection is hastened by fatigue, excesses, prolonged standing, walking, or riding.

Sometimes prodroma precede the inflammation, such as sexual excitement, seminal emissions, pain in the inguinal or lumbar regions. The patients also not unfrequently complain of a sense of uneasiness in the testis itself. The symptoms are increased by standing or walking, while in the horizontal or resting position they cause but little inconvenience. When they have lasted for a day or two the patient complains of severe pain in one testis, and especially in the epididymis, and the pain may extend along the spermatic cord, or even down the thigh. The skin of the scrotum becomes reddened, hot, and swollen; the epididymis is swollen, very sensitive, and hard, and the testis is pushed forward and upward, is but slightly sensitive, only slightly swollen, and not at all hard. The vas deferens and the parts around it, as well as the whole spermatic cord as far as the abdominal ring, are hard, painful, and twice or thrice as thick as in the normal state. The patient can neither stand nor walk. During the first few days there is often a slight amount of fever. The pain and swelling increase during the first four or five days, then remain for a time stationary, and so far disappear in the course of the second week that the patient suffers but little inconvenience; but for some time to come sensitiveness on pressure remains, and longer still, it may be for the rest of the patient's life, the epididymis remains hard. The disease is much more slow in its progress, and more painful, if the inflammation attacks the opposite epididymis, or, to speak more correctly, extends along the other ejaculatory duct. It is but rarely that we observe any considerable participation of the testis in the inflammation; it is more common for it to be accompanied by inflammation of the tunica vaginalis. The pain and swelling then become more marked, the tumor of the tunica vaginalis is more pear-shaped, and there is distinct fluctuation. As a rule, this inflammatory effusion quickly subsides, but occasionally it may remain for some time. I have never, however, seen a true chronic hydrocele result from this inflammation of the tunica vaginalis.

When suppuration occurs in the course of epididymitis, as it does in rare cases, it will be found, according to my experience, that in not a few of these tubercular disease of the prostate exists at the same time, and commonly that it has existed previously. I have, however, met with exceptions. Occasionally we observe extensive induration result, which is very intractable, and not unfrequently ends in atrophy of the testis, and if this occurs on both sides, complete, wholly incurable impotence results. I have often observed this, and it is due, at any rate occasionally, to obliteration of the vas deferens, which has been demonstrated anatomically by Gasselin and Duplay.

Owing to this induration, which may remain a long time, and the possibility of such obliteration, I always in my clinic attach special importance to the necessity for energetic treatment of the disease and its results, which, as the pain often passes away spontaneously in the course of a few days, is often regarded too slightingly by the practitioner. A rare form of the disease, but one of a very troublesome character and attended by much pain, is that in which the inflammation attacks a testis retained in the inguinal region, and which has not passed through the inguinal canal. Here, in addition to the painful symptoms otherwise met with, we have those due to strangulation. Usually, however, recovery follows. It is scarcely possible for epididymitis to occur when the testis is retained within the abdomen, for it is then usually atrophied.

We have already mentioned that protracted and in any way neglected gonorrhœa may lead to orchitis. It is, therefore, a great error to suppose that the use of injections, or of cold, will excite the inflammation formerly regarded as metastatic. On the whole, young and vigorous healthy men are at least as much predisposed to it as those who have a scrofulous or tubercular tendency. The influence of occasional causes has been already dealt with.

Prognosis.

This is not *per se* by any means unfavorable, as the patients are able to resume their ordinary avocations again, as a rule, in the course of a few weeks. The epididymitis has but a slight tendency to terminate in suppuration, unless tubercular deposits are present. Even the inflammatory hydrocele becomes absorbed as a rule; but the induration which remains subsequently, demands the greatest attention, and may lead to obliteration of the vas deferens and atrophy of the testis. In rare cases we may meet with recurrences, especially in careless patients and those who have been neglected.

Treatment.

Prophylactic measures are here of the utmost importance. Early and energetic treatment, rest, and the application of cold, in the inflammatory form, specifics in ordinary gonorrhœa; wearing a suspender, which I recommend to all my private patients affected with gonorrhœa; rest as far as possible in a horizontal position; the avoidance of much walking, and especially of riding; a moderate and scanty diet; the careful avoidance of sexual excitement, are, as a rule, sufficient to prevent the occurrence of epididymitis, and I have very seldom met with it in private patients when they could or would take care. Fathers of families often cannot, and young, thoughtless people will not take care.

Rest in the horizontal posture is particularly necessary in the treatment of the disease, and the scrotum should be elevated by a thick conical cushion placed under it. Cold applications, or, if there is great pain and considerable swelling, the application of leeches to the corresponding inguinal region is serviceable. Warm poultices or fomentations diminish the pain after the first intensity has passed away. The induration remaining should be carefully treated, and I generally administer iodide of potassium internally for some time in doses of from nine to eighteen grains (0.6–1.2) daily, and use an ointment externally of iodide of potassium or iodide of lead, in the proportion of a drachm (4.0) to the ounce (30.0) of lard. If an abscess forms, which is often of a tubercular character, it must be opened as soon as fluctuation can be detected. I only employ compression, which has been so much recommended, when intractable induration remains, and by means of strips of strapping applied so as to overlap one another; a layer of them is first applied horizontally, and then a vertical layer superficial to and crossing the other.

Usually the gonorrhœal discharge ceases as soon as the epididymitis commences, and it is indeed a great mistake to try to excite it anew. If it does return again after the inflammation, it is simply an ordinary gonorrhœa to be treated by balsam of copaiva and injections.

Diseases of the Bladder, Ureters, and Kidneys Dependent on Extension of Gonorrhœal Inflammation. Cystitis, Pyelitis, Cystopyelitis Pyorrhoica.

That contagious gonorrhœa, which usually extends as far as the immediate neighborhood of the neck of the bladder, should reach this, and, by further extension, the kidneys, is far less remarkable than that it should not happen much oftener.

It is exceptional for the catarrh of the bladder to occur early; as a rule, it only comes on after the urethritis has lasted for weeks, and if, as is so often the case, the catarrh of the neck of the bladder is then neglected, the disease steadily spreads till at last, in the most extreme prolongations of the mucous membrane of the kidneys, it reaches the limits of the urogenital mucous tract. Though the catarrh of the neck of the bladder generally commences acutely, and only becomes chronic and extensive from neglect, yet it may, from the first, be of an insidious character and latent. In the ordinary acute form more or less severe dysuria comes on unexpectedly, the desire to pass water is not merely troublesome, severe, but also comes on very frequently. Each time micturition is attempted only a small quantity of urine is voided with great trouble and much pain; and, in the intervals, a sense of uneasiness continues to be felt in the neighborhood of the neck of the bladder, and the irritation is not unfrequently accompanied by fever. The urine is also sometimes mixed with blood when voided, and when collected deposits a brownish, blood-colored, muco-purulent sediment. The urethral discharge diminishes, and becomes sero-mucous; the sensitiveness and pain do not merely extend over the ano-perineal region, but also not unfrequently over the base of the bladder, which is painful when pressure is made over the pubes. Still more troublesome is the affection when it becomes aggravated to complete ischuria, and the introduction of a catheter, when the bladder is distended, is rendered very difficult by the great amount of spasm and inflammatory irritation of the neck of the bladder, so that only an elastic catheter can be introduced.

The moderate amount of fever present, and its short duration in even severe cases of this sort, have struck me as remarkable, while the gastric symptoms, loss of appetite, coated tongue, retching, occasional vomiting, hiccough, etc., often attract greater attention. As a rule, the vesical tenesmus begins to diminish considerably as early as the sixth or eighth day, no more blood escapes, the quantity of muco-pus diminishes, and convalescence dates from the second or third week, to go on steadily to recovery. The malady may, however, easily recur, or become very protracted, and finally utterly chronic. The proliferation which may then take place in the neck of the bladder may subsequently give rise to those evil consequences which the conical excrescence, often wrongly called third lobe of the prostate, excites. Subsequently, also, there may be a very troublesome, painful sensation on emission of the semen whenever intercourse takes place. In rare cases, according to Zeissl, there may be a chronic catarrh, a spermatorrhœa, of the vesiculæ seminales, and the catarrh may also spread to the ducts of the prostate. In these cases, on strong pressure, on straining at stool, etc., mucus escapes, which is mistaken for semen. Chronic vesical catarrh may originate from the neglected acute form with protracted gleet, beginning with symptoms of spasm of the neck of the bladder, with occasional hæmaturia, and later being associated with comparatively slight dysuria, but with a constant purulent condition of the urine, which gives a neutral or alkaline reaction. For further details I must refer to the description of chronic vesical catarrh. After some months under appropriate treatment, this affection may disappear completely, but in other cases may be very intractable.

Prognosis.

As regards prognosis, we may say that acute catarrh of the neck of the bladder is much more painful than serious, and as the patients suffer too much to allow of their neglecting themselves, they submit much earlier to curative treatment than those suffering from chronic vesical catarrh, which, indeed, often resists the most appropriate treatment for a long time, and has added to it, as a very unfortunate complication, stricture of the urethra with its consequences, the removal of which expedites the cure of the vesical catarrh considerably.

If the inflammation spreads to the ureter and the pelvis of the kidneys, the patient complains of pain in the loin of the affected side, but this symptom may be absent. The purulent discharge will be increased, and we shall find epithelial cells from the ureter and the mucous membrane of the kidney in the urine. Any certain pathognomonic signs whereby we may recognize this renal catarrh are not forthcoming, but the diagnosis is more easy in those cases in which renal catarrh coexists with but slight vesical catarrh. If blood escapes from the kidney, it is not unlikely to take the form of cylindrical, worm-like clots during its passage down the ureter, and may be voided in this form sometimes with great pain, or even with symptoms of renal colic and ischuria. Renal catarrh in consequence of contagious pyorrhœa is, on the whole, of rare occurrence and only transitory, but it may exceptionally be aggravated to protracted pyelitis, and subsequently to pyelo-nephritis.

Treatment.

In the first place, I must refer to what has been said in reference to catarrh of the neck of the bladder. I need only add that on the commencement of the catarrh of the neck of the bladder all treatment, by means of balsams or injections, must be discontinued. The spasmodic symptoms may be alleviated by warm fomentations, poultices, and baths, and the use of preparations of opium, especially morphia, internally, hypodermically, or in suppositories. The spasmodic symptoms may also be relieved, if we keep to the use of morphia at night, by lupulin, the preparations of cannabis indica, or bromide of potassium. We keep the bowels open by means of enemata of castor-oil. During the acute stages I usually order the baths to be repeated twice daily, and allow the patient to remain for an hour or an hour and a half in a lukewarm bath, and where difficulty is experienced in providing lukewarm baths so frequently, I substitute hip-baths. As nourishment and a drink at the same time, there is nothing so suitable as milk; we may, however, also allow pure drinking-water, almond emulsion, and acid drinks, such as lemonade; whereas we forbid all water containing carbonic acid. It is only when a frequent desire to pass water and uneasy sensations in the region of the neck of the bladder remain after acute inflammation has subsided, that we try to alleviate this irritability by continuous and very careful treatment with bougies, and I have usually succeeded quite satisfactorily in such cases. In the treatment of chronic vesical catarrh all the means mentioned under that head are applicable; but in these cases great attention must always be specially paid to the question of the existence of a stricture, which, if present, must by all means be treated and cured. The same treatment is suitable for the most part in renal catarrh, but here astringents are most efficacious.

Stricture of the Urethra.

Stricture of the urethra results so almost exclusively from gonorrhœa, that our account of gonorrhœal affections would certainly be imperfect if we did not give a short description of it and its proper treatment, though, from want of space, we cannot enter into the question of operative surgical treatment, which, indeed, would be foreign to the purpose of the work.

The starting-point of a non-congenital stricture of the urethra

is usually an ulcer of the urethra, which may either not have cicatrized and may narrow the calibre of the urethra by its projecting
border, or after cicatrizing may have left a hard cicatrix behind,
which, it is true, but seldom projects into the channel as a cicatricial growth, but by its contraction may cause the adjacent
parts to project like a roll. Growths from the mucous membrane
or from the glands in connection with it may form the starting-
point of the stricture. According to their form, we distinguish
these projections and contractions as comb-like, semicircular,
circular, and valvular. They may be some millimetres, even a
centimetre (⅔ inch) or more in length; they are most frequently
situated in the membranous and bulbous portions of the urethra,
next at the fossa navicularis, and extremely rarely in the prostatic portion; occasionally there may be several of them. We
may further distinguish those which involve only the thickness
of the mucous membrane, and those in which the submucous
connective tissue is deeply involved. In the latter case the induration projects beneath the skin.

The secondary changes dependent on these strictures are
numerous and of the greatest importance in regard to symptomatology. We shall not be going too far if we assert that there
is hardly any other part of the body in which anatomical changes
of so slight a character, comparatively, are followed by such
manifold and severe results. In the first place, a chronic inflammation of the mucous membrane of the urethra is set up, which
is attended by a muco-purulent discharge and may easily again
assume the characters of acute gonorrhœa under the influence of
irritation and excesses; chronic inflammation also becomes developed behind the stricture and may gradually spread to the
neck of the bladder, to the bladder itself, and even to the pelvis
of the kidney and the kidney itself. We thus meet with extensive catarrh of the bladder and of the kidneys, and in consequence a deposit of phosphates, the formation of concretions and
calculi, thickening of the mucous membrane, distention of its
follicles, induration of the submucous cellular tissue, and particularly great hypertrophy of the muscular coat, which, as soon
as the hypertrophy commences, begins to expel the urine when
it has only collected in small quantity, and thus, the capacity of

the bladder is diminished.   On the other hand, we also find that if the bladder is but imperfectly emptied, the urine overcomes the resistance of the muscular coat and the bladder becomes distended.   The muscular bundles, then, often become separated from one another and depressions form between them, which may even be developed into diverticula in which gravel and concretions are deposited; it is in this way that encysted vesical calculi are often formed.   Rupture of the bladder, followed by extravasation of urine, fatal peritonitis, and septic or uræmic poisoning may also result.   Another but less disastrous occurrence is rupture of the urethra in front of the neck of the bladder, which is followed, usually, by the formation of circumscribed urinary fistulæ.   Lastly, the prostate and testes may be involved, the emission of semen prevented, and the testes may gradually atrophy.

In the first place, the stream of urine becomes smaller, somewhat tortuous, and cannot be projected to the usual distance. If excoriations are present, pain, increased during micturition, ejaculation of the semen, and the introduction of instruments, and often accompanied by slight bleeding, is frequently complained of at the points where they are situated.   If the contraction increases, the stream steadily becomes smaller and is projected a shorter distance, so that by degrees the urine only escapes drop by drop, and subsequently there are added the exceedingly troublesome symptoms of catarrh of the bladder, tenesmus, and purulent, alkaline, offensive, and even bloody urine.   The urethra should be carefully examined at an early period.   A soft bougie is best adapted for the purpose.   The "model bougies" of Decamp, which were formerly used so much, have of late fallen into disuse as untrustworthy.

The examination should, of course, always be conducted in a very gentle and careful manner.   When we come to the stricture, we encounter a certain amount of resistance which is gradually overcome, the bougie feeling gripped, as it were; we, however, persist till we have reached the bladder in order to ascertain whether there are not several strictures present.

The smaller and the more feeble the stream, the more frequent becomes the desire to relieve the bladder, so that, ultimately, the patient is compelled to pass water every half-hour or quarter of an hour, or even oftener, and thus after some years' duration, and usually only after inappropriate treatment, he is deprived of all rest and is perpetually reminded of his troublesome malady. The bladder can then be detected by palpation and percussion above the symphysis pubis, and is felt to be hard, almost always full, and more or less bulky. The prostate is comparatively rarely enlarged. Of great importance in the later stages of the disease is the circumstance that while the bladder is often so enormously distended that it reaches the umbilicus, the urine constantly dribbles away as if from a vessel running over, and this may easily mislead a practitioner who is shy of using the catheter, into the belief that no retention exists in the very cases in which catheterization is of the utmost importance. Phosphates frequently pass in the form of gravel.

If inflammation of the retro-peritoneal connective tissue of the pelvis comes on in cases in which infiltration of urine has occurred, the patient suffers from severe fever and pain in the pelvic region, and either abscesses form, which burst outwardly, often lay bare the lower part of the rectum, lead to the separation of sloughs of connective tissue, gradually empty themselves and close, often, however, causing death by septicæmia and pyæmia; or, the inflammation spreads at an early period to the peritoneum, and so causes death quickly; or, owing to extension of the inflammation to the connective tissue behind the kidneys, nephritis and suppuration from the kidneys may follow. If a perineal abscess forms, this results, as a rule, from a more circumscribed inflammation and ends in an urinary fistula, which can usually only be cured by relieving the stricture; urinary fistulæ occasionally, but rarely, involve the lower part of the rectum. If urine constantly escapes through fistulæ of this sort, great irritation of the surrounding parts is produced; under these circumstances they communicate with the bladder, for, if they open into the urethra, urine only flows through them occasionally. If the urine has been retained in the bladder a long time and in large quantity, if the inflammation has become chronic, and has extended to the kidneys, the patient becomes emaciated, hectic comes on, or he sinks gradually into a comatose condition, interrupted by slight delirium, or accompanied by signs of partial paralysis or by convulsions, and dies with all the symptoms of complete uræmia or ammoniæmia. In the later stages of stricture of the urethra it is also tolerably common for digestion to be interfered with; the patient becomes dyspeptic and suffers from constant vomiting. All these symptoms, and the impotence which comes on subsequently, owing at first to the semen passing into the bladder and then to its being no more secreted, make the patient highly hypochondriacal and melancholic, or may even occasionally lead him to commit suicide.

Diagnosis.

The diagnosis is not, as a rule, by any means difficult, but it is highly important to recognize the affection early. We therefore examine the urethra early, in every case of gleet, with a catheter, and, if we find evidence of stricture, with bougies; it is useless to give diagnostic details for any one who does not know how to handle these instruments. Otherwise, we shall soon be led to suspect the existence of stricture by the stream of the urine becoming diminished in length and volume, weaker, and more tortuous; if all the other signs of deep-seated disease of the urinary organs make their appearance. there can no longer be any doubt.

Prognosis.

The earlier the stricture is recognized the better the prognosis. It is obvious that spasmodic stricture, consisting in a quite transitory dysuria, which is partly spontaneous and partly evoked by the passage of instruments, is easy of cure. The longer the stricture has existed, the narrower the calibre of the urethra, the harder, more resistant, longer and extensive the contraction, the more serious the complications which will be developed in the urinary organs; at length there is added to the great inconvenience of the malady the steadily increasing danger to life.

Treatment.

If we have merely to deal with a transitory spasmodic stricture, accompanied by signs of simple dysuria, lukewarm continuous baths, emollient cataplasmata over the region of the
bladder, opium internally and in the form of clysters, are to be
tried first of all. If these remedies do not suffice, we take a
bougie of moderate size, about 3–5 millimetres (from ⅛ to ¼ of an
inch) in diameter, well oiled, and try to introduce it slowly, carefully, and without using any force, and if this does not succeed,
we carefully try a catheter, most suitably a flexible one.

When we have satisfied ourselves of the existence of an
organic stricture, dilatation is undoubtedly the best treatment,
and, as a rule, it can be accomplished by appropriate means.
Wax bougies or flexible ones are most suitable. We always
begin with a good-sized one, 3–4 millimetres (from ⅛ to ¼ of an
inch) in diameter, and only fall back on the small and thinnest
ones when the larger ones will not pass. When I have to use the
very finest, I prefer those made of catgut to the wax bougies.
As soon as the urethra has become accustomed to bougies, we
may use firmer ones made of gutta percha, and gradually increase
the size. We should never be in too great a hurry, for it often
happens that the bougie is stopped by the obstruction; but if
we press gently for awhile, and at the same time try to divert the
patient's attention by conversation, the instrument suddenly
passes on. We support the bougie by the finger as far as we can
follow it along the urethra, or else the wax bougie readily bends
on the slightest pressure and doubles on itself, so that one is liable at first sight to imagine one has reached the bladder. When
we have found the bougie which corresponds to the calibre of the
narrowed urethra, we introduce it once daily and let it remain for
awhile, at first five, then ten, and subsequently fifteen minutes
each time. During the first few days a slight discharge occurs,
but this is not of any material importance. Every four or five
days we may pass a large bougie, increasing its size by ½–1 millimetre (.02–.04 of an inch) in diameter. (We prefer to indicate the
size of the bougies by half millimetres or millimetres rather than

by the ordinary numbers, the intervals between which vary very much.) This treatment, even in average cases, generally takes from four to six weeks, and in very narrow strictures must be continued for two or three months, and for some time after the stricture is well dilated, in order to prevent recurrence. I order a bougie to be passed at first every two days, then twice a week, and then once a week.

It is only when a long time has elapsed since leaving off treatment without any renewed diminution of stream, that we can regard the cure as complete. In hard, callous strictures, bougies of gutta percha, at first introduced only every two or three days, later more frequently, are more serviceable than wax bougies, and we may also employ iodine both locally and internally, with a view to the ultimate diminution of the induration.

If the urine only dribbles away, or is wholly retained, and bougies cannot be passed, we try patiently with a small catheter, using some little force in order to overcome the constriction, which usually becomes torn somewhat, and a little bleeding of no moment occurs. Forced catheterization is, however, only safe in the hands of skilful and experienced surgeons. We then substitute a larger catheter for the thin one, allow the inflammatory condition to subside, and then complete the cure by dilatation by means of bougies. In the most extreme cases of severe ischuria, infiltration of urine, etc., puncture of the bladder has been recommended formerly, but is only to be employed in case of need, and is then most suitably performed above the symphysis pubis by means of a slightly curved trocar. Of late, however, by the incision of hard and long strictures, by urethrotomy, practised long ago by Amussat and improved by Reibard and others, by the so-called "boutonnière," the division of the indurated parts from the perineum, as recommended especially by Civiale and Syme, and by this means obtaining entrance to the bladder, a cure may be effected in cases in which formerly the bladder would have been punctured without hesitation; the details concerning these operations belong to the domain of operative surgery, and we refer our readers especially to the excellent treatise by Pitha on Strictures of the Urethra, in Virchow's Pathology.

Contagious Pyorrhœa in Females.

We have already stated plainly that the spotless fame of women suffering from gonorrhœa is founded on the self-love of their affected lovers much more than on their spotless mode of life, and that, as a rule, ordinary leucorrhœa does not communicate gonorrhœa—it is only actually existing gonorrhœa which does so ; the only possible exception is when a woman infected by a man suffering from gonorrhœa communicates the disease to another before it has had time to develop in herself; this is, however, of very rare occurrence.

We may distinguish the following forms of gonorrhœa in woman according to the parts affected : gonorrhœa of the urethra, a part which is only exceptionally the chief seat, of the vulva, of the vagina, and of the uterus. By extension, the inflammation may cause cystitis and ovaritis ; the latter, however, is somewhat doubtful.

As regards the urethritis of females, we may say that for the most part it possesses the same character as in males, but is far less intractable and painful. The patient complains of more or less severe scalding and of a purulent discharge with the urine, and by pressing with the finger underneath the neck of the bladder from behind forward, we can squeeze out a drop or more of a purulent fluid. If the inflammation spreads to the neck of the bladder, there is dysuria or frequent desire to pass water, with incomplete emptying of the bladder, vesical tenesmus, even complete retention, and blood and pus may be mixed with the urine. In the worse cases, the inflammation spreads to the neck of the bladder and excites all the symptoms of vesical catarrh. If we have to examine such women for legal purposes, it is not always easy to arrive at a diagnosis ; by ablution and by passing water just previously, the pus may for a time be washed away. By pressing with the finger from behind forwards, however, and by the inspection of the reddened and swollen meatus, we may, as a rule, arrive at the true state of affairs. At the commencement of the disease, the patients experience some sexual excitement, but, as soon as the purulent discharge appears, intercourse is very painful.

The ordinary gonorrhœa of the vulva produces similar symptoms; and the loss of a quantity of epithelium, in consequence of the sudden onset of the inflammation, accounts for the fact that, even without any catarrh of the urethra, micturition and also any contact with the genitals are very painful, and in addition to the very copious purulent secretion we find superficial irregular excoriations on the labia minora and the entrance of the vagina. All these parts, and especially the nymphæ, may also become swollen from inflammatory œdema. If the discharge at first is sero-mucous, the purulent character becomes comparatively quickly developed, and as suppurative inflammation of the large sebaceous glands of the vulva is also often present, a peculiarly offensive odor is imparted to the discharge by admixture with the volatile fatty acids, and in corpulent women the parts in the neighborhood of the vulva, especially below and at the sides, become erythematous. If we wash the part we find individual sebaceous glands greatly swollen, and we can squeeze a drop of pus out of the openings of their ducts. The inflammation may also spread to the large vulvo-vaginal glands of Bartholini, and I have several times, under such circumstances, had to open abscesses of these glands which had enlarged to the size of a chestnut. If the inflammation is limited to their ducts, a peculiar, occasional, localized, and marked hypersecretion may occur, which we may sometimes squeeze out by pressure. Simple vulvar catarrhal gonorrhœa may be cured quickly by proper and early treatment, but becomes protracted by neglect in proportion to the extension of the gonorrhœal inflammation to the vagina which then usually occurs.

Vaginal gonorrhœa sometimes arises from the preceding, and sometimes *per se*. The uneasy sensations at first are the same as in the vulvar form, and so is the scalding on micturition. The discharge is only at first of a sero-mucous character; it quickly becomes purulent and remains so, and the vagina becomes painful throughout its whole extent, and its temperature is raised. In favorable cases, however, the disease throughout its whole course may be of the character of a slight, superficial catarrhal inflammation. By admixture with free fatty acids, the secretion may have a somewhat acid reaction. The peculiar parasite, trichomonas vaginæ, which Donné discovered thirty-five years ago, is not peculiar to gonorrhœa. Now and then a chancre may be the source of vaginal gonorrhœa; this can only be determined by the use of the uterine speculum, if this does not cause too much pain, and at the same time we may also discover the papillary growths of granular vaginitis which occur sometimes in gonorrhœa, but are not peculiar to it, or we may find evidences of the gonorrhœal catarrh having spread to the uterus. As a rule, gonorrhœa affecting the vagina has a disposition to spread from the vulva to the uterus. When the inflammation is severe, there may be some fever at first. By proper treatment and judicious conduct on the part of the patient the disease may be completely cured in a few weeks, but may easily be again excited by the next menstruation, and it may be necessary to examine again carefully, and even to employ energetic treatment once more. Irritation of the genitals by intercourse at too early a stage will protract the disease considerably, and leads either to a chronic vaginal gonorrhœa or to a chronic leucorrhœa which gradually loses its infecting character, but may sometimes lead to a permanently indurated, hypertrophic condition of the vaginal mucous membrane, which then loses its customary soft, velvety condition.

When gonorrhœa spreads to the uterus, it usually affects the cervix, and can only be detected by examination with the speculum. In addition to redness, slight swelling, and occasionally superficial erosions around the os uteri, we also observe a mucous, viscid, or purulent secretion escaping, which is sometimes mixed with gelatinous mucus, and sometimes is more distinctly purulent; a certain amount of sanguineous discoloration is also not unfrequently visible. The uterine secretion is always alkaline. Erosion of the lower lip of the os uteri gives rise to the streaks or spots of blood sometimes seen. *Per se*, however, gonorrhœa of the cervix uteri, which seldom spreads to the mucous membrane within the uterus, affords no pathognomonic signs throughout its whole course, which may be very protracted.

Occasionally we may see granular spots of a deep red color, greatly developed and hypertrophied papillæ, which have been described as granular ulcerations, and on which undoubtedly the epithelium is deficient; also simple erosions, especially of follicles, are situated in the neighborhood of the os uteri, and these not unfrequently extend into its cavity; sometimes the whole cervix uteri appears swollen, and of a somewhat dark red color.

Gonorrhœa in women, therefore, shows all the signs of an inflammation attended by purulent discharge and power of infection, and extending from the vulva and meatus urinarius into the cavity of the uterus. The last and rare extension through the uterus and along one of the Fallopian tubes to the ovary is characterized, according to the authors who describe it, by a painful tumor, which makes its appearance suddenly on one side, at the lower part of the abdomen, and which usually terminates in resolution at the end of two or three weeks, the pain ceasing and the tumor disappearing.

Diagnosis.

The onset of gonorrhœa is very easily detected both by the physician and by the patient. Most important are the pain, the acute onset, the marked swelling, the offensive purulent discharge, and the marked scalding on micturition. I have, however, exceptionally, twice met with a similar state of things directly after marriage in women with small genitals, and who had previously never had sexual intercourse. In these cases rest, abstinence, cold applications, and lukewarm baths suffice to remove this state of simple irritation quickly, whilst contagious gonorrhœa goes through its different stages. If we can squeeze a muco-purulent fluid out of the urethra, we obtain valuable evidence as to diagnosis; but this symptom is not present, as a rule. If the early and more painful stage has subsided, and there is less pus in the discharge, while the quantity of mucus has increased, it is almost impossible to establish a certain diagnosis, unless the women come spontaneously to consult the medical man; and it is just such cases, as they are usually neglected, which remain infectious for a long period. The affections of the glands of Bartholini have no decisive diagnostic value, for all sorts of diseases of these glands occur in women who have no gonorrhœa, and even in virgins.

Prognosis.

When gonorrhœa in the female is unattended by any complications, it is, as a rule, much more readily cured than in the male subject. If it is treated early, it often remains confined to the vulva, or the entrance of the vagina ; if it has once spread to the neck of the uterus, it is generally intractable ; and it is especially so if neglected, and then often remains for as many months as it would have done weeks if it had been properly attended to. Even when neglected, however, it is not by any means attended by any such ill consequences as in the male subject.

Treatment.

This closely resembles the treatment employed in the male subject, only when the urethra is affected ; when the inflammation is acute, it should be of a soothing character, consisting of rest, attention to diet, cold applications, lukewarm hip- or immersion-baths, at a temperature of from 86° to 89.6° F. (30-32 C.). It is only in this form that cubebs and balsam of copaiva are of use ; they may be given in the manner already sufficiently indicated.

In the usual form of vulvo-vaginal and uterine pyorrhœa we must adopt more energetic procedures. On the one hand, women may prevent the development of gonorrhœa by cleanliness, frequent ablutions, the use of injections after any intercourse attended by the least suspicion ; and, on the other hand, the abortive treatment is much less painful and attended by much less danger if tried in the earliest stage of the disease, before severe inflammation has been already set up. It is often sufficient to inject a solution of nitrate of silver of the strength of from four to nine grains (0.3-0.6) to an ounce (30.0) of water once or twice daily, and introduce sponges and pieces of charpie of moderate size, surrounded with thread, and which can be withdrawn by means of a thread hanging down. Care should be taken not to leave stains on the linen.

If, however, severe inflammation has once set in, it is manifest that such treatment would do harm, and be too irritating. Under these circumstances we must try rest in the horizontal position, cold wet applications, and, at a later period, the use of mild fomentations and injections of infusion of marshmallow or decoction of flaxseed, with hyoscyamus or with decoction of poppy-heads, repeated five or six times daily, long-continued lukewarm baths, lukewarm, or, if they can be at all borne, cold hip-baths several times a day, continued for 5–10–15 minutes, friction of the parts irritated with almond oil, simple cerate, marshmallow ointment, and the application of cold lead lotion. During this time the diet must be strictly attended to, and drinks of lemonade, orange sherbet, the diluted juices of fruits and syrups, etc., are necessary, and all sexual intercourse, or, indeed, excitement, must be most carefully avoided. We always take the precaution of separating the labia from one another by the introduction of strips of linen or charpie dipped, in the early stage, in cold water, and subsequently, in astringent fluids.

If by these means we have converted the acute symptoms into the subacute and painless stage, astringents are indicated. The preparations of zinc, lead, tannin, and alum are useful in the form of injections, or applied by means of small sponges in doses of from four to nine grains (0.3–0.6), or more, to an ounce (30.0) of water. The lead preparations are most suitable in cases in which the inflammation is still subacute. I have used the acetate of lead in gradually increasing doses of from twenty to thirty grains (1.25–2.0) to an ounce and a half or an ounce (50.0–30.0) of water. Alum is also of great service, and as these injections have to be continued for a long time, in order to diminish the cost as much as possible, I usually order the patient to procure from two to four ounces (60.0–120.0) from the apothecary, in a box, and to dissolve from one-half to two teaspoonfuls in four or five ounces (120.0–150.0) of water for an injection. Of late I have often substituted tannin for the alum in the proportion of a drachm (4.0) to an ounce (30.0). While the injection is being given, the pelvis should be raised and sloping backward; it is most conveniently given over a bed-pan, so that the bed-clothes may not be saturated. By far the best astringent for injection at this stage is the nitrate of silver, beginning with from two to three grains (0.12–0.18) to the ounce (30.0), and gradually increasing to from four to nine grains (0.3–0.6). I generally order a drachm (4.0), dissolved in two ounces (60.0) of water, and direct the patient to add a teaspoonful to the usual quantity for an injection. This is undoubtedly the most rapid and certain of all the remedies in use ; one injection at night before going to bed is sufficient ; whereas if the lead and alum solutions are used, two injections must be made daily, and some cotton-wool, dipped in the fluid, must be introduced between the labia.

In uterine gonorrhœa and in erosions and granular ulcers of the cervix uteri, I know no better means of treatment than cauterization with a stick of nitrate of silver, applied externally and also within the neck every three or four days.

If the case is complicated by an outbreak of herpes vulvæ, lukewarm baths and lead lotions are useful. If abscesses form, they should be opened early, and when they are situated in the glands of Bartholini, I usually cauterize them several times subsequently with nitrate of silver, or else they are liable to form again.

The internal treatment, when the urethra is not involved, should be of an expectant character. As soon as the inflammatory stage has passed I order nutritious, substantial food, and if the gonorrhœa is intractable, we should not only try to discover any uterine complications which may exist locally, but we should also attend to the general state of the system ; the use of the preparations of iron in chlorotic or anæmic conditions is often advantageous, and in scrofulous subjects, tonics, acorn coffee, decoction of walnuts, cod-liver oil, iodide of potassium, and iodide of iron especially, etc. We shall only, in fact, treat these or any other diseases of the female genitals successfully by combining accurate observation of the general indications with the use of the modern aids to diagnosis and continuous local treatment.

Gonorrhœal Affections which are Common to Both Sexes.

Under this head are gonorrhœa of the rectum, gonorrhœal ophthalmia, and gonorrhœal rheumatism; doubts as to the latter, however, arise for several reasons.

Gonorrhœa of the Rectum.

This disease, which is of rare occurrence, mostly arises from unnatural gratification of the sexual impulse. Simple contamination of the anus, such as occurs so frequently in women owing to the secretion running down, is a very exceptional cause, and is more likely to come into play when, owing to hemorrhoids or prolapse of the rectum, parts of the latter are brought into direct contact with the infecting material, than when the lower part of the rectum and the anus are healthy.

This gonorrhœa of the rectum causes congestion and swelling of the mucous membrane, and is attended by a purulent rather than a mucous discharge. The constant sense of pressure, burning and itching in the anus is much increased on each evacuation of the bowels, and sometimes there are very troublesome spasmodic attacks in the anus, and extending even to the bladder. Excoriations and fissures are very liable to form in the folds of the anus and render the evacuation of the bowels still more painful. Gonorrhœa of the rectum has, however, happily a decided tendency to heal in a few weeks. Exceptionally, the inflammation may spread to the submucous connective tissue, and in this way give rise to the formation of abscesses, or even fistulæ in the neighborhood. Much more frequently we observe slight erythematous irritation of the skin around the anus. Sometimes pointed papillary outgrowths subsequently develop.

Treatment.

If we see the case at an early period, we may try the abortive treatment and inject seven and a half grains (0.5) of nitrate of silver, dissolved in an ounce or an ounce and a half (30.0–40.0) of water, followed quickly by a copious clyster of cold water.

The pain excited by the nitrate is often considerable, but is generally transitory. As a rule, we only see such cases when they have already attained their full development. If the pain is very persistent and severe, we may order cold applications or lukewarm hip-baths, a small enema of two ounces (60.0) with ten drops of laudanum which must be retained by the patient, or insert a suppository of cacao-butter with a sixth of a grain (0.01) of morphia from time to time. Occasionally it may be necessary to apply six or eight leeches around the anus, and they may be of service if some congestive condition of the rectum has existed previously. In order to avoid hard stools, small quantities of castor oil or compound liquorice powder should be ordered. If the first inflammatory stage, which hardly lasts a week, has passed, we inject a solution of alum, from forty-five to seventy-five grains (3.0–5.0) to from two to three ounces (60.0–100.0) of water once or twice daily, and in the intervals insert charpie dipped in the solution, according to the rules followed in the treatment of diseases of the rectum. The smallest fissure whatever must be cauterized every two days with a stick of nitrate of silver, which must be passed within the anus, and of course is very painful. Abscesses in the neighborhood of the anus must be opened as early as possible. Gonorrhœa of the mouth and nose have been accepted in various quarters on theoretical grounds, but have never been actually demonstrated by clinical observation so far as I know. Gonorrhœal ophthalmia, on the other hand, is of more frequent occurrence and often of a very rapidly destructive character.

Ophthalmia Pyorrhoica—Gonorrhœal Ophthalmia.

This is undoubtedly the most terrible complication of gonorrhœa. If, on the one hand, it is true that specific gonorrhœal ophthalmia arises in the majority of cases from direct transference of the specific poison, yet, according to Ricord, this is not by any means the sole mode of origin. Of the first mode of direct contagion there exist very many undoubted examples. Ricord cites the following: A woman, who did not herself suffer from gonorrhœa, bathed her eye with a lead lotion in which her husband washed his penis affected with gonorrhœa, and was attacked with very severe gonorrhœal ophthalmia. A man suffering from gonorrhœa was attacked with gonorrhœal ophthalmia, and soon afterwards a brother, who slept with him but was not suffering from gonorrhœa, had a very severe attack of gonorrhœal ophthalmia. In the hospital at Zürich were two ophthalmic patients lying close together, who washed themselves with the same sponge. One had gonorrhœa and gonorrhœal ophthalmia; the other, who was free from the disease throughout, was attacked with a very severe gonorrhœal ophthalmia, resulting in the destruction of one eye. The self-infection of the patient is often taken for granted, but is not always easily proved. Whether this gonorrhœal ophthalmia may occur in patients long after an attack of urethral gonorrhœa, and without direct contagion, as Ricord believes, seems, to me at least, doubtful.

Symptoms.

Usually the inflammation begins in one eye only, but quickly makes its appearance in the other. The patient is suddenly attacked with severe burning and itching in the eyelids, the whole orbital region becomes very painful, the palpebral and ocular conjunctiva become hyperæmic, assuming a red, velvety appearance. At the very commencement there is an overflow of tears, and the discharge is of a serous character, but soon becomes purulent, and does not merely glue the eyelids together, but flows uninterruptedly from between the eyelids. Externally, the eyelids look swollen and red, and sometimes are even everted. On the inner surface an extreme degree of chemosis is rapidly produced. Occasionally the eyelashes may be turned inward and cause irritation. The cornea, which at first is quite intact, lies at the bottom of a pit formed by the greatly swollen, bright red, and œdematous conjunctiva, and is partly bathed in pus. Subsequently the cornea becomes affected. At first it is slightly less transparent, then ulcerations occur, followed either by extensive leukomata or by collections of pus between the corneal lamellæ, softening, perforation, escape of the fluid contents of the eyeball, and total loss of vision. In the bad cases both eyes may be lost. In the worst cases of very severe contagion the progress may be so rapid that the result just mentioned may occur in twenty-four hours. Usually, however, the symptoms progress rapidly, but less destructively. In twenty-four hours the chemosis and purulent discharge are well marked, but the cornea is not affected for some days, so that at the end of the first or in the beginning of the second week there may be well-marked opacities or ulcers of the cornea, or the latter may have become perforated—results which commonly follow if the disease has been left to take its course, or has been inefficiently treated. Under appropriate treatment, on the contrary, improvement follows usually in the course of three or four days. The swelling of the eyelids and of the conjunctiva diminishes slightly, the redness becomes less intense, and the cornea, in the most favorable cases, remains wholly free, or, more usually, is slightly opaque and ulcerated ; but perforation does not occur, nor is there any onyx. When the inflammation is very severe it may extend to the iris. If the improvement continues, the swelling and the discharge of pus quickly diminish during the next few days, and the pain is much less severe. The fever, which at the height of the disease may sometimes be severe, disappears, and the disease commonly terminates in from ten to fourteen days, some hyperæmia of the conjunctiva continuing for a while longer, and the opacities of the cornea diminishing in the course of time.

Diagnosis.

It is hardly necessary to say much as to the diagnosis, for it is scarcely possible to confound gonorrhœal ophthalmia with any of the ordinary superficial inflammatory affections of the eye; and the ordinary form, the so-called Egyptian, and the ophthalmia neonatorum, differ more on account of the causes which give rise to them than on account of their symptoms, and even from this point of view the ophthalmia neonatorum is not so distinct as is generally believed, for it not unfrequently depends really on the existence of an infectious discharge from the female genitals at the time of the birth of the child. The differential diagnosis of diphtheritic ophthalmia is much more important, but it would take us out of our way to go into the question here.   According to v. Graefe,[1] not only may gonorrhœa be followed by catarrh and granular conjunctivitis, etc., but also by true diphtheria of the conjunctiva, an important fact in regard to treatment.

Prognosis.

Of all forms of acute ophthalmia, the group designated by the term purulent, and especially the form known as gonorrhœal, are the worst, with the exception of the diphtheritic ophthalmia, but vary according to their progress.   The more rapid and acute the latter is, the less does energetic and proper treatment avail, whilst, when the progress is less rapid, as is commonly the case, our skill has at least time to produce an effect.   I have never, as yet, had the misfortune to see blindness result from an attack of purulent ophthalmia in adults or in new-born children when the patient came under care early, but, as a rule, have been fortunate enough to save both eyes ; only once has one eye been totally lost, and, in that case, I do not distinctly recollect whether the eye had shrivelled up or was merely affected with extensive opacity.   I cannot divest myself of the suspicion that the unfavorable results formerly met with have depended, in part, at least, on inefficient treatment.   This does not apply to diphtheritic conjunctivitis after gonorrhœa, for I have never had an opportunity of treating a case.

Treatment.

It is of the utmost importance to prevent the onset of the disease.   Every person suffering from gonorrhœa should be warned of the liability to infection by careless contact of fingers, sponges, towels, etc.   The most trustworthy prophylactic measure is to treat the gonorrhœa as energetically as possible ; of late years, since the idea has been given up that we ought to let the disease run its course for a while, for fear of driving it in by interference,

---

[1] Deutsche Klinik. 1858. Nr. 21.

purulent ophthalmia has become much less frequent. In the department for syphilis at the Zurich hospital, I never knew the infection to occur once, and all the cases I had to treat came from outside, and showed the disease in an advanced stage. If one eye is affected, every precaution should be taken by means of the position in which the patient lies, care in washing, etc., to prevent the inflammation being communicated to the other, and, for this purpose, a close-fitting protective bandage should be applied, and the patient placed in a suitable position. As long as there is any danger of infection, it is well to close the sound eye with strapping.

As to indications in reference to the treatment of the inflamed eye, we do not waste any time in trying to bring back a urethral gonorrhœa which has already disappeared. The slighter forms are to be treated in the same way as ordinary catarrhal ophthalmia, but must be very carefully watched. In the severer forms complete rest in a darkened room, general and local antiphlogistic remedies, and the energetic employment of nitrate of silver are necessary. A copious venesection should be accomplished, and from fifteen to twenty leeches should be applied to the temple or behind the ear, and repeated, according to circumstances, every eight or twelve hours. From the first, in gonorrhœal ophthalmia, we cauterize the conjunctiva quickly and superficially with the nitrate of silver in stick, or in the form of a concentrated solution—in children, of the strength of one part to four or six of water, and in adults, of one part to two or three of water. After each cauterization cold water or a weak solution of salt should be injected. If the inflammation is very severe, or if the discharge has only ceased or abated for a few hours, a second cauterization should follow the first in eight to ten hours, and, if necessary, a third should follow after a similar interval. In addition, a copious cold injection should be made every hour with a glass syringe or the well-known curved tube of the eye-douche, the eyelids being, of course, sufficiently separated from one another. If the inflammation has already begun to subside, it is well, as a rule, to apply weaker caustics every day or two, cold applications to the eyes being employed in the intervals.

If the chemosis is very considerable and intractable, it is

advisable to snip off large folds of conjunctiva with Cooper's curved scissors, the bleeding which follows from the greatly congested vessels being also beneficial. If it is necessary to use any caustic, this should be applied before excising any portion of the conjunctiva. When the inflammation has somewhat abated, I am in the habit of substituting tannin for the nitrate of silver, and I order it in the form of a solution of the strength of from four to nine grains (0.3 to 0.6) to the ounce (30.0), to be dropped into the eye three or four times a day. When the disease is at its height, I have had good results from the application of large blisters behind the ears or at the back of the neck. Ricord recommends the local abstraction of blood, on the plan advocated by Gama, which consists in applying only two or three leeches at a time, but replacing them by others as soon as the first fall off, for a period of twelve hours or longer. Internally, I generally give calomel in moderately large doses, from one and a half to two grains (0.10 to 0.12) every two hours, and in addition order mercurial ointment to be rubbed into the forehead at a sufficient distance from the eye. If the calomel is not borne, or if salivation occurs quickly, I administer nitrate of soda in doses of two drachms or half an ounce (8.0 to 16.0) daily, or vigorous purgatives, extract of colocynth in doses of from two to three grains (0.12 to 0.18) in the morning while fasting, or a glass of Seidlitz or Püllna or Ofen bitter water. In short, only energetic treatment is likely to be attended by any good results. In diphtheritic conjunctivitis, antiphlogistics and mercurials are useful, while caustics and vesicants are to be avoided entirely.

Diseases Occurring as Accidental Complications of Gonorrhœa or having an Indirect Connection with it.

Under this head we shall treat of the so-called gonorrhœal rheumatism and of the papillary cutaneous outgrowths designated "pointed condylomata."

Articular Rheumatism Occurring in the Course of Gonorrhœa.

Since the appearance of the work of Swediaur, we have been aware that articular rheumatism not unfrequently attacks patients who are suffering from gonorrhœa, or who have only just recovered from it, while physicians of great authority were not willing to accept any intimate relationship between the two diseases, and regarded the connection as accidental; other physicians, owing to their humoral pathology tendencies, considered the so-called gonorrhœal arthritis a true metastasis of the disease, and the fact, which undoubtedly occurs sometimes, that some patients complain of pains in the joints on each fresh attack of gonorrhœa, was taken to be an incontestable proof of the truth of the theory. A third party, starting from the fact that the mere introduction of a catheter in the male is sufficient occasionally to excite pains in the joints, and that these may also occur in puerperal women, argued the existence of a genital rheumatism, and an otherwise excellent investigator, Lorain of Paris, supported this view. However, rigors and other accidents occur more frequently after the introduction of a catheter than do pains in the joints; the arthritic pains complained of by puerperal women not unfrequently have a pyæmic origin. The knowledge which we at present possess, therefore, merely allows of our being certain of the fact that articular rheumatism frequently occurs during the course of gonorrhœa, or very soon after its cure. I have also several times met with neuralgia, especially in the hip, inflammation of the sheaths of tendons, etc., during or soon after an attack of gonorrhœa. That the latter, therefore, predisposes to a certain extent to the occurrence of rheumatic affections, and especially articular rheumatism, may consequently be granted. I shall abstain, however, from offering any explanation as to the way in which the urethritis of the male or the gonorrhœa of the female sets up the joint-affection or other rheumatic complication, all the more readily because none of the theories, or, more strictly, hypotheses hitherto suggested, are tenable.

The arthritis shows a certain preference for the knee-joint, and is attended by considerable effusion. In the case of one patient in Paris this struck me as so remarkable that I put the question directly to the patient, a young girl, whether she was not suffering from gonorrhœa, and at first received an indignant denial; but when a local examination left no doubt on that point, she then confessed. On the whole, this kind of rheumatism is by far less frequent in the female than in the male sex.

Symptomatology.

It is exceptional for rheumatism to make its appearance at an early period; it generally comes on at the end of a few weeks, and in cases of neglected gonorrhœa especially. The onset of the articular pains is generally sudden and accompanied by considerable swelling, and for the most part by fever; in the knees, which are often affected, there is not unfrequently considerable effusion. As in other kinds of rheumatism, sometimes only a few joints are affected and sometimes several, sometimes only the larger ones and sometimes the smaller ones: it may disappear in a few weeks, or may have a much longer duration; characters which are commonly met with in articular rheumatism uncomplicated with gonorrhœa. I have several times been struck with the rapidity with which the acute inflammatory effusion into one or both knee-joints has become absorbed. The suppuration which occurs with extreme rarity in the joints can scarcely, *per se*, be due to the gonorrhœa. It is asserted that this articular rheumatism, which has a distinct tendency to attack certain localities, never excites endo- or pericarditis. I know of no exception to this, but the peculiarity in the course of the disease must be established on more definite evidence than at present exists before we shall be justified in deducing any theories from it. The neuralgia and inflammation of the sheaths and of the bursæ mucosæ, which occur in patients affected with gonorrhœa, have no special characters.

Prognosis.

This is, as a rule, of a favorable character, and it is but seldom that any sequelæ are left, and it is also exceptional for the rheumatic pains to be protracted or to become chronic. The prognosis, therefore, is in general that which pertains to ordinary rheumatism. It is so far of a more favorable character that there is no, or but little, tendency to affections of the heart, and I have never known a case of sudden death in this disease when com plicated with gonorrhœa, while in other forms of rheumatism this untoward result has not been of such great rarity, and especially in Breslau. We may justly, however, object as regards both these points, that many patients suffering from acute articular rheumatism may have had gonorrhœa or a gleet of no long standing, without the physician suspecting it. At one period, during which I examined the urethra of every male patient suffering from articular rheumatism admitted into the Zurich Hospital, I several times found urethritis and its consequences, which otherwise I should not have discovered. Until the urethra has been carefully examined in hundreds of cases of articular rheumatism, and the history carefully taken, with a view to gonorrhœa, we shall not be in a position to speculate and draw conclusions on the subject.

Treatment.

Irrespective of the treatment of the gonorrhœa, the articular rheumatism, *per se*, is best treated expectantly, for none of the reputed anti-rheumatica are of any avail in definitely shortening its duration. Inunctions of fatty materials into the joints, cold applications if the pains are severe, hypodermic injections of morphia at night if the pains persist, and rest in the horizontal position, form the chief means of treatment. If the disease persists locally, painting with iodine and the internal administration of iodide of potassium, alone, or in combination with colchicum, may be of service. As a drink, I order for all such patients plenty of lemon-juice, as much as from three to four ounces (100.0 –120.0) daily, sufficiently diluted with water and sweetened. If the rheumatism becomes chronic, it must be treated on the principles which guide us in other forms of the disease.

Papillary Outgrowths in Patients Suffering from Gonorrhœa.

I have already, some years ago, in my large work on Pathological Anatomy, stated what I still believe to be a fact: that the papillary outgrowths, which are called pointed condylomata,

have no direct connection with any venereal disease, but occur
much more frequently in those who have often suffered from such
affections and are dirty in their habits, than in those who are
cleanly and have either never suffered from venereal disease, or
only slightly so. The number of cases also is not by any means
small, in which I have found similar growths in men as well as
in women, without the slightest connection with gonorrhœa; indeed, I have several times, and even recently, met with such in
chaste virgins. The repeated but scarcely demonstrated contagion of these so-called pointed condylomata would, at the most,
only prove their transferability, but not by any means that they
originated from gonorrhœa. Still less is there any connection
between the multiple tumors due to hypertrophy of the sebaceous glands, which have been very inappropriately named subcutaneous condylomata, and any gonorrhœal disease whatever.

It would lead me too far out of my way were I to treat in
detail of these localized hypertrophies of the skin, which not
only affect the deepest layers of the epidermis, but also the papillæ. The situations in which they are met with show that
they occur where sebaceous products accumulate and disinte-
grate: on the glans and at its base; on the prepuce, especially
when this is tight; in women, on the labia, in the urethra, in the
vagina, on the os uteri, around the anus, etc; when their surfaces
often undergo change and renewal, owing to friction, irritation,
and contact with fluid secretions, they somewhat resemble granulations, while at other times they are drier and more horny on
the surface. By pressure they may become flattened, or else
otherwise; they rather resemble strawberries or a cauliflower.
If they obstruct the flow of urine or the passage of the fæces,
owing to their position, they are also liable to be irritated by
these excretions and may become inflamed, or in rare cases the
surface may even slough or become gangrenous.

As I do not consider that they have any direct connection
with our subject, I shall only deal shortly with the question of
treatment. I have always found it best to snip them off early
and thoroughly with curved scissors. We may also sometimes
get them to shrivel up, if they are but small, by the application
of perchloride of iron or tincture of iodine. Astringents, as well

as caustics, however, cause much more pain and are much slower in their action than the simple plan of cutting them off. When they occur in large numbers massed together, such free bleeding may be caused by their extirpation that it may be necessary either to destroy them with the galvanic cautery, or get rid of them by degrees by trying different parts in succession. In my work on Pathological Anatomy, illustrated by copperplates, I have given the histories of cases of such large cauliflower-like growths from the skin, accompanied by drawings taken both before and after operations, and which demonstrate the thorough efficiency of this plan. The whole of this group of hypertrophic and neoplastic formations, however, rather belongs to the domain of surgery, and has but an indirect connection with the subject of gonorrhœa, as I have already pointed out.

FUNCTIONAL AFFECTIONS

OF THE

MALE GENITAL ORGANS.

———

CURSCHMANN.

THE FUNCTIONAL AFFECTIONS OF THE MALE GENITAL ORGANS.

The diseases of the male genital organs will be described in the following pages, so far as they belong, by a custom which is daily becoming more established, to the physician's province. Obviously, no sharply defined line of separation from surgery can be drawn; but, since in practice the great majority of these cases are more akin to surgery than to medicine, we find no reason to depart from the customary boundaries of our subject. We shall here treat, therefore, only of morbid seminal losses, as well as of impotence and sterility, in the male.

The general title alone—"Functional Diseases"—under which we have collected these conditions implies that, although this is a manual of special pathology, we are compelled to give a merely symptomatic section instead of sharply defined and precisely characterized descriptions of disease.

Unfortunately, we are at present unable, and probably shall be unable for a long time, to present our knowledge of the subject in any other manner. There can hardly be any other section of clinical medicine as incomplete and neglected as this, and it makes an author feel his subject the more thoroughly thankless the farther he advances with it.

The existing literature on this subject must be described as extremely imperfect, not a few even of the works which are often quoted scarcely rising to the right of being called scientific. The older treatises fail in this, that, having no basis in anatomy and physiology, they have no decided direction; unimportant points are exaggerated, important ones slurred over, incompleteness and gross errors are met with to an unusual extent, even in those works which, in their day, had the highest reputation.

In the last fifteen years (probably as a reaction after the previous flood of literature produced by Lallemand's work) very little, relatively, has been done in this matter; and the best recent authors have sought to criticise what had been formerly done, by the help of the notable progress of modern physiology, without introducing anything really new.

Lallemand's spacious and haughty edifice, fancifully completed even to the smallest details, has thus been changed into a fragmentary and neglected structure, based here and there only upon very poor foundations.

The following study of the subject will be nothing more; it only claims to be a superficial statement of what (according to my own observation and that of others) is probable or certain, and it particularly endeavors to bring out the obscurity and gaps still existing; for a systematic exposition of the subject will only guard the student against mistakes, and urge the physician to further progress, when it has been scientifically established to the last point.

Abnormal Seminal Losses.

(Pollutiones nocturnæ et diurnæ.   Spermatorrhœa.)

A. Cooper, Obs. on the Structure and Diseases of the Testis. London, 1830.—Kobelt, Die männl. und weibl. Wollustorgane. Freiburg, 1844.—Kohlrausch, Zur Anatom. und Physiol. der Beckenorgane. Leipzig, 1854.—Valentin, Phys. des Menschen. Vol. 2. III.—Casper, Gerichtl. Medicin. Biol. Th.—Donné, Nouv. expér. sur les anim. sperm. Paris, 1837.—Frerichs, Todd's Cyclopædia. Vol. IV. —Duplay, Rech. sur le sperme des vieillards (Arch. Gén. Déc. 1852).—Koelliker, Physiol. Stud. über d. Samenflüssigkeit (Zeitsch. f. wissenschaftl. Zoologie. VII. pp. 252 sqq., und Würzb. Verh. VI. pp. 80 sqq.).—Schweiger-Seidel, Arch. f. Mikrosk. Anat. I. p. 309.—La Valette St. George, Ibid. p. 403; and in Stricker's Histology. Cap. XXIV.—P. Mantegazza and Bozzi, Anat. patol. dei testicoli. Milan, 1865.—Mantegazza, Gaz. med. Lombard. Aug. 1869.—Langerhans, Die access. Drüsen d. Geschlectsorgane. Virchow's Archiv. Vol. LXI.— A. Dieu, Sperme des vieillards. Journ. d'Anat. et Physiol. 1867. pp. 449 sqq. —Liégeois, Veränderungen des Samens in Krankh. cf. Virchow's Jahresb. 1870. Vol. I. p. 257.—La Valette St. George, Centralblatt. 1871. p. 342.

Peter Frank, Behandlung der Krankh. des Menschen. (German translation by Sobernheim.) Vol. VII. (A treatise on spermatorrhœa which is still classical.)— *Naumann*, Handb. der med. Klin. (A very complete survey of the literature which had appeared up to that time.)—*Trousseau*, Clinique médicale (Second edition, translated into German by Culmann). Vol. II.— *Canstatt-Henoch*, Spec. Pathol. und Therap.—*Pitha*, Krankh. der männl. Genital. in Virchow's Handbuch.—*Kocher*, in Pitha and Billroth's Handb. der Chirurgie. Vol. III. 2.— *Benedict*, Electrotherapie. First edition.

Wichmann, De pollutione diurna, frequent. sed rarius observ. tabesc. caus. Göttingen, 1782. (A work much esteemed in its time, and even now worth reading.) —See also the very complete account of the literature of spermatorrhœa, up to Lallemand's time, in *Kaula.*—*Lallemand*, Des pertes séminales involontaires. Paris et Montpellier, 1836.—*Civiale*, Traité prat. sur les maladies des org. génit.-urin. II. Cap. 2, des maladies des vésicules séminales, etc. Paris, 1841.—*Pauli*, Ueber Pollutionen mit besond. Bezieh. auf Lallemand's Schrift über diese Krankh. Speyer, 1841. (An unsparing criticism of the first volume, and of the first part of the second volume of Lallemand's work.)—*Kaula*, Der Samenfluss, by Eisenmann. Erlangen, 1847.—*Bergson*, Zur Diagnose und Ther. der unfreiw. Samerverluste. Med. Ztg. 1845. No. 10.—*Clemens*, De semine urinæ intermixt. Frankf. 1849.—*Id.*, Deutsche Klin. 1860.—*Pickford*, Ueber wahre und eingebildete Samenverl. Heidelb. 1851.—*Milton*, Spermatorrhœa. Med. Times, March, 1852.—*Benedict*, Spermatorrh. Oesterr. Zeitschr. f. prakt. Heilk. X. 1864. Nos. 3 and 4.—*L. Mandl*, On the Genito-Spinal Neuroses Connected with Spermatorrhœa. Union méd. 3 and 5. Dec. 1863.—*Skoda*, Ueber Spermatorrhœ. Allgm. med. Centralzeitg. 1869. Nos. 46 and 47.—*Gross*, De la prostatorrhée. Arch. Gén. Sept. 1860.—*Guerlain*, De la prostatorrhée dans ses rapports, etc. Paris, 1860.—*Lazarus*, Wiener med. Presse. 1870. No. 19. (Treatment by Means of the Bougie.)—*Lafonte-Gouzi*, Efficacité du brom. de potass. dans la spermatorrh. Bull. de Thérap. Sept. 1861.—*Nepveu*, Note sur la présence de tubes hyalines partic. dans le liquide spermatique. Gaz. méd. de Paris. 1874. No. 3.

Tissot, Von der Onanie. Translated from the French by Kerstens. Leipzig, 1874.— *Deslandes*, De l'onanisme et des autres abus vénér., etc. Paris, 1835.— *W. A. Johnson*, Lancet. 7th April, 1860. (The same case also quoted by *Behrend*, Ueber Reizung der Geschlechtstheile, besonders über Onanie ganz kleiner Kinder. Journ. f. Kinderkrankh. 1860. Parts 11, 12).—*Lisle*, On the Influence of Spermatorrhœa in the Production of Insanity. Arch. gén. Sept., Oct., 1860.— *R. Ritchie*, Masturbation as a Cause of Mental Disturbance. Lancet. Feb., March, 1861.—*Schroeder van der Kolk*, Pathol. und Therapie der Geisteskrankh. Braunschweig, 1863. Pp. 191, sqq.—*Plagge*, Geschlechtsgenuss und Geistesstörung. Memorabilien. VIII. 8. 1863.

Under this heading we shall describe the long series of conditions connected with abnormal seminal losses, beginning with mere nocturnal pollutions which are still within the limits of health, and reaching their climax in what is called spermatorrhœa.

Many authors will be found who treat impotence and sterility in the male in the same chapter, and with some reason, inasmuch as the two subjects are very closely connected ; but, for the purposes of a general survey of the subject, I shall here separate them.

Before proceeding farther, we must recall to our recollection the most important properties of normal semen, since no account can be given of pathological seminal losses, unless these are known.

In a healthy male who has reached the age of puberty, semen when ejaculated is a colorless, opalescent mass, of alkaline reaction, of the consistence of white of egg, and with a specific odor, which has been compared to that of the flowers of the common barberry, or of the sawing of fresh bone. Soon after ejaculation the almost gelatinous consistence it had at first becomes more fluid (Koelliker). In water fresh semen forms a whitish, flocculent, tenacious sediment. The chemical composition of the seminal fluid has been very little studied. According to Vauquelln, it contains 90 per cent. of water to 10 of solid matter : of which last 4 per cent. consists of inorganic compounds, especially phosphate of lime, the rest being an albuminous body which this author called spermatin.

Semen, as ejaculated, is known not to be a simple secretion of the testicles, but to be a mixture of this with the secretions of the seminal vesicles, of the prostate, and of Cowper's glands. These last in particular contribute the fluid portion of the semen, the secretion from the testicles alone being a whitish, tenacious, inodorous mass. The specific odor is obviously also derived from the secretion of the accessory glands, of which we know little more than that it is strongly albuminous.[1] It is, therefore, erroneous to consider that the peculiar odor is one of the necessary criteria of fertile semen. The only true test of this is to be discovered by the microscope, and is the presence of the so-called "spermatozoids."

The contents of the vas deferens, derived directly from the testis, consists almost entirely of these interesting bodies (about nine-tenths), on the presence and integrity of which (so far as we at present know) the impregnating power of the semen depends. A complete knowledge of these is not merely interesting theoretically, but, as we shall see later on, when treating of sterility in the male, is of practical importance.

Each spermatozoid is made up, as will be remembered, of an oval head, and of a thread-like appendage, which is divided into a middle portion and a tail. The head is broadest at the point of insertion of the appendage, being smaller and

---

[1] Compare *Bruxmann*, Beiträge zur Kenntniss des Prostatasaftes. Giessen, 1864. (A dissertation under Eckhard's direction.)

flatter anteriorly. We need not dwell here upon the minutest structure of this body.

In the vas deferens the seminal bodies are still and motionless, but in recently ejaculated semen they are seen to move actively, and this is a necessary criterium of their functional activity. It is at present uncertain whether the secretions of the accessory sexual glands promote these movements merely physically, by supplying a fluid for their suspension, or whether their action is also chemical, by their alkalinity. The movement is produced only by the thread-like appendage, the head having no appearance of independent motion. After evacuation, the movements may be observed to continue for hours under certain circumstances, and in the dead body for 12 to 24 hours (Koelliker), or even 84 hours (Valentin). In the female genitals when their secretion is normal, this phenomenon may be noticed after eight days, a fact of the highest importance in the theory of impregnation.

Koelliker in particular has given a detailed account of the behavior of these bodies towards various reagents. For our purpose it is enough to know that alkaline fluids excite the movements, while acids paralyze and arrest them; acid secretion from the female genitals would, therefore, have the same effect. Pure water stops the movements, which can be again excited by the addition (even after they have ceased for some time) of sugar, salt, albuminous solutions, etc. Even when semen has been frozen, if not to too low a temperature, the spermatozoa again move on being thawed.

The amount of semen ejaculated on one occasion by a healthy man varies considerably, under the influence of circumstances which are of many different kinds, but some of which are peculiar to each individual. According to Mantegazza it is from 0.75 to 0.6 cubic ctm. in healthy persons.

The frequency of evacuation has a great effect upon the quantity and composition of the semen: the oftener this is repeated, the less is the amount and consistency of the secretion, and, in particular, the fewer the spermatozoa present. A case related by Casper is worthy of note in this respect: a scientific man, sixty years of age, examined for a long while, with Casper, his semen after each coitus, so as to ascertain that it was thinner and poorer in spermatozoids the oftener the act was repeated; if he had connection every day or every other day, these bodies were entirely absent. This last observation, which by no means stands alone, probably applies equally to a large number of men who are capable of the generative act, and has very great practical importance in the investigation of doubtful cases of sterility in the male; for in such cases one has always to bear in mind the possibility of what may be called a physiological temporary absence of seminal bodies in persons who are quite healthy, and to form one's opinion only after repeated inquiry into the different conditions of the sexual act.

It is of equal importance to be informed as to the age when semen is first produced, and when it ceases to be formed. It is well known that fertile semen is not secreted at the same time as the first distinct signs of puberty appear; but at what age this is first produced can hardly be ascertained, even approximately, on account of the difficulty of the inquiry, and also because manifold extraneous circumstances, such as temperament, mode of life, education, determine the greatest differences in this respect. Thus it seems to be possible to anticipate materially the normal period of its formation by masturbation, and by precocious indulgence in lascivious ideas.

The age up to which fertile semen (viz., that which contains spermatozoids) can be formed is decidedly greater than one would à priori be inclined to suppose. The investigations of Duplay and Dieu have established this with tolerable constancy even up to a very great age; only finding the seminal bodies invariably absent after the age of eighty-six. These two authors together dissected the bodies of 152 old men, and found spermatozoa in

25 of the age of	60	....	68.5 per cent.	
76 " "	70	....	59.5	"
51 " "	80	....	48	

In one-third of the cases in which spermatozoa were found they were fewer in number than usual, and were also variously altered in shape, their appendages were shortened or absent, and they were of different sizes.

As to the production of semen in disease, we shall have much to say in the section on Sterility.

Almost every healthy adult male, during the years of sexual activity, loses from time to time a certain quantity of semen at night during sleep, generally with erotic dreams accompanied by erection and special sensations; unless seminal evacuation be produced by coitus or other mechanical cause (masturbation), this kind of loss is called a *pollution*. They of course occur most frequently during the years of greatest sexual activity; but the period of their first occurrence varies extremely in different individuals according to their mental and bodily conditions (such as training, temperament, mode of life, and direction of thought). The same circumstances also determine the frequency of the pollutions, which occur in some persons once a week or oftener, in others once a month or less frequently. Even in the same individual they occur with no regularity, but greatly vary from temporary causes.

Usually the day after these seminal losses there is a feeling of relief and lightness, or, at any rate, an absence of any subjective or objective suffering; and from this alone it can be determined whether the pollution is to be considered as normal. It is a complete mistake to try to decide whether they are healthy or not simply by enumerating them, as some of the best authors (*ex. gr.*, Trousseau) are inclined to do, for what will be very injurious to one man, requiring medical intervention, will in another be quite within the bounds of health.

Next to the feeling of ease after a pollution, the most essential test of its being normal is that it occurs *at night during sleep*, therefore, in the absence of consciousness and of that power of the will which is the chief moderator of the sexual function. The accompanying erotic dreams appear to be not so much the proximate cause as the consequence of that excitement of the genital organs which precedes ejaculation. Even at the present day normal pollutions are ascribed with the greatest probability to a condition which the older authors called somewhat singularly "seminal plethora." It is to be supposed that in healthy men the secretion of the genital glands, if never or too seldom evacuated, naturally accumulates and produces a certain tension of the passages, and particularly of the vesiculæ seminales, which leads to their reflex contraction, and so to ejaculation. To put it teleologically, nature compensates by nocturnal pollutions for the absence of normal evacuations.

This natural occurrence of pollutions may in various ways exceed the bounds of health, and, firstly, *by being more frequently repeated than is suitable to the peculiarities of the individual.* Even when there is not the least irregularity about the act itself, it yet proves itself to be excessive, if, instead of leaving no trace behind, or a feeling of relief, it is followed the next day by a general dulness and weakness, headache, diminution of mental activity, and the like. In this way most cases afterwards known as spermatorrhœa, even the most severe ones, begin by a relative increase in the number of pollutions, which continue for a time to be perfectly normal as far as their following erection and orgasm. The difference in this stage of the disease is not a qualitative one, but consists rather in the increased relative[1] frequency of the occurrence, and in its consequences. It is clear from this that *no sharply defined limit can be drawn between normal and abnormal nocturnal pollutions.* At any rate, there will be cases in which it must depend upon the indi-

---

[1] Particular stress must be laid upon this word "relative," or I might be convicted of inconsistency in what I shall say farther on.

vidual judgment of .the medical attendant whether such seminal losses are to be looked upon as natural or as unhealthy.

If matters become worse, although the frequency of natural pollutions is subject to great individual variations, their number at last reaches a point which we must undoubtedly consider pathological. Patients then have pollutions every other night, or, indeed, once or several times each night. They may still occur without any essential anomaly in the manner of their occurrence; but soon erection and the specific sensation are diminished, and cases sometimes occur in which ejaculation takes place during sleep without being perceived, and is first recognized in the morning by the traces it has left behind. The amount of secretion lost is often much less (as seems, moreover, always to be the case with pollutions as compared with coitus), and it must also be changed in quality, as is proved by its decidedly less consistence.

In spite, however, of the actual loss being less in quantity, and the nervous excitement being much less marked than in ordinary pollutions, the patient on awakening is troubled to a much greater degree with the same general symptoms we have mentioned above. Considerable torpidity of mind and body, pains in the back, palpitation, shortness of breath, weakness of memory, and even affections of speech are here particularly to be remarked.

The malady assumes a much more serious shape when, *even in the daytime, or* (*to speak more precisely*), *when awake, without the usual mechanical causes* (coitus, masturbation), *or as a result of any trifling external cause, seminal losses occur.* These are called *diurnal pollutions,* and are always to be looked upon as pathological, since they imply a serious state of irritable weakness of the genital organs for the ejaculation to take place in spite of perfect consciousness and voluntary power. *A healthy man never loses true semen, when awake, except as a result of coitus, or of some equally intense mechanical cause.* It is necessary to insist upon this in opposition to other authors, for instance, Lallemand, who asserts that true pollutions are quite possible, and, indeed, are frequently produced, in perfectly healthy persons by the mere shaking in riding or driving.

These diurnal pollutions occur in different forms. In what are relatively the most favorable cases, as we have already implied, mechanical action upon the genitals is necessary to produce ejaculation by reflex action—for instance, certain positions and movements which produce some amount of friction or concussion of the generative organs. The pollution then occurs with tolerably complete or partial erection, and also with specific sensations, although these are usually less intense than is natural.

In a yet further degree of the same malady, simple movements of the penis under excitement is sufficient, and soon the patient reaches a stage in which *mechanical causes, even the slightest, are no longer necessary, but the evacuation is produced by mere psychical irritation.* Reading lascivious books, erotic pictures, the mere sight of women, and obscene ideas, are followed by seminal losses, usually with little or no erection and orgasm ; but, on the contrary, sometimes with a burning sensation in the penis, which is completely flaccid.

The case will generally be considered still more serious when *patients pass semen with urine or fæces, without any thought of sexual matters.* The existence of this form of spermatorrhœa (which Hippocrates long ago described) cannot be denied, and if attempts have occasionally been made to do so in too skeptical a spirit, these have been the natural reaction against the exaggerations into which Lallemand and his school have fallen. But it is necessary to be particularly careful to avoid several sources of confusion, which will be more closely examined when we come to treat of diagnosis. Whether *true semen* can be lost *by perfectly healthy, strong men* of normal sexual excitability, under such circumstances, as even some authors of note are inclined to think, I must for the present leave undecided; but I believe that even single ejaculations in these conditions imply a state of morbid irritability. We shall return to the subject again.

Finally, I am also doubtful whether we are to receive quite literally the accounts given of cases in which semen is said to have flowed continually from the penis. Nothing at all approaching this has come before me in the course of a not inconsiderable experience, and the best authors express themselves with great reserve on the subject. Probably cases are described in this language where the irritable weakness has been so great that the very slightest causes, hardly even felt, produce flow of the genital secretion, which therefore takes place *with extreme frequency.*

We have been, therefore, brought to recognize three forms in which abnormal loss of semen is observed. Between the two first (nocturnal and diurnal pollutions) there is a sharp boundary line, according as they occur during consciousness and when the power of the will is active, or not. It is more difficult to distinguish "spermatorrhœa" (a term usually applied to the highest degrees of the malady) from diurnal pollutions, for the definition of the term varies in different authors, some using it only for cases (at the least, very rare) of frequent or almost constant flow of the secretion from the genital glands, while others consider its characteristic to be the absence of erection and orgasm, and others, again, employ it generally for all the varieties of abnormal seminal losses.

We consider all attempts to distinguish minutely between diurnal pollutions and spermatorrhœa as useless, and in what we are about to say shall use the latter term *merely for the worse degrees of the former;* while occasionally, for the sake of brevity, the word must serve as a generic name for all pathological evacuations of semen.

Etiology.

Although so much has been written, with a semblance of great accuracy, on the causation of abnormal seminal losses, yet, on going into the subject, we find it generally obscure, and with considerable gaps in it. On the whole, those authors have done most harm who have violently tried to force the subject into an arbitrary, narrow scheme, as did Lallemand (who was for some time almost omnipotent in this matter) and most of his disciples and admirers.

We must, above everything, remember (what those authors overlooked) that *abnormal seminal losses by no means constitute a separate disease, but are only a symptom, which may be traced partly to local, partly to general affections, and partly to both of these together.*

This leads at once to the conception that *the collection of general disturbances of nutrition, and of nervous symptoms, which some authors ascribe to spermatorrhœa, are not caused by it, but are co-ordinate with it, and owe their origin to the same conditions as produce it.*

Direct observation confirms this in by far the greater number of cases, by teaching us that, under influences of very various kinds, first general or local disturbances are produced, which then either directly cause spermatorrhœa (a new, very prominent, and, in its turn, very important link in the chain of symptoms), or, by means of other assisting causes, bring it about immediately or after they have been at work for some time.

These general conditions, which precede the severer forms of spermatorrhœa, are better known to us in their symptoms than in their own nature. Even at the present day we, like the older writers, are obliged to content ourselves with vague descriptions of them, finding perhaps some consolation in the very fact that we are more conscious of our ignorance than our predecessors were. We mean that there is, in connection with anæmia, *a debility of the whole body, and in particular of the nervous system, which consequently becomes unduly excitable.*[1]

Some persons—fortunately, very few—are unusually predisposed to this condition, either from hereditary influence or as a result of previous disease, so that slight causes, which in others could hardly be called excesses, are capable of so far disturbing the general health and genital functions as to bring about abnormal pollutions, and even spermatorrhœa. We frequently learn that these unfortunate individuals have many insane or epileptic relations, or that they have themselves been for a long while very excitable or even epileptic. Trousseau has particularly pointed out that many of them have been subject to nocturnal enuresis, and that, in place of the earlier irritability of their urinary passages, a similar condition of the genital organs comes on with puberty.

---

[1] See the detailed description of this condition below, in the Symptomatology.

Many chronic diseases and convalescence from some acute diseases — particularly infectious ones — very decidedly predispose to this state, which fortunately hardly ever goes farther than nocturnal pollutions ; we need here only mention the early stages of pulmonary phthisis, convalescence from enteric fever, etc.

But in by far the greater number of cases, patients who were previously in perfectly good bodily health, have, by their own act, induced a state of which spermatorrhœa is a result. In this respect the most important causes are *the various forms of sexual excess.*

Before going farther, we must remember that the limits of excess are more extensive in the case of the genital functions than of any others in the body. Sexual activity and the tolerance of it are well known to be so extremely variable, that we constantly see persons who commit what, according to ordinary ideas, would be the greatest excesses, without any ill results.[1] The principal reasons for these individual diversities are constitution (heredity), temperament, age, education, mode of life, and occupation.

Masturbation plays a particularly prominent part among the abuses of the genital organs.

To speak plainly, the majority of those who suffer from spermatorrhœa either are, or have been, masturbators. Either they have abandoned themselves to this vice alone, or they have indulged in it after giving way to ordinary sexual excess.

Masturbation is of the greatest importance as a cause, not merely of spermatorrhœa, but of the other functional diseases of the genital organs. Undoubtedly, it does much more harm than ordinary sexual excess ; and, at first sight, this might appear strange. It might be said that masturbation and coitus are, mechanically considered, precisely similar acts, with the same results, and that the reaction on the constitution must therefore be the same. This may be granted of each individual act of both kinds, for certainly the moralizing phrase, so often heard—"The infraction of the laws of nature revenges itself severely "—needs no serious refutation. The very weighty reasons why masturbators suffer so much more severely are of quite another kind. In the first place, masturbation *begins much sooner in life,*

---

[1] In this respect I am always reminded of one of our most able literary men, who, according to his own admission, masturbated to a very great extent from his ninth to his twentieth year, without suffering in body or mind, as his literary success proves.

even in early childhood, and, on an average, long before coitus is possible.[1] Again, masturbators *indulge in this vice much more frequently* than is possible in the case of natural sexual excess. The opportunity (so to speak) is always present, and every erotic impression may be followed immediately by the unnatural act. Even an erection is not required for its completion, as may be learned from masturbators if they give their full confidence to their medical attendant. These unfortunate individuals, then, set no bounds to their indulgence. I have myself known patients who, for a long time together, have masturbated from four to six times in each twenty-four hours, and other writers give still more shocking particulars.

As the masturbator is quite independent of external circumstances, and has no other check than his own will, which rapidly grows weaker, he is cured of his habit with far greater difficulty than one who exceeds "in venere vera," and who has therefore much to do with external factors. We have just seen, that even without erection (and therefore in impotent patients) masturbation is possible, and many persons who have sought to rid themselves of this habit by natural coitus in marriage, on finding this to be impossible, relapse again into it.

The force of habit in this regard is completely irresistible to many persons. Some time since a merchant consulted me, who had been married for years, and yet could not abandon the practice of masturbation, although he rightly ascribed to it a number of serious nervous ailments. The case strongly reminded me of one related by Schroeder van der Kolk:[2] a clergyman, even as a young man, strove against this vice, married early in life for this reason, and yet could never overcome it, although he was the father of five children.

Next after masturbation, natural sexual excess is also a frequent cause of spermatorrhœa.

But it must not be forgotten that many of such patients either have been, or are still, masturbators; and one cannot help believing that, but for this habit, the constitution of many of them would have shown greater tolerance of the results of natural excess. The bodily power of resistance in this respect is, of course, extremely variable in different individuals; indeed, the limits of variation are probably wider than in the case of masturbators, although determined by the same external and individual conditions.

---

[1] Erections are well known to be observed in quite young children; I have myself observed them at the age of six months, when infants are warmly clad, and lie on their backs. The youngest child I have seen who masturbated was four years old; I have often afterwards seen it attacked by epileptiform convulsions. Other writers have assigned three years, and even less, as the earliest period at which masturbation is begun. (See *Johnson* and *Behrend*, loc. cit.)

[2] Pathol. und Ther. der Geisteskrankh. p. 195, note.

It is often important to inquire into the external circumstances under which a patient has practised sexual excess; it may be found that frequently these greatly favor the production of abnormal pollutions. I have had under my care, for very frequent pollutions, an upholsterer, an extremely strongly built young man, twenty-nine years of age. For many years, while living in the same house with his mistress, he had connection with her at least four times a week without the least injury to his health. He then removed to another dwelling which was about a league from her house, and continued to have connection with her as frequently as before, walking home each night soon after the act. After six months very serious pollutions came on, at first only by night, but later also by day, which ceased very soon on his giving up this mode of life, and being put under tonic treatment.

Let us now ask *in what way sexual excess, whether natural or unnatural, produces its effect upon the genital functions; what conditions are the specially injurious ones; and how spermatorrhœa is thereby established?*

Formerly, by far the most injurious part of the harm done by sexual excess was sought to be ascribed to the loss of semen, which is admitted to be a highly concentrated and composite secretion;[1] but at the present day, this view of the question has been almost entirely abandoned. For, in the first place, the semen ejaculated on each occasion had been previously collected in the vesiculæ seminales, and was therefore out of the circulation, and of no further account in the economy. And, if it be objected that with increased frequency of excess a much larger quantity is secreted and so withdrawn from the body, it may be replied that the amount of material thus lost is so small that any notable alterations of nutrition cannot be explained thereby.

The most important source of mischief is apparently rather to be found in the *conditions which precede and accompany ejaculation, and especially in certain phenomena connected with the nervous system*, which have a two-fold effect—on the genital organs in particular, and then on the general health. In most patients, at any rate after some time, both these classes of effects are observed together; but they are very variously combined, according as in one person the tolerance of the system at large is greater, or in another the genital organs are more resistant.

---

[1] See above, in the Introduction, the chemistry of the seminal fluid.

As far as sexual excess *especially affects the genital* organs, it is clear that their frequent excitement by often-repeated erections and ejaculations must give rise to an irritability, and then to a diseased condition of the parts. At first, this consists in an increased secretion from the genital glands,[1] which in turn, by increased pressure on the walls of the genital canals, leads reflexly to more frequent erections and ejaculations (see above, the description of normal pollutions). Moreover, the ejaculations are greatly favored by a much higher state of irritability of the expulsive apparatus, which responds to central and peripheric stimuli with an ejaculation far more readily than usual; the older authors not inaptly called this condition one of "irritable weakness." Beyond this irritability, or habit of ejaculation under abnormally slight causes, a relaxation and enlargement of the ejaculatory ducts may also exist, removing an important obstacle which in health prevents spontaneous flow of semen when the passages are full.

A further influence, and one very injurious to these patients, is that the ejaculations themselves always have a stimulating effect on the genitals, increasing thereby both the amount and the readiness of excretion, so that these unhappy persons, under the influence of this vicious circle of cause and effect, pass sooner or later (especially when their constitution and mode of life is unfavorable) from ordinary nocturnal pollutions to diurnal ones, and finally to actual spermatorrhœa.

It seems to me more than doubtful whether true inflammation of the urinary passage, prostate, ejaculatory ducts, and testicles, is ever produced by excessive coitus or masturbation, as Lallemand and his disciples consider to be certain, and even not very uncommon. No doubt the theoretical possibility of this occurrence cannot be denied; but we never witness anything of the kind in masturbators, in

---

[1] Whether the testicles and the other glands of the sexual apparatus share proportionately in this increase of secretion, is not established; it seems more probable that they do not, at any rate in the severer forms of spermatorrhœa. It is usually found in such cases that, while the quantity of fluid ejaculated undergoes little or no diminution, it is notably thinner, less coagulable, and almost destitute of its peculiar odor. The microscope shows that the number of spermatozoids is considerably diminished, so that the conclusion is suggested, that in such cases the secretory activity of the testicles, relatively to that of the other glands (prostate, seminal vesicles, etc.), is diminished.

whom it should be most frequently observed.   On account of the intensity of the cause, and in cases of natural sexual excess it is scarcely possible to exclude gonorrhœal infection, which (as we shall afterwards see) favors the development of spermatorrhœa in persons already predisposed to it.

Let us now ask *how sexual excess acts on the constitution at large, and how it leads, through this, to spermatorrhœa ?*

It has been already shown that the mischief does not consist in the loss of semen; by far the most important influence of sexual excess is upon the nervous system and (secondarily?) upon nutrition.   The act of copulation, and those mechanical irritations which have the like effect, are well known to be connected with a very intense excitement of the nervous system, which reaches its highest point just before ejaculation, and ends by the reflex discharge.   Even in a state of health the act is followed by a notable degree of relaxation, which, however, soon passes away without any trace; but, if it be repeated too often (relatively to the strength and tolerance of each individual) the physiological effects on the nervous system become more enduring.   This view has been met with the objection that women, undergoing the same nervous excitement in coitus as men do, scarcely suffer in their general condition, and as to their nervous system in particular, from sexual excess. · It is argued thence, that this cannot be the source of its injurious effects in men, and that some other mode of action must, therefore, be looked for. The conclusion would be valid if the premises were true; but, in the first place, the intense agitation which in the male precedes erection is absent in the female; and secondly, the excitement of the nervous system during coitus seems to increase more slowly in women, and seldom to reach the same pitch as it attains in men just before ejaculation.   Daily experience accords with this, as showing that women are decidedly less affected by each act than men, and can repeat it much more frequently without injury.[1]

Unfortunately, the intimate connection between the nervous system and the genital functions is very little known, so that we are still almost completely in the dark as to the special manner in which its changes bring about spermatorrhœa.

---

[1] See *J. Mueller's* Physiology. Vol. II. p. 643.

We have most information as to the relation of the spinal cord to the genital organs. According to Eckhard,[1] certain spinal nerves have been shown specially to govern erection; and Goltz[2] has established that its primary centre is in the lumbar portion of the cord; the movements of the seminal vesicles and ducts seem also to be connected with the same part (Budge, Eckhard-Loeb). The secretion of semen seems likewise to be governed by the spinal cord; at least, it is arrested by injury of that organ (Longet).

We are also indebted to Eckhard for some highly interesting particulars as to the relation of the brain to this function. In rabbits, he has produced erection by electrical stimulation of the pons and of the points where the crura cerebri enter the cerebrum, while similar irritation of the cerebellum had no such effect;[3] whence he concludes that the "nervi erigentes" have their origin in the cerebellum.

Starting from these physiological data, we can very readily understand that the too frequent irritation of the peripheral ends of the spinal nerves, caused by sexual excess, may gradually lead to an "irritable" condition of the reflex centres in the brain and spinal cord, which would cause abnormally slight central (mental) or peripheral impulses to bring about contraction of the seminal vesicles and ejaculation.

The assumption that there is some *functional anomaly of the spinal cord* is supported by the existence of those nervous symptoms which we shall by and by more fully describe, especially the sensory and motor disturbances observed in bad cases, and the occasional occurrence of difficulty in micturition and defecation.

But we cannot agree to the supposition that *actual and intense degeneration of the spinal cord* can be produced by sexual excess alone. We shall have to return to this point later, and will here only remark that this erroneous belief must be due (besides the external resemblance between the two conditions) frequently to this, that in the beginning of diseases of the spinal cord, among other symptoms of the congestion thus produced, patients often complain of violent erections amounting even to

---

[1] *Eckhard's* Beiträge. Vol. VII. pp. 67, sqq. Compare also the other essays of this author, who has opened the way to our knowledge of erection.

[2] See, in the chapter "Impotence," a more detailed account of the physiology of erection.

[3] Precisely the contrary of the ordinary supposition, that the centre of the sexual passion (as *Gall* taught) is in the cerebellum.

priapism, and frequent pollutions. These symptoms may then readily mask other less striking ones, or may so far impose upon the patient as to lead him to consider them to have been the earliest, and to have been the cause of his malady.

I remember the case of a merchant, a married man, and very discreet in his sexual relations, in whom very frequent erections (almost amounting to priapism) and pollutions occurred at a time when only very vague symptoms suggested to his medical attendant a suspicion of some commencing spinal affection. Only by degrees, and later, did the phenomena of ataxia become clearly developed.

Physiological experiments prove that the *brain* has a two-fold influence over the sexual function, partly by the existence of a reflex centre for erection, which has been shown to exist here also (Eckhard), and also by those parts of the brain which are connected with the so-called psychical functions.

Even in the case of abnormal seminal losses, mental conditions play a very important part, as such patients are, sooner or later, completely dominated by extravagant sexual ideas. Very dissolute men (and this is especially true of masturbators) gradually fall into a state of mind in which all serious mental occupation becomes difficult and even impossible, their former energy is paralyzed and their memory enfeebled. Their thoughts and desires turn essentially on sexual matters, and things which are almost indifferent to men of sound mind are a sufficient occasion for them to indulge in wild fancies. Of course, this "mental masturbation" has a very decided effect upon the genital organs, and leads to sexual excess, or, when this is not indulged in, the genital irritation excites in its turn the diseased state of mind. A mutual interchange of cause and effect is thus gradually produced, which is most injurious to the patient, between the almost continual stimulation of the genital organs and immoral thoughts. These patients always go from bad to worse, so that, while at first only frequent nocturnal pollutions occur, they are soon produced in the daytime by very slight causes.

This incontinence of mind is decidedly more injurious, as a cause of irritation of the sexual organs, than mere excess in venery, even to persons of otherwise sound mind, exposing them to very great risk of becoming masturbators.

Physicians and students should pay particular attention to

this condition, which is very readily developed in youths who are deficient in force of character and strength of will, but, after it has lasted some time, can only be eradicated with great difficulty, and becomes at last almost incurable.

Psychical conditions play a part—and one not to be too much neglected—in those cases, which are certainly very rare, where *absolute or relative continence* has led to morbid pollutions. If, in strong men of lively, sanguineous temperament, no natural satisfaction of the sexual appetite is obtained, frequent erections and increased flow of blood to the part may result, and pollutions (which were before not too frequent) gradually increase under the persistent influence of genital irritation.

Lallemand, who usually tends to exaggerate, has laid undue stress on continence as a cause of morbid seminal losses; while others, especially English authors, err on the opposite side, by giving a very positive denial to this statement. The truth lies between the two opinions: such cases do occur,[1] but, as I have already said, very rarely indeed, and only under a combination of specially favorable circumstances, of which the chief are generally nervous temperament, whether congenital or acquired, and strong sexual instincts kept up by external impressions.

It is necessary, however, to be on one's guard against too great credulity in this matter. For the most part these cases are more complex than they seem, and the majority of the patients who assign this as the cause of their illness are masturbators, who either still practise the vice, or were for a long time addicted to it.[2] They have urgent need of making their ailment known to their medical attendant, but only go half-way, and speak of their seminal losses, without mentioning that they had themselves, in an unnatural manner, produced them. This common psycho-

---

[1] Certain observations on stallions afford almost an experimental proof of the possible occurrence of these cases. According to the statements, particularly, of French veterinarians, stallions which on account of their bad points are only used for the purpose of ascertaining whether the mares are ready for covering, but are not allowed to cover them, suffer from spermatorrhœa. This statement, which I found originally in Kaula's work, has been confirmed to me by Privy Councillor Gurlt, who, however, also told me that these animals are much addicted to masturbation.

[2] These latter patients, in particular, cannot with truth ascribe their pollutions to continence, but to the irritability and weakness of the genital organs produced by the evil habit in which they had long indulged, though afterwards abandoned, and which must be considered the principal cause of seminal losses afterwards favored by continence.

logical peculiarity must always be borne in mind when examining suspected masturbators.

Lallemand has much to say of diurnal pollutions as a result
of continence in persons who, generally slightly built, have particularly flaccid, small, undeveloped genital organs, and in whom
seminal loss would appear, as a rule, to occur unconsciously
when passing motions or urine. Since the days of Lallemand
and his enthusiastic followers, these statements have received no
very positive confirmation ; while, à priori, one would expect to
meet with a less intense sexual passion in such persons, and, at
the same time, diminished genital activity ; besides, not a few of
these patients may be masturbators.

We have now to mention a series of conditions which are usually termed *local causes of abnormal pollutions. These include
certain affections of various parts of the genito-urinary and
neighboring organs, and alterations of their contents.*

But it is not to be supposed that these conditions always, or
even in the majority of cases, produce spermatorrhœa *alone, and
without other changes in the body*—a plausible but one-sided
view, which has been particularly adopted by the school of Lallemand, and the one which chiefly led him to describe spermatorrhœa due to local causes as an almost self-existent disease.

Lallemand's lively imagination was under the guidance of theories, and, therefore, made him attach himself too exclusively to these local states, causing him
often to ignore coexisting general conditions of great importance. The argument
used by his followers, that he had every reason, from the results of his treatment,
to take the view he did, is a poor one. Recent independent observers have by no
means so frequently seen good results follow local treatment; and when they are
noted, they may be partly due, not to the mechanical, but to the moral effect of
these manipulations upon patients who place reliance upon them; for we learn by
experience that the influence of the mind is greater over diseases of the genital organs than over those of any other part of the body.

Moreover, it is to be remarked that Lallemand certainly fell into many errors in
diagnosis. This was first pointed out by Pauli, who was, however, too sceptical;
but it can be shown that Lallemand frequently took what were obviously cases of
gleet for spermatorrhœa. He also gives histories of patients whom he examined
minutely for spermatorrhœa, although they had no suspicion of its existence, and
perhaps complained of very different ailments; the seminal losses were not exactly
proved to exist, but were looked upon as the cause of all their other maladies.

Again, in other cases, where there certainly was spermatorrhœa, we find Lallemand ascribing it to very unimportant local causes, as a scrotal or perineal eczema, or a hemorrhoidal tumor, while *sexual excess is mentioned quite incidentally, or not reported at all, although it might have been discovered.*

It cannot, indeed, be denied that local changes in the parts mentioned above may be sufficient causes of pollutions, which may, by degrees, become abnormally frequent ; but this is by no means the case so often, and so independently of other causes, as Lallemand supposed. It will always, however, be an undoubted merit of this brilliant author that he called particular attention to the etiological relation of these local affections to spermatorrhœa. *They are, however, always essentially exciting causes, giving the last impulse to morbid seminal losses, to which there had long been a predisposition, by the action of more general conditions of another kind.*

We will first mention one of the most important of these causes, viz.: *a chronic inflammatory state of the neck of the bladder, and of the urethral mucous membrane adjoining the orifices of the ejaculatory ducts* (the prostatic portion of the urethra, and particularly the caput gallinaginis).

The very merit of Lallemand's account of this affection, which has obtained a certain historical celebrity through his brilliant style, makes it a danger in the study of our whole subject. Being the discoverer of this cause of spermatorrhœa, he thought he found it in almost every case, and as universally employed his one-sided treatment (cauterization of the caput gallinaginis).

No doubt the possible existence of this condition must be seriously considered in every case of morbid seminal losses.[1] Sometimes a gleet may be discovered which has remained after gonorrhœa has either died out or been checked by active treatment, and may be rendered more obstinate, or even increased, by the production of a stricture, leading to increased irritation of the mucous membrane from obstruction to the passage of urine and secretion from the inflamed part.

---

[1] *Benedict* (Electrotherapie, 1st ed. p. 447) states that the Austrian soldiers inject brandy into the urethra in order to check gonorrhœa, and thereby frequently produce spermatorrhœa. This is extremely interesting as an almost experimental proof of the possible propagation of this disease from the urethra.

The particular mode in which this produces pollutions is this: the mucous membrane is inflamed and in a state of increased irritability, and so more readily produces the reflex discharge of ejaculation. In many cases seminal losses may be particularly facilitated by a result of this inflammation—a flaccidity of the ejaculatory ducts and the surrounding tissue, which, in health, is very elastic.[1] An enlargement of the seminal passages is thus brought about, allowing the semen to pass into the urethra in response to a less stimulus, and with less expulsive force than usual. This very plausible theoretical supposition is supported by the results of treatment—by the action of astringents, for instance, but still has much need of further anatomical proof.[2] As we shall hereafter see, Trousseau has based a peculiar mechanical treatment of spermatorrhœa upon this theory of the relaxation of the seminal vessels, which has been successful in suitable cases.

It would, however, be erroneous to set up two distinct forms of spermatorrhœa on the basis of the facts just mentioned—viz.: a form due to increased irritability of the seminal vessels, and an atonic form—for neither of these exists separately, but they are almost always so combined that the evidences of the one are much more prominent than those of the other.

It is almost necessary to assume the existence of flaccidity and enlargement of the ejaculatory ducts to explain the extreme cases of seminal loss known as spermatorrhœa (in the strict sense); for, when semen escapes from the slightest causes—sexual impulse being not increased or even diminished—the passage must be considerably dilated.

It is not, however, to be forgotten that abnormal pollutions do not follow upon every case of gleet, even if complicated with

---

[1] The ejaculatory ducts become notably narrower towards their orifices, as may be seen on mere external inspection (they are 4 mm. thick in their course, and 1 mm. at their terminations). In the prostate they are surrounded by a cavernous tissue, which, by its elasticity, usually closes the urethral orifices of the ducts, so that, in order to allow the passage of semen, a much greater pressure than that of mere secretion is needed. Compare *Luschka* (Anat. der Beckenorgane) and *Henle* (Nachr. v. d. Königl. Gesellsch. d. Wissensch. zu Göttingen. 1863. No. 9).

[2] Hitherto a condition of this kind has only once been found post-mortem, by *Lallemand.* See the section below on "Pathological Anatomy."

stricture; they only occur in very few instances, from which alone we might conclude that other predisposing causes must also exist in such patients. It will most frequently be found that, before the local symptoms occurred, the general symptoms (particularly of the nervous system) due to sexual excess might be recognized.

The conclusion of the whole is that we must look upon chronic inflammation of the prostatic portion of the urethra as being pre-eminently a condition which favors spermatorrhœa, and must give it a very important place in this respect. But it is needful to urge minute care in the diagnosis of this affection, remembering that the example of Lallemand and his followers is to be shunned, as well as the treatment based upon their views, being by no means harmless to the patient in its results, as much unfortunate experience has shown.

Affections of the vesiculæ seminales very rarely cause abnormal seminal losses, being themselves not common. The extremely rare *acute inflammation* of those organs is a very distinct example of spermatorrhœa produced by purely local causes; such patients are tormented by very frequent and painful losses of semen, which sometimes—a symptom much dreaded by non-professional persons—is mixed with blood. The pollutions, of course, cease on the disappearance of the disease, which, by the way, is not one admitting of a very favorable prognosis.

Chronic inflammation of the seminal vesicles also produces pollutions, probably not always, but especially when it is connected with gleet; for the form which accompanies hypertrophy of the prostate seems hardly ever to lead to spermatorrhœa, although no doubt the age of the patient has much to do with this difference. Those cases in which a single or repeated contusions of the perineum have been followed by seminal losses must be considered as belonging to affections of the vesiculæ seminales, and perhaps also of the prostate and ejaculatory ducts, the condition being one either of acute inflammation or of morbid irritability as a result of concussion.

The way in which these affections of the seminal vesicles produce pollutions is always to be explained by a reflex contraction of their walls in response to the irritated mucous membrane.

Another very rare anomaly of the seminal vesicles, which we only mention here for the sake of completeness in enumeration, also produces pollutions by reflex action, viz.: *pressure and traction upon them* brought about by union with neighboring organs (as after lithotomy), by vesical hernia,[1] or by tumors.

The condition of the *prepuce* is also important as a cause of spermatorrhœa; special attention has been called to it by Lallemand (though with exaggeration), Pauli, Pitha, and others. *Too great length and narrowness of the foreskin,* which makes it difficult or impossible to uncover or clean the glans, may produce inflammatory irritation of that part by decomposition of the accumulated preputial smegma; and it is clear that pollutions may thus be produced by reflex action in persons already predisposed thereto, and may afterwards become habitual if the cause continues.

It is to be noted that in specially irritable persons a phymosis, which appears only moderate when the organ is flaccid, may, during erection, produce such a mechanical pressure on the penis as to cause pollutions. Compare the case, related by Pitha, of a young medical man thus affected, and whom he cured of spermatorrhœa by circumcision.

It is also very important to bear in mind that phymosis is very often the first cause of masturbation. Children are very readily led to form this habit by the violent irritation so produced; and when they reach the years of manhood, they suffer from spermatorrhœa, which is to be ascribed at least as much to masturbation as to phymosis.

Abnormal states of the rectum and anus are likewise correctly assigned as causes favoring spermatorrhœa. This is then brought about in one of two ways: either sympathetic contraction of the vesiculæ seminales is produced by the intimate connection between the nerves of the pelvic organs, or the contents of the rectum when set in movement press out a portion of the fluid in the vesicles.

The effect of *constipation* has been much discussed; it can

---

[1] *Peter Frank* long ago mentioned these causes; his account of spermatorrhœa is far superior to that given by almost all modern authors. (Behandlung der Krankh. des Menschen, übers. v. Sobernheim. Berlin, 1835. Vol. II. p. 133.)

act only when it is *habitual,* for when merely transitory, the pollutions it may produce can, of course, not be habitual. It may be readily explained as a sympathetic effect, according to which view the vesiculæ seminales would be set in action at the same time as violent contraction of the rectum, and in particular of the sphincter ani, occurs; on the other hand, many authors urge energetically that the influence of costiveness in producing abnormal pollutions is *merely mechanical.* Some believe that actual semen may be lost, under these circumstances, by strong, healthy men, particularly when they live continently. They consider that hard fæcal masses, which distend the rectum, may in their downward passage press out some of the contents of the seminal vesicles; and they consider that they remove every objection to this view by proving that the fluid evacuated contains spermatozoa.[1] In five such cases of perfectly healthy men, who passed fluid from the urethra, sometimes frequently, with or after a stool, I examined the fluid microscopically, and never found spermatozoa, so that I am led to the conclusion that these discharges are not to be looked upon as true semen, but probably as a prostatic secretion.

When real semen is lost (and we have no reason to doubt the statements made on this subject), there may, of course, be diseased conditions, although not fully developed; but I should be rather inclined to believe that the seminal loss is produced by sympathy, and not merely mechanically. For, as a matter of theory, the alleged action of pressure from the rectum upon the vesiculæ seminales is by no means so plausible as might at first sight appear. These organs, between the bladder and rectum, are tolerably mobile, and can easily give way in one direction or another, under any pressure; so that pressure would act much more readily upon the orifices, which lie close together and are relatively more fixed, than upon the very divergent cæcal ends of those organs; now, pressure upon the orifices of the vesicles

---

[1] *Pickford,* Ueber wahre und eingebildete Samenverluste. Heidelberg, 1841.—*Davy,* Edinb. Med. and Surg. Journ. Vol. I. 1838. It is singular that this latter author appears generally to have found the spermatozoa dead, which is scarcely consistent with the character of the recently evacuated semen of a healthy man, and must therefore rather cause grave suspicion of some previously existing disorder of the genital system.

would be much more likely to produce obstruction than evacuation.

There is much more anatomical probability in supposing the fluid in question to be prostatic secretion. The prostate is known to be very firmly fixed in the pelvis, and to be so placed between the fundus of the bladder and the rectal pouch immediately above the anus (which is particularly well marked anteriorly), that during defecation hard masses must almost inevitably be pressed against the prostate by the backward action of the sphincter ani.

We repeat, then, that we look upon those cases in which actual semen is lost as pathological, and ascribe the loss to a sympathetic influence upon the ejaculatory apparatus, which could hardly be possible in perfectly healthy men.

Hemorrhoidal tumors, painful fissures, itching eczema, and *other eruptions about the anus* may, of course, as frequent accompaniments of habitual constipation, materially assist in the production of pollutions by the violent local irritation to which they give rise.

It will often be worth while to ascertain whether *ascarides* are present. If they are very numerous, they may keep up a chronic irritation of the rectal mucous membrane, which is sometimes very intense, and may, by sympathy, produce frequent pollutions in persons already predisposed thereto. As is well known, they are most commonly met with in children, and then, indeed, frequently lead to masturbation, and therefore indirectly to spermatorrhœa in later life.

Peter Frank mentions among the exciting causes of pollutions the use of *irritating clysters, too hot or too cold*. The possibility of this in strongly predisposed persons cannot be denied, and may, no doubt, be explained also by sympathetic action.

In the same way many *affections of the bladder*—above all, lithiasis—may give rise to spermatorrhœa. To the same category belongs the often-observed effect of certain *medicines*, improperly employed for too long a time, *which irritate the mucous membrane of the urinary organs, particularly cantharides.* However, the mere fact that the individual is taking such remedies

would in most cases suggest a degree of sexual feebleness sufficient to predispose greatly to spermatorrhœa.

I am not quite clear how syphilis, as such, can conduce to
spermatorrhœa, as Lallemand considers to be a very possible and
frequent occurrence. In such cases it is far more likely that the
general results of previous excess are to blame, and perhaps, in
addition to these, acquired chronic inflammations of the genital
organs (gonorrhœal affections).

To the category of psycho-pathological curiosities belong
those cases in which intense mental excitement (often of a totally
different kind, as violent terror, fear, anger, or shame), though
of course transient, produces seminal losses and even diurnal
pollutions. Our literature records many such instances, which
are, of course, of no practical importance.[1]

Mental strain may also sometimes lead to morbid pollutions.
When this is the case, it must always be in persons with greatly
disordered nervous systems, or otherwise highly predisposed.

Pathological Anatomy.

There hardly exists any special anatomical information as to
the conditions of which we are treating. One reason for this is
that such cases are either never examined post-mortem, or only
when extensive disease of other kinds has completely masked
the particular anatomical characters. Moreover, even when circumstances are favorable to post-mortem examination, this
would generally lead to no result, as we may conclude from
what has been said above, under the head of Etiology ; for we
find that various conditions play a very important part as
causes, which could hardly leave any anatomical traces at present appreciable by us.

In a small number of instances, namely, where certain local
affections of the urinary and pelvic organs have been the causes
of morbid seminal losses, special results will certainly be found
on dissection. We obtain thereby, however, nothing more than

---

[1] Occasionally, no doubt, conditions of sexual excitement, produced under these abnormal circumstances, are of practical account from a medico-legal point of view.

simple descriptions of the local changes in the organs involved, and so far do not advance our knowledge of the subject. Kaula has collected a number of such accounts of port-mortems,[1] to which we may here refer those who value obscure descriptions of disease. The following are the morbid appearances observed: the results of chronic inflammation, with suppuration and induration in the prostatic portion of the urethra, extending towards the ejaculatory ducts and seminal vesicles. These last are atrophied or notably enlarged, and partially adherent to neighboring organs; sometimes the orifices of the ducts are fissured and dilated, their walls are thinned and their lumen enlarged. Besides these changes, there may be found strictures of the urethra, inflammations of the bladder (particularly of the neck); while the prostate may be wholly or partially hypertrophied, or, on the contrary, atrophied.

There have hitherto been no systematic examinations, in cases of spermatorrhœa, of the whole genital apparatus and of the nervous structures in direct relation therewith, which are on a level with the present state of science. They have probably not been made because far more important matters delay their solution.

Preceding and Accompanying Symptoms.

Diagnosis.

We must above all never lose sight of the fact that spermatorrhœa is only a symptom, and never a special malady, as Lallemand and his school endeavor to prove; we cannot therefore head this section with the phrase "symptoms of this disease."

We will, merely for the sake of completeness, begin by describing those alterations of the genital organs and their secretions which are connected with these morbid conditions; next pass on to those disorders of other organs which most frequently precede seminal losses, and seem to stand in the relation of causes to them; and finally, treat of the series of symptoms accompanying them. Most of these last are *co-effects* with the

---

[1] Loc. cit. pp. 134 sqq.

pollutions (as cannot be sufficiently insisted upon in opposition to Lallemand's teachings), while a few may be ascribed to the immediate influence of spermatorrhœa upon the nervous system and the mind. We shall see in the therapeutical section of our work how important it is to be quite clear upon these points, the physician being thereby spared many mistakes, and the patient much useless and even injurious manipulation.

We have already sufficiently informed ourselves as to the various conditions and ways in which spermatorrhœa occurs, and as to the various terms founded thereon—nocturnal and diurnal pollutions, and spermatorrhœa in the strict sense of the word. What we then stated we must again repeat: that *no certain diagnosis of the loss of true semen can be made without the use of the microscope*,[1] neither the color, odor, nor consistence of a discharge, nor the manner in which it is evacuated, being a sufficient test of this. We shall further see that seminal loss is very easily and frequently confused with other states ; for, on the one hand, the physical characters just mentioned are common to true semen with certain other secretions ; and, on the other hand, the seminal fluid in spermatorrhœa is very different from its normal state. A familiar knowledge of healthy semen, and particularly of its microscopical character, is of course absolutely necessary for understanding these morbid changes, and for this we must refer back to the information we have given above.

Our knowledge of normal semen (at least as to its histology) is very exact and detailed, but our present knowledge of its condition in cases of spermatorrhœa is as incomplete and uncertain. The information at present current (Lallemand's, Donné's, and others'), which partly contradicts older statements, has great need of a new and more extensive examination. Let us first mention that even in healthy men there is no fixed amount for the quantity of fluid lost at each pollution, or for the number of

---

[1] *Lallemand*, and after him *Trousseau*, have given certain signs as means of discovering by the naked eye the presence of semen in the urine. They consider small, round globules in the cloudy sediment as characteristic, looking upon these as products of the seminal vesicles. In spite of abundant opportunities for the examination of urine containing semen, I have never discovered, with any certainty, bodies of this kind.

spermatozoids contained in the fluid which holds them in suspension, and also that the characters of the spermatozoids may notably vary according to the stages of their development. Individual peculiarities, as to genital power and the frequency of repetition of the sexual act, have the most important part in producing these differences.

When pollutions just begin to be morbid, the fluid ejaculated does not generally present any abnormal characters, and this is, of course, the case sometimes for a long (although very variable) time. The quantity is the same as in natural pollutions, being probably (as we have seen above) less than is lost in coitus ; the microscope, too, shows no important change.   But, as the pollutions occur more frequently, the fluid evacuated is wont to be diminished both in quantity and consistence ; the spermatozoa diminish in number, often very considerably, are (it would appear) smaller,[1] particularly in the tail ; according to some authors they are more transparent and more destructible.

It is extremely probable that we are then concerned, not with somewhat abnormal and (so to speak) "diseased" spermatozoa, but rather with earlier stages of their development, owing to their being discharged too soon from the increased activity of the genital organs.   The same idea is suggested by what may be frequently observed, that cap-like membranous appendages adhere to the head of the spermatozoön (particularly to the central portion and to the thread-like end) ; according to Koelliker, these are obviously remains of the parent cell.   It is still uncertain whether the seminal bodies undergo any diminution of their mobility, although such has been asserted ; and on account of the difficulty of examining them when freshly evacuated in these cases, this question is not likely yet to be decided.

According to Bence-Jones, and Nepveu,[2] who corroborated the observations of the former author, peculiar hyaline cylinders are to be described as existing in the semen of persons suffering from spermatorrhœa. These are notably long and of varying diameter, the narrowest being twice as broad as the largest urinary tube-

---

[1] *Mandl* (loc. cit.) gives definite measurements in this respect.

[2] *Nepveu*, Note sur la présence de tubes hyalines particuliers dans le liquide spermatique. Gaz. Méd. de Paris. 1874. No. 3 ; Centralbltt. 1874. No. 18.

casts;[1] the largest so broad that, according to Nepveu, they can only originate in the deferent, and not in the secretory canals of the testis. According to the same author, there is nothing absolutely characteristic about them, since they are also found under other circumstances.

As we have already remarked of physiological seminal evacuations (Casper, Lewin), so in the case of abnormal pollutions, spermatozoa may be almost entirely or entirely absent. In such cases—which are certainly rare—a too hasty negative conclusion is to be avoided; but these bodies are to be sought for on repeated occasions, when they will in some rare cases be found to be sometimes present and sometimes absent. In the extremest degrees of spermatorrhœa, when the semen is quite watery, and especially when it passes away at the same time as the urine, Lallemand first described what he supposed were malformed spermatozoa—small, shining bodies of the size of the head of these structures, but showing no sign of tail.

In Lallemand's school these "aborted spermatozoa" play a great part, and even Trousseau corroborates their existence and Lallemand's explanation of them; but very soon manifold objections were raised, and even now their existence is not satisfactorily established.

Perhaps an observation which I have made may throw some light on the matter. In the case of a clerk, who suffered from abnormal nocturnal pollutions, I was able to examine when fresh the urine passed after them. I found in the cloudy sediment well-developed spermatozoa in abundance; but if I let the urine stand, by the second day only a few were still recognizable, and these with their tails already broken off or rolled up. On the other hand, *there were a number of small, shining corpuscles*, which were proved beyond a doubt to be the spermatozoa, that had been meanwhile destroyed, by the remains of a tail which still adhered to many of them.[2]

The medical man has not only to be on his guard against the sources of error already mentioned; if he is not sufficiently cir-

---

[1] We must not omit to mention here certain urinary cylinders of very unusual size (the thickness of a hair) which Eichhorst found in the urine in one case of granular kidney (Berlin klin. Wochenschr. 1874. No. 7). These might give rise in diagnosis to some uncertainty, which could, however, easily be cleared up.

[2] This might seem to contradict Donné's statement that the seminal bodies retain their characters unaltered for months in the urine; but there is a question whether, in the case of *abnormal* seminal losses, the power of resistance of the spermatozoa against any action of the kind may not be diminished.

cumspect or sceptical in the examination of his patient, he is liable to fall into still greater mistakes. He must always bear in mind, that, however strange it may at first sight seem, by no means all the patients who consult him for "seminal losses" really suffer from abnormal pollutions. Perhaps only a minority do so, some seeking to deceive intentionally their medical attendant, while others give him what is intended to be a correct account, but is really a misleading description of their state. The former are masturbators, of whom not a few are wont to complain of excessive seminal losses in order to conceal onanism, which is the real cause of their trouble. They believe that if they only impress their physician with the loss of semen they will receive suitable medical treatment for it, and will thus be spared the humiliating confession that each loss is produced entirely by their own act. But, in the first place, these persons are very different to a practised eye from really spermatorrhœic patients in all respects, and particularly in the way they describe their malady, and they can also be easily brought to confess, and are even obviously relieved by doing so, if the matter be sufficiently insisted on.

There is a totally different source of error arising from this, that actual spontaneous discharges from the genital organs of a mucous fluid resembling semen may easily be mistaken for spermatorrhœa.

It is not very unusual for healthy young men, especially if they are for some time exposed to frequent sexual excitement without satisfying it (as is particularly the case with those engaged to be married), to consult a medical man, complaining that during and after violent erections a transparent, viscous fluid is discharged from the part. These patients are usually greatly distressed, looking upon such discharges as diurnal pollutions, and generally, under the influence of fear, describe the quantity of fluid as much greater than it really is. I have carefully examined two individuals on several occasions after this had occurred, and am able to say that the quantity of fluid visible at the apex of the glans, and expressed from the urethra, scarcely amounted to two drops. It was viscous, albuminoid, and contained no spermatozoa, but merely mucus-corpuscles and urethral epithelium-cells in large numbers. It appears to be secreted from the urethral mucous membrane, and perhaps also from Cowper's glands.[1]

Another not unusual cause for erroneously supposing spermatorrhœa to exist occurs in certain cases where strong, healthy men, at the time of going to stool, usually after lasting constipation, or with the last drops of urine, pass a tenacious, inodorous, alkaline, albuminoid fluid by the urethra, sometimes in not inconsiderable quantity. The amount may be about the same as that lost in a pollution, and the patients' fear that it is semen will be confirmed by its leaving stiff spots upon their linen. Added to which many of them do not feel quite secure in the matter of sexual excess, have indulged in masturbation, or have suffered from inflammatory conditions of the genital organs, chronic gonorrhœa, or the like. If their medical man takes all these points into account, he may readily, for the moment, be in some uncertainty, or even in error; but if he brings the microscope to his aid, he will discover no trace of spermatozoa, but only urethral epithelium, mucus-corpuscles, and prismatic or rounded amyloid bodies, which last are characteristic of the prostatic secretion (Pitha, Guerlain, Gross). In fact, we have to do in these patients with a secretion from the prostate, especially from its somewhat enlarged follicles, probably also with the assistance of Cowper's glands. These patients are (as we have said) usually healthy and strong, and when the state of the case is satisfactorily explained to their somewhat hypochondriacal fears, an examination of the prostate, and, indeed, of all the genital organs, proves them to be in a normal condition.

But although these cases are the more frequent, such a favorable prognosis is not always to be given, when prostatic secretion is diagnosed mainly from the negative results of microscopical investigation, without a careful examination of the gland itself. In some (certainly rare) instances, hypertrophy of the prostate is discovered, particularly where there is a history of frequent violent irritation, or chronic inflammation of the genital organs still existing. These forms of disease have been especially described

---

[1] See below, under the heading of "Impotence," the physiology of erection.

under the name *Prostatorrhœa ;* and the prognosis is then doubtful, though usually rather favorable than the reverse.

As for the mechanism by which the .prostatic secretion is evacuated, we need here only refer in passing to what has been explained above ; it is easily conceivable, from the relative positions of the parts concerned, how it may be produced by the pressure of hard scybala passing through the rectum.

We wish here to call special attention to the fact that, notwithstanding the labors of Gross, Guerlain, and others, the whole subject still deserves a minute study based upon numerous cases, particularly with repeated and careful microscopical examinations. No doubt one reason why so little has been done in this way is because hospitals rarely supply any material of the kind, and in private practice, although more common, it often cannot be precisely proved to exist on account of the doubly great difficulties in the way.

Impotence, which is very frequently associated with abnormal pollutions, is to be mentioned as a further symptom on the part of the genital organs ; but we only refer to it here for completeness' sake, as a special chapter will be assigned for its more detailed description.

As far as regards *the external condition of the genitals,* in many (perhaps in most) persons suffering from spermatorrhœa, nothing abnormal can be detected. I must leave it undecided whether in masturbators (who form so large a proportion of these patients) the penis is remarkable for its special size, or hardness of the corpora cavernosa, as many authors suppose ; there are certainly many instances to the contrary.

Flaccidity of the scrotum, and anæsthesia of its skin, small size and softness of the testicles, are often mentioned, and correctly, among the symptoms in advanced cases. Under the electric stimulus, sensibility is often found to be very notably diminished, particularly in the testicles, while on the contrary the urethra is often in a state of hyperæsthesia (Benedict).

A certain number of patients suffer from neuralgia of the testicles ; of course, there is nothing absolutely characteristic in this ; on the contrary, it often affects perfectly sound, healthy men, whose genital functions are otherwise normal.

We next pass on to those phenomena which are · usually known as the *general* symptoms of spermatorrhœa, because they cannot, as yet, be strictly localized. We need only here briefly remark that they are for the most part not originally produced by spermatorrhœa, but are *co-effects with it of other* causes, particularly of sexual excess and masturbation, often in persons with some inherited or acquired predisposition.

A tolerably detailed account of the state in question can hardly be given, for the group of symptoms to which spermatorrhœa belongs presents itself under the most diverse forms, and refuses to be forced into the strait waistcoat, which systematic writers, since Lallemand's time, employ. Some symptoms will be more prominent in one patient, some in another; or they will appear earlier or later, and accordingly the gravity of the whole disease will (in part at least) vary, being, as a whole, different in each individual, according to each patient's constitutional or local state. For instance, it may happen that one masturbator presents at first a preponderance of symptoms connected with the nervous system and nutrition, abnormal pollutions occurring relatively only very late or to a very slight extent; while in other patients very frequent seminal losses are the earliest symptom, and they may continue so long in the foreground that the patient, and even the medical attendant, may look upon them as the real cause of the other symptoms, which are only gradually developed; and yet it is this last form which Lallemand and the great majority of his followers have set up as the type of their whole system.

Certain *phenomena connected with the nervous system and with nutrition* are usually very constant and early in their appearance. As yet we know almost nothing certain of the special manner in which these are produced under the influence of sexual excess or anomalies of the sexual organs; indeed, the present standpoint of physiology hardly enables us to see how this question can be solved. A few elements towards its solution can, however, be given, and here and there found to harmonize.

We have relatively more data at our command in respect of the affections of the nervous system than of altered nutrition. It is extremely probable that the disturbances of nutrition depend upon those of the nervous system, and are, therefore, apparently to be looked upon as the result of abnormal innervation of the parts in question, the nutrition of which is still further injured by disturbed digestion, which may also in its turn be ascribed to perverted innervation. We must once more repeat that we can in no instance share the opinion of those authors who refer the altered nutrition to mere loss of semen as such.

We must not omit one general remark before passing on to describe the nervous symptoms in detail; in these cases, we must always be careful not to ascribe such symptoms at once to sexual abuse (even when this is admitted by the patient or put prominently forward), without first *excluding the possibility of other local changes in the parts of the nervous system concerned.* The demonstrable relations of the genital organs, to the symptoms of which we are speaking, are at present so vague that it is *only by way of exclusion* that we can proceed to connect them. Thus alone can one avoid the fanciful ideas (in part so erroneous) of Lallemand, who ascribed the most diverse forms of disease to a spermatorrhœa which was often very difficult of detection, although, according to his own account, they were capable of some much more natural interpretation.

Among the earliest and most constant symptoms on the part of the nervous system, which usually precede the occurrence of abnormal pollutions by a more or less long time, are *a sense of bodily weariness and sinking, mental depression,* and *loss of sleep.*

The sense of unnaturally great fatigue, which represents the earliest disturbance of the motor system in the beginning, usually only occurs after the sexual act or a pollution, and is the first thing which characterizes these last as abnormal. These patients, on awaking in the morning after a seminal loss, complain of a stiffness in the back and limbs, and feel the need of stretching them; and, as the disease progresses, the feeling of fatigue lasts all day long, even if adequate rest be taken. In spite of this weariness, many experience a very troublesome sensation of restlessness, a continual urgency to move hither and thither; Lallemand and Trousseau were probably only mistaken in describing this as a particularly constant and early symptom. In advanced cases, trembling of the limbs, and at the same time trembling of the hands, usually occur; and even—but this is only in the worst instances—stronger involuntary muscular twitching is observed in the limbs, particularly in the lower extremities. Happily it is much more seldom the case than might be supposed from the gloomy and fanciful descriptions given by Lallemand, that these troubles go so far as to limit the patients' movements to slight stretching, and to suggest to a superficial observer the idea of some chronic disease of the spinal cord.

These motor disturbances are often accompanied by *sensory troubles*, which, however, more frequently occur rather later in the development of the disease.

We then hear complaints of numbness along the spinal cord, in the lower extremities, or in the fingers, but which cannot be thoroughly localized, being sometimes more intense in one part, sometimes in another, and then completely disappearing, to return again in some fresh place. Or, on the contrary, these patients may suffer from hyperæsthesia of any part of the skin, lasting likewise only a short time, or passing from one spot to another. Cases are observed in which merely touching the skin, percussion, or even pressure on a hair, are felt in the keenest and most painful manner. Besides these troubles, we find many patients complain of cold in the back or some other part, often in some very limited part, as the hands; these sensations of cold may alternate suddenly with a feeling of heat ("flushes"). Often there is no objective sign corresponding to either of these sensations; at any rate, in uncomplicated cases, pyrexia can never be proved to exist.

Happily all these symptoms are, in the great majority of cases, neither very complete nor very highly developed in any one patient. It is extremely rare, at any rate in our own experience, for any patient to combine the various troubles described above so completely and to such a degree as to be in a condition bearing a certain resemblance to tabes dorsalis. But, even then, the transitory and mobile character of the symptoms and their definitive disappearance, as a rule, when their cause is removed, should prevent any erroneous idea that a deep-seated disease of the cord exists. The troubles of that organ must be "functional," or (to speak more precisely) dependent on such alterations of structure as are undiscoverable by our present means of investigation.

Another point which may contribute towards producing a certain superficial resemblance to tabes dorsalis is, that almost all these patients, when affected to such a high degree, suffer from obstinate constipation, and difficult micturition (generally traceable to some local affection) makes the simulation more complete. *Vertigo, headache*, and *mental depression*, as we have already remarked, are the earliest and relatively the most frequent phenomena connected with the *brain*. They are often the first evidences of the morbid character of pollutions, when they follow seminal losses which have appeared perfectly normal ; and as the disease progresses they continue during the whole interval, though usually worse after each pollution.

Headache varies extremely both in its seat and intensity, but in no characteristic manner ; those who suffer from it ordinarily complain also of "determination of blood to the head," which may be either purely subjective or accompanied by the outward evidence of transitory redness of the face. Many patients, particularly those who have been consulting popular books on the subject, complain of a sensation of heat and weight in the occiput.

The *alterations in the mental condition of these patients* take two principal directions, according as they affect the intellectual faculties or the character and mode of thought. When these disturbances occur, they almost invariably precede, by a longer or shorter time, the first appearance of abnormal seminal losses, being an earlier result of sexual excess than they are. They are wont to occur unusually early in masturbators,[1] and, above all, in persons who have given themselves up to sexual excess very early in life.

At first, these patients feel dull and depressed only after the sexual act, as we have seen is the case with the other cerebral symptoms. But, as matters grow worse, this condition becomes more and more continuous, so that sooner or later the patients'

---

[1] The symptoms of mental depression are here generally so charactersistic, in many ways, that experienced schoolmasters and tutors are often able to conclude from this symptom, with tolerable certainty, that the vice exists in their pupils.

previous energy and power of thought are decidedly lessened ; they lose all courage and desire for serious work, and any confidence they may have had previously in their own powers. Either the acuteness of their minds is notably diminished, or else the will has lost its former power of concentrating mental activity upon any determinate object. The memory is also very often impaired, and this alone is sufficient to increase greatly the mistrust of such persons in their own powers.

The disturbed self-consciousness impresses itself also upon the external behavior and demeanor of these patients ; they appear more indolent and undecided than they once were, and evince remarkable shyness, which may develop sometimes into a positive dislike for the society of others. On the other hand, they are often irritable and quarrelsome with those who are habitually about them.

It is not uncommon for the speech to be rather stuttering, so that words cannot be found by these persons with sufficient quickness to express their ideas ; this state usually becomes worse the more painful it is to them. In some instances, moreover, the mobility of the tongue is somewhat affected : it trembles, and certain sounds (particularly the consonants) are therefore produced incompletely and irregularly.

In bad cases the sleep is ordinarily restless, much interrupted, and troubled by harassing dreams and wild sexual fancies ; happily, complete insomnia is rare. The whole of this condition is accompanied by a hypochondriacal habit of mind which causes these patients to feel their symptoms very intensely, and to be very anxious with regard to them. They soon begin to despair of the possibility of recovery ; an ordinary erection (which may still occur), or still more, a seminal loss, produces the greatest alarm. They seek counsel from such works as "The Silent Friend," or worry their medical attendant for every trifle. Many talk of suicide, and even seriously think of it, but usually have not sufficient energy to put their design into execution.

Finally, cases occur (particularly where there is an hereditary tendency) where actual insanity is at last developed. The commonest form for it to assume is melancholia, especially with fanatical religious delusions and tendency to self-accusation.[1] Lallemand professes to have often observed actual paralytic dementia ; but it is more than doubtful whether this disease is ever merely the consequence of spermatorrhœa and is not due to the sexual excess which has gone before, or rather, even this last can only be looked upon as exciting the germs of disease which had long lain dormant in the body.

The hypochondriacal state to which I have referred makes it more difficult in many cases to form a correct opinion as to the other nervous symptoms, especially when these are mainly subjective. This should be borne in mind particularly when affections of sensation, vertigo, etc., have to be judged of, and it also deserves great weight in respect to certain affections of the sensory nerves ; although it is certainly not thereby suggested that such symptoms are merely illusory.

Most frequently these patients complain of *deafness* and of *noises in the ears ;* on the contrary, hyperæsthesia is rare. *The keenness of sight* is occasionally diminished, and, combined with this, or sometimes alone, there may be double vision. In Lallemand's fanciful descriptions, complete amaurosis is several times mentioned ; but criticism is silenced when we are told that it disappeared speedily after cauterization of the caput gallinaginis.

Epilepsy may accompany abnormal seminal losses, in the same manner as it does sexual excess. But it seems to be extremely doubtful whether it is an immediate result of spermatorrhœa ; and it becomes the more necessary to insist on this because, in America, cases of epilepsy which were ascribed to spermatorrhœa have been on this principle treated by castration ! (See Holthouse. Lancet. 1859.)

Before passing on to another group of symptoms, we must once more warn the reader who may have formed his idea of the disease from Lallemand's work, that the symptoms we have hitherto described are *only partially constant and severe in all cases of abnormal pollutions.* Happily, *the melancholy picture drawn in that book is rarely indeed realized,* and most patients complain only of some of these symptoms, or at least only some of them are prominent. A hypochondriacal cast of mind is per-

---

[1] See *Ritchie* and *Schroeder v. d. Kolk*, l. c.

haps the commonest of them, no other affection in the male hav.
ing anything like the same influence on the character as diseases
of the genital organs.

The great diversity in the nervous symptoms accompanying
spermatorrhœa, and *the absence of any proportion between the
severity of both*, are to be explained simply by this : that the
pollutions are generally not the cause of these symptoms ; but
are, on the contrary, rather a consequence of the nervous condition. This (whether general or locally affecting the sexual
organs) is produced (as we said under the head of Etiology) by
many different causes, among which inherited nerve-troubles and
sexual excess of various kinds play the chief part.

But, if abnormal pollutions once become established, they
may have a very notable effect in aggravating any nervous
symptoms which already exist—above all, hypochondria. The
influence of diseases of the sexual organs in general, and of
spermatorrhœa in particular, on the character, is so marked and
constant that no other affection of any other organ approaches
it in this respect. The slightest symptoms about the sexual
organs, which a healthy person would hardly be conscious of,
will greatly agitate our patients, so that sometimes at last their
whole mind and attention are directed to their genital organs.

The *disturbances of nutrition* which occur in many patients,
and are then observed relatively early, are very prominent and
remarkable. They may often be observed *before the occurrence
of abnormal pollutions*—a proof that they are not produced
or increased by these, but are co-effects, with them, of other causes.

These patients become pale and thin, the muscles are flaccid,
the skin sallow and dry ; in many instances there is not much
emaciation, but rather a pasty and bloated appearance.

The alterations of sanguification and assimilation which are
the primary causes of these disturbances of nutrition are practically unknown to us. Their causes are no doubt to be sought
for in nerve-affections, which may act in two different directions : firstly, by affecting injuriously those processes of innervation which directly influence sanguification and assimilation (by
means of the vaso-motor and trophic nerves) ; secondly—and this
is probably the more important point—*by first producing morbid*

changes in the process of digestion, which are followed by perverted nutrition.

Dyspepsia is one of the commonest symptoms in persons who suffer from functional diseases of the genital organs, and its "nervous" origin is proved by these points : that it varies extremely in the same person at different times without any errors of diet; that it may come on very suddenly, change without cause, and completely disappear without any real treatment.

Many patients have at first no complaint to make of loss of appetite; on the contrary, they state that it is notably increased, and that they suffer from sudden fits of true bulimia connected with abnormal sensations in the epigastric region, such as pressure, dragging, burning, etc. In the earlier stages of the disorder, this increased desire for food may be beneficial to the patients by increasing the supply of nourishment,[1] and the extra amount thus taken may be thoroughly digested. But gradually eructations and a discomfort after eating come on, and a sensation of weight in the stomach, which is often followed by abdominal pain and sudden action of the bowels, a portion of the food that has been taken being then usually recognizable in the stools, thus proving that the stomach-digestion has been incomplete, and that the undigested food has had an irritating effect upon the intestines. This diarrhœa very rarely lasts long ; on the contrary, it usually alternates with very obstinate constipation, which in turn reacts injuriously on digestion. We will here once more remind the reader that this constipation may also become a cause assisting in the production of seminal losses.

These patients are also very frequently troubled with *palpitation* and *shortness of breath.* It is true of these, as of the digestive disturbances, that *they occur not only in persons suffering from spermatorrhœa, but as a result of sexual excess in general.* Masturbators who have long given way to that vice are especially in the habit of complaining of these symptoms,

---

[1] When they become pale and thin at this stage, without any evidence of the least disturbance of digestion, this can only be accounted for by the suggestion we have made above, of processes of innervation directly influencing sanguification and tissue-change.

and often put them before all others. I might, indeed, give palpitation a prominent place among the results of sexual excess.

In these persons the action of the heart, which is normal while they are at rest, is unusually excited by moderate movements which would have no effect on healthy individuals. During their consultations with a medical man these patients are generally hardly free from their palpitation, which is very annoying to them, however quiet they endeavor to be. I have sometimes observed also an irregularity of the pulse ; and in one young man, who had been much reduced by masturbation, this came only by paroxysms to such an extent that he was always made aware of it, without feeling his pulse, by the disagreeable and extremely anxious sensations in the cardiac region and carotids.

If the heart be examined, it is not found to be enlarged, and no organic mischief about the valves and orifices is discoverable ; a systolic murmur, *notably increased by excited action of the heart*, is, however, often audible at the apex.

The palpitation we have just described is certainly to be looked upon as "nervous" in character ; although, in patients who already show signs of anæmia, it is more natural to ascribe it to this condition. Even here *direct disturbances of innervation* (not produced by anæmia) play their part. It is, indeed, well known that, in perfectly healthy men, intense sexual excitement and the acts connected therewith are associated with violent palpitation ; and we thus find masturbators, and those suffering from pollutions, complain seriously of palpitation for some time before there can be any question of anæmic symptoms.

The *shortness of breath* which these patients suffer from— particularly if they walk quickly, make any effort, go upstairs, or climb mountains—is partly to be ascribed to the altered composition of the blood, partly to the mechanical influence of palpitation on the respiratory organs. *Both these symptoms, however—palpitation and dyspnœa—require great caution in diagnosis.* These patients are often in the habit of looking upon themselves as consumptive ; and even if the physician at once excludes this, he may allow himself to be misled into supposing that a slight heart-disease exists, if he has not remarked the manner in which the symptoms came on ; and the mistake is the more natural, because (as we have observed above) inorganic murmurs may be remarkably intense when the heart's action is excited. A further source of error sometimes exists in the irregularity of the pulse, which has been mentioned already, and which appears to me not to have been sufficiently insisted upon in this respect.

Before concluding this section we must not omit one general remark of great importance in diagnosis. We have seen that a great number of very diverse symptoms occur in our patients, producing very different types of disease, according to individual and other circumstances. If, therefore, no great care be taken, severe diseases of various organs may readily, but wrongly, be supposed to exist; but, on the other hand, diseases which present these symptoms may really exist, and yet, if we are told there are also pollutions, there may be danger of ascribing the symptoms to these, and mistaking their real significance. Not a few examples of this latter error are to be found in Lallemand's celebrated work, in which cases are described of obviously different nature, where the proof of the existence of spermatorrhœa, which is to explain everything, is almost dragged in by force. Indeed, in other cases, detailed particularly in the first part of the book, not the slightest decisive proof is given that spermatorrhœa really existed; at any rate, it was not established by microscopical examination.

Course and Terminations. Prognosis.

Not much can be said on the prognosis of spermatorrhœa, taken as a whole, and as little of its course and terminations, the simple reason for this being that—as we have before shown—spermatorrhœa, as such, is not a disease which has a separate existence. These questions are, therefore, to be answered chiefly by considering the *causes* of the seminal losses, which, as we have seen under the head of Etiology, vary extremely.

One general remark only we can make: that the forecast in these cases is undoubtedly far from being so gloomy as the older writers, and especially the school of Lallemand, supposed. The miserable circumstances which, according to Lallemand's description, came daily before him, must be set down by us as very rare; and if we ever see such cases, we usually find, on closer examination, that they depend on other less obvious causes, and are only referred to spermatorrhœa as the most striking symptom.

It is undoubtedly incorrect that death from exhaustion ever occurs as a result of continued pollutions alone. We have already seen that the loss of semen is by no means the most important factor—perhaps it is the least important—in the action of spermatorrhœa upon the general system. If death, with the appearances of general asthenia, ever does occur, complications will be found sufficient to explain it, or some primary disease will be discovered of such gravity that the loss of semen falls quite into the background when contrasted with it.

The influence of seminal losses is of more importance when they occur during convalescence from severe acute diseases (as typhus and variola), or in the course of chronic ones, as in the early stages of phthisis. They may then materially delay recovery, and hasten the termination, which would, in any case, be inevitably fatal.

There are other results of spermatorrhœa, however, far more frequent than its shortening life, the chief of these being its *influence on the generative faculty.* We have already remarked that *impotence* is very frequently developed after seminal losses have persisted for some time.

The reactions of the various states connected with seminal losses, on *the general health,* are not less important, particularly in their bearing on *nutrition, the nervous system,* and *the mental faculties;* but we have dwelt upon them sufficiently in the account we have given of the symptoms.

Before describing the prognostic importance of the various morbid states which are the bases of spermatorrhœa, we will endeavor to find some *general points of view* which must be particularly borne in mind when forming an opinion as to prognosis.

The individual constitution of each patient is of special importance in this respect. Men who were previously robust and healthy, of course, offer far more resistance than those who were already sensitive, sickly, and nervous. Among these last the outlook is particularly bad in cases where any nervous disease, or a tendency to insanity, is hereditary, for they fall all the more easily and speedily into that state of hypochondria which, we have seen above, is an extremely frequent accompaniment of sexual diseases, even in non-predisposed persons. On the other hand, men of good constitution often do not escape from hypochondria, but fall deeper and deeper into it, in spite of the most earnest and sensible efforts to set themselves straight. Many fall into actual melancholia, and the number of suicides due to this cause is not a small one.[1]

I consider it, however, quite unproved that these conditions connected with spermatorrhœa can ever lead to true paralytic dementia. The not very rare belief that they do is based upon the fallacy "post hoc, propter hoc," a pitfall which is to be most carefully avoided in forming an opinion as to the relations of all sexual anomalies to insanity. *Very often—perhaps, indeed, in most cases—the mental symptoms, although not obvious at first, constitute the primary condition, and the sexual phenomena depend upon them.* This is especially to be borne in mind in regard to epilepsy; in almost every case where it is supposed to be a result of masturbation and spermatorrhœa, the relation of cause and effect is precisely the opposite.

Next after the constitution, the *age* of the patients is of great importance in determining the course of spermatorrhœa. When it is developed very early in life, or, at any rate, during the period of greatest sexual activity, the prognosis is generally much more unfavorable than when we have to do with older persons in whom the function is already physiologically diminished. Lallemand, indeed, adduces cases of severe spermatorrhœa in men of sixty, and even of more than seventy years of age, apparently in order to show that age is of no importance in this relation; but even if we are to assume that these cases are well founded and proved, they can only be looked upon as curiosities.

The *duration and severity* of the disease are, almost as a matter of course, most important in forming an opinion as to a case of spermatorrhœa, and from this point of view pollutions

---

[1] See *Schroeder v. d. Kolk*, Pathology and Treatment of Mental Diseases; *Plagge*, Sexual Indulgence and Insanity; and *Ritchie*, loc. cit.

occurring only by night admit of a more favorable prognosis than those which take place in the day. Yet it is erroneous to consider diurnal pollutions so serious as Lallemand's school is disposed to consider them ; if we can remove the causes producing them, the pollutions also in most instances cease.

Let us now glance at *the bearing of the various causes of spermatorrhœa on prognosis.* Those cases are to be considered as relatively most favorable where the morbid seminal losses are either produced or materially favored by *certain local conditions.* By this I mean the forms of chronic gonorrhœa, phymosis, varicocele, and the various anomalies of the rectum and its contents, described above. Such abnormal conditions of the genital organs or of neighboring parts, which are capable of easy removal, contribute the greater number of the frequently described, and often very striking, cures of spermatorrhœa ; and to them Lallemand owed most of his brilliant successes, save where there are other grounds for doubting the correctness of his descriptions.

Unfortunately, the prognosis of these forms of abnormal pollutions is often obscured by the co-existence of unfavorable constitutional states, so that the local affections only play the part of exciting causes.

More serious and obstinate forms of spermatorrhœa are frequently produced under the influence of *sexual excess—masturbation* here again playing the most fatal part, and for the following reasons : it has usually been practised from a very early age and very frequently, has had a very intense effect upon the patient, and his struggles to overcome the evil habit are either extremely difficult or without any result, according as it has lasted a shorter or a longer time. The influence of the form of disease produced by masturbation on the psychical condition of the patient is far greater than in the case of natural sexual excess, and must be very seriously weighed ; but, to avoid repetition, we refer the reader to what we have previously said on this subject.

Treatment.

The chief difficulty in the treatment of spermatorrhœa consists in rectifying its ultimate causes and those accompanying conditions which either produce it or favor its development. For this reason we have thought it necessary to bestow particular care upon the etiology of this morbid state; and from the account we have given it follows that the causes of abnormal seminal losses are very manifold, and that we must proceed with great care in order to treat these conditions rationally and successfully.

Lallemand, by his one-sided conception of the etiology of his subject, and by his recommendation (based upon this) of only one or a few methods of treatment, has rather damaged than advanced the question. Of course, his assumptions and inferences have received no confirmation, or very little, from most subsequent observers, except his pupils and immediate followers; and this disillusion led rather to an ill-grounded scepticism than to a search for any better treatment.

It was supposed that spermatorrhœa belonged to the class of diseases which can be cured only with difficulty, or hardly at all.[1] No doubt there are forms of the disease which can only be treated with difficulty by the means at present at our disposal; nay, indeed, often defy all treatment, as might be foretold from a knowledge of the causes producing them; but, on the other hand, in many instances, however serious they may at first sight appear, we may do much that is important if we duly bear in mind the primary causes of the affection.

Before describing the treatment (in the narrower sense of the word), we must first consider the *prophylaxis*.

We have seen that the general state which precedes and causes abnormal seminal losses—one of disturbance of the nervous system and of nutrition—may be traced in many, probably in most cases, to sexual excess, and especially to masturbation. Education, therefore, supplies a powerful means for combating

---

[1] Even in the eighth edition of Niemeyer's Hand-book we find this statement: "Therapeutics are almost powerless to resist a tendency to abnormal pollutions."

the evil, if careful consideration be bestowed upon all the sexual relations, and especially if rational means be taken to oppose the widely-spread vice of masturbation. It may be safely affirmed that watchfulness over the sexual relations during childhood and adolescence is one of the most important problems of the education and hygiene of youth. The great difficulties which surround this subject, and the need for extreme care and thought in dealing with it, are generally recognized; a more minute consideration of this interesting question does not come within our scope.

It is necessary to be extremely sceptical when enquiring into masturbation. One must be prepared to meet with the vice in quite little children, and also not to abandon too readily our suspicions of its existence in adults. We have already remarked that many men do not free themselves from this vice after marriage, and every practitioner must have observed that patients have admitted practising masturbation, whom he would never in the least have suspected of it.

But, even when there can be no question of natural sexual excess or of masturbation, we must not dismiss the subject from our minds without remembering that, in many cases where neither of these vices still exists, there is an immorality of thought which has a very powerful influence in keeping up genital excitement, even in those who are physically continent.

If other circumstances allow of it, many patients are greatly benefited by being advised to marry, particularly when pollutions do not occur frequently. Matrimony has the greatest effect in regulating the unruly passions, and often does more than the most decided treatment.

hen marriage is impossible, we are of opinion that it does not fall within the physician's province to recommend ordinary coitus, and to regulate the frequency with which it should be practised. Even if the moral side of the question be completely excluded from consideration, the dangers connected with illicit intercourse (syphilis, gonorrhœa, etc.) are too great and too difficult to guard against. The cynical manner in which these matters are treated, down to the most disgusting details in a well-known manual of electro-therapeutics, is in every way thoroughly unworthy of medical science.

The *special treatment* of each case must be based upon a study of the general state of the patient, and of those local changes which are connected with the disease.

We have seen that disturbances of the general nutrition of

the body and of the nervous system are observed in a large number of persons who suffer from morbid seminal losses, and usually precede these for a longer or shorter time. In such cases good results are often obtained by a *tonic* plan of treatment ; but it is necessary to be prudent at first in its employment, and careful in the choice of the remedies we use, for sometimes (especially in the early stage of the disease) a tonic and excitant treatment does considerable harm by increasing the irritability which already exists.

An easily digestible diet, mainly composed of animal food, and excluding irritating substances, spices, etc., has a chief place among the means of renewing the strength ; for this reason the milk-cure has sometimes produced excellent results. The use of alcoholic drinks is not to be altogether condemned, being often of great use in suitable cases.

At the same time tonic medicines may be administered—the preparations of cinchona and iron. A residence in the country or in a mountainous district sometimes materially promotes recovery, and patients may often combine these advantages by visiting some chalybeate spring. A change of scene and absence from the cares and troubles of daily life are all the more serviceable to these patients, because they so frequently suffer from hypochondria.

It is always important for the physician to study the character of these patients. As a result of the very powerful influence of the mind on the genital functions, many patients are exceedingly alarmed by what they hear, or by reading popular works on the subject, and any one who is able to gain their confidence and bring their fears within reasonable limits does them the greatest service.

Besides these means of treatment, moderate bodily exercise will be of service, and the patients should be advised to occupy their minds proportionately to their individual capacity.

Much attention should be paid to the *process of digestion*, as many patients suffer from considerable disturbance of that function. We have seen above that dyspepsia, gastric and gastrointestinal catarrh, are among the most frequent results of the condition which we described ; and we also learned that obstinate constipation is one of the commonest causes favoring the production of pollutions.

Hydropathy, combined with other suitable treatment, often has a good effect, especially when the nervous excitability is highly developed, the very striking advantages which may often be seen to result from its use in properly selected cases being referable to the diminution of the increased reflex excitability of the genital organs when that of the whole body is relieved; of course it follows from this that recent cases have a relatively better chance of recovery than those in which general or local loss of power appears to be connected with degenerative processes. It is best to begin with cold sponging of the whole body, or with the wet pack, especially at bedtime, and when these act well, to go on to a methodical use of the cold-water cure.[1]

Sea-bathing represents to a certain extent a higher degree of the cold-water cure, and may be of great benefit, particularly in robust patients; but in persons who are of feeble constitution, much reduced by illness, or suffering from some hereditary nerve-defect, much care is to be recommended, for in such cases sea-water baths seem to act much too violently, and may notably increase both the general weakness and the nervous excitability.

Derivative treatment has been praised as a result of experience (Trousseau) in cases where the spinal symptoms become most prominent. The cold douche may first be applied to the vertebral column; dry cupping, or cupping with abstraction of blood, along the back, painting with tincture of iodine, and flying blisters, have all been occasionally employed with advantage. These means may no doubt be considered as quite rational, especially where an excited condition of the spinal cord is implied by motor and sensory disturbances, which we already know to be connected with the most important genital functions.

Among available internal remedies physicians have employed.

---

[1] According to my own experience, I can only recommend cold sitz-baths and cold douches to the genital organs with great reservations; indeed, where there is great irritability of those parts, I find it advantageous to forbid simple washing with cold water. In cases of an opposite kind, where cold applications to the genitals seem desirable, as patients are often instinctively led to think, I have not unfrequently found the irritability is increased.

all that class of medicines which are reputed to have a sedative, cooling, or resolvent effect, particularly in the beginning of the disease, when the seminal losses have been supposed to be connected with increased irritability of the sexual organs.

To this category the following medicines belong: the acids, cream of tartar, valerian, mixtures containing cherry laurel-water or opium, extract of henbane and extract of belladonna, which has an almost exactly analogous effect.

Of late, bromide of potassium has been greatly praised as a remedy for spermatorrhœa, first by Tiedemann, and afterwards by Lafont-Goyzy, Morin, and Monot. I think further inquiries in this direction are very desirable, especially since physiological researches made formerly (in 1850 by Puche and Huette) lead one to suppose that this drug has an effect upon the genital functions. I look upon the dose recommended by Lafont-Goyzy (from fifteen to thirty grains once a day at bedtime) as too small, and in adults would prescribe at least from one to one and a half drachms in the twenty-four hours.

A remedy which has been very frequently employed in all forms of genital excitement, and especially in spermatorrhœa, is *lupuline*, of which the dose is from seven to fifteen grains. In spite of all recommendations, the sedative effect of this substance upon the sexual organs is still wholly unproved. I have never myself gained anything from its use, and believe that the favorable results occasionally ascribed to it by patients are to be attributed rather to the knowledge that something is being done for them than to any specific effect of the medicine. *Camphor* used formerly to have the same reputation as lupuline for abnormal seminal losses ; [1] but this has also considerably suffered. It used almost always to be given in combination with opium, and then a sedative effect was ascribed to it which far more probably belonged to the other drug. When employed alone, even in large doses—which may, indeed, have some sedative effect—no decided result has been obtained ; while in small doses an excitant rather than a sedative effect might be expected from it.

---

[1] Avicenna long ago vaunted this property of the drug, and the monks are said formerly to have worn camphor-bags to assist them in keeping their vow of chastity.

Next to the general treatment hitherto described, it is of the greatest importance *to take account therapeutically of the special condition of the genital organs, and of such other local affections as may stand in the relation of causes to the spermatorrhœa.* The local treatment of the genital organs will consist in diminishing their irritability, in relieving the state of relaxation which is supposed sometimes to exist, or in removing such definite diseases as may be thought to cause or favor the seminal flow. Excessive irritability of the urethra, particularly in its prostatic portion, has been occasionally treated with great success by the systematic *introduction of bougies,* of which the size is gradually increased, and which are at first left in only a short time, but gradually longer and longer (even for hours in the case of the "sonde à demeure"). In suitable instances we can only heartily recommend the cautious employment of this mode of treatment, but its routine use (as was the case some time ago) is to be avoided ; and it may be said that where urethral strictures —which of themselves require this treatment—do not exist, the use of bougies in spermatorrhœa is not often indicated.

Where there is reason to suppose the existence of an inflammatory condition of the prostatic portion of the urethra and neighboring parts, *the local application of astringents* is called for. Most will be gained by injections of nitrate of silver injected into the part affected by means of a catheter made for the purpose. The necessary manipulations require great skill and practice, and perhaps might be much more efficiently carried out with the assistance of the endoscope. Guyon[1] has described a peculiar "injecteur uréthral" for this object which may be strongly recommended to instrument-collectors.

I think it doubtful whether strong solutions of lunar caustic should ever be used with the intention of producing an acute inflammation, and so modifying "the state of the mucous membrane, and arresting chronic inflammatory processes." We are never completely masters of such a mode of treatment, and may often do the greatest mischief by it.

Still more heroic is the celebrated treatment of the same kind

---

[1] Bull. de thérap. 1867.

employed by Lallemand, which I have already mentioned—I mean *the cauterization of the prostatic portion of the urethra with solid nitrate of silver*. It is well known that he has assigned most extraordinarily extensive indications for this method, since he one-sidedly considered that almost all cases of abnormal seminal losses could be traced to chronic inflammatory conditions in the region of the caput gallinaginis. Even if we believed Lallemand's treatment indicated in all cases of the kind, it would nevertheless, according to our present views, be applicable only to the minority of cases of spermatorrhœa, since we suppose that state to be much more rarely due to these inflammatory conditions than the older authors thought. But even in cases where inflammation can be proved to exist, the use of lunar caustic is by no means always advisable. Usually the milder treatment—the use of astringent injections—is decidedly to be preferred. From our present standpoint there will probably only remain a few instances in which a trial of Lallemand's cauterization is justifiable, viz., where, after an insidious inflammation of the prostatic portion of the urethra, relaxation and enlargement of the ejaculatory ducts and their orifices may be supposed to exist. The cauterization must then be performed *extremely lightly and quickly, and must not be repeated too frequently or at too short intervals*, as English authors especially are to blame for doing.

We cannot here go into the details of the operation. In the few cases where the medical attendant considers it to be indicated, a much more careful preparation would be needed than our limited space would here allow of our describing. We must refer the reader to Lallemand's own work. His instrument, in the opinion of a competent judge (Pitha), is well adapted for the purpose, and the technical details he gives appear to be extremely minute and practical, as are also all his recommendations for after-treatment when cauterization has been performed.

Lallemand's caustic-holder was very variously modified in his day, just as now almost every one who devotes himself to diseases of the throat and mouth feels bound to connect his name with a new laryngoscope or rhinoscope. According to Pitha, a graduated stylet, to which the nitrate of silver has been attached, is sufficient without any other apparatus. This is introduced through a gum-elastie catheter open at the end.

The *electrical treatment of spermatorrhœa* rightly plays a more important part at the present day than cauterization. Lallemand, indeed, had already made some trials of the kind with the wholly inadequate means then at his disposal, seeing that he applied one pole of a *voltaic* pile (afterwards Bunsen's battery) to the neck of the bladder and the other to the perineum, or even to the prostatic region in the rectum. But even his mind, which was so sensitive to therapeutic success, obviously was not specially impressed in its favor, as the enthusiastic but very careful Kaula only mentions that his master employed this method without recording its results.

More recently Schulz,[1] and, above all, Benedict,[2] have gained a great reputation by this mode of treatment. Both employ almost exclusively the *constant current*, in opposition to Duchenne, who recommended faradic electricity, particularly in severe cases. They are able to say they have obtained very good results; thus Benedict, considers that, in both slight and severe cases, the prognosis under treatment by galvanism is "tolerably favorable."

Schulz recommends the application of the positive pole of a battery containing from twenty to thirty Daniell's elements, to the spine, while the negative pole is applied to the pubis or perineum; each sitting lasts two minutes, and is repeated three or four times in the week. He believes that by this means the reflex excitability of the cord is lessened.

Benedict, who, as we have already said, also employs the constant current by preference, places the copper pole over the lumbar vertebral region, and passes the zinc pole successively and repeatedly over the spermatic cords, penis, and perineum. On an average, he recommends that the treatment should be continued from six to ten weeks, with daily sittings of two or three minutes each; he employs currents so weak that they can only

---

[1] Wiener med. Wochensch. 1861. No. 34.

[2] Oesterr. Zeitschr. fur prakt. Heilk. X. 3, 4. 1864; and Electrotherapie, pp. 446 sqq.

just be felt. In obstinate cases he recommends that galvanic catheterization (which Lallemand, as we have seen, had already arrived at) should be added to the other treatment, but that it should not be performed so often (about three times in a fortnight), and in many cases, when the irritability of the urethra is great, it should be preceded by the methodical use of bougies. The special means adopted for galvanic cauterization are these: the copper pole, which is formed into a catheter, is introduced as far as the caput gallinaginis, while the zinc pole is drawn over the spermatic cords.

Benedict finds the sensibility of the skin very different over different parts of the genital organs ; wherever it is unusually diminished, he uses also the galvanic or faradic brush.

Although we still meet with many expressions of incredulity when we recommend the treatment of spermatorrhœa by electricity, in the present state of our knowledge its trial may be strongly urged. And yet it is necessary to be clear on this point, that experience has so far not justified our forming any definite opinion on the subject. Just as we have seen was formerly the case with cauterization, so now there is a tendency to employ galvanism much too indiscriminately. The first problem to be solved, is to seek for *more precise indications* of this method of treatment ; the cases in which it is unnecessary, because they can be cured without it, must first be excluded, and then those must be distinguished in which it may prove injurious. For, if no harm can well follow the mere application of one pole of a weak battery to the skin, this can hardly be supposed always the case with galvanic catheterization, although, in many severe cases, if carefully chosen, this procedure may be very effectual.

Trousseau introduced what seems at first sight a very singular method of treating spermatorrhœa, namely, the application of the so-called *"prostatic compressor,"* which is a plug, at one end olive-shaped and of the size of a pigeon's or hen's egg, but tapered away gradually at the other end to a diameter of about one-quarter inch. This instrument is introduced into the rectum so that the enlarged end may press upon the prostate, while the smaller end projects from the anus, and is fixed by means of a T-bandage or some such means. It is made of slightly different lengths, according to individual variations in the position of the prostate.

Trousseau bestows extraordinary praise upon this instrument, by the use of which he states that he has cured speedily even cases which before seemed hopeless. He explains its action by its compression of the ejaculatory ducts in the prostate so as to prevent the contents of the abnormally contractile seminal vesi· cles passing too readily through the ducts when they are relaxed and dilated.

This plan has been very little noticed in medical literature, Pitha alone praising it highly from a trial he made of it in one case. Yet it would be unfair at once to condemn it; it would always be worth a trial in advanced and obstinate cases of sper-matorrhœa where there was good reason for believing the ejacu· latory ducts to be enlarged and relaxed.

We may here most suitably remark that when this state of relaxation is proved to exist, cold sitz-baths should be prescribed, and internally, the preparations of nux vomica, or perhaps of ergot, which has been again lately recommended by Italian phy· sicians. However, too much confidence must not be placed in these remedies, of the efficacy of which no positive evidence can usually be obtained.

We shall here mention, only in order to warn our readers against them, certain mechanical means which have long been employed and have come down to our own day with many modi-fications. Such are the lacing up of the organ (recommended, indeed, by Stoll and Morgagni) and certain instruments called "pollution-hinderers," which are intended to close temporarily the urethral orifice, particularly at night. To the same category belongs also the "warning girdle" (Warnungsgürtel) of Ten-derini, which has often been recommended. The absurdity of such contrivances is much too obvious for us to dwell longer upon them.

In some cases, as we have seen, a condition materially favor-ing spermatorrhœa exists in a narrowing of the prepuce, which produces irritation of the glans during erection, or by means of balanitis. The credit of having suggested the successful treat-ment of such cases by operation is due to Lallemand. Pauly,

Pitha, and other recent authors, speak in equally high terms of the operation for phymosis in suitable cases. Circumcision is also frequently of service indirectly by checking the practice of masturbation in persons who have fallen into that vice as a result of phymosis.[1]

Ravoth[2] has lately reported very good results in certain cases of spermatorrhœa which he was able to trace to varicocele as a cause, when this last was cured by a peculiar pressure-apparatus.

The treatment of any varicocele that may exist is always an indication worth noting in cases of abnormal pollutions; but we must avoid the fallacy of assuming that, because two affections are coexistent, one is therefore the cause of the other.

Castration, which has been repeatedly proposed in England, and supported by medical men in America, is thoroughly objectionable, and the same may be said of the ligature of the spermatic arteries. This last operation is not of much more use than shooting an arrow into the air.

It is very important to treat the *constipation* which exists in most patients and is generally very obstinate, since it certainly has a very decided effect in increasing the spermatorrhœa. When it has only lasted a short time and is not very obstinate, it may usually be removed by properly regulating the diet and mode of life, by pedestrian excursions, bodily exercise, etc. If these means fail it will be necessary to have recourse to purgatives; but, as far as possible, drastics are to be avoided, or at any rate employed with great caution, for, in the first place, they tend to injure the already weakened digestive powers, and we also find by experience that they often favor the occurrence of seminal losses by the violent contractions of the rectum and anus which they cause. The same is true of irritating enemata; indeed, in particularly excitable persons, injections, which are merely too hot or too cold, may produce pollutions (Peter Frank). The preference among purgatives should therefore be given to the milder saline aperients and to castor-oil.

---

[1] See Johnson's case, Lancet, April 7, 1860. Related by Behrend. Journal für Kinderkrankh. Vol. 35, parts 11 and 12.

[2] See Berl. klin. Wochenschr. 1874 and 1875.

In order to omit nothing, we will mention a few more conditions which may occasionally suggest indications for treatment; such are: *diseases of the bladder*, especially *catarrh* and *gravel*, and *worms* when they inhabit the rectum. We need not dwell further on the remedial measures; they will be determined in each instance by the nature of the disease.

To conclude: the chief point in the after-treatment of these patients, when they have been either greatly improved or cured of their seminal losses, is to watch over their sexual relations with the greatest care. For the majority of convalescents, coitus, if moderate and well regulated, is not to be forbidden, but, on the contrary, recommended when other circumstances permit. They are to be most earnestly warned to avoid every occasion of useless and incomplete sexual excitement; and if they once happily succeed in overcoming that impurity of thought in which they had previously indulged, and which is so extremely injurious, they should be induced never to give way to it again.

IMPOTENCE.

The literature of impotence is almost wholly the same as that of spermatorrhœa. The most important causes of both affections are identical, and in all other respects we find so many points of close contact, that if we were to give here a list of writers on the subject, we should be open to the charge of repeating almost entirely that prefixed to the last section.

For like reasons we are able to abbreviate considerably our account of impotence, seeing that we dwelt with all possible detail upon the etiology and symptomatology of spermatorrhœa. Even the prognosis and treatment have so very much in common that we shall need but little space for our present chapter.

By the term impotence is meant a diminution or complete loss of the power of sexual intercourse.

If this state is not due to defective formation or mutilation of the genital organs (these being structurally normal), there must be some *incompleteness, too short duration, or complete absence of erection*, which is the essential condition for natural coitus.

Hence it follows that most men who are impotent are also *sterile, unable to procreate*, although possibly their genital glands may yield a perfectly normal and fruitful secretion. Yet it would be a great error to look upon sterility as an absolute consequence of impotence; indeed, we know that, even when erection is incomplete or absent, ejaculation may take place, and that this may prove fertile (under specially favorable circumstances) without any penetration of the female genitals (as in cases of impregnation with imperforate hymen).

The permanent power of complete and sufficiently lasting

erection is connected with the functional activity of the testes, *or at least one of them.*

Credible cases are, indeed, recorded (by Astley Cooper and Curling), in which erections occurred after castration, and even the sexual act could be accomplished ; but even these are only apparent exceptions, since all remains of former virile power diminished more or less speedily, and finally completely disappeared.

In order to a fuller understanding of our subject, we must first recall to our readers' recollection the most important points in the *physiological production and nature of erection.*

This phenomenon is to an eminent degree under the control of the nervous system, and can be originated from three parts of it: firstly, from the nervous centres, which is the way in which mental causes produce erection ; secondly, from the peripheric ends of certain nerves, especially those in the skin covering the penis, and in the glans ; finally, from any part of the nerve-trunks in the course of those nerves.

Eckhard has shown as clearly as possible which are the nerves producing erection in the dog, and they no doubt have their analogues in the other higher animals and man. According to this physiologist, they arise in the spinal cord, and can thence be traced up into the brain, so that, by (electrical) stimulation of the pons and of the point at which the crus cerebri enters the brain, he produced distinct erection of the penis ; whence he concluded that the fibres conveying the impulse required for erection arise in the cerebrum, and pass downwards through the crus and pons to the spinal cord. In the cord he found that stimulation of various parts, especially of the upper cervical region and of the lower section of the divided lumbar portion, produced erections. Goltz has extended these details by discovering that after section of the spinal cord in the lumbar region, erection of the penis can still be produced by peripheric irritation (of the glans) ; this he explains by assuming that an independent centre for erection exists in the lumbar cord. A further discovery made by this author is very interesting and (as we shall afterwards see) practically important, viz. : that this supposed centre in the lumbar cord may be acted upon inhibitorily from the upper part of the medulla, and still more from the brain, so that, after the spinal cord has been divided between its dorsal and lumbar portions (thus removing the influence of the brain and upper part of the spinal cord), reflex erection is generally produced more speedily and completely.

The existence of these three principle points in the nervous system for the production of erection is apparently confirmed by observation on human beings ; thus, in the first place, obscene ideas cause erection ; secondly, irritation and injury of the spinal cord (particularly in the cervical region) may produce erections ending in ejaculation, sometimes even going as far as priapism, which is a common symptom of the primary (hyperæmic) stage of certain diseases of the cord. Finally, those morning erections which usually occur when the bladder is full and the body in the recumbent position, may be ascribed to peripheric irritation of the "nervi erigentes," although they certainly also admit of being explained by reflex stimulation of the centre for erection, by tension and pressure of the irritated bladder and seminal vesicles.

The special mechanism of erection is, particularly in the human subject,[1] not yet fully known in all its details; but the following general sketch gives all that is at present most certainly established.

The essential condition of erection is *an increased fulness of the meshes of the corpora cavernosa with blood, owing to a disproportion between the blood entering the part and that leaving it.* Diminution of the outflow of venous blood cannot be the only cause, as some physiologists formerly supposed; this may be proved experimentally by showing that mere ligature of the veins of the penis never produces erection. The arterial blood must also enter the part more abundantly, as is put beyond doubt by finding that in animals during erection the manometer shows a diminution of arterial pressure in all the pelvic vessels, which Eckhard even found to extend to the crural arteries. This increased arterial inflow may be brought about in two ways: firstly, by increased cardiac action, which we may either exclude altogether or look upon as of very subordinate importance. The principal, and probably the only way in which it is produced is by *the arteries of the penis being rendered more permeable as a result of the nervous impulse producing erection, and so allowing a larger quantity of blood to enter in a given time.* This dilatation may, ordinarily speaking, be produced in one of two ways; either actively, by an arrangement of muscular fibres in the walls of the vessels, or passively, by their relaxation (Hausmann). Which of these two modes is the one actually producing erection, or whether they both act at once, is not yet thoroughly proved.

Still greater uncertainty surrounds the question of the diminished venous outflow. Koelliker and Kohlrausch ascribe it, not to the veins themselves, but to certain changes in the cavernous bodies; they suppose that, under the influence of the nervi erigentes, the unstriped muscular fibres of the cavernous tissue are relaxed, and therefore offer less resistance to the increased entry of blood into the part. These authors have carried out this general theory into details in different directions; an impartial critic can hardly yet pronounce in favor of one or the other; perhaps they do not exclude each other; at any rate, special arrangements of the vessels are not to be observed in all parts of the corpora cavernosa.

We have still to remark, concerning the more obvious phenomena of erection, that it begins at the root of the penis and gradually extends towards the glans,

---

[1] It appears that the minute structure of the penis (especially the arrangement and mode of ending of the vessels) varies much in different species, the same object being attained by various means. We need here only instance the clubbed terminations of the arteries shown by *Eckhard* to exist in the horse, to which he assigns the same function as *J. Mueller* does to the helicine arteries in man, supposing, at present, these last not to be artificially produced, as some authorities (*Valentine*) believe.

which part is thus the last to be completely distended. During erection the reticulate structure of the caput gallinaginis becomes filled, so closing the urethra on the side of the bladder, and preventing the semen flowing back into it during ejaculation (Kobelt).

Ejaculation is, no doubt, rendered easier by the urethral passage remaining open during erection, and by its mucous membrane being lubricated with a glandular secretion (query, whether from Littré's glands alone, or also from the prostate and from Cowper's glands). It is this fluid which passes from the urethra in some quantity under sexual stimulation in very excitable or over-excited persons, and often leads them to fear erroneously that they are suffering from spermatorrhœa.

The causes of impotence are as variable as its degrees and forms. First of all, of course, come *certain congenital or acquired malformations and defects of the genital organs*, which are accompanied by impotence, usually permanent, though occasionally only temporary. We may mention first, *absence of the penis, or considerable diminution in its length, either congenitally, or as a result of operation.* The absence of the glans only does not completely destroy the power of copulation, although it is the principal organ for the reflex production of ejaculation—cases enough being on record in which connection was possible as long as sufficient of the penis remained for the purpose of copulation when erect. One variety of temporary or permanent absence of the penis is afforded by *hydrocele or hernia*, in which the skin of the penis is taken up by the coverings of the gradually enlarging scrotal tumor, which also conceals the corpora cavernosa.

Tumors of the penis, when very large or in unfavorable situations, may in like manner render the sexual act impossible ; and in this case there is little to be hoped from any operation, since carcinoma is far more common than benignant tumors (fibroid, aneurismal, lipomatous, etc.).

Changes in the corpora cavernosa and their results play an important part in the etiology of impotence. As an effect of partial inflammation of the cavernous bodies, *indurations* and *knots* form in them, and these, by hindering uniform enlargement of the penis during erection, lead to its being disturbed in various ways, and so render the introduction of the penis into the vagina impossible ; moreover, in such cases, erection is often extremely painful. External injuries are the commonest causes of these

conditions, which may more rarely be produced by severe gonorrhœal inflammations of the urethra.

I may here relate very briefly a remarkably interesting case of the kind. A railway official, a robust man, twenty-six years of age, endeavored, on awaking one
morning with a strong erection, to force the penis downward. It gave way suddenly with violent pain, and such an abundant extravasation of blood took place
under the skin of the organ, that when I saw it, it was of a dark blue color, and
almost the size of a fist. On recovering from this condition, it was found that the
right corpus cavernosum had been ruptured by the injury, and as a result of the
induration that remained, the penis was twisted upward and to the right when erection occurred, in such a manner that coitus was mechanically impossible.

Under much rarer circumstances, *ossifications in the septum,*
or *fibrous casing of the corpora cavernosa* (the so-called "bones
in the penis" of Malgaigne and Velpeau), may have the same
effect as the indurations in the cavernous bodies, if they are of
some size or unfavorably situated. The prognosis is, however,
often more favorable in these cases than in the former, simply
because they may be more frequently removed by operation.

More important, because more frequent, than changes in the
cavernous bodies, are *congenital or acquired affections of the
frænulum, its shortening, contraction, or thickening,* in consequence of ulceration, usually syphilitic. These states may produce a twisting of the penis during erection, which is often
accompanied by severe pain, and which completely prevents
intercourse, or makes it very difficult.

*Loss of the testicles, or such disease of them as is equivalent
to their loss,* is, of course, followed by impotence. As we have
already remarked, erections have, indeed, been observed after
castration, but only for a certain time after the removal of the
genital glands, and then the power definitively ceases. Bilateral
atrophy of the testes only destroys sexual power when it has
reached its highest degree, and is therefore equivalent to castration. The not very unusual diminution in size and softening of
the testes, which is observed, for instance, in varicocele, appears
scarcely to affect virility.

Cryptorchism (of course, when of both testes) produces impotence, but only when the retained glands are completely atrophied and unable to perform their function. The power of

copulation has been almost always found to be unaffected when the testes are in the inguinal canal, and not unfrequently when they are in the abdomen (Cloquin, Curling, and others); whether the power of impregnation is affected is a question to which we shall return by and by.

When the testicles have been completely atrophied from a very early age, or have even completely disappeared (anorchism), there will be very distinct evidence of it in the development of the genital organs and in the whole habit of body.

I had the opportunity of making a post-mortem examination of a very striking case of this kind in 1870. The person in question, who was thirty-one years of age, had died suddenly from fracture of the vertebræ, with concussion of the spinal cord. The general conformation was unmistakably that of a woman; he was beardless, the voice had been thin and high. The extremities were slender, the hands remarkably small, with long, thin fingers; the panniculus adiposus was extraordinarily thick, and the nipples, which were very large, were attached to masses of fat of such an unusual size as to simulate actual mammæ. There was no hair on the body—in particular, none on the chest or in the linea alba—and that upon the mons veneris, which was very scanty, had a decidedly feminine character in its amount and extent. The penis was hardly thicker and longer than that of a child of one year old, measuring from the root to the apex about one and one-quarter inches; the glans was disproportionately small, and covered by a narrow foreskin. The shallow, small pouch of skin which represented the scrotum was empty, and the seminal ducts could be traced up into the abdomen, where they gradually became smaller, and ended in some fatty tissue in which no trace of testicular structure could be detected even by the microscope.[1] According to information I received, and as might have been supposed a priori, this individual had never exhibited any trace of the sexual instinct.

Many cases of so-called hermaphroditism are nothing more than cryptorchism with a great amount of hypospadias and fissure of the scrotum. It would be a great error to consider at once such persons impotent; if there is not also complete atrophy of the testicles, the malformed member is quite capable of erection, and the patient will, under certain circumstances, be able to have connection.

Chronic inflammation of the testes and bilateral epididymitis do not, as a rule, lead to impotence, but usually to that form of sterility termed "azoöspermism," to be hereafter described; in twenty-one cases of the kind Liégeois only found virility diminished eight times.

---

[1] The preparation is in the pathological collection at Giessen.

Tumors of the testicles only destroy the power of copulation with any certainty when the whole glandular substance is compressed and destroyed by them.

Again, impotence may be *a symptom of certain acute or chronic diseases*. The question is of no practical importance as far as concerns acute diseases, but may become so, under special circumstances, in the case of chronic affections. Among these are *disorders of the digestive organs and kidneys*, but, above all, certain *diseases of the brain and spinal cord*, particularly tabes dorsalis and spinal meningitis with their consequences. Impotence first shows itself in the early stages of tabes, sometimes alternating with excessive sexual excitement, and even priapism, so that these are often mentioned among the prodroma of the disease. The primary cause of the loss of power in such cases is supposed to be a direct action upon the sexual nerve-centres, as would, indeed, seem plausible on physiological grounds.

It is more difficult to explain impotence when it occurs as a consequence of *chronic diseases of the organs of nutrition*. In many instances the chief fault seems to lie in the bodily exhaustion produced by them; yet, there are chronic disorders which appear to contradict this explanation, for in them, although there is notable weakness and emaciation, the sexual desire and power are completely retained—sometimes, indeed, increased. Pulmonary phthisis is the only disease we need mention in this respect.

The impotence of diabetic patients is a far more interesting example of this subject. It is well known that diminution or loss of sexual power is frequently one of the *earliest symptoms* of this mysterious disease. It is not unusual for men who still appear quite healthy and robust, and have not even any suspicion of the existence of diabetes, to notice a decided loss of sexual power.[1] It follows from this that the change is not merely to be considered as dependent on exhaustion produced by the disease.

---

[1] Compare *Seegen*, On Diabetes Mellitus (second ed. pp. 117 sqq.). The numerous observations of this author are the more important because until quite recently very different statements as to the relation of impotence to diabetes are to be found in the text-books, and its frequency has been exaggerated (see, for instance, *Cunstatt*).

In other diabetic patients, however, the sexual power is undiminished during the whole course of the disease (except, probably, its latest period); sometimes it is even increased.

From these variations in the sexual functions it must be concluded (and this is confirmed by direct examination of the urine) that the quantity of sugar excreted bears no direct proportion whatever to the degree of impotence. Some other causes must here be at work, which are at present wholly unknown to us, and which probably coincide with variations in the nature of diabetes.

Certain *medicines* and *articles in common use* have, more or less deservedly, the reputation of diminishing virile power, so that some of them have been employed therapeutically, as we have seen above, under the treatment of spermatorrhœa. We need here only mention camphor, bromide of potassium, and lupuline, remarking, however, once more, that the information we have on this subject rests hitherto upon a weak foundation.

Many persons state that, after drinking much beer, they have experienced a certain degree of frigidity. Whether this fact, which is tolerably certain, is to be explained by the presence of the active principle of hops (lupuline) found in beer, is still uncertain. It is, at any rate, much more improbable that the alcohol in the beer should have this effect, because the use of other alcoholic drinks—of wine, in particular—seldom or never has this effect, but rather the opposite.

The long-continued use of arsenic would seem to have produced occasionally a diminution of sexual power. Rayer formerly published an account of a patient, who suffered from lepra, in whom he observed this; and Charcot has since related two confirmatory cases, in which the persons, who had been for a long time treated with arsenic for psoriasis, became impotent, but (what is to be particularly noted) regained their virile power on leaving off the medicine. There is absolutely no evidence with regard to many other drugs, such as the preparations of opium and nicotine (in the case of tobacco), which have been supposed to have an injurious after-effect of this kind.

It is obvious that *before and after a certain age the power of copulation is always absent.* The period at which virility first occurs is subject to variations, which are comparatively unimportant; but, on the other hand, its natural diminution and cessation in old age has very wide limits, which are different in each individual.   Many retain their power, almost unaltered, to a very great age; while in others the senile condition comes on unusually early in life, under the influence of diseases of all kinds, or even without any material disturbance of health, and, so to speak, physiologically.[1]

Individual circumstances, the state of the constitution, and, above all, the sexual relations in earlier life, play a great part in determining the age at which virility ceases.

The *measure of sexual power* is well known to vary as much *quantitatively* as in its duration ; and, without a careful consideration of this point, it is almost impossible to come to a just conclusion as to the existence of impotence in individual cases. Of course our definition of the term cannot be so narrow as only to include those cases in which every sexual act is impossible ; we are in the habit, rather, of applying the word "impotence" to those instances where, during the period of virility, a man becomes aware of a temporary or permanent loss of the sexual power he previously possessed.

The power of copulation varies extremely, not merely in different individuals, but even in the same person (of course we mean independently of age), according to bodily and mental disposition, and other circumstances.   We shall return, hereafter, to certain peculiarities of this kind.

Among all these influences of different kinds, the effect of the mind upon the sexual functions is pre-eminent, as is proved by the existence of that common and well-known form of impotence which has been specially termed "*psychical.*"

As every practitioner knows, a considerable proportion of those who suffer from this form of impotence are recently-married men.   They come to their medical attendant a few days after marriage in great trouble, and tell him that their first attempts at connection, and all subsequent ones, have been complete failures, and that absolutely no erection has occurred ; on the contrary, many of them state that the more excited they have been,

---

[1] Compare what has been said above (p. 828) on the secretion of semen ; we must, however, warn our readers against the mistaken conclusion that the presence of spermatozoa proves the power of copulation.

and the more earnestly they have desired an erection, the greater has been the local frigidity.

Others, again, may have had slight erections, but lasting so short a time that they entirely ceased, on attempting coitus, before ejaculation could occur. Most of these patients further tell us that, before their marriage, and particularly during the time of their engagement, they have experienced the most decided and complete erections; indeed, many mention further, as an unfortunate circumstance, that, even after marriage, they have had now and again erections which were completely normal, but only at times when they could not have connection.

Many consider their ill-luck the more inexplicable, because they have been, for many years, in the habit of having intercourse with prostitutes, and always without difficulty.

For the most part these patients ascribe their first failure to an excess of excitement in their earliest attempts to have connection with their wives; while others, on the contrary, attribute it to timidity, nervousness, or the fear of failure.

The painful remembrance of this first mischance, and the shame and fear of its recurrence, play the most important part in the succession of failures which follow it. We are told by communicative patients — and most of them soon become extremely confidential on this subject — that, however inexperienced and ignorant of such matters women may be before marriage, yet they at once perceive that something is wrong, and are extremely disturbed by it. The knowledge of this naturally increases the husband's confusion, he becomes more and more anxious, and, in many cases, falls almost into despair.

If we investigate the remoter causes of these conditions, we arrive at very diverse, and sometimes almost diametrically opposed conditions.

In the first place, some persons are thus affected who previously very rarely had sexual intercourse, or had even been completely continent. The former seem to be the more exposed to this misfortune, if they have been previously in the habit of intercourse with prostitutes, with whom they have been particularly brought into contact.

On the other hand, by far the larger number of our patients

are those who had been formerly given to sexual excess, and of these, again, the majority have been addicted to masturbation; indeed, if we were to assume that three-fourths of these temporarily impotent persons had been greatly given to this vice, we should hardly be putting the proportion too high; we shall be the more convinced of this if we bear in mind that an assertion of absolute chastity is intended by patients to apply only to ordinary sexual intercourse, and—sophistically enough—not to masturbation.

Natural sexual excess far more rarely precedes this form of impotence; not, perhaps, because it is in itself less injurious, but rather (as we have several times before remarked) because masturbation leads to much earlier and greater excesses.

Among those who have previously given way to natural sexual excess, those most frequently become impotent who—under the influence of a perverted imagination, and encouraged by dissolute women—have been accustomed to have intercourse in all kinds of unnatural and ingenious ways and attitudes. In these patients it has, so to speak, become a matter of habit, and they do not succeed when they cease practising these artifices.

We have no certain idea of the intimate nature and mechanism by which this mode of impotence is brought about. But a very interesting indication of the direction in which we are to look is supplied by the proof given by Goltz, to which we have referred above, of a direct influence of the brain upon the reflex centre of erection in the lumbar portion of the spinal cord. This observer has proved indisputably the inhibitory influence of the brain over this centre by showing that, after the cord has been transversely divided above its lumbar portion (by which all connection with the brain is cut off), irritation of the glans generally determines much more speedy and permanent reflex erections. It is reasonable, therefore, to suppose that in men likewise a similar inhibition of the brain over the reflex centre of erection may be induced by excessive mental stimulation.

With this psychical form of impotence those rare cases are to be connected, in which the impotence only shows itself in regard to certain women, either because they present bodily peculiarities disliked by the man, or because of some aversion based on mental causes.

However rare this state may be, it has a certain medico-legal importance, so that the text-books of medical jurisprudence go into it more fully. It is enough for our purpose to show that the affirmation of impotence, in respect of one woman in particular, is not always to be put aside as false, because intercourse with other women is possible.

A much more unusual form of psychical impotence, and one which appears completely paradoxical, is when a man can only have connection in certain states of mind which are ordinarily opposed to sexual excitement. One of the most striking examples of this is a case related by Schulz,[1] of a man, twenty-eight years of age, who could have connection with other women under the influence of the normal sexual impulse, but could only do so with his wife by first rousing in himself intentionally the passion of anger.

Another frequent and important form of impotence is that usually termed *irritable weakness.*

In these cases, usually after very great desire and violent mental excitement, there is more or less complete erection, but ejaculation occurs immediately upon attempting coitus, before penetration is possible. It is obvious that this form of impotence is more akin to spermatorrhœa than any other, and, indeed, in its highest development may be included under the one term as well as under the other. As a rule, these patients have suffered before from abnormal pollutions (nocturnal or diurnal), and they may still be troubled with them.

Sexual excess, and particularly masturbation, is here also of the greatest importance as a cause. These individuals have generally indulged immoderately in that vice, and even when under the influence of good advice they have checked themselves; frequent erections have been produced by irregularities of fancy. We have said enough already on the invariably evil effect of this uncleanness of mind. As is the case with psychical impotence, these patients also become more and more doubtful of their virile

---

[1] Wiener med. Wochenschrift. 1869. No. 49.

power after each failure, and speedily lose all confidence in themselves.

The form of impotence in which erection is complete, but ejaculation occurs before penetration of the vagina, trenches upon the limits of the normal state, being in close connection with cases of precipitate ejaculation (which are not to be looked upon as pathological) where connection is possible, and coitus is begun as usual, but terminates very speedily by the occurrence of ejaculation. In some persons of a very lively temperament this is the rule; in others too rapid evacuation only takes place occasionally, especially when they have been continent for a long time; as, on the other hand, in most healthy persons ejaculation is retarded when the sexual act is very often repeated, or under the influence of certain articles of food or drink, as beer.

Until recently, precipitate ejaculation could only be a very unimportant subject of inquiry to the physician, since (according to the theories of impregnation then current) it was almost immaterial under what conditions the semen was deposited in the genital organs of the female, provided only it was introduced there. But since it has now been shown to be more probable that during coitus certain movements of the cervix and os uteri are produced by reflex action in the female, which favor the reception of the seminal fluid, it may well be asked whether conception would not be rendered more difficult by a hasty ejaculation, always occurring in coitus before the orgasm in the female has reached the degree needed for the production of these reflex movements.

The two forms of impotence hitherto described, which, although they run into each other, we have distinguished as psychical impotence and irritable weakness, have this character in common, that *erections, and even ejaculations, occur from time to time*, although these are not produced when most desired, which may be insufficient for the purpose, or end too hastily in seminal discharge.

The case is quite different with the category of patients of which we are now about to speak : *erections are absent, not merely temporarily, but permanently, and under all circumstances.* At the most, some signs of erection may occur under the influence of very special causes, but sexual intercourse is wholly impossible.

This *permanent* form of impotence is the expression of a

functional weakness of the genital organs and of the nervous apparatus connected with them ; it has been not inaptly termed the *paralytic form of impotence.*

It is relatively not very common, is generally acquired, not congenital, and has been usually preceded by one of the varieties already described. Sexual excess here also plays the same part as a cause, and to an overwhelming extent masturbation ; the latter probably for this special reason that it is quite possible, and is frequently practised when erection is only partial or null, and therefore, *when impotence already exists.*

When erection continues to be impossible for some time, the psychical relations of the sexual instinct are often materially diminished, or altered in various — often very peculiar — ways. Things which would have produced notable excitement in a patient before his illness, now have hardly any effect upon him. Some of these individuals are quite unable to arouse any sexual excitement whatever, while others (and they are by far the greater number) need the most extraordinary things, often unintelligible to healthy men, to excite momentarily the feeble sparks of passion. These last are often psychological enigmas, and supply most of the examples of the manifold loathsome forms of sexual abuse ; many of them may safely be looked upon as of unsound mind.

The genital organs are found, even by the closest examination, hardly to depart in the least from their normal state, except perhaps that they may have a withered and a kind of senile appearance. In some patients atrophy of the testes may be discovered ; they are then small, soft, and flaccid, have lost, wholly or partly, their peculiar tenderness under pressure, and are relatively or absolutely insensible under the galvanic current. Relaxation and smoothness of the scrotum, which is very pendulous, is mentioned as a very characteristic symptom. The sensibility of the skin of the scrotum, as well as that covering certain portions of the penis, under the galvanic stimulus, is also sometimes materially diminished.[1]

---

[1] In order to judge of these states, it is, however, necessary to be aware that the galvanic excitability of different parts of the skin of the genital organs varies notably in the state of health. According to *Benedict* (loc. cit. p. 447) the right spermatic cord

The *congenital variety* of this paralytic impotence is much rarer than that which has been acquired. A few cases have been observed in which well-built men, of good health in every other respect, and with naturally formed and apparently sound genital organs, are absolutely without any sexual desire, or have it so slightly that only feeble traces of erection occur, and sexual intercourse is, therefore, completely impossible. Such cases, as we have said, are very rare, so that even medical men of experience may not have seen one in their whole lives, yet they are met with every now and then. At present we are far from being able to explain this condition; it need hardly be remarked that we are not to confuse it with the congenital atrophy of the sexual organs (and particularly of the testes) described above.

Prognosis and Treatment.

Our prognosis in impotence, and the means by which we are to oppose it, vary extremely according to its various forms ; for, as we have seen above, the ways in which this affection may be produced are very numerous.

Where the *local anomalies of the genital organs* we have described above are in fault, the prognosis will entirely depend upon their nature, and the possibility of their successful treatment. A few of them are very satisfactory, as the primary affection can be entirely removed ; we need here only mention those cases of voluminous hernia or hydrocele, which as they develop take up the skin of the penis into their own coverings, and conceal the corpora cavernosa. Such few tumors of the penis as are happily non-malignant have also a very favorable prognosis, when their size and position enable them to be extirpated. We may remark under this head that even where the whole glans has to be removed, complete sexual intercourse by no means becomes always impossible ; although the glans is the principal peripheric organ for producing the reflex act of ejaculation, a whole

---

and the right half of the penis are less sensitive than the left side ; the upper surface of the penis is more sensitive than the under, and sensibility diminishes gradually, but notably, from the apex of the glans to the root of the organ.

series of records of operations prove that this may be excited from other parts of the penis.

Less favorable results have, on the whole, been obtained in the case of those distortions of the penis which indurations of the corpora cavernosa produce during erection. In most cases treatment is very fruitless, owing to reproduction of the cicatricial tissue; and good results have only been occasionally obtained in recent cases. In the distortions due to partial ossification of the penis, the chances of treatment may be better, inasmuch as these can be sometimes completely extirpated. A series of cases cured in this way have been published by Velpeau.[1]

The prognosis and treatment of impotence occurring as a consequence of certain acute and chronic diseases are the same as those of the primary disorder.

The course of the variety which has been described as *psychical impotence* is usually far more favorable than many writers on the subject, and almost all patients affected by it, suppose. When recently married men, who have not been previously addicted to sexual excess, nor suffered from morbid pollutions, are unable to have the erections necessary for coitus simply as a result of anxiety or over-agitation, the medical attendant will usually not be consulted, but will first learn the difficulty that occurred long after it has disappeared under the influence of habit.

Psychical impotence is usually more obstinate when it occurs in men who have previously been masturbators, as is frequently the case. Until this vice has been completely eradicated, and the patient has even acquired a thorough detestation of it—and this, as we have seen, is not always to be completely attained by marriage — a positive cure is hardly to be expected. And even when this has long since been done, there are very great difficulties in the physician's way in the usually hypochondriacal character of such patients and in their complete want of energy and courage; and these difficulties increase with each fresh failure. The moral treatment of these cases is of particular importance, and for this purpose the individual peculiarities of each patient

---

[1] Nouv. élém. de méd. operat. Paris, 1839. Vol. IV.

must be taken into account. As a general rule, we have to endeavor to rid them of the despairing idea which is often impressed on their minds that nothing can be done to relieve them; they should be as far as possible encouraged, each according to his own character, although it is not to be forgotten that they should usually be warned that several failures in the next attempts at coitus are possible and even probable, so as to lessen the injurious after-effect of these failures as much as possible. They are to be particularly cautioned against practising any unnatural attitudes or manœuvres, with the object of producing an erection; these almost always have an opposite effect. We have seen above that erections are very easily prevented by too earnest a desire for them; on the contrary, many authors recommend the absolute prohibition of coitus as the surest way to render it possible, and in many cases this is very successful. By this artifice many patients acquire the necessary freedom from anxiety, they have intercourse in the ordinary manner, and their supposed infraction of the rules laid down for them is rewarded by complete recovery.

Where the constitution of the patient requires it, the use of certain remedial measures may be added to the moral treatment. Tonic medicines, change of air, hydropathy, or sea-bathing are often of great use. In very timid persons (and, unfortunately, even energetic men are only too liable to fall into such a condition) medicines often have an effect, simply from the consciousness that something definite is being done for them; and the patients feel that this is a material assistance to their failing confidence.

Moral treatment will often do an extraordinary amount of good to those persons in whom impotence takes the form of "irritable weakness," which is for the most part due to the same causes as the variety just described (viz.: sexual abuse and masturbation), and has the same effect upon the character and energy. When it is thought this abnormal state can be traced to local irritation of the genital organs, this latter is to be treated in the manner described in the chapter on Spermatorrhœa. We will mention once more irritation of the urethra, particularly its prostatic portion; when this exists the local application of astringents, or the systematic use of bougies, is sometimes as successful in the treatment of impotence as in that of spermatorrhœa.

The prognosis is most gloomy in the "*paralytic*" varieties of impotence.

The congenital cases, happily extremely rare, scarcely afford any point at which they may be attacked by treatment. The most important advice which can be given on this subject to medical men who have had little experience of it is not to allow themselves to be induced to give too favorable an opinion by the appearance of the patient, which is often very robust, and by the seemingly complete integrity of the genital organs. This form of impotence is the only one in which we do not think a trial of the so-called aphrodisiacs objectionable; these include, as is well known, cantharides (in the form of tincture), phosphorus, nux vomica, and sometimes ergot. Nothing certain is known of these last two remedies in this respect; as to cantharides, it is well known to cause an increased flow of blood (which may even go on to severe inflammation) to the genito-urinary organs, and so to produce erection.[1]

It is precisely this irritating action of the drug (the individual tolerance of which varies extremely) that, in our opinion, absolutely forbids its use in the *acquired* form of "paralytic" impotence. In an affection which is almost always due to ver-excitement of the genital organs, every kind of artificial irritation should be avoided; any apparent improvement would soon disappear, and be followed by an increased weakness.

On the contrary, after such patients have abandoned their vicious practices, they should, at first, be enjoined abstinence from every occasion of sexual excitement. A period of repose must, above all things, be insured for the weakened constitution and relaxed genital organs, during which an attempt should be made to restore the general health and the tone of the sexual organs by the use of tonic remedies (bark, iron, etc.), baths, and general and local hydropathy, adapted to the peculiarities of

---

[1] The often-asserted action of phosphorus upon the genital organs is explained in a similar manner.

each case. We do not here go into any detailed account of the mode of treatment which we have but now been considering under the head of psychical impotence, especially as everything of importance has been fully dwelt on under the Treatment of Spermatorrhœa.

To conclude, we may refer again to the treatment by galvanism, introduced into Germany by Schulz and Benedict, the special rules for which are the same as those laid down for spermatorrhœa.

STERILITY IN THE MALE.

Aspermatism. Azoöspermism.

Lapeyronie, Mém. de l'académ. de chir. Nouv. ed. Paris, 1819. Vol. I. p. 316.—
  Gosselin, Arch. gén. de méd. Aôut. Sept. 1847.—*The same*, Gaz. méd. de Paris.
  1850. No. 42.—*The same*, Gaz. des hôp. 1853. III. Compare also *Canstatt's*
  Jahresb. 1853. Vol. IV.—*Demarquay*, Mém. de la soc. de chir. de Paris. T. II.
  p. 324.—*Roger*, Thèse. Paris, 1857.—*Hirtz*, Gaz. de Strasbourg. 1861. No. 5.—
  Hiquet, Allg. med. Centralztg. 22. Jan. 1862.—*The same*, Bull. gén. de thér. 15.
  Sept. 1862.—*Schmitt*, Würzburg. med. Ztsch. Vol. III. 1862. p. 361.—*Schulz*,
  Wiener med. Wochensch. 1862. Nos. 49 and 50.—*Demeaux*, Gaz. des hôp.
  1862. No. 21.—*Cosmao, Dumenez* (pupils of Demarquay), Gaz. méd. de Paris.
  1863. Nos. 12 and 14.—*Amussat*, Gaz. des hôp. 1866.—*Liégeois*, Annal. de der-
  matol. 1809. No. 5.—*The same*, Med. Times and Gaz. Oct., Nov., 1869. pp.
  381, 511, 541.—*Virchow's* Jahresber. 1869. Vol. II. p. 185.—*Kocher*, Krankh.
  des Hodens, in Pitha and Billroth's Handb. Vol. III. 1875.

An accurate knowledge of male sterility is an acquisition of
recent date. Formerly, the reason why no children were born of
a marriage was, almost as a matter of course, ascribed to the
wife; but later investigations have taught us that, even *in otherwise healthy men, of apparently good sexual development, and
without any diminution of the power of copulation, the power
of procreation may be temporarily or permanently lost.* Sterility
in the male must often have been overlooked, because formerly
no distinction was made between the power of having connection
and that of begetting children, while, as we have sufficiently
shown above (in the introduction to Impotence), the absence of
the one does not necessarily entail complete loss of the other.

To be precise, we include under the term *sterility, those cases
in which no semen, or, at least, no fertile semen, is produced,*

or in which, although the secretion is formed, *it cannot be ejaculated, at any rate in its normal composition.*

According as the one or other of these conditions exists, sterility has been divided into two forms, and this is fully justified by practice—viz.: the so-called *Aspermatism* or *Aspermism*, and *Azoöspermism.* *The former term is applied to those cases in which coitus takes place naturally, but no seminal ejaculation occurs.* *"Azoöspermism,"* *on the other hand, is employed when the faculties of coition and ejaculation are preserved, but the semen contains no spermatozoa, and is, therefore, not fertile.*

Aspermatism.

The name aspermatism (absence of semen) expresses strictly, according to the definition given above, something more than is generally understood by it.

It is not usually supposed to include a variety of conditions in which no semen is formed (as certain malformations or injuries of the genital organs, especially absence or malposition of the testes), its most important distinguishing mark being found in this, that the semen is more or less completely formed, and only its evacuation during sexual intercourse is hindered.

Until quite recently aspermatism has been reckoned among medical curiosities, and this is still true of some forms of it; but others are much more common than used to be supposed, and need, therefore, very great attention on the part of the practitioner.

The various conditions which lead to aspermatism, and the different forms thus produced, may be arranged, as Schulz first showed, in two groups. In the former those cases are to be included in which the power of ejaculation has been always (congenitally) absent, or has been completely lost for some time without ever returning during the period—*permanent or absolute aspermatism.* The second group contains those where coitus only occasionally and under certain circumstances does not end with an ejaculation, which at other times occurs normally—*temporary or relative aspermatism.*

From the point of view of their causation, the separation of these two groups may also be justified, inasmuch as absolute aspermatism can be almost exclusively traced to local changes, demonstrable clinically and anatomically, while the temporary form is connected with transitory disturbances, affecting for the most part the nerve-centres.

Absolute (or permanent) aspermatism generally occurs when certain alterations in the seminal passages prevent the passage of the *combined secretions* of the genital glands into the urethra; or, if it arrives there, hinder their escape from the orifice of the glans.

The obstacle is usually situated in the neighborhood of the common orifice of the genital gland-ducts — more rarely it is between that point and the apex of the glans. If the obstacle lies in the genital passages behind the caput gallinaginis, in the vasa deferentia or epididymis, only certain constituents of the semen (the testicular secretion) will be thus excluded, and the result will be rather "azoöspermism," for the sexual act will no doubt still end in the ejaculation of a secretion, often not inconsiderable in quantity and resembling true semen.

According to the particular situation of the obstacle, different cases are possible which will be of importance in diagnosis. Either no semen whatever may enter the urethra, because its passage is barred by changes in the substance of the prostate, or in the ejaculatory ducts embedded in it, or the semen escapes from the ejaculatory ducts, but remains in the urethra because the passage is blocked, and is then diverted into the bladder, so that spermatozoa are afterward found in the urine. It is therefore important in all cases of aspermatism, or where it is suspected, to make a microscopical examination of the urine at suitable times. For the details of this examination we must refer the reader to what we said on the subject of urine containing semen, under the head of Spermatorrhœa. A third case, possible, but very rare, is that the obstacle lies somewhat farther forward in the urethra than the caput gallinaginis, or is even in the neighborhood of the external orifice, so that in coitus the semen passes into the urethra and as far as the orifice, but cannot be evacuated.

Let us now endeavor to study the special causes which ordinarily produce these obstacles and so bring about aspermatism.

The various inflammatory processes connected with gonorrhœa, and their consequences, must be mentioned first here as being decidedly the most frequent. They are the usual causes of strictures of the urethra, which produce the various forms of aspermatism, according to their different seats, in the way we have already described. Those strictures which are at some distance from the prostatic portion of the canal, between it and the glans, if they ever cause any difficulty at all, which seems to be very rare, lead to that form of aspermatism which is a retention of semen in the strict sense of the words, i. e., to its arrest in the urethra behind the narrowed part.

It is difficult to understand how an opening, which, although narrowed, is quite permeable to the urine, should not allow the semen to pass; but there are other points to be considered which would make this seem possible. In the first place, it is at any rate conceivable that in these rare cases the strictured part may be completely yielding and permeable when the organ is flaccid, and yet during erection its condition may be so changed, owing to some unfavorable disposition of the exudation-matter, that it would less readily allow of any passage. Moreover, semen is of considerably greater consistence than urine, and the force of ejaculation is decidedly less than that employed in the expulsion of the urine.

So much being premised, the following case (a very remarkable one, I think), which I had the opportunity of observing in 1873, becomes intelligible. I was consulted by an engineer, thirty-five years of age, who had been married for five years without children, and who ascribed the unfruitfulness of his marriage not to his wife, but to himself. According to his own account he had formerly had several attacks of gonorrhœa which had been very carelessly treated; moreover, up to the time of his marriage, and even afterward, he occasionally masturbated. For some weeks after his marriage he was impotent (psychical impotence), but was afterward able to have connection in a perfectly normal manner, ending as usual with the ordinary specific sensation and with the production of ejaculatory movements, but no trace of semen escaped from the urethra; a short time afterward, however, as the organ became relaxed, there flowed from the urethra a viscous fluid, which I once had the opportunity of examining, and found to contain many spermatozoids.

An exploration of the urethra showed that there was a very tight stricture situated exactly under the pubic symphysis, which admitted a No. 3 bougie. The patient unfortunately, after I had seen him several times, withdrew himself from further observation (I know not why), and from the cure which would very probably have followed the systematic use of bougies.

I have met with one other case in medical literature, related by Lapeyronie (loc. cit.), which closely resembles my own. A man, who likewise had no particular difficulty in micturition, and was able to have sexual intercourse as usual, found that the reflex ejaculatory movements, which were normally produced, did not end in evacuation of *seminal fluid, which only escaped from the urethra when the penis began to relax ; the amount was the same as used previously to be lost.* Here, on dissection, a deposit of cicatricial tissue in a particularly unfavorable position was found to be the cause.

Such cases are closely related to those others in which a very tight phimosis has produced aspermatism. A very striking example of this is afforded by a case of Amussat's (loc. cit.), in which aspermatism which had lasted five years was cured by an operation for phimosis.

Aspermatism is much more frequently caused by strictures *in the neighborhood of the orifice of the ejaculatory ducts* than by those we have so far spoken of ; in this case the semen generally flows back into the bladder, and is only evacuated mixed with the urine which is next passed.

These cases do not appear to be very rare, and scarcely call for any further description here. We will only briefly mention a case related by Hirtz,[1] which is remarkable for a kind of spontaneous cure which took place, and which has often been quoted. A man, who otherwise had connection normally, but could never ejaculate and afterward always passed cloudy urine containing semen, felt on one occasion during coitus a very violent pain, but which was *this time followed by seminal evacuation.* At the same time a severe hemorrhage occurred and the sterility ceased, as was afterwards proved by his wife being delivered of a child. In this case some obstacle due to a previous gonorrhœa was suddenly removed, under circumstances of which we know nothing more.

In a third form of aspermatism, which is also most frequently a result of gonorrhœal inflammation, *no semen at all may enter the urethra from the seminal passages.* Here there is either contraction, obstruction, or complete occlusion of the ejaculatory ducts, or various changes in surrounding parts. In this last respect the *prostate* demands especial consideration ; under the influence of chronic gonorrhœa it may undergo secondary contraction, or abscesses may form in it, which either directly narrow or occlude the ejaculatory canals by the formation of cicatricial tissue, or masses formed by the gradual thickening and calcification of the pus may, if so placed, close the ejaculatory ducts by pressure from without.

---

[1] *Hirtz's* other cases, which he describes under the somewhat singular title of "primary sterility," belong, we may remark in passing, not to aspermatism, but to azoöspermism.

As we are here recording all the other *affections of the prostate* which ever produce aspermatism, we may mention first that *prostatic calculi*, which are not so very rare, may, if of a certain size and position, close or deviate the ejaculatory canals. New formations in this organ can hardly have any relation to aspermatism ; seeing that benignant tumors are exceedingly uncommon, and malignant ones run so rapid a course, and are attended by so many other painful symptoms, that any question as to the existence of aspermatism falls completely into the background.

On the other hand, there have been cases in which apparently *congenital atrophy of the prostate* (accompanied, indeed, by that of the seminal vesicles) has been a mechanical cause of aspermatism. Schmitt has published a case of the kind in his very instructive account of the subject.

Traumatic or *intentional wounds in the perineal region* may have the same result as gonorrhœa. Our literature contains a tolerable number of cases, in which abscesses of that part have followed contusions, and have left behind permanent aspermatism (Demeaux, Demarquay, Kocher). In such instances there have either been cicatricial strictures in the prostatic portion of the urethra, or without any narrowing of the urethra, there is some *deviation* of the ejaculatory canals and their orifices, so as to direct the semen into the bladder instead of taking its usual course.

The following case of Demeaux's will serve as an instance of this last form : a healthy man, twenty-three years of age, had, as the result of a fall, a violent inflammation of the perineum with formation of an abscess, which healed after being opened. Some months later the patient remarked that coitus (which was in other respects quite normal) was not followed by any evacuation of semen. On examination with the catheter no stricture could be discovered, but the urine passed after connection contained many spermatozoids. On examination by the rectum, the perineum was found to be diminished in size, and the prostate drawn down lower than usual, from which Demeaux concluded (apparently with reason) that some displacement of the seminal passages had occurred in consequence of the injury.

Certain intentional injuries by *operation* (of which lithotomy is the most important) may have precisely the same bad results as accidental injuries of the perineum.

There are some cases of aspermatism which hold an inter-mediate position between the so-called absolute and temporary varieties of the affection ; Schulz was the first to lay due stress upon them.

They seem to be always congenital : *the persons affected never have during their whole lives an ejaculation when awake, although sexual desire is normal, erection is sufficient in degree and duration, and the mechanical part of coitus can be completely performed.* It seems the more remarkable to these patients that *sexual intercourse never ends with an ejaculation, because in sleep they not unusually have seminal losses of normal quantity and character with the ordinary specific sensations.*

The main distinction, therefore, between such cases and those previously described is this, that in the former actual semen passes into the urethra, or, at any rate (when the ejaculatory ducts are closed), the movements of ejaculation are produced with normal sensations, while in those we are now speaking of *the whole of the final period of the sexual act is completely absent.* The penis is withdrawn from the female genitals after long-continued but useless friction,[1] either in a state of erection or flaccid, but without any discharge, and without any voluptuous sensation.

A further distinguishing mark is to be found in the absence of all post-mortem appearances. In all cases hitherto recorded organic changes in the genital organs could be completely excluded ; they were always found to be completely intact, and especially without any obstacle to the passage of semen.

It is not possible at present to give an explanation of this form of aspermatism, which appears to be very rare. Schulz thinks that there must be an absence of excitability in the reflex ejaculatory centre ; but such a supposition does not seem to advance us at all until we are better informed as to the seat and relations of that centre. As yet we are even unable to come to a definite conclusion whether the centre for ejaculation is the same

---

[1] Cases are on record where men have been able to continue the mechanical act of coitus for an hour and more without ejaculation being produced.

as that for erection.[1] Moreover, in such cases it may also be asked whether, instead of some disorder of the reflex centre, there may not rather be a disturbance of the reception or propagation of the stimulus normally produced by friction of the glans and other parts of the penis.

The cases described as *temporary* or *relative aspermatism*, rare in comparison with the so-called organic form of the same condition, have much in common with the variety just described: there is, in the first place, absence of any cause which can be anatomically shown to exist, and also the impossibility of producing the ejaculatory movements, although coitus can be practised as usual, and nocturnal pollutions are not uncommon. The principal distinctive mark is that *these persons are not always unable to produce an ejaculation, but only sometimes and under certain circumstances.* There are great individual variations in this respect. Many patients only experience it with regard to certain women—not a few with regard to their wives—while coitus with other women is not merely possible, but ends with ordinary ejaculation, which sometimes occurs more speedily than usual. In other cases the difference is found to depend less upon the person with whom intercourse is had than upon particular situations and conditions of mind of the patient.

Any one who is familiar with the essential phenomena of impotence will see at once that there is a very interesting connection, going almost as far as identity, between this form of aspermatism and psychical impotence.[2] A very valuable basis for the physiological explanation of this might be obtained if we could be certain that there is but one centre for erection and ejaculation. The special causes and occasions of temporary asperma-

---

[1] We are quite aware that physiology at the present day and certain clinical facts are rather in favor of this supposition than opposed to it. For the rest, it may be objected that, if the centres are supposed to be identical, the absence of ejaculation should not stand alone, but should always be accompanied by the loss of power of erection. *Schulz*, who endeavors to prove that the two centres are identical, sees this difficulty, and strives to escape from it by assuming that erection occurs under a *less degree of excitement* of the centre, to the highest degree of which ejaculation corresponds, and that these patients are not able to produce this.

[2] *Gueterbock*, who deserves the greatest credit for his account of this state, in Canstatt's Jahresbericht, terms it, not inaptly, psychical aspermatism.

tism, and particularly the causes of each attack, are almost entirely the same as those of psychical impotence. We have to deal with individuals with hereditary. neurotic taint, who have formerly been masturbators, or have very greatly exceeded in venery, in whom the fear of failure in coitus (very materially increased by a single fiasco), shame, and want of confidence in their own powers, give the last impulse to the disorder. Why these conditions should result in impotence in one patient and in aspermatism in another is a question which we cannot at present solve. Those cases are very interesting in which the patients either alternately or during successive periods present the symptoms of impotence and of aspermatism.[1]

It is not at present possible to explain the mechanism of temporary or psychical aspermatism. Schulz has examined the subject very carefully, and, by the exclusion of other explanations, is induced to assume that there is a spasmodic condition of the seminal passages, particularly of the ducts and vesiculæ seminales; but we must consider the cogency of his argument as more apparent than real. At present one would be much more disposed to look for the solution of the problem to quite another quarter, in which a possible explanation is suggested by the valuable experiments of Goltz on the inhibitory action of the cerebrum over the centre for erection.

Prognosis and Treatment.

The prognosis and treatment of aspermatism may be dismissed in a few words.

In organic aspermatism they will depend upon the form in which it occurs, whether the disease producing it is curable, and the rules laid down for the treatment of such disease must be followed.

Where simple strictures are the cause, the prognosis will often be favorable, because they often yield to treatment, whereas the cases in which it has been produced by pressure of neighboring organs, or diseases of the walls of the ejaculatory ducts

---

[1] *Schulz* relates an instructive instance of this kind.

leading to their occlusion or deviation, offer only few chances of cure.

It is difficult to say what was the character of the obstacle which suddenly broke down during coitus in Hirtz's case, quoted above. At any rate, it is quite an exceptional one.

Cases of complete congenital aspermatism without any discoverable organic hindrance, where ejaculation has never occurred during connection, are of absolutely bad prognosis; they offer at present no point available for treatment.

The so-called temporary or psychical aspermatism is very closely related to psychical impotence in its prognosis and treatment, as well as in its causation. In the one case as in the other, the first point is to consider the general health, to go thoroughly into the history and mental characteristics of the individual, and to base the treatment upon the information thus acquired; the details required for carrying it out coincide entirely with those laid down under the head of Impotence. Many authors have much to say in favor of galvanism. Schulz thinks that we are only justified in trying it very cautiously; since he cannot doubt the antispasmodic action of the constant current, and is inclined (as we have said above) to ascribe psychical aspermatism to a spasmodic condition of the seminal passages.

Azoöspermism.

Since Gosselin's study of the subject, this form of male sterility has been distinguished from aspermatism; and in actual practice the two states can usually be diagnosed with tolerable precision.

Here, again, the power of coition is not materially altered; ejaculation is possible, *but the individual affected is sterile, because the seminal fluid contains no spermatozoa.*

Speaking generally, the absence of these bodies may be due to two different conditions; *either no seminal bodies are produced, owing to some abnormal state of the testicles, or (these glands being more or less functionally active) the passages which conduct their secretion are blocked.* Even this latter form is sharply distinguished from aspermatism by the site of the obstacle, since it is due to occlusion of the epididymis or seminal passages as far as their entry into the seminal vesicles, while the impediments causing organic aspermatism are always to be looked for between the vesiculæ seminales and the urethral orifice. What we said was the case with aspermatism is equally true here : it has become more and more the custom among writers to include under the term azoöspermism only those cases which may be traced to some impediment to the passage of the testicular secretion, to the almost complete exclusion of the series of conditions we mentioned first, in which no spermatozoa are formed at all. Strictly speaking, this — as every one will see at once — is inconsistent ; and all that can be said for it is that, since absence of the seminal elements is always accompanied by impotence, the subject may as well be treated of under that head. In order to avoid repetitions, we have here conformed to the custom, and will only very briefly dwell upon it, referring for further details to the chapter on Impotence.

The variety of azoöspermism due to obliteration of the seminal passages has usually been originally caused by *inflammatory conditions of the epididymis and vasa deferentia. Gonorrhœal affections* play by far the most important part in this. Traumatic inflammations may, indeed, give rise to azoöspermism, but extremely seldom compared to the frequency with which they cause aspermatism ; the simple reason for this being that in order to produce complete azoöspermism, the passages for the testicular secretion must be *closed on both sides,* and only some very singular accident could do this. Daily experience teaches us that indurations of the epididymis or vas deferens of one side do not produce azoöspermism, but it has never yet been thoroughly established whether the functional activity of the testis that is intact is thereby affected. We must not, however, omit to mention that Liégeois (loc. cit.) has under these circumstances observed a decided lessening of secretion, which he, somewhat vaguely, ascribes to a sympathy between the two testicles.

The labors of Gosselin (whom we must look upon as the founder of our knowledge of azoöspermism) supplied the first starting-point to a study of the obliteration of the seminal passages caused by bilateral gonorrhœal inflammation. Liégeois has presented us with a precise idea of the gravity of double epididymitis in this respect, based upon a considerable number of cases (83 in all) collected by him,[1] inasmuch as he showed that spermatozoids were only found to reappear in the semen in eight of these patients.

In spite of this, the secretory activity of the testicles does not seem to be generally lost. At any rate, anatomical examination has several times (Gosselin) established that there was enlargement of the vas deferens behind the obliteration;[2] and Curling in two cases made the very interesting observation that after each coitus there was a sense of tension and pressure in the testicles, and the region of the epididymis was notably enlarged. Liégeois, in twenty-one cases, found virile power completely unaffected thirteen times, and diminished only eight times, but never completely destroyed.

As we remarked in the beginning, these patients ejaculate almost always in, apparently, a completely normal manner. The fluid evacuated, of which, according to Liégeois, the quantity is usually equal to that lost by healthy men (1–3 grms.), and is sometimes more, has the peculiar odor of normal semen, very much the same color and consistence,[3] and even microscopically exhibits all the formed elements belonging to semen, except the spermatozoa.

The *prognosis* of all cases which can be traced to obliteration of the seminal passages, as is plain from what precedes, is an extremely bad one in respect of the procreative power of the patient. Perhaps traumatic cases offer a somewhat better chance of treatment, as we have here only to deal with an exudation deposited outside the canal and compressing it, whereas in the

---

[1] Twenty-five cases of Gosselin's, thirty-five of Godard's, and twenty-three of his own.

[2] In one case of the kind the epididymis had reached six times its natural size, and was filled with a thick yellow fluid containing countless spermatozoa, while the testis itself appeared healthy.

[3] *Liégeois*, indeed, thinks he has observed some changes in this respect, but these are tolerably indefinite, and in any case of little value so long as authors are not agreed as to these peculiarities in normal semen.

blennorrhagic forms, where the disease begins in the mucous membrane of the vas deferens and epididymis, and the external exudation is secondary, there will almost always be adhesions of the walls of the canal which can hardly ever be removed. Following the analogy of the nomenclature of aspermatism introduced by Schulz, this variety may be termed "*permanent or absolute azoöspermism.*"

We must here mention those obscure cases, rarely observed, of which Hirtz has given two detailed descriptions. The cases were those of two strong young men, who, without having ever previously suffered from any disease of the genital organs, lost, otherwise naturally, at each ejaculation a fluid completely void of spermatozoids. They both agreed in the remarkable statement that they never experienced any trace of the exhaustion felt by other men after coitus.

To the same category all those cases are to be added in which the seminal bodies are not developed, owing to disease, malformation, or complete absence of the testicles, if they are not described in detail in connection with the impotence which is combined with them, as we have remarked above, and as we have, for practical reasons, done in this work.

The contrary to the absolute variety—*temporary* or *relative azoöspermism*—is found in those instances where spermatozoa are not found in the fluid ejaculated, either for a short time or under certain circumstances. This has been observed in the course of various diseases, and also, not very rarely, in healthy men who have died suddenly (Casper).

It would appear that even in perfectly healthy men when · living a kind of temporary azoöspermism is not so very uncommon when they practise coitus too frequently, in proportion to their individual capacity. The case observed by Casper, and already fully described by us, is a sufficiently detailed example of this physiological condition.

INDEX.

Lightning Source UK Ltd.
Milton Keynes UK
UKHW041200300119
336362UK00017B/245/P

9 78152